D1112374

Geriatric Psychiatry

Geriatric Psychiatry

Edited by

Ewald W. Busse, M.D.

*President, North Carolina Institute of Medicine; and
Dean Emeritus, Medical and Allied Health Education,
Duke University Medical Center,
Durham, North Carolina*

Dan G. Blazer, M.D., Ph.D.

*Professor of Psychiatry; and
Director, Affective Disorders Program,
Duke University Medical Center,
Durham, North Carolina*

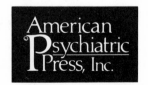

1400 K Street, N.W.
Washington, DC 20005

Note: The authors have worked to ensure that all information in this book concerning drug dosages, schedules, and routes of administration is accurate as of the time of publication and consistent with standards set by the U.S. Food and Drug Administration and the general medical community. As medical research and practice advance, however, therapeutic standards may change. For this reason and because human and mechanical errors sometimes occur, we recommend that readers follow the advice of a physician who is directly involved in their care or the care of a member of their family.

Books published by the American Psychiatric Press, Inc., represent the views and opinions of the individual authors and do not necessarily represent the policies and opinions of the Press or the American Psychiatric Association.

The paper used in this publication meets the minimum requirements of American National Standard for Information Sciences—Permanence of Paper for Printed Library Materials, ANSI Z39.48-1984 ∞

Library of Congress Cataloging-in-Publication Data

Geriatric psychiatry / edited by Ewald W. Busse, Dan G. Blazer. — 1st ed.
    p.   cm.
  Includes bibliographies and index
  ISBN 0-88048-279-6
  1. Geriatric psychiatry I. Busse, Ewald W., 1917–
II. Blazer, Dan G. (Dan German), 1944–
  [DNLM: 1. Geriatric Psychiatry. 2. Mental Disorders—in old age.
  T 150 G3686]
C451.4.A5G469 1989
18.97' 689—dc19
  NLM/DLC
  r Library of Congress   88-7432
                        CIP

Contents

Contributors

Dan G. Blazer, M.D., Ph.D., Professor of Psychiatry; Director, Affective Disorders Program, Duke University Medical Center

Andrew L. Brickman, Ph.D., Department of Psychiatry, University of Miami

Ewald W. Busse, M.D., President, North Carolina Institute of Medicine; Dean Emeritus, Medical and Allied Health Education, Duke University Medical Center

Caron Christison, M.D., Assistant Professor of Psychiatry, Loma Linda University Medical Center

George Christison, M.D., Assistant Professor and Chief of Inpatient Psychiatry, Jerry L. Pettis Memorial Veterans Administration Hospital, Loma Linda Medical Center

Wade E. Craighead, Ph.D., Professor, Affective Disorders Program, Duke University Medical Center

Jonathan Davidson, M.D., Associate Professor of Psychiatry, Duke University Medical Center

Carl Eisdorfer, Ph.D., M.D., Professor and Chairman of Psychiatry, University of Miami

Don Evans, M.A., Department of Psychiatry, Duke University Medical Center

Dolores Gallagher, Ph.D., Geriatric Research, Education and Clinical Center, Palo Alto VA Medical Center

Linda K. George, Ph.D., Professor of Sociology and Social Psychiatry; Associate Director, Center for the Study of Aging and Human Development, Department of Psychiatry, Duke University Medical Center

Thomas A. Glass, M.A., Department of Sociology, Duke University

Carolyn C. Hoch, Ph.D., Program Coordinator, Geriatric Sleep Research, Western Psychiatric Institute and Clinic, University of Pittsburgh School of Medicine

Lawrence W. Lazarus, M.D., Assistant Professor of Psychiatry, Rush Medical College; Psychiatric Consultant, Johnston R. Bowman Health Center for the Elderly

George L. Maddox, Ph.D., Professor of Medical Sociology, Duke University; Chairman, Council on Aging and Human Development, Duke University Medical Center

Timothy H. Monk, Ph.D., Director, Human Chronobiology Research Program, Western Psychiatric Institute and Clinic, University of Pittsburgh School of Medicine

Charles B. Nemeroff, M.D., Ph.D., Professor of Psychiatry and Pharmacology; Center for the Study of Aging and Human Development, Duke University Medical Center

Leonard W. Poon, Ph.D., Director, Gerontology Center; Chair, Faculty of Gerontology, University of Georgia

Murray A. Raskind, M.D., Professor of Psychiatry and Behavioral Sciences, University of Washington School of Medicine

Charles F. Reynolds III, M.D., Departments of Psychiatry and Neurology; Director, Sleep Evaluation Center, Western Psychiatric Institute and Clinic, University of Pittsburgh School of Medicine

John W. Rowe, M.D., President, Mt. Sinai Medical Center, New York

Ilene C. Siegler, Ph.D., Associate Professor, Division of Medical Psychology, Department of Psychiatry, Duke University Medical Center

Robert J. Sullivan, Jr., M.D., Assistant Professor of Medicine, Associate Professor, Community and Family Medicine; Medical Director, Geriatric Evaluation and Treatment Clinic, Duke University Medical Center

Larry W. Thompson, Ph.D., Associate Director, Geriatric Research, Education and Clinical Center, Palo Alto VA Medical Center; Division of Gerontology, Stanford University School of Medicine

F. Stephen Vogel, M.D., Professor of Pathology, Duke University Medical Center

Alan D. Whanger, M.D., Professor of Psychiatry, Duke University Medical Center

Preface

The editors of this volume previously produced *The Handbook of Geriatric Psychiatry,* and for several years it has been evident that a new book was in order. After careful thought, this multiauthored publication emerged. By definition it could be a handbook, since it is concise and devoted to a specific subject. However, it is not a second edition of our earlier *Handbook.* It is a totally new publication. The contents of this book reflect the rapidly expanding base of our scientific knowledge of aging and geriatrics. It is designed to provide the scholar and the clinician with the scientific facts and the applied skills and knowledge that are so needed in dealing with the mental disorders of late life. Consequently, this volume not only covers the wide range of important mental diseases of late life, but also covers the so-called normal age changes that result in biologic and behavioral changes in late life.

The chapters are ordered to present the fundamentals of geriatric psychiatry in a sequential and integrated pattern. The carefully selected contributors are scientists and scholars who have demonstrated that they can present very complex material in a manner that is understandable to the health professional.

The phenomenal growth in geriatric psychiatry has been accompanied by a significant change in American psychiatry with the gradual implementation of the various editions of the *Diagnostic and Statistical Manual of Mental Disorders.* The changes that are found in DSM-III-R are reflected as fully as possible in this book.

In developing this new book we adhered to an eclectic orientation to the theory and practice of geriatric psychiatry. Although the contributors are predominantly psychiatrists, it was believed appropriate to include biomedical and behavioral scientists. This is particularly true of the chapters that are concerned with the basic sciences since such knowledge must be incorporated into a comprehensive approach to patient care.

The primary target of this educational publication is the psychiatrist who has an interest in and commitment to geriatrics. Our previous experience suggests the frequent use of this book by a broad spectrum of health professionals and science writers. This book will be of value to the candidates seeking certification in geriatrics from the American Board of Internal Medicine and the American Board of Family Practice, since that board examination has announced that there will be a considerable emphasis on geriatric psychiatry and the behavioral aspects of aging.

We wish to express our deepest appreciation to our secretaries — Ms. Dina Grinstead, Dr. David Knight, and Ms. Denise Dixon — for their long hours typing, editing, and organizing the manuscript.

Ewald W. Busse, M.D.
Dan G. Blazer, M.D., Ph.D.

The Basic Science of Geriatric Psychiatry

Chapter 1

The Myth, History, and Science of Aging

Ewald W. Busse, M.D.

For thousands of years scholars, physicians, theologians, philosophers, and others have written on the subjects of life, aging, and death. Some of their observations and conclusions are casual, a few are frivolous, and some are based on careful study and considered judgment. Some of the older writings are interesting because they provide information regarding social values, the influence of political and economic factors, the level of scientific knowledge, and, in particular, the interpretation of the significance and application of existing knowledge. This summary includes selections from the literature (ancient and past), prose and verse, and myths and events relevant to geriatric psychiatry. Additional examples and details can be found in publications such as those by Gerald J. Gruman (1966) and Osborn Segerberg, Jr. (1974).

The Prolongation of Youth and Life

Attempts to prolong youth or to restore sexual vigor and physical vitality have existed for many centuries and are still found today. Many such attempts at rejuvenation carry a distinct risk. In fact, Greek mythology teaches that the risk is greater than the gain. The goddess Aurora (also called Eos) with great effort persuaded Zeus to grant her husband Tithonus immortality. Regretably, she neglected to mention that she also wanted him to remain eternally young. As the years passed, Tithonus became more and more disabled, praying frequently for death. In one account Tithonus escaped his misery by turning into a cicada. The male of this insect produces a shrill sound similar to the voice of a demented person.

3

Ancient Greek tales do contain one success story. The sorceress Medea claimed to hold the key that unlocked the door to eternal youth. She mixed a ram's blood, a snake's skin, an owl's flesh, roots, herbs, grass, and other ingredients and then proceeded to fill the veins of King Aeson with this potion. The king promptly leaped from his sick bed, bursting with energy and youthful vitality; how long his energetic state lasted is unclear.

Centuries later, a similar injection ended in catastrophe. Pope Innocent VIII (1432–1492) was appropriately named, since he requested his physicians to transfuse the blood of young men into his veins. Obviously the blood types were incompatible, for he died almost immediately.

During the 19th century there were a number of famous rejuvenists. Dr. Charles Edouard Brown-Sequard was a distinguished physician who described a syndrome known as the Brown-Sequard syndrome. This syndrome consisted of damage to one-half of the spinal cord that resulted in ipsilateral paralysis and loss of discrimination with contralateral loss of pain and temperature sensation. In 1889 at a scientific meeting in Paris, Brown-Sequard announced that he had discovered a way to make old men young again. He accomplished this by injections of mashed-up dog testicles. He claimed that he had personally taken the injections and they had improved his potency. Following this announcement, rumors of this incredible discovery flowed through Paris and spread around the world. His office was besieged for rejuvenation treatment. However, this passed out of favor as adverse reactions developed (Zeman 1967). The Brown-Sequard effort in rejuvenation does not appear to be so bizarre if one appreciates the status of medical science at that time. Knowledge of internal secretions and their impact on physiological function had been enhanced by the work of Claude Bernard (1813–1878). Addison gave an account of the disease named after himself and its relationship to a disease of the super renal capsule. Brown-Sequard in 1856 demonstrated that excision of the adrenals in animals was followed by fatal symptoms similar to those of Addison's disease. Numerous other advances were made regarding the functions of the thyroid gland and the substitution of extracts or chemical substances from organs. Regardless, it appears that Brown-Sequard was overly enthusiastic and may have abandoned the scientific standards he had employed in other experiments and observations.

A similar incident occurred early in the 20th century. John Romulus Brinkley, who advocated transplanting goat testicles into men, was forced to close his offices in the United States, but he moved to Mexico. He reputedly transplanted the testicles of 6,000 billy goats into the scrotums of aging men (Zeman 1967).

Serge Voronoff (1866–1951), a Russian physician in Paris, continued in his efforts to restore youth. He claimed great success by grafting testicles of a monkey into an aging male. Elie Metchnikoff (1845–1916), another Russian, had a different approach to the prolongation of life. He advocated the removal of the large intestine and the ingestion of large amounts of yogurt. Advertising seen on television for more than two decades suggests that long-lived Cossacks achieved this status by consuming large amounts of yogurt (Zeman 1967).

During the past 30 years an injection rejuvenating technique has been given considerable publicity. The technique was developed by Paul Neihans of Geneva, Switzerland. He injected living cells derived from a lamb embryo into his clients. Considerable success was claimed, and the technique continues to be used; however, there is no doubt that the introduction of a foreign protein into a human body can result in disaster.

The Hyperborean Theme

The idea that in remote parts of the world there are people who enjoy remarkably long lives appears in the mythology of people throughout the world. The Greek legend of the Hyperboreans held that there was a group of people who lived beyond the north wind in a region of perpetual sunshine. These fortunate people were free from all natural ills. They were extremely happy and "aloof from toil and conflict." Pliny wrote, in the first century A.D., that they lived to an extreme old age until, "sated with life and luxury, they leaped into the sea."

It is interesting that this idea of people living in remote parts of the world who enjoy a long life persists in the mythology of the centenarians that occurs periodically in news media and scientific literature (see section titled "The Centenarians," p. 12).

Antediluvian Theme

The idea that people lived much longer in the past has support from the Old Testament. In Genesis are recorded the life spans of 10 patriarchs who lived before the flood. The ages range from the 365 years of Enoch to 969 years for Methuselah (Genesis 5:3–32). They are (listed in length-of-life order):

Enoch	365 years
Lamech	777 years
Mahalalel	895 years
Enosh	905 years
Kenan	910 years
Seth	912 years
Adam	930 years
Noah	950 years
Jared	962 years
Methuselah	969 years

Because these longevity records appear in the Old Testament, they have posed a problem of interpretation for theologians. Three types of explanation have been put forth—mythical, metaphorical, and literal. The mythical interpretation denies any historical validity. The metaphorical interpretation reasons that each patriarch symbolized a tribe or group that existed for that period of time that carried the name of the founding patriarch. The literal interpretation is that before the Great Flood these patriarchs pursued a moral and proper behavior as well as diet conducive to long life. They were "beloved of God." Not only are such long-lived individuals reported in the Bible, but also Greek and Roman historians refer to a number of persons who attained extremely long lives. Pliny (23–79 A.D.) claimed to identify a number of individuals whose ages ranged from 150 to 800 years (Gruman 1966).

Other opinions have been expressed regarding the longevity of the patriarchs. Roger Bacon deduced that if after the fall precipitated by Adam and Eve humans were still able to live almost a thousand years, then the short life span of his own time must be the result not of the will of God but of human ignorance.

The Fountain of Youth

In America the myth of the fountain of youth is well known because it was instrumental in Ponce de Leon's discovery of the state of Florida. The fountain of youth legend is traced by scholars to several possible origins. Two ancient myths involve the Hindu Pool of Youth and the Hebrew River of Immortality. The reading of ancient manuscripts as well as a travel guidebook for Greece prepared by Pausanias apparently played a role in renewing interest in the fountain of youth in the 14th and 15th centuries. In ancient Greek and Roman writings there are two interesting references to fountains with prolongevity properties. Hera, the wife of Zeus, bathed each year in a spring that renewed her maidenhood. In another classical reference, Herodotus recounts a search for a spring and pool whose constant use made people live longer. The water was most unusual; nothing would float on it (neither wood nor anything lighter than wood), but all sank to the bottom. The water was strangely oily and had a fragrant quality. An Ethiopian king attributed his life of 120 years to using this water (Segerberg 1974).

The Hindu Pool of Youth is linked to the legend of Cyavana, which is at least as old as 700 B.C. and probably considerably older. Cyavana was an aged and venerable priest who was highly respected by the king. Sukanya, the daughter of the king, was given to Cyavana to be his wife. After some tribulations, the dutiful wife remained loyal to her senile husband. He in turn resolved to correct the situation and was able to negotiate the site of the Pool of Youth. After bathing in it, he emerged divinely fair, youthful, and wearing brilliant earrings. This Hindu fable was probably transmitted to medieval Europe by either the Arabs or the Nestorian Christians of the Near East (Gruman 1966).

The Myth of Gilgamesh

One of the principal heroic tales of antiquity is the Gilgamesh epic. The Babylonian clay tablets were discovered among the remains of the library in Nineveh by George Smith of the British Museum. Although the clay tablets were made about 650 B.C. the origin of this story traces back to the Sumerian civilization about 3,000 B.C. Translations were difficult but eventually produced the longest and most beautiful Babylonian poem yet discovered in the mounds of the Tigro-Euphrates region, one that ranks among the great literature masterpieces of mankind.

Gilgamesh was a vigorous young king who not only was exuberant, but also was arrogant and bullied his overburdened subjects. To divert him from his tyrannical behavior, the gods created Enkidu, a man of wild appearance and enormous strength. Gilgamesh and Enkidu engaged in a long, bitter struggle with neither being able to overcome the other. Recognizing each other's power and skill, they became close friends and decided to travel together to combine their strengths and abilities to seek fame and fortune. These overcompetent superhumans violated divine law by killing sacred animals and by hurling insults at a goddess. The gods decreed the death of Enkidu, who became sick and died. Gilgamesh realized that regardless of his abilities and enormous strength, he too someday would die and he became obsessed with the desire to obtain the secret of immortal life. He first decided to seek out the prophet Utnapishtim, a Babylonian-type Noah who lived far away. After traveling over land and sea, Gilgamesh finally located Utnapishtim. Utnapishtim told Gilgamesh that he must stay awake for 6 days and 7 nights in order to master sleep; Gilgamesh was unable to do this. He was then told that there was one last hope and that was to retrieve from the bottom of the sea a thorny plant which possessed powers of rejuvenation. Gilgamesh succeeded in retrieving the plant from the bottom of the ocean, but on the way home he saw a pool of water and decided to bathe. After bathing, he was unable to resist sleep and while he slept a serpent appeared and ate the precious plant. By eating the plant, the serpent gained the power of shedding its own skin and renewing its life. In addition, the serpent became the symbol of a number of gods of healing.

Alchemy

Alchemy was the medieval chemical science and speculative philosophy whose objective was to achieve the transmutation of base metals into gold, the discovery of an elixir of life, a universal cure for disease, and a means of indefinitely prolonging life. The seeds of alchemy had emerged centuries before. Some can be traced back into Egyptian and Babylonian civilizations. The opportunity to see material change provided basis for alchemy speculation. Alchemists wondered, If a bluish stone treated with fire becomes the red metal (copper), what is the true nature of the substance? Obviously, water is an excellent example since it can evaporate or freeze into ice or snow. In the 10th century, Ibn-Snia, one of the most famous physicians to emerge between Galen and modern times, worked diligently to find the elixir of life although he rejected the idea that metals could be turned into gold and silver.

The twin goals of alchemy filtered into Europe during the 12th century. Roger Bacon, in the 13th century, accepted the tenets of alchemy and believed that the life span of his day, which usually was not more than 45 to 50 years, could be tripled with alchemy's help. His reasoning was in part based on the long life spans of Methuselah and Noah, because he believed if life had been that long, some reversal was possible. Bacon became a Franciscan monk in order to pursue a moral and physically clean life. He did recommend the rejuvenating breath of a young virgin, but as a monk cautioned against any accompanying licentiousness. He reasoned that if disease were contagious, why not vitality? Clearly Bacon's views were related to gerocomy.

Gerocomy

Rejuvenation efforts were abundant in the Near and Far East centuries ago. One that persisted in many societies is called "gerocomy." Gerocomy is the belief and practice that a man, particularly an older man, absorbs virtue and youth from women, especially younger women. King David in the Old Testament believed in gerocomy and practiced it accordingly. There is clear evidence that Romans had a similar view. In recent times, gerocomy is believed to have been associated with the downfall of Mahatma Ghandi. In his extensive view of Ghandi's life, Erik Eriksson (1969) indicates that in spite of Ghandi's expressed preference for celibacy, he was accused of gerocomy and that this contributed to his political demise.

The Myth of Cell Immortality

Alexis Carrel (1873–1944) was born in Lyon, France, and received his medical education and surgical training in France. Carrel was a very skillful and creative surgeon who encountered frustrations in his career. He left for America in May 1904. At the University of Chicago and later at the Rockefeller Institute he devoted his work to vascular and cardiac surgery and wound healing. This interest in wound healing led him to an interest in growing tissues outside the body. For his surgical contributions, he won the Nobel prize for physiology and medicine in 1912. He rapidly developed his studies in tissue culture, and on the basis of some of his own apparent successes, he became convinced that some human cells grown in culture were immortal. This claim of possible cell immortality was emerging and was reported by Carrel and Ebeling beginning in 1912. In spite of numerous objections to his work, Carrel was very persuasive and his belief was accepted. Subsequently it was demonstrated that these respected investigators had made an error in their methodology that resulted in improper conclusions. In January 1912, Carrel established a series of chick heart fibroblast cultures. One of these cultures was destined to become the immortal cell strain. Both Ebeling and Carrel continued to publish and apparently maintained excellent public relations. Their claimed success of maintaining cell culture was such that the *New York World Telegram* made periodic inquiry about the health of the cells and reported on their status.

The Carrel-Ebeling cell culture was fed an extract taken from chick embryos. This extract actually contained a very few but significant number of new viable cells; hence, the introduction of new cells permitted the culture to survive. It was found that if the extract was carefully prepared, removing all new cells, the cell colony would die.

Although other experiments have suggested that animal and human cells have the capacity to be immortal, it has been demonstrated that all such immortal cell colonies are abnormal in one way or another. At the present time the only human cells that are apparently immortal are transformed or abnormal cells such as the HeLa cells which were originally taken from the cancerous cervical tissue and grown in glass culture by George O. Gey in 1950 at Johns Hopkins University School of Medicine. Normal human cells are diploid; that is, they have two sets of 23 chromosomes or a total of 46. HeLa cells are mixoploid and may have anything from 50 to 350 chromosomes per cell with the chromosomes differing considerably in size and shape from the 46 chromosomes found in the normal diploid human cell.

Prior to 1961, the accepted dogma was that cells and tissue culture were potentially immortal. The death of a cell line was usually attributed to failure to utilize proper laboratory methods. In 1961 Hayflick and Moorhead first described the finite replicative capacity of cultured normal human fibroblasts and interpreted the phenomenon to be aging at the cellular level. They demonstrated that even when normal human embryonic cells were grown under the most favorable conditions, death was inevitable after about 50 population doublings. Thus, the death of the cell line was the inherent property of the cells themselves. Until this demonstration, the death of a cell line was not attributed to aging, but was considered some sort of an artifact in that the cell cultures were not being properly taken care of. The belief that cells could divide indefinitely if the investigators could only find the proper way of growing them was so entrenched that when Hayflick and Moorhead first submitted their original manuscript it was rejected on the grounds that they must have made an error in providing the right milieu for the dividing cells. Hayflick referred to Carrel's belief that he had been able to culture chick heart cells indefinitely. Hayflick and Moorhead concluded that normal cells do not have an intrinsic finite capacity to replicate and that immortal cell populations consist of abnormal cells.

In 1965, Hayflick reported that culture fibroblasts derived from older human donors divided fewer times than those derived from embryos. Since then a number of investigators have replicated the work of Hayflick, finding that the number of population doublings of cultured human cells is inversely proportional to donor age. Subsequently it has been demonstrated that freezing viable normal human cells at subzero temperatures does not alter the memory in the cells for the number of doublings that had previously transpired. These cells have been held for over 24 years in a frozen state and when thawed have a remarkable memory and only double the amount that would be in the remaining doublings.

Through a series of experiments, Hayflick (1977) and others (Tomkins et al. 1974) reached the conclusion that changes in the immune function of the cell do not change the density of human lymphocyte antigen determinants on normal human diploid cells throughout their in vitro lifetime. They also looked at the idea of production errors in essential proteins and the accumulation of these errors. They studied the biosynthetic capabilities of young and old cells, focusing on DNA, RNA, protein, and lipids. They found some slowing in the incorporation of a number of precursors, and discovered that lipid synthesis is affected to a lesser degree than protein and nucleic acid synthesis in cellular aging.

Although Hayflick has admitted that many of the studies are not conclusive, he has continued to hold the belief that the death of diploid cells is under genetic control (Hayflick 1986).

Gerovital H₃

Gerovital H_3, an exceedingly controversial compound, has been sold in Europe for many years. It is claimed by its predominantly European advocates to have a variety of curative and restorative powers for disabilities and diseases affecting the elderly. The most active advocate of Gerovital H_3 was Professor Anna Aslan of the Geriatric Institute of Bucharest, Romania. Although procaine hydrochloride has been used in Europe as a general tonic for over 60 years, it was not until 1945 when Professor Aslan began to use and proclaim its value that this particular drug began to receive considerable attention. Gerovital H_3 has been used by political and religious leaders in Europe. Many of Aslan's claims are probably exaggerated, and this may mask its potential usefulness. She reports beneficial results in a wide variety of conditions including depression, degenerative arthritis, hypertension, angina pectoris, reversal of graying of the hair, and improvement in texture and appearance of the skin. Recently she has reported animal experiments supporting the use of Gerovital H_3 (Aslan et al. 1985). Originally Aslan used a commercially available 2 percent solution of procaine hydrochloride. In 1955, she dropped the treatment with commercially available procaine and started to make and treat with Gerovital H_3. Gerovital H_3 is a solution of 2 percent procaine hydrochloride with benzoic acid added as a preservative and potassium metabisulfite as an antioxidant. The solution is buffered at pH 3.3 in order to ensure maximum (shelf) stability (Food and Drug Administration 1973). Each 5-ml ampule contains 100 mg of procaine hydrochloride. Assuming that it does have some pharmaceutical effect, the question is, How is this accomplished? One explanation is that the solution is an effective inhibitor of monoamine oxidase. Another explanation involves the presence of benzoic acid, which positively influences the availability of the needed substances to cell. An alternative is that presence of benzoic acid enhances the action of the metabolic products, which include paraaminobenzoic acid and at least one other substance that is believed to have favorable effects upon the organism (Busse 1973).

Ostfeld et al. (1977), in a review of 285 articles and books addressing the subject of procaine hydrochloride, concluded that except for the possible antidepressant effect, there is no convincing evidence that procaine or Gerovital H_3 has any value in the treatment of disease of older patients. Inasmuch as its sole capability may be a mild antidepressant effect, it is possible that the reported improvements may be the relief of complaints associated with the depressive condition.

Limited efforts have been made to produce Gerovital H_3 in the United States. A small amount was sold in two western states, but the drug has not been widely marketed in the United States. The major source of Gerovital H_3 is the Bahama Islands.

Rejuvenation in the Soviet Union

Zhores Medvedev is a distinguished Russian scientist who has made many contributions to biologic aging, including the redundant theory of aging—that the amount of DNA reserve within the genome that can be called upon to maintain vital function plays an important role in determining life span (Busse 1983). He has published two books that are important and are relevant to geriatric psychiatry. Medvedev wrote a historical account of pseudoscience entitled *The Rise and Fall of T.D. Lysenko,* which first appeared in the science underground of the Soviet Union in 1961 and was published in the United States in 1969. The second book, *A Question of Madness,* which Medvedev coauthored with his brother Roy, was published in the United States in 1972. This book is a vivid account of the problems of using psychiatry for incarcerating and harassing political dissenters (Busse 1984).

Medvedev's first book vividly recounts how between 1937 and 1964 Lysenko used a false doctrine and fabricated scientific data to achieve fame and power. Of particular interest to the geriatric psychiatrist is the account by Medvedev of a technique of rejuvenation advocated by a disciple of Lysenko, a woman by the name of O.B. Lepeshinskaya. Around 1949 Lepeshinskaya began to advocate the use of soda baths to prolong life and restore vigor. This practice was warmly supported by Lysenko. This approach quickly moved to the drinking of soda water and finally to the introduction of soda into the body by enema. Apparently the latter two techniques were used as substitutes for those who were unable to take frequent soda baths. Lepeshinskaya also claimed that she could make living matter from nonliving material. Geriatrics is vulnerable to the pseudoscientist.

The Centenarians

Reports have involved three wide-ranging pockets of people. One group (the Viejos) lived in Vilcabamba, a small mountain village in Ecuador. The other two pockets were in widely separated regions of Asia—the Hunzukuts of the Karakoram region in Kashmir and the Abkhazians of the Republic of Georgia in the Soviet Union. Over the past decade, a number of individuals visited the two groups in Ecuador and Georgia. In February 1978, the National Institute of Aging brought together a number of scientists who had visited Vilcabamba. After three visits to Vilcabamba they concluded that the oldest person in the community was 96 years of age. Similar visits to the Soviet Caucasus and reevaluations found the longevity had been grossly exaggerated (Palmore 1984).

An interesting publication of the Soviet Institute of Gerontology (Chebotarev 1984) reported no individuals beyond the age of 114 years. The Soviet scientists concluded that longevity was promoted by physical labor during the course of life, regimens of work alternating with rests, and characteristics of nutrition promoting longevity. The study of Soviet centenarians included data of functional ability. Twenty-five percent of the Soviet centenarians were unable to "self serve," 2 percent showed psychic disorders, 50 percent had hearing loss, and 24.3 percent suffered from impaired vision. In 1985 of the 28.5 million Americans over the age of 65 years, 32 percent were between 75 and 84 years old, 10.5 percent were 85 years and over, yet less than 1 percent had attained the age of 100 years or more.

During the same era, a brief flurry of publicity centered on the "long-lived" Hunzukuts. Hunza is a 2,000-year-old country that has remained virtually isolated from the rest of the world. The statements in the news media claimed that this civilization originated in 330 B.C. when an army division of Alexander the Great of Macedonia broke away, took Persian wives, and purposely lost themselves in the vastness of the Himalayas. These individuals supposedly lived from 120 to 140 years, and men aged 100 years and older fathered children. Hunza women, at age 80, supposedly looked like American women of 40 years. Their longevity was attributed to a number of factors including exercise, diet, periods of relaxation, and moderation in many things including the consumption of wine. In 1978, a biocalendar health system appeared supposedly based on information attained from the Hunza. In recent years, no additional information has appeared. Consequently, we can only assume that these reports were a fabrication or a distortion of fact.

There is widespread agreement that maximum human life span does not and will not in the foreseeable future exceed 116 years.

Attitudes Toward Aging

Marcus Tullius Cicero, the Roman orator and statesman of the first century (106–43 B.C.), incorporated into his elegant speeches and writings the philosophical views and social values of his time (Gruman 1966). Cicero, at the age of 62, produced an essay on senescence ("de Senectute"; 44 B.C.), suggesting that old age was not welcomed equally by different human races. The status the elderly held within a society apparently made a difference. The Spartans capitalized on the experience of older men, and the gerotes, a council of 28 men past 60 years of age, controlled the city–state (Thewlis 1924). Cicero argued that successful aging was obtainable if one developed an appropriate attitude and dealt effectively with the four major complaints associated with aging. It is interesting that these same four complaints exist today.

The first complaint was that society excluded the aged from important work of the world. Cicero replied by saying that courageous elders can find a way to make themselves useful in various advisory intellectual and administrative functions.

The second charge was that aging undermines physical strength and reduces the value of the individual. Cicero answered that bodily declines count for little compared with the cultivation of mind and character.

The third complaint was that aging prevents or reduces the enjoyment of sensual pleasures, particularly sexual enjoyment. Cicero replied that such a loss has some merit because it allows the aged to concentrate on the promotion of reason and virtue.

Finally, to the charge that old age brings with it increasing anxiety about death, Cicero followed Plato by saying that death could be considered a blessing, freeing individuals and their immortal souls from their bodily prison on this very imperfect earth. He added that if one does not believe that the soul is immortal, death remains a virtue as all things must have limitations and the limitation on the duration of life is not unlike the end of a play in the theater.

Cicero concluded by saying that the wise individual is one who submits to the dictates of nature and passes through the vicissitudes of life with a tranquil mind. He implied that the prolongation of life seemed undesirable. He indicated that the prolongation was particularly undesirable, if, in old age, he was to go back to being "a crying child in the cradle." He also indicated that he had no desire to relive his life or to be summoned back to some starting point.

How It Feels to Grow Old

Walter E. Barton, professor emeritus of psychiatry of Dartmouth Medical School and former president of the American Psychiatric Association, was asked to reflect on how it feels to grow old. His response (1986), at which time he was 80 years of age, is a remarkable report and is consistent with clinical experience in dealing with elderly persons. It is also very similar to reports that have appeared in the literature for many centuries although some of those who have reported in the literature apparently experienced the ravages of aging at a younger age. Barton, in his self-observation of aging, comments on visual problems including glare and the hazards of night driving, the decline in manual dexterity, and the fear of loss of mental acuity. In spite of these and other concerns, Barton observes that "We [Dr. and Mrs. Barton] suffer no depressed mood" and "We have developed the ritual which we observe each Friday when we toast our survival through another week" (p. 192). In answer to the question, how does it feel to grow old, Barton responds that it feels "disgusting, disagreeable, and terribly terminal" (p. 192). If one is blessed with an intact mind, according to Barton, one can find satisfaction in life and erect defenses against undesirable feelings. However, he does conclude, "The years of the seventies are not so bad, but the eighties with the rise in chronic illness are mostly downhill" (p. 192).

Another famous psychiatrist, Francis Braceland, also a past president of the American Psychiatric Association, commented about aging, "When it's quiet I can almost hear brain cells drop out" (Braceland 1978).

Maximianus was a Latin poet contemporary with Boethius in the time of Justinian the Great (483–565), a Byzantine emperor. Maximianus wrote six elegies on old age and love that are, according to Lind (1988), "unmatched in ancient or modern poetry" for their explicitly detailed realism and their almost clinical descriptions of the visible and psychological phenomena of aging.

Maximianus preferred to refer to himself as the Etruscan, but this was a misnomer because the Etruscan race no longer existed and he was probably a Tuscan. There is nothing prudish about Maximianus' elegies as he reflects on the four major loves that occurred during his life. The first was Lycoris, who was either his concubine or a live-in partner and who remained the longest with him but finally left him in their old age. After two subsequent loves, Maximianus met his fourth love, an unnamed Greek performer in Constantinople, with whom he had the most humiliating of all of his sexual experiences—a collapse into impotency.

Lind, in his introduction to Maximianus, quotes from a number of other medieval poems. The poems contain very negative statements about old age and particularly dwell on how older people become ugly. It is evident that most of the older persons living in medieval times lost their teeth and did not have false teeth. This not only interfered with their ability to chew "with toothless gums," but was a major contributor to their ugliness. It is also very likely that exposure of the face to sun and weather not only increased those skin changes associated with aging, but also increased skin lesions. One poem states that old men become "so revolting . . . to wife and children and themselves that even fortune hunters pass them by."

Gerontocomia was published by Gabriele Zerbi in 1482 in Latin. Zeman (1967) reported finding this fascinating volume and said that Zerbi's work had not previously been quoted by any medical or lay writer since its original publication. Lind (1988) attests to the fact that this lengthy manuscript had previously not been translated into English and had been largely overlooked. Lind describes *Gerontocomia* as "the first practical manual on the problems of old age" (p. 7). Zerbi deals with the care of the aged in a rest home, especially selected with regard to climate, exposure, equipment, and staff. He covers all of his ideas regarding longevity and maintaining health. He advocates exercise, bathing, massage, rest, and diet. He refers to medications that are useful to old people and discusses their ingredients and dosages. One of Zerbi's most fascinating recommendations is the continuing use of human milk for the aged. Zerbi emphasizes the proper characteristics of the wet nurse and advises that the patient take the milk directly from the nipple. This custom, which was deeply rooted in antiquity, continues to appear periodically in recent times. In Steinbeck's *Grapes of Wrath* a dying old man is nursed by a young girl who has just lost her baby. As to clothing, Zerbi recommends silk over linen. Silk garments are soft and warm while linen is flat textured and therefore cold. He says that clothes woven with wool and silk are warm and dry and keep one moderately warm. Recognizing that death and old age are inevitable, Zerbi states, "It is impossible therefore to prevent the wasting away of old, but it is possible to combat and resist it considerably."

According to Zerbi, there are two kinds of causes of old age: extrinsic and intrinsic. The extrinsic are in the realm of the astrologers. The first perod of old age is governed by Jupiter while the last stage of old age is governed by Saturn. He observes that there are very few humans who live beyond 100 years. Those who do live that long are said to pass from the leadership of Saturn to that of the moon, which is, in effect, a reversion to the moon which was important to humans at approximately 25 years of age. His comments indicate that since no one can do much about the astrology component, physicians should be more concerned with the intrinsic processes of old age. He further states that the human body has the beginnings of its generation from the sperm of both men and women, but apparently the fetus grew as a result of both blood and sperm. Apparently the idea was that when something goes wrong with the composition of the two fluids, then problems develop. These problems are both claimed to be in the areas of astrology and medicine; therefore, Zerbi says, "These two masters, the physician and the astrologer, must in particular consult and provide for human nature" (Lind 1988, p. 35).

Almost 400 years later, Alfred Worchester published a book, *Care of the Aged: The Dying and the Dead.* Worchester (quoted in Zeman 1967) observes that not all persons are suitable to practice the health professions and states, "I have maintained that a young woman's fitness for the nurse's calling can be determined by the reaction of babies to her care of them. In a like manner, I maintain that a young physician's fitness can be gauged by the reaction of his aged patient as it evolves in his care of them. No surer measure can be of this tact and courtesy and his sympathy and devotion. These are the indispensable qualities of the physicians" (p. 152).

The Advantages of Aging

Most people seem to have difficulty thinking of the advantages of aging. Palmore (1979, p. 220) quotes this example from Kanin's *Remembering Mr. Maugham*:

> W. Somerset Maugham was being honored by the Garrick Club as part of his eightieth birthday celebration. He spoke the customary salutations, paused for a moment and said, "There are many . . . virtues in . . . growing old." He paused, he swallowed, he wet his lips, he looked about. The pause stretched out, he looked dumbstruck. The pause became too long—far too long. He looked down, studying the tabletop. A terrible tremor of nervousness went through the room. Was he ill? Would he ever be able to get on with it? Finally he looked up and said, "I'm just . . . trying . . . to think what they are!"

Palmore believes he has documented some major advantages of aging. These include the fact that the aged are the most law abiding of all age groups, except for young children. The aged are much better citizens and are interested and active in public issues and political affairs. They make an enormous contribution to society by maintaining voluntary participation in community organizations, churches, and recreational groups. Although many are not gainfully employed, they are quite capable of participating in performance tasks. Older workers are stable and dependable workers and have less absenteeism. Although older persons are equally exposed to crimes of certain types, they are much less likely to be the victims of crime in general than other age groups. Although some of their apparent advantages are under constant pressure, it is obvious that Social Security and other pension systems have improved their economic status, as have lower taxes and other economic benefits such as reduced rates in many hotels, motels, and recreational facilities. Medicare, inspite of its limitations, provides health insurance for many older people who would not otherwise be covered. Undoubtedly there are other advantages. The disadvantages, as is true in all medical publications, repeatedly appear throughout this book.

A Definition of Aging

Aging in living organisms usually refers to the adverse effects of the passage of time, although occasionally the term refers to the desirable processes of maturation or acquiring a desirable quality. The multiple processes of decline that are associated with growing old can be separated into primary and secondary aging (Busse 1987). Biological aging is not necessarily confined to the latter years of life; some declines begin with conception. In general, the term does designate those physical changes that develop in adulthood, result in a decline in efficiency of function, and terminate in death. Primary aging is held to be intrinsic to the organism and the decremental factors are determined by inherent or hereditary influences. The rate of aging as a functional decline varies widely between individuals. Further, there are extreme aging variations in systems, organs, and cells. Secondary aging refers to the appearance of defects and disabilities that are caused by hostile factors in the environment including trauma and acquired disease.

This operational separation of primary and secondary aging processes has limitations since both the inherent (hereditary) and the acquired decremental age changes are often of multiple etiology. Inherent defects that make the organism vulnerable may not appear unless and until the organism is exposed to hostile precipitating events.

Aging definitions, including those for primary and secondary aging, that have been offered are not consistently accepted and applied. The aging of living organisms is a universal phenomenon, but the rate of aging can vary between individuals and groups. In humans, aging differences are in part genetically determined but are substantially influenced by nutrition, life-style, and environment. There are some scientists who define primary aging as first cause, and secondary aging as the pathologic processes that ensue from the first cause.

Many age changes are relatively benign and allow a person to continue to function, meet personal needs, and maintain a place in society. Age changes are recognized as a decline in efficiency or performance but in the extreme are often labeled a disease. Examples of age changes that can become sufficiently severe to be a disease include kidney function (creatinine clearance), respiratory performance (forced expiratory volume), an increase in systolic blood pressure (isolated systolic hypertension), and the response to oral glucose tolerance tests (non-insulin-dependent diabetes) (Tobin 1984).

The chronological age of a person is often estimated by changes in appearance and the person's ability to perform tasks associated with activities of daily living and working. As one ages, skin often becomes wrinkled, dry, and seborrheic, and actinic keratosis appears. Hair becomes gray and thinner; baldness increases. Teeth decay and are lost. As one ages, height tends to decrease, as does weight. Chest depth and abdominal depth both increase. The ear lengthens and the nose broadens. Fat cells invade muscle and muscle strength decreases. Posture and height are affected by musculoskeletal changes. Bone densities, influenced by sex and race, decrease with age; some bones are more vulnerable than others.

The metabolic dimensions that are affected by age include absorption, distribution, destruction, excretion, the kinetics of drug binding, and alterations in biologic rhythms. Drugs are therefore metabolized in old people differently from the way they are metabolized in younger adults.

One important age change is the loss of irreplaceable cells, most noticeable in the brain, heart, and muscle.

Striated musculature diminishes about one-half by approximately 80 years of age. As these muscle cells disappear, they are replaced by fat cells and fibrous connective tissue. Hence the storage capacities are increased of certain drugs that are stored in fat cells. The loss of brain cells alters important aspects of body metabolism and affects circadian rhythms. Aging also produces a decrease in heart cells resulting in alterations in certain cardiac functions. Pulmonary changes take place.

In the brain, neurons are lost and there are alterations of neuronal synapses and networks. The loss of nerve cells, particularly those in vulnerable areas of the hypothalamus, may contribute to placing the elderly at risk for certain physiologic changes and associated mental and emotional aberrations. Aging results in a decline of neurotransmitters such as dopamine, norepinephrine, serotonin, tyrosine hydroxylase, and cholinesterase. The activity of monoamine oxidase increases with age.

Selected Biologic Theories of Aging

There are many theories and processes of aging. A satisfactory, unified theory of aging does not exist. In part this is explained by the fact that the body is composed of three major components, namely, cells capable of dividing, cells not able to undergo mitosis, and an interstitial noncellular material. Similar age changes have been identified in one or two of the body components, but rarely are seen in all three. A number of theories of aging lack adequate scientific proof. For example, at the present time, although not proved, there is substantial evidence that intrinsic cellular or molecular aging changes underlie many of the neuronal or endocrine changes associated with the brain.

Classification of theories. In a review of biologic theories of aging, Hart and Turturro (1985) categorized theories into cellular, organ, and population based; integrative approaches; and meta-aging. The cellular-based theories are those that emphasize the importance of the inherent limited potential proliferation of cells. These theories are consistent with the fact that animals have decreased cellularity in a number of organs as aging advances. Consequently, stem cells as they age exhibit a progressively limited ability to repopulate differentiated daughter cells. The capacity for limited proliferation is linked to some experiments that have demonstrated that the limited proliferation of cells is the result of stochastic changes. Other experiments have been concerned with somatic mutation theory of aging and the closely associated "error theory." Finally, cellular aging may be attributed to accumulated effects of damage from the expression of "cell death genes" important to development. This is linked with the observation that during embryogenesis the number of cells retained for further development is reduced by some genetic mechanism. Since cells are reduced in late life, it would be important to understand the underlying mechanism that early in life is needed by the organism but late in life may be detrimental. In a similar manner, this review identifies those theories of aging that are properly related to the category under discussion. The final category of aging theories mentioned by Hart and Turturro is meta-aging. This encompasses what the authors refer to as "the theory of the theory of aging." The complexity of such a discussion is obvious, and the development of a unified theory of aging will be extremely difficult since such a theory of biosenescence would take into consideration all of the processes an individual undergoes as well as the sequence of interactions that transpire within the individual over a lifetime.

Watch spring theory. One early biologic explanation of aging rested on the assumption that a living organism contained a fixed store of energy not unlike that contained within a coiled watch spring. When the spring of the watch was unwound, life ended. This is a type of exhaustion theory.

Another simple theory relates to the accumulation of deleterious material. This particular theory is given some support by the observation that pigments such as lipofuscin accumulate in a number of cells throughout the life span. Although these two simple theories may make some contribution to the aging process, there is little evidence that they have any substantial role.

The "aging clock." The hypothalamus is said to be the location of the "aging clock." Age changes within the hypothalamus play a particularly important role in losses of homeostatic mechanisms in the body. Cell loss, the common event in late life, occurs within clusters of cells within the hypothalamus. The disappearance of a few critical cells in the hypothalamus may have far-reaching consequences. The remaining aging cells may become less efficient. The hypothalamus undoubtedly affects important changes within the pituitary that in turn have impact on other glands and organs within the body. As a consequence, there are many endocrine changes. Alterations within the hypothalamus affect numerous connections within the brain and play a major role in age changes associated with chemical messengers of the brain.

Stochastic theories. Processes of aging that are associated with random changes such as cell loss or mutation are often termed "stochastic" theories. Stochastic implies "a process or a series of events for which the estimate of the probability of certain outcomes approaches the true possibility as the number of events increases" (Busse 1977).

The atomic scientist Leo Szilard advanced a stochastic theory based on what he termed "a hit." A hit was not solely the result of radiation, but rather could be considered any event that would alter a chromosome. In addition, Szilard believed that every animal carries a load of what he termed "faults." A fault is a congenital absence or impairment of one of the genes essential to cell function. A cell is capable of operating as long as one of the pair of genes continues to function; however, when both members of a pair of essential genes are incapable of functioning, the cell declines and dies. Therefore, a cell will cease to function effectively if one of the pair carries the fault and the other is the victim of a hit or if both of the pair are the victims of hits. One reservation in Szilard's theory is that it is applicable only to irreplaceable cells. The second objection to the fault/hit approach is that individuals having pairs of like (homozygous) genes should survive hits much more readily than heterozygous individuals having many dissimilar gene pairs. Yet hybrids, that is, heterozygous individuals with dissimilar genes, live consistently longer than inbreds or homozygous individuals (Busse 1977).

Holliday (1986) observed that stochastic processes may also be under genetic control, since the frequency of defects in macromolecules or the ability to remove defects is known to be determined by the genotype of the organism.

Deliberate biological programming. The theory of deliberate biologic programming has received considerable attention. This theory holds that within a normal cell are stored the memory and the capability of determining the life of a cell. This theory is consistent with the research and conclusions of Hayflick. The memory capacity to terminate life is found in all normal human diploid cells. In mixoploid or cancer cells this memory or capacity to be carried out apparently is destroyed and the cells can duplicate indefinitely.

Cristofalo (1972) reports that the number of doublings is not different in male or females cells. (Female cells are easily identified by the presence of a bar body, the second sex chromosome.) This observation suggests that the difference in life expectancy between the male and female human cannot be attributed to intracellular differences (Weiss 1974).

The free radical theory. A free radical is a chemical molecule or compound that has an odd number of electrons (an unpaired electron) and is highly reactive, in contrast to most chemical compounds, which have an even number of electrons and are stable. Often considered molecular fragments, free radicals are highly reactive and destructive, but they are produced by normal metabolic processes and are ubiquitous in living substances. They can also be produced by ionizing radiation, ozone, and chemical toxins such as insecticides. Free radicals can be produced as the intermediate byproducts of normal metabolic processes. The free radical molecule O_2 is an important agent of oxygen toxicity and the aging process. Scavengers of free radicals exist within cells. Enzymatic defenses involve superoxide desmutase, catalases, and perioxidases. Free radicals have been linked to DNA damage, the cross-linkage of collagen, and the accumulation of age pigments (Busse 1983).

Immune system. The immune system performs both surveillance and protective tasks. It is a complex, widespread bodily function that is essential for the preservation of life (Suskind 1980). The destruction of the immune system is well known to people because it is identified with acquired immune deficiency syndrome (AIDS) (Laurence 1985). Traditionally the immune system has been considered to have two major components. One is the humoral immune response, characterized by the production of antibody molecules that specifically bind the introduced foreign substance. The second is the cellular immune response. Cells are mobilized that can specifically react with and destroy the invader. Considerable evidence has accumulated that a decrease in the immune competence and alterations in the regulation of the immune system are associated with aging. With aging, surveillance is impaired and there is a decline in the efficiency of the protective mechanism. Furthermore, there is a loss of control so that immune functions become so distorted that they are self-destructive. The impairment of the immune system results in an increased incidence of certain diseases in the aging population. Certain tumors in the aged appear to be related to the failure of the body to recognize and eliminate abnormal cells. Autoantibodies increase with the passage of time, and the presence of autoantibodies identifies subpopulations at risk of early death. The older body has an increased susceptibility to infection, and, in general, effective immunization cannot be induced in late life (Finkelstein 1984).

Cells that cannot divide (i.e., neurons and cardiac muscle cells) may be particularly vulnerable to alterations in the immune system. The loss of nondividing cells in the aging body has been previously mentioned. It may be that this loss is the result of the inability of the immune system to protect these nonreplaceable cells or that the death of the cells may be the result of autoaggressive processes.

Eversion (cross-linkage). The cross-linkage or eversion theory of aging is based on the observation that there are changes in collagen structure associated with aging. Collagen is probably the most important protein in the human body. There two types of collagen—interstitial and basement membrane. With the passage of time the ester bonds from within the collagen molecule switch to binding together individual collagen molecules. This aging chain alters the characteristics of connective tissue. Cross-linkage may, in addition, be caused by glycosylation.

Glycosylation. Glucose is the body's most abundant sugar and is important to cell metabolism, particularly neurons. Glycosylation is a nonenzymatic reaction between glucose and protein (Cerami et al. 1987). It is known as the browning reaction or the Maillard. This reaction has been known to food chemists for years, but it was not understood that it could take place within the body. The process has long been known to discolor and toughen foods.

Normally within the body when enzymes attach glucose to proteins, they do so at a specific site on a specific molecule for a specific purpose. In contrast, the nonenzymatic process adds glucose haphazardly to any of several sites along any available peptide chain. The nonenzymatic process apparently increases with aging and culminates with the formation and accumulation of irreversible cross-links between adjacent protein molecules. Cerami et al. (1987) also propose that the nonenzymatic addition of glucose to nucleic acids may gradually damage DNA.

The end products of glycosylation are yellowish-brown and fluorescent and have specific spectrographic properties. Most important for the body is that many of these end products can cross-link with adjacent proteins. The realization that the browning reaction could occur in and potentially damage the body emerged from studies of diabetes. Now it appears that the glucose changes could also play a role in the tissue changes associated with normal aging.

Although additional research is needed to understand the importance of glycosylation, it is a promising theory since it appears that treatments could be developed to prevent some of the changes that connect glycosylation with aging.

Genetics of human aging. Brown and Wisniewski (1983) stated that the genetic nature of the aging process is reflected by the wide range of maximal life span that animal species may attain. Among mammals, the life span range is from 1 year in the smoky shrew to over 114 years in humans. This wide variation in life span emphasizes that the aging process is likely to have an underlying basis that is in part encoded in our genes. The genetic basis may involve two types of inherited species-specific differences. The first type relates to development of the organism. This mechanism governs program timings in developmental stages as well as rates of maturation. The second genetic determinant relates to self-maintenance. This mechanism influences the efficiency of enzymatic systems as well as protection and repair of internal and external insults to the machinery. If the DNA process in itself is damaged or declines in efficiency, the functioning capacity of the organism is severely impaired. It is obvious that the numerous biologic changes that transpire over the life span are very complicated. It is likely that many interacting genes are involved. However, specific genetic defects have been identified that are particularly relevant to certain life-shortening conditions. It is possible there are other genes that contribute to a longer life; however, at this stage of our knowledge, only rarely have specific genes been identified that consistently increase life expectancy, while there are many genetic defects that contribute to reducing life expectancy.

McKusick (1982) listed over 3,000 specific human gene conditions that are known to result in defects within the human organism. These 3,000 recognized human gene conditions are genetically considered to be autosomal, dominant, or recessive and/or X-linked. It appears that there are rare autosomal, dominant genetic conditions that may increase the average life expectancy. One of these is the condition of serum lipids involving hypo-beta-lipoproteinemia and hyper-alpha-lipoproteinemia that decrease susceptibility to atherosclerosis and hence may prevent the occurrence of heart disease.

In Chapter 12 the genetic determinants in dementia are discussed. In brief it is evident that senile dementia of the Alzheimer's type (i.e., at least certain subgroups) does have a genetic component. Creutzfeldt-Jakob's disease appears to be related to both a virus and a familial tendency. Two important factors are involved, and it may be that heredity produces a susceptibility to infectious viruses. A relatively rare syndrome, Gerstmann-Straussler syndrome, is a dementia accompanied by spinocerebellar ataxia that has been shown to have an autosomal dominant inheritance. Interestingly, from a neuropathologic viewpoint, this syndrome has neuritic and amyloid plaques, which of course are very common in senile dementia of the Alzheimer's type and are related to chromosome 21 (Barnes 1987).

Martin (1977) reviewed a long list of human genetic conditions to select out those that had physical and physiologic changes usually associated with senescence. He identified the 10 genetic disorders that had the highest number of senescent features and thus were considered to be associated with the aging process. These 10 genetic diseases included Down's syndrome, Werner's syndrome, Cockayne's syndrome, progeria, ataxia telangectasia, Seip syndrome, cervical lipodysplasia, Klinefelter's syndrome, Turner's syndrome, and myotonic dystrophy.

Length of Life: The Sex Differential

In humans and in many other animal species, females outlive males. It is easy to assume that the differences between the two sexes are genetically determined by the presence or absence of the male Y chromosome. It has been suggested that the greater constitutional weakness of males may be due to their having only one X chromosome.

Prior to 1900 in those nations where data are available, it appears there were slightly more older men than women. After the turn of the century, this situation gradually changed, and by 1940 the situation had reversed itself. Thereafter, the preponderance of older women grew rapidly. In 1985 in the population over 65 years the sex ratio was 147 women for every 100 men; this discrepancy is increasing.

Contrary to the reasonable expectation of the equal balance in males and females at birth, there are in the United States approximately 106 to 110 white males born for every 100 white females. Among the United States blacks, there are approximately 104 black males born for every 100 black females born. It is reported, but not confirmed, that in black populations of several islands in the West Indies, there are fewer males than females at birth (American Association of Retired Persons 1987).

Numerous environmental factors have been investigated to determine their influence on sex ratio at birth. In England and Wales it has been reported that upper socioeconomic groups are likely to have a higher ratio of males to females than do lower socioeconomic groups. During World War II many European countries observed that the ratio of males was higher than during times of peace. It is possible this is due to the births occurring in younger parents as opposed to older parents during peace time.

At birth the female in the more developed nations has a life expectancy of as much as 8+ years beyond that of the male. In 1978 France had the most extreme male–female differences for life expectancy at birth, 8.21 years. Canada was second with a difference of 7.59 years. In 1981 Japan had the best life expectancy at birth. For females it was 79.1 years and males 73.8 years, a difference of 5.3 years. In Japan this male–female difference is increasing rather than decreasing since in 1970 there was a difference of 4.4 years and in 1952 a difference of 3.4 years.

Geriatric psychiatry is particularly concerned with the remaining years after the age of 65. In the United States in 1985 the female aged 65 years could expect to live another 18.6 years, but the male only 14 years (American Association of Retired Persons 1987). This sex imbalance in late life has important social and medical implications. Most older men are married, while most older women are widowed or single (divorced or never married). The sex imbalance is enhanced by the practice of men marrying younger females, thus expanding the pool of older, unmarried women. The recognition of the preponderance of women in modern society undoubtedly affects socioeconomic planning and programs in health care.

Waldron (1986) reviewed the literature as to causes of sex differences in mortality. She noted that in contemporary industrial societies the single most important cause of higher mortality for males has been greater cigarette smoking by males. Other sex differences are related behaviors that contribute to the males' higher mortality. Such behaviors include heavier alcohol consumption and employment in hazardous occupations. In many nonindustrial societies, these factors play a less important role where, in many instances, the sex differences in mortality are not as great as in the industrial societies.

In the nonindustrial societies, females are more vulnerable to infectious diseases. This may be related to less adequate nutrition and health care for females. Waldron described a wide variety of factors that influence sex differences in mortality. In contrast to males in undeveloped nations, males in the United States tend to have a higher death rate than do females for infectious and parasitic disease; American males were more vulnerable in 1930 than in 1978. However, one must be cautious in interpreting this information since Waldron pointed out that sex differences do vary somewhat for different types of infections and parasitic diseases.

The sexes show differences in their immune capacities; for example, females have higher levels than males do of one of the major classes of immunoglobulins (IgM). In theory this may be attributed to the differences in the sex chromosomes. It appears that the female X chromosome carries one or more genes that influence the production of IgM. The pair of X chromosomes in females could result in higher production of IgM than in the single X chromosome of the male. It is also true that sex differences may be the result of exposure to infectious disease. Both work and recreational types of exposure may expose the males to greater contact with infectious diseases.

Death rates by accidents and other violent causes are much higher for males than for females. Motor vehicle accidents account for a significant percentage of these differences. Although Waldron did not mention it, the differences caused by motorcycle accidents in young males is a factor that appears in other U.S. statistics. Males have a much higher death rate than do females from accidental drownings and fatal gun accidents. Suicide is also more prevalent among males and increases with age. Other factors that may play in roles in the male's higher death rate are heavier alcohol consumption and other types of male risk-taking behavior. This may or may not have a biologic component; there also may be a cultural factor.

Ischemic heart disease has been consistently higher for men than for women in almost all available international and historical data. However, the magnitude of sex differences for ischemic heart disease has varied considerably in different regions, historical periods, and ethnic groups.

That a relationship of cigarette smoking to heart disease exists cannot be ignored. Of interest is the fact that women who smoke do not have the same risk as men. This is attributable to different smoking habits. Not only do men smoke more cigarettes per day, but they inhale more deeply. As to smoking, an often overlooked consideration is that females "may often feel sick as a result of smoking their first cigarette" (Waldron 1986, p. 64) and this may be a deterrent to their smoking.

Coronary-prone behavior also plays a significant role. There is a greater prevalence of type A coronary-prone behavior among men than among women. Type A behavior is marked by impatience, competitive drive, and hostility (Busse and Walker 1986).

As to the influence of menopause, there is contradictory evidence regarding the risk of women before or after menopause. There continues to be a debate regarding early onset of menopause. Early natural menopause may be encouraged by smoking, and this may account in part for the increased risk of myocardial infarction for women with early natural menopause (Waldron 1986).

Mortality due to malignant neoplasms or cancer is more frequent among males than females over most of the age span. Because of the large variety of cancers, the patterns and causes of sex differences vary for many different types of malignant neoplasms. Furthermore, occupational exposures contribute to men's higher cancer rate.

Behavioral factors cannot be ignored for either sex. Consequently, there is a complex interaction of cultural, anatomical, physiologic, and behavioral characteristics.

Waldron discusses "Mortality of older adults." This category includes all adults aged 40 and over. Ordinarily this would be considered middle-aged, with old age beginning at 65 years of age. In this age group a reversal of certain trends is beginning to show, for example, the gradual decline of ischemic heart disease.

Waldron (1987) added some additional statistical information as to causes of sex differential in longevity. Of deaths from ischemic heart disease, 50 percent are attributable to smoking. Ischemic heart disease is the major cause of death linked to atherosclerosis, but the atherosclerosis linked to cerebrovascular disease accounts for only 2 percent of the sex differential in total mortality (National Center for Health Statistics 1984). Waldron concluded that smoking's effects on hormones and on atherosclerosis are responsible for, at most, 25 percent of the sex differential and total mortality in the United States. She concluded that other observations point to behavioral factors as more important causes of sex differences in mortality. Taking high-risk behavior as a group, the behaviorial differences appear to be responsible for at least 50 percent of the sex differential in total mortality in the United States. What remains unanswered is, What are the important factors that influence this difference in behavioral risks?

Psychologic Theories of Aging

Birren and Renner (1977) expressed the opinion that there was no pressure on the field of psychology to formulate a unified theory of aging or to explain how behavior is organized over time. They did offer a definition of aging for the behavioral sciences that recognizes that there can be incremental functions as well as decremental changes that occur over the adult life span. "Aging refers to the regular changes that occur in mature, genetically representative organisms living under representative environmental conditions" (Birren and Renner 1977, p. 4). Later, Birren and Cunningham (1985) said, "The psychology of aging is concerned with differences in behavior, changes in behavior with age, and patterns of behavior shown by persons of different ages in different periods of time" (p. 18). They also note that "much of contemporary psychology of aging is a collection of segments of knowledge" (p. 18). Further, this implies that most theories in the psychology of aging are actually microtheories because they do not embrace large amounts of data derived from various domains of behavior.

Baltes and Willis (1977) reached a somewhat similar conclusion saying, "All existing theories [of psychologic aging and development] are of the prototheoretical kind and are incomplete" (p. 148). The psychologic theories that have appeared are often the extension of personality and developmental theories into middle and late life. Personality theories usually consider the innate human needs and forces that motivate thought and behavior and a modification of these biologically based energies by the experience of living in a physical and social environment. Schaie (1977–1978) has recently advanced what he calls "a stage theory of adult cognitive deveopment." His tentative scheme involves four possible cognitive stages. These sequential stages are denoted as acquisitive (childhood, adolescence), achieving (young adulthood), responsible and executive (middle age), and reintegrative (old age). During middle life he postulates two overlapping cognitive patterns—a "responsible" component and "executive" abilities—neither of which can be judged by common psychometric testing. He suggests that during the life span there is a transition from "what should I know" through "how should I use what I know" to "why should I know" phase of life. Schaie (1977–1978) believes that numerous new strategies and techniques will have to be developed in order to fully test a stage theory that alterations in the theory will emerge.

Kalish and Knudtson (1976) recommended the extension of the concept (theory) of attachment common in infant and child psychology to a lifetime conceptual scheme for understanding relationships and involvements of older people. They further believed that the concept (theory) of disengagement is not functional and that it should be eliminated. Attachment is a relationship established and maintained by "social bonds" and is distinguished from social contact. Elderly people lose significant early objects of attachment. New attachments are often much weaker and frequently not mutual and therefore vulnerable. Kalish and Knudtson (1976) argued that an appreciation and understanding of attachments will provide a better approach to explaining the psychologic changes in elderly people. Relevant to the attachment concept is the finding by Lowenthal and Haven (1968) that more than any other single factor, having a confidant appeared to discriminate between elderly persons who were institutionalized and those who could remain in the community.

There are obvious realistic limitations in the psychologic theories of aging; however, these are quite realistic in view of the complexity of the research. Furthermore, recognizing the complexity of psychologic experimentation and theory is essential to be aware of the considerable psychologic investigations that have contributed to a better understanding of human aging. Consequently, the material by Siegler and Poon presented in Chapter 7 ("The Psychology of Aging") is essential to achieving an adequate knowledge of human aging.

Social Theories of Aging

Palmore (1981) proposed five social categories of social theories. These include (1) disengagement activity and continuity theories, (2) age stratification, (3) minority group theory, (4) life events and stress theory, and (5) homogeneity versus heterogeneity.

Disengagement theory states that aging invariably causes physical, psychologic, and social disengagement (Cumming and Henry 1961). Physical disengagement is attributable to a decline in physical energy, strength, and the slowing of responses. Psychologic disengagement refers to the withdrawal of concern from a rather diffuse interest in many people to those who are directly related to the individual. Some describe this as a shift of attention from the outer world to the inner world of one's own feelings and thoughts. Social disengagement means the reduction of all types of social interaction including such activities as those related to family, friends, community actions, church participation, and so forth. This theory of disengagement originally held that it was actually good for the older person and for society for the older person to disengage. It was held that the disengaged older persons tend to be happier and healthier than those who remain active.

Shortly after the appearance of the disengagement theory the activity theory appeared (Havighurst 1963). This theory holds that remaining active is good for the aging individual and society. Activity is believed to affect health, happiness, and longevity.

The continuity approach is something of a compromise position between the disengagement and activity theories (Neugarten 1964). This maintains that older people tend to behave in a pattern that has been established prior to late life. At times the person may disengage and other times remain active. It is also apparent that some elderly people will drop one type of activity only to replace it by something that is more suitable to their health status and environment.

Age stratification is really a model of life span development, but obviously includes late life as a part of the conceptualization. According to Palmore (1981), age stratification considers that society is composed of different age groups with different roles and different expectations. Each age group must move up through time while responding to changes in environment. Age stratification focuses on distinguishing between age, period, and cohort effects.

The minority group theory relates to differences such as those attributed to race and ethnic groups. It asserts that the aged are a minority group and are frequently discriminated against by society just as other minorities are (Busse 1970).

The theory of life events and stress maintains that those major events usually associated with advancing age are particularly important to health and well-being in late life. A study utilizing this approach must distinguish events that may be welcomed or resisted and those that do not affect all people in a similar manner. Some people resist retirement while others welcome it. Some are unhappy in retirement and others see it as an opportunity to attain life satisfactions.

Some social theories are related to the age distribution of the population and economic influences. One of these theories holds that the status of the aged is high in static societies and tends to decline with the acceleration of social change (Ogburn and Nimkoff 1940). Another theory is that the status of the aged is inversely related to the proportion of the aged in the population. The aged are mostly highly valued in societies in which they are scarce and their value and status decrease as they become more numerous. The modernization theory of Cowgill and Holmes (1972) suggests that elderly persons are more highly respected in agricultural societies than they are in urbanized societies, and that the status of the aged is inversely proportionate to the rate of social change. A recent study suggests that in some societies in the process of modernization, the status of the aged goes through phases. During a developmental phase toward modernization there is an increase in family control of resources, but as modernization continues the status of elderly people is likely to decline (Gilleard and Gurkan 1987).

Homogeneity and heterogeneity are concerned with the issue of whether individuals become more like each other or more different from each other as they age (Maddox and Douglass 1974). One interesting consideration is the possibility that those who survive into late life (i.e., 85 years old and over) have identifiable characteristics that are very similar, while in contrast, they may have been quite different from the other people in the same age group 10 to 15 years earlier.

There is also the controversy as to differences between men and women. Do they become increasingly different, or increasingly similar?

All of these theories have been demonstrated to have varying degrees of validity. No satisfactory composite theory of social aging is available that is applicable to all aging people.

Models of Early Aging

The progerias are syndromes that are linked with premature aging. The victims of these disorders do, to a limited extent, provide an opportunity to study accelerated bodily changes that resemble those attributable to aging. Because Werner's syndrome differs from normal aging in several respects, Martin (1985) classified this condition as a "segmental progeroid syndrome."

The appearance of these individuals is indeed striking since the initial impression is that the person is very old. Although all of these syndromes are quite rare, two have received the most attention. These are the Hutchinson-Gilford syndrome (Hutchinson 1886; Hastings 1904) and Werner's syndrome. The early-onset Hutchinson-Gilford syndrome is characterized by dwarfism, physical immaturity, and pseudosenility. These individuals have a peculiar form of hypermetabolism and generally die during their mid-teens of coronary heart disease. Progeria affects both sexes and has been described in white, black, and Asian races. The affected individuals look like very old, wizened, small distorted humans. This is because their heads are comparatively large, while the face is small, and the ears and nose are small. Scalp hair, eyebrows, and eyelashes are lost. Some of the features that are commonly associated with aging are not increased in Hutchinson-Gilford syndrome. These include tumors, cataracts, and osteoporosis.

The search for the mode of inheritance of Hutchinson-Gilford syndrome continues. It has been considered to be a rare autosomal recessive condition, but it has been argued that is it more likely a sporadic autosomal-dominant mutation because of several observations including (1) a lower frequency of consanguinity than expected, (2) the low frequency of reoccurrence in families, and (3) a possible parental age effect. The vast majority of cases occur with no siblings affected. For this reason, progeria (particularly Hutchinson-Gilford syndrome) may be a sporadic dominant-type mutation.

Although the life span of fibroblasts of progeria is affected, there have been variations in reporting whether the life span reduction is modest or severe. Furthermore the suspicion that a basic defect in protein synthesis fidelity is a basic defect in progeria lacks confirmation (Goldstein et al. 1985). Similarly there is confusion regarding the existence or nonexistence of definitive immune abnormalities. As to DNA repair capability, although such a defect is not uncommon, it is not a consistent marker for progeria. Because of this deficiency in knowledge, one must conclude that the basic metabolic defect is, at this time, unknown.

Werner's syndrome is a later onset type of progeria. Werner (1904) described in his doctoral dissertation for graduation from Ophthalmological Clinic in Kiel an unusual disorder under the title "Cataract in Connection with Scleroderma." Werner reported the condition in siblings, two brothers and two sisters, between the ages of 36 and 40 years of age. Parents, grandparents, and one sister were healthy. As the disease develops, the individuals look 20 to 30 years older than their actual years, and their life span is shortened. Since the disease usually appears before growth is completed, individuals frequently will have thin limbs and are of smaller stature and less developed than would be expected. Their appearance is striking in that the face develops a tightly drawn pinched expression. There is a pseudoexophthalmos, a beak nose, protuberant teeth, and a recessive chin. Cataracts develop early, and in addition to hypogonadism individuals are likely to have diabetes. Not infrequently they develop cancer, which contributes to their shortened life expectancy. The connective tissue cells and fibroblasts of these patients have been studied. For instance, Hayflick (1977) mentions that the fibroblast cells derived from such individuals and cultured in vitro undergo significantly fewer doublings than their age-matched controls. Progressive mental deterioration is not commonly associated with the progerias, and there are few neuropathologic studies of their brains. The usual microscopic changes associated with aging, senile plaques, and neurofibriliary tangles are not a characteristic of Werner's syndrome (Ishii et al. 1985). Sumi (1985) reports that Marinesco found small, round eosinophilic inclusions in the nuclei of the neurons in the substantia nigra. According to another review, approximately 25 percent have mild neurologic defects such as loss of distal deep tendon reflexes, but no systematic psychologic or electroencephalogram studies have been reported. It is highly likely, however, that psychologic problems are common (Omenn 1977).

Since 1904, at least 250 patients have been reported with similar clinical findings and have been labeled "Werner's syndrome." Goto et al. (1978) reported 15 patients with progeria—12 males and 3 females—ranging from 17 to 59 years of age. All patients showed the following signs and symptoms: short stature and light body weight, slender extremities with a stocky trunk, beak-shaped nose, high-pitched and weak voice or hoarseness, juvenile bilateral cataracts, flat feet, and hyperreflexia of the patellar and Achilles tendons. Thirteen of the 15 patients had parents who were consanguineously married, although the article does not indicate any further information regarding their consanguineous relationship. It was noted, however, that a consanguineous marriage is common in Japan. Goto et al. were able to collect a total of 100 cases in Japan and found that the sex ratio was one to one. They do note that the patients were so similar in their facial characteristics that they could be easily mistaken for identical twins. In an attempt to determine the genetic causation, they found no chromosomal abnormalities.

As to the immunologic data, only in one patient did Goto et al. find any differences in the titers of IgG, IgA, IgM, and IgE. The only deviation occurred in one patient who had an elevated IgE. They also note that the ratio of the T-cell subpopulation has been reported to decrease with age; that is, it declines in a normal aging group. However, utilizing the method of Nakai, they found there was a decrease in the T-cell subpopulation. Goto et al. (1978) do not report the age of death of any of the subjects studied.

Werner's syndrome seems to be somewhat different than Hutchinson-Gilford syndrome in that 10 percent of Werner's patients develop neoplasms with a particularly high frequency of sarcomas and meningiomas.

References

American Association of Retired Persons: A Profile of Older Americans, 1986. Washington, DC, American Association of Retired Persons, 1987

Aslan A, Ionescu T, Bordea M, et al: The influence of Gerovital H_3 on the immune cell response in x-rayed Wistar rats. Presented at 13th International Congress of Gerontology, New York, July 12–17, 1985

Baltes PA, Willis SL: Toward psychological theories of aging and development, in Handbook of the Psychology of Aging. Edited by Birren JE, Schaie KW. New York, Van Nostrand Reinhold, 1977

Barnes DM: Defect in Alzheimer's is on chromosome 21. Science 1987; 235:846–847

Barton WE: How it feels to grow old. Integrative Psychiatry 1986; 4:191–192

Birren JE, Cunningham WR: Research on the psychology of aging: principles, concepts, and theory, in Handbook of the Psychology of Aging (second edition). Edited by Birren JE, Schaie KW. New York, Van Nostrand Reinhold, 1985

Birren JE, Renner VJ: Research on the psychology of aging, in Handbook of the Psychology of Aging. Edited by Birren JE, Schaie KW. New York, Van Nostrand Reinhold, 1977

Braceland FJ: Aging ourselves tomorrow, in The 18th Carrier Foundation Symposium. Edited by Garber RS, Sugerman AA. Nutley, NJ, Roche Laboratories, 1978

Brown TW, Wisniewski HM: Genetics of human aging. Review of Biological Research in Aging 1983; 1:81–99

Busse EW: The aged: a deprived minority. North Carolina Journal of Mental Health 1970; 4:3–7

Busse EW: Longevity and rejuvenators, in Mental Illness in Later Life. Edited by Busse EW, Pfeiffer E. Washington, DC, American Psychiatric Association, 1973

Busse EW: Theories of aging, in Behavior and Adaptation in Late Life (second edition). Edited by Busse EW, Pfeiffer E. Boston, Little, Brown, 1977

Busse EW: Biologic and psychosocial bases of behavioral changes in aging, in American Psychiatric Association Annual Review (Volume 2). Psychiatry Update: Washington, DC, American Psychiatric Press, 1983

Busse EW: The political abuse of psychiatry. Perspectives 1984; 4(2):22–24

Busse EW: Primary and secondary aging, in The Encyclopedia of Aging. Edited by Maddox G, Roth G, Atchley R, et al. New York, Springer, 1987

Busse EW, Walker JI: Heart and neuropsychiatric disorders, in The International Text of Cardiology. Edited by Cheng TO. New York, Pergamon Press, 1986

Cerami A, Vlassara H, Brownlee M: Glucose and aging. Sci Am 1987; 256(5):90–96

Chebotarev DF (ed): Longevity: Medical and Social Aspects. Kiev, USSR, Institute of Gerontology AMS USSR and USSR Gerontological and Geriatric Society, 1984

Cowgill D, Holmes L (eds): Aging and Modernization. New York, Appleton-Century-Crofts, 1972

Cristafalo VS: Animal cell cultures as a model for the study of aging, in Advances in Gerontological Research. Edited by Strehler BL. New York, Academic Press, 1972

Cumming E, Henry W: Growing Old. New York, Basic Books 1961

Eriksson EH: Ghandi's Truth on the Origin of Militant Nonviolence. New York, W.W. Norton, 1969

Finkelstein MS: Defenses against infection in the elderly: the compromises of aging. Triangle 1984; 23(2):57–64

Food and Drug Administration: Gerovital H_3 Injectable (prepared by Rom-Amer Pharmaceuticals, Ltd.). Washington, DC, Food and Drug Administration, 1973

Gilleard CJ, Gurkan AA: Socioeconomic development and the status of elderly men in Turkey: a test of modernization theory. J Gerontol 1987; 42:353–357

Goldstein S, Wojtyk RI, Harley CB, et al: Protein synthetic fidelity in aging human fibroblasts, in Werner's Syndrome and Human Aging (Advances in Experimental Medicine and Biology, Volume 190). Edited by Salk D. Fujiwara Y, Martin GM. New York, Plenum Press, 1985

Goto M, Horiuchi Y, Tanimoto K, et al: Werner's syndrome: analysis of 15 cases with a review of the Japanese literature. J Am Geriatr Soc 1978; 26:341–347

Gruman GJ: A History of Ideas About the Prolongation of Life: The Evolution of Prolongevity Hypotheses to 1880. Philadelphia, American Philosophical Society, 1966

Hart RW, Turturro A: Review of recent biological research theories of aging. Review of Biological Research in Aging 1985; 2:3–12

Hastings G: Progeria: a form of senilism. The Practitioner 1904; 73:188–217

Havighurst R: Successful aging, in Processes of Aging. Edited by Williams R, Tibbitts C, Donahue W. New York, Atherton Press, 1963

Hayflick L: The limited in vitro lifetime of human diploid cell strains. Exp Cell Res 1965; 37:614–616

Hayflick L: Cellular basis for biological aging, in Handbook of Biology of Aging. Edited by Finch CE, Hayflick L. New York, Van Nostrand Reinhold, 1977

Hayflick L: Foundations of cytogerontology, in Dimensions of Aging. Edited by Bergener M, Ermini M, Stähelin HB. New York, Academic Press, 1986

Hayflick L, Moorhead PS: The serial cultivation of human diploid cell strains. Exp Cell Res 1961; 25:588–621

Holliday R: Testing molecular theories of cellular aging, in Dimensions of Aging. Edited by Bergener M, Ermini M, Stähelin HB. New York, Academic Press, 1986

Hutchinson J: Case of congenital absence of hair and mammary glands with atrophic condition of the skin and its appendages. Lancet 1886; 1:473–477

Ishii T, Hosoda Y, Hamada Y, et al: Pathology of the Werner syndrome, in Werner's Syndrome and Human Aging (Advances in Experimental Medicine and Biology, Volume 190). Edited by Salk D, Fujiwara Y, Martin GM. New York, Plenum Press, 1985

Kalish, RA, Knudtson FW: Attachment versus disengagement: a life-span conceptualization. Hum Dev 1976; 19:171–181

Kanin G: Remember Mr. Maugham. New York, Athenum, 1966

Laurence J: The immune system in AIDS. Sci Am 1985; 84–93

Lind LR (trans): Gabriele Zerbi, Gerontocomia: On the Care of the Aged and Maximianus, Eligies on Old Age and Love [translated from the Latin]. Philadelphia, American Philosophical Society, 1988

Lowenthal MF, Haven C: Interaction and adaptation: intimacy as a critical variable, in Middle Age and Aging. Edited by Neugarten BL. Chicago, University of Chicago Press, 1968

Maddox GL, Douglass E: Aging and individual differences. J Gerontol 1974; 29:555–563

Martin GM: Genetic syndromes in man with potential relevance to the pathobiology of aging: genetics of aging. Birth Defects 1977; 14:5–39

Martin GM: Genetics and aging: the Werner syndrome as a segmental progeroid syndrome, in Werner's Syndrome and Human Aging (Advances in Experimental Medicine and Biology, Volume 190). Edited by Salk D. Fujiwara Y, Martin GM. New York, Plenum Press, 1985

McKusick VA: Mendelian Inheritance in Man, Catalogs of Autosomal Dominant, Autosomal Recessive and X-linked Phenotypes (sixth edition). Baltimore, Johns Hopkins University Press, 1982

National Center for Health Statistics: Monthly Vital Statistics Report 1984; 33(9)

Neugarten B: Personality in Middle and Later Life. New York, Atherton Press, 1964

Ogburn WF, Nimkoff MF: Sociology. Boston, Houghton Mifflin, 1940

Omenn GS: Behavior genetics, in Handbook of the Psychology of Aging. Edited by Birren JE, Schaie W. New York, Van Nostrand Reinhold, 1977

Ostfeld A, Smith CM, Stotsky BA:The systemic use of procaine in the treatment of the elderly: a review. J Am Geriatr Soc 1977; 25:1–19

Palmore E: Advantages of aging. The Gerontol 1979; 19:220–223

Palmore E: Social Patterns in Normal Aging: Findings from the Duke Longitudinal Study. Durham, NC, Duke University Press, 1981

Palmore EB: Longevity in Abkhasia: a reevaluation. The Gerontologist 1984; 24(1):95–96

Schaie KW: Toward a stage theory of adult cognitive development. Journal of Aging and Human Development 1977–1978; 8:129–138

Segerberg O Jr: The Immortality Factor. New York, E.P. Dutton, 1974

Sumi SM: Neuropathology of Werner syndrome, in Werner's Syndrome and Human Aging (Advances in Experimental Medicine and Biology, Volume 190). Edited by Salk D, Fujiwara Y, Martin GM. New York, Plenum Press, 1985

Suskind GW: Immunological aspects of aging: an overview. Presented at National Institute on Aging conference on Biological Mechanisms of Aging, Washington, DC, 1980

Thewlis MW: The history of geriatrics, in The Care of the Aged. Edited by Thewlis MW. St. Louis, C.V. Mosby, 1924

Tobin JD: Physiological indices of aging, in The Baltimore Longitudinal Study of Aging (NIH Pub. No. 84–2450). Edited by Shock NW. Rockville, MD, National Institutes of Health, 1984

Tomkins GA: Stanbridge EJ, Hayflick L: Viral probes of aging in the human diploid cell strain W1-38. Proc Soc Exp Bio Med 1974; 146:385–390

Waldron I: What do we know about causes of sex differences in mortality: a review of the literature. Population Bulletin of the United Nations 1986; 18:59–76

Waldron I: Causes of the sex differential in longevity. J Am Geriatr Soc 1987; 35:365–366

Weiss AK: Biomedical gerontology: the Hayflick hypothesis. Gerontologist 1974; 14:491–493

Werner O: Uber Katarakt im Verbindung mit Sklerdermie. Doctoral dissertation, Ophthalmological Clinic, Kiel, 1904

Zeman FD: Some little known classics of old-age medicine, JAMA 1967; 200:150–152

Chapter 2

The Clinical Impact of Physiologic Changes with Aging

John W. Rowe, M.D.

The Physiology of Aging

Over recent decades, increasing interest in aging and the medical problems of older persons has fueled substantial growth in physiologic, psychologic, and sociologic research on aging. Investigators involved in such studies recognize the critical importance of separating pathologic from age-related changes. Thus, for physiologic studies careful guidelines are developed to exclude individuals whose results might not represent "normal" aging, but would be contaminated with changes related to specific disease processes (Rowe 1985; Shock et al. 1984). Results on the remaining population are felt to represent "normal" aging, with confidence regarding the age specificity of the findings resting more on longitudinal studies of age changes than on cross-sectional comparisons of age differences, which are sensitive to cohort effects. Numerous carefully conducted cross-sectional and longitudinal studies on well-screened, well-characterized populations have demonstrated major effects of age on a number of clinically relevant variables, including hearing, vision, renal function, glucose tolerance, systolic blood pressure, bone density, pulmonary function, immune function, sympathetic nervous system activity, and a variety of cognitive and behavioral measures. Such nonpathologic aging effects are important to understand not only as reflections of the aging process but, since they serve as a physiologic substrate for the influence of age on the presentation of disease, as reflections of response to treatment and the complications that ensue.

The decline in most variables that change with age is linear into the

35

eighth and ninth decade. While healthy 80-year-olds are more aged than their younger counterparts, having accumulated more of the changes secondary to age, they are not losing function at a more rapid rate.

While many important physiologic variables, including cardiovascular, immune, endocrine, renal, and pulmonary functions, show fairly substantial losses with advancing age, an important characteristic of these data sets is the substantial variability (Rowe 1983, 1985; Shock et al. 1984). The variability often increases with advancing age so that older people become less like each other, not more like each other. In many data sets, one can easily find older persons with minimal or no physiologic loss when compared to their younger counterparts, while the average change in the aged group is a very substantial decrement from the results seen in youth.

Changes in one organ are not necessarily predictive of changes with age in other organs. If an apparently healthy 60-year-old is found on serial prospective measurements to have a cardiac output that is falling at a certain rate, this information is of no value in predicting the rate at which the individual's kidneys, thyroid, sympathetic nervous system, or any other organ is changing with time. This apparent failure of various organs to be synchronized in their age-related changes rules against the presence of a basic biologic clock. Currently one cannot construct a variable termed "functional age" that predicts performance on a physiologic or psychologic test better than the individual's chronologic age.

The variability in human aging from individual to individual is also substantial. In studies of functions that undergo major changes with age, the variance is often large, and one can easily identify apparently healthy 40-year-olds who perform at the same level as the average 80-year-old. Likewise, many 80-year-olds can be found who perform like the average 40-year-old.

Successful and Usual Aging as Subtypes of Normal Aging

The prior focus of research on dichotomizing findings into either disease or "normal" aging categories has important limitations. This approach tends to neglect the substantial heterogeneity among older persons with regard to many physiologic and cognitive variables, it tends to imply that the physiologic changes that occur in older individuals in the absence of disease are harmless and do not carry a significant risk, and finally, the identification of certain physiologic changes as "normal" suggests that these changes are the natural state of affairs and thus cannot or should not be modified.

The physiologic changes that occur with "normal" age, in the absence of disease, are very variable, are in many cases associated with attributable risk for adverse health events, and are potentially modifiable. The contribution of the intrinsic aging process to decrements observed in aged population may be substantially less than previously recognized, with factors such as personal habits, diet, exercise, nutrition, environmental exposures, and body composition playing more important roles.

Rather than focusing purely on differentiation of the effects of disease versus "normal" aging, gerontologic studies should recognize that the "normal" aging group includes two important subsets. One subset is composed of those individuals who demonstrate minimal age-associated losses in a given physiologic function (e.g., immune function, bone density, carbohydrate tolerance, renal function, cognitive function). These individuals might be viewed as aging "successfully" with regard to the particular variable under study. Individuals who demonstrate "successful" aging in a constellation of physiologic functions rather than just one present a state of minimal physiologic loss and robust physiologic function in advanced age—a pure aging syndrome. This successful aging group represents a small but potentially increasing portion of the overall "normal" aging population, the bulk of which is represented by the group that might be termed "usual" aging. For a given physiologic variable, the usual aging group has significant impairments compared with their younger counterparts, but do not qualify as diseased. As noted previously, the physiologic losses in the usual aging group display large interindividual differences and those individuals with the greatest "age effect" are at increased risk for the emergence of a specific disease or disability.

The pathways of physiologic or psychologic change that individuals take with advancing age are influenced by the intrinsic aging process and a variety of extrinsic factors, including genetic and environmental influences, personal habits, diet, psychosocial factors, and diseases. We should also be aware that older persons who display "usual aging" for a given function may be able to improve their function and thus potentially reduce their risk of adverse outcomes. Thus, the focus of study moves gradually from the evaluation of the emergence of diseases in an aging population to elucidation of those factors that regulate the transition of individuals from successful to usual state of aging and vice versa.

With these general considerations in mind, the specific physiologic changes associated with aging will be reviewed from two perspectives. First, the types of changes will be discussed, since they represent a continuum in the interaction of intrinsic aging and pathology. Second, detailed information will be presented on specific clinically relevant physiologic changes in the major organ systems.

The Continuum of Interaction Between Physiology and Pathology in the Elderly

The interaction of age and disease varies from a lack of interaction on one end of the spectrum to the extreme example where the changes that occur with age and are often aggravated by extrinsic factors actually represent disease inasmuch as they have direct, predictable, adverse clinical sequelae. Several specific, clinically relevant points along the continuum can be identified.

Variables That Do Not Change with Age

Perhaps the most important physiologic change that occurs with age, from a clinical standpoint, is no change at all. Too frequently clinicians are apt to ascribe a disability or abnormal physical or laboratory finding to "old age," when the actual cause is a specific disease process. An example of this lack of change may be seen in hematocrit. Frequently elderly individuals will be found to have low hematocrit levels, and the clinician will categorize the patient as having "anemia of old age." The physician may fail to pursue the underlying basis of the anemia, believing that the normal aging process has induced the anemia and that no investigation or treatment is warranted. However, data from several sources, including the Framingham study, indicate that in healthy community-dwelling elderly people there is no change with age in hematocrit (Gordon and Shurtleff 1973). Thus, a lower hematocrit in an elderly individual cannot be ascribed to "anemia of old age," but deserves a proper investigation and treatment.

Physiologic Changes by Which Specific Diseases Become Less Likely or Severe with Age

Although aging is characteristically considered to be associated with a greater prevalence or severity of disease, it is quite possible that the physiologic changes associated with normal aging result in many diseases being less likely or less severe in advanced age. Clearly some disorders that appear to be based, at least in part, in altered immune system response, such as systemic lupus erythematosus, myasthenia gravis, and multiple sclerosis, are seen much more commonly in younger individuals than in older individuals. It is feasible that the changes that occur in the immune system with age might result in a less robust immunologic response to the inciting agent or event in these disorders (Gillis et al. 1981). In this regard, recent findings of increased auto-anti-idiotypic antibody production with age suggest a basis for lessened autoimmune disease in the elderly.

Similarly, some diseases that occur in old age as well as in younger adults clearly run a less virulent natural history in the elderly. One example may be carcinoma of the breast. Many cancer specialists feel that carcinoma of the breast runs a more virulent and more aggressive course in premenopausal than postmenopausal women. In addition, the likelihood of breast carcinoma responding well to hormonal therapy increases with the number of years after menopause. Thus, elderly individuals with this disease might be expected, on average, to enjoy a more favorable clinical course than their younger counterparts.

Physiologic Changes That Alter the Presentation of a Disease

This poorly understood area has long been recognized as of major importance to the practice of geriatric medicine. Many diseases that occur in both young and old adults have manifestly different clinical presentations and natural histories in the two age groups. These disorders should not necessarily be looked on as either less or more severe in the elderly, but just *different.*

One example of a common disorder that presents very differently in the elderly compared with the young is uncontrolled diabetes mellitus. In children and young adults uncontrolled diabetes is generally manifested by diabetic ketoacidosis, with elevations of blood glucose to levels between 300 and 500 mg/dl and coincident severe metabolic acidosis associated with markedly elevated levels of circulating ketones. Conversely, elderly individuals with uncontrolled diabetes will frequently present with hyperosmolar nonketotic coma, altered consciousness, striking elevations of blood glucose (often to levels exceeding 1,000 mg/dl), and a relative or absolute lack of circulating ketones or acidosis.

Impaired Homeostasis in the Elderly: Physiologic Changes That Increase the Likelihood or Severity of a Disease

This category encompasses age-related reductions in the function of numerous organs that place the elderly person at special risk of increased morbidity from diseases in those organs.

Cross-sectional and longitudinal studies in carefully screened subjects across the adult age range indicate that increasing age is accompanied by inevitable physiologic changes that are separable from the effects of diseases. There is no pleasant plateau of the middle years during which physiologic function is stable; instead, there is a progressive age-related reduction in the function of many organs, including major losses in renal, pulmonary, and immune functions. Simultaneous linear reductions in homeostatic capabilities in several organs result in a geometric reduction in the total homeostatic capacity. When coupled with the functional impairments associated with disease states, this constricted homeostasis is responsible for the markedly increased vulnerability of the elderly to morbidity during acute illness or trauma (such as burns; see Figure 1), major surgery, or administration of medications.

Normal aging is associated with a marked reduction in pulmonary function, as reflected in the forced vital capacity and other measures of lung function. Healthy individuals in the ninth decade of life frequently will have lung function equal to only one-half that of their 30-year-old counterparts. Thus, an acute pulmonary disease, such as bacterial pneumonia, will be more likely to induce a serious clinical manifestation in the elderly because of the markedly lessened pulmonary functional reserve. Over the past decade very

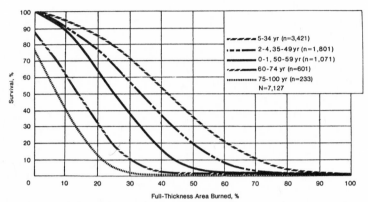

Figure 1. Survival of patients as a function of the total percentage of body surface burned and age. (Reproduced with permission from Feller I, Flora JD, Bawol R: Baseline results of therapy for burned patients. JAMA 1976; 236:1943–1947.)

significant advances have been made in our understanding of the marked reduction in immune competence that occurs with age. Immunosenescence is likely responsible, in some ways, for the increased severity of infections in the elderly. Thus, an elderly individual with pneumonia may be less likely to contain and control that infection in the respiratory tract than a young individual. Failure of immune function may result in dissemination of that infection to many organs, and a much more serious if not life-threatening clinical illness may develop.

An additional example of a mechanism whereby age-related alterations in function increase the prevalence of a disease relates to the development of accidental hypothermia in frail elderly. This disorder has a high mortality rate and can be seen not only in individuals exposed to unheated rooms in the winter, but in individuals in heated rooms who appear to spontaneously develop marked lowering of body temperature. This disorder is essentially absent in healthy young individuals and occurs with increasing frequency with advancing old age. Although the mechanisms of accidental hypothermia are poorly understood, alterations in sympathetic nervous system responsiveness seem likely to be a major contributor.

Physiologic Changes That Mimic Specific Diseases

Some changes that occur with aging may be seen to mimic specific clinical entities, thus causing confusion regarding the diagnosis of specific diseases in the elderly. Perhaps the best and most widely recognized instance of this is the decrease in carbohydrate economy, reflected in decreased performance on oral or intravenous glucose tolerance tests, that occurs with advancing age in the absence of diabetes mellitus (Davidson 1979). This is discussed in detail later in this chapter.

Physiologic Changes That Have a Direct Clinical Impact

For decades gerontologists and geriatricians have drawn a clear line between changes that occur with age and those that are associated with specific disease states. We have staunchly defended the view that aging is not a disease, but a normal process that must be clearly understood to adequately diagnose and treat the increasing burden of illness that will befall a rapidly growing population. Substantial data suggest that this approach is no longer tenable. There is no question that some physiologic changes of aging have clearly adverse clinical sequelae. Although a change may represent "normal aging" inasmuch as it is present in the entire population and cannot be avoided, one should not assume that "normal" change is necessarily harmless.

Although one can argue about the specific criteria for the definition of a "disease," one generally acceptable definition would include any process that results in clear adverse clinical sequelae measured as either morbidity or mortality. Under this definition there are clear changes that occur with advancing age that appear to be normal characteristics of the aging process and that would also qualify as diseases. Of the potentially long list of such processes, three will be briefly reviewed.

More than any other biologic changes, menopause seems clearly to be accepted as age related. Although menopause is thus clearly "normal," it has become abundantly clear that this normal change is associated with increased risk for certain diseases such as osteoporosis and atherosclerosis as well as for symptomatic clinical manifestations such as hot flashes, which are associated with sleep disturbances and are so frequent and severe as to be disabling in many individuals (Hannon 1927; McKinlay and Jefferys 1974).

A second change that occurs with normal aging and that has direct adverse clinical consequences is cataract formation. Posttranslational modifications of central lens proteins with advancing age result in increasing opacity as well as decreasing flexibility of the lens, which is manifested in decreasing capacity to accommodate to near vision (Weale 1963). The reasons for development of cataracts in some individuals and not others are poorly understood. Lens opacification or cataract is a common cause of blindness in older Americans. Thus, this normal age-related change, in its most extreme form, would seem to clearly represent a disease.

A third characteristic type of change with advancing age that would appear to have direct clinical consequences is arteriosclerosis. This thickening of the walls of major arteries must be distinguished from atherosclerosis, which represents the development of plaques on the vessel intima that encroach on the lumen. Arteriosclerosis appears to be a normal consequence of age-related changes in the extracellular material in arterial walls and is reflected in decreased compliance and increased stiffening of vessels with advancing age (O'Rourke 1970). This is manifested in increased systolic blood pressure, which is discussed in detail later in this chapter.

Age-Related Physiologic Changes in the Major Organ Systems

Endocrine Systems

Gerontologic interest in endocrine systems has been based in part on the view that senescence is an incapacity to regulate the internal environment in response to changes in the internal or external milieu. Endocrine systems display a broad spectrum of effects during aging that are of major clinical relevance (Minaker et al. 1984). This rich variety provides the opportunity to increase the understanding of specific common illnesses and evaluate general mechanisms underlying physiologic aging.

Evaluation of endocrine systems has generally emphasized anatomical studies and measures of circulating hormone levels under basal conditions and during physiologically relevant stresses. Similar normative changes occur with age in the anatomy of most endocrine glands. Each gland appears to decrease in weight and to develop a patchy, atrophic appearance accompanied by vascular change and fibrosis. Most glands have a tendency to form adenomas.

Basal hormonal levels in animals and humans are generally not influenced by age. Several hormones, however, clearly have reduced serum concentrations of their active form after changes in binding hormones are taken into account. These include renin, aldosterone, and dihydroepiandrosterone. Secretion rates of most hormones decline with advancing age whether lean body mass is adjusted for or not. Substantial declines in the secretion of testosterone, insulin, adrenal adrogens, and thyroid hormone are well established. The maintenance of near normal circulating hormone levels in the face of decreased secretion rates necessarily implies that hormone clearance rates are decreased similarly with age. While it is not presently known whether the primary defect lies in hormone secretion or in hormone clearance, the implication is clear that the capacity to adjust hormone secretion or to maintain stable levels of plasma hormones is maintained with age. The generation of active metabolites, where examined, suggests there is decreased rate of production of these with advancing age.

Receptor binding during aging appears to show no systematic changes. While some receptors are clearly decreased, either in affinity or number, the majority are unchanged (Minaker et al. 1984). Postreceptor responses to hormone action appear to decrease with advancing age. This is the case with somatomedins, insulin (particularly with regard to glucose metabolism), catecholamines, and steroid hormones. Elucidation of the mechanisms by which age decreases postreceptor hormone action and the relative contributions of aging per se and extrinsic factors to these effects represent the next major frontier of gerontologic endocrine research. The following section deals with specific changes that occur with age in the physiology of a number of clinically relevant endocrine systems.

Carbohydrate Metabolism

An age-related impairment in the capacity to maintain carbohydrate homeostasis after glucose challenge has been recognized for over 60 years. Over the past two decades a number of studies have focused attention on elucidation of the underlying mechanisms and a general consensus is now emerging. Increasing age in individuals without clinical evidence or family history of diabetes is associated with a progressive decline in carbohydrate tolerance, a modest (approximately 1 mg/dl/decade) increase after maturity in fasting blood glucose levels, and a rather striking increase in blood sugar after oral glucose challenge (8 to 10 mg/dl/decade at 1 hour) (Davidson 1979). Recent studies indicate that at least 22 percent of Americans aged 65 to 74 demonstrate impaired carbohydrate tolerance that is not severe enough to warrant a diagnosis of diabetes mellitus (Harris et al. 1987). The increases in postprandial glucose levels seen with aging are also reflected in increased levels of hemoglobin A_{Ic}.

Pathogenetic mechanisms postulated to underlie these changes in carbohydrate tolerance include age-related changes in body composition, diet, activity, and insulin secretion and action. In response to oral or intravenous glucose challenges, elderly on high carbohydrate intakes have repeatedly been found to have circulating insulin levels that are equivalent to, or in many cases greater than, levels found in their younger counterparts. This is due in large part to the fact that clearance of insulin is impaired in the elderly. Insulin release is either not influenced or is mildly impaired with age. The major effect of age under these conditions is decrease of the effectiveness of insulin to induce glucose metabolism in peripheral tissues. On diets low in carbohydrate content, older persons demonstrate impaired insulin release as well as insulin resistance.

There is no effect of age on basal hepatic glucose production or the regulation of hepatic glucose production by insulin. There is also no age effect on insulin receptor number or affinity. It appears that the insulin resistance of aging is due to a postreceptor defect in glucose transport into cells.

The carbohydrate intolerance of aging may be an example of "usual" aging rather than "successful" aging and may carry substantial risk. A recent report from the Honolulu Heart Study evaluated a 12-year risk of stroke in 690 diabetic and 6,908 nondiabetic individuals free of stroke at study entry (Abbott et al. 1987). Diabetes was associated with a clearly increased risk of stroke. In addition, in nondiabetic subjects, the risk of stroke was moderately age related and was statistically significantly higher for those at the 80th percentile serum glucose when compared to those at the 20th percentile. Studies focusing on postprandial hyperinsulinemia, a cardinal feature of the insulin resistance of aging, have shown increases in insulin levels to be a significant independent contributor to the incidence of coronary artery disease. In addition to these effects, increases in insulin level are associated with increases in triglyceride level and decreases in high-density lipoprotein choles-terol levels, both of which are known risk factors for heart disease.

A number of studies have attempted to identify the relative contributions of aging per se and a number of extrinsic factors to the noted carbohydrate intolerance associated with advanced age. Zavaroni et al. (1986), studying factory workers aged 22 to 73, evaluated the contributions of obesity, physical activity, family history of diabetes, and the use of diabetogenic drugs to age-related increases in glucose and insulin levels after an oral glucose tolerance test. The initial strong correlations among age, postprandial glu-cose, and insulin level increases became much weaker when the effects of these other factors were taken into account, so that the correlation between glucose and age was limited to marginal statistical significance and there was no longer an effect of age on insulin levels. In addition, other studies have shown a significant direct relationship between physical fitness as reflected in maximal oxygen consumption and insulin-stimulated glucose metabolism in nonobese older men. Other studies have shown that the capacity to metabo-lize glucose is markedly improved in those older persons who are physically trained compared with their less well-trained counterparts.

These findings clearly suggest that much of the observed glucose intoler-ance and insulin resistance of older people may be caused by factors other than biologic aging per se. In addition, the available data suggest that the carbohydrate intolerance of aging may not be "normal" in the sense that it is not harmless. More aggressive approaches to modifying the extrinsic factors associated with impairment of glucose metabolism would be in the best interest of many elderly individuals.

Parathyroid Function

The general consensus of a number of careful studies of healthy men and women across the adult age range is that human aging, in the absence of disease, is associated with the development of a very mild form of hyperpara-thyroidism. There is clear evidence of a gradual and very variable increase in circulating levels of parathyroid hormone with advancing age. As parathyroid hormone is metabolized, fragments accumulate in the blood that are gener-ally excreted by the kidneys. It is not surprising, in view of the marked decrease in glomerular filtration rate (GFR) with age (discussed later in this section), that radioimmunoassays that detect intact hormone, as well as these inactive fragments, indicate an 80 percent increase in circulating levels of parathyroid hormone between ages 30 and 80 years. However, when assays sensitive only to intact hormone are employed, a persistent increase of 30 percent is still observed over the adult age range. The modest increase in circulating levels of parathyroid hormone is not accompanied by change of total serum calcium but rather by a slight reduction in ionized calcium that probably represents a stimulus from parathyroid release. This increase in parathyroid hormone is clearly physiologically relevant since it is reflected, in the elderly, in increased levels of urinary cyclic AMP.

The major physiologic mechanism contributing to a slight decrease in ionized calcium with age and the attendant slight increases in parathyroid hormone level is a well-documented decline in intestinal calcium absorption (Bullamore et al. 1970). This decline is probably due, in turn, to decreases in 1,25-dihydroxy-vitamin D levels, which have been well documented with age and which, in turn, are probably related to decreases in renal mass. Thus it would appear that the primary abnormality with advancing age is a decrease in renal mass.

While this is very variable, as discussed later in this chapter, in those individuals in which it is physiologically significant, it leads to a progressive cascade of alterations in endocrine and gastrointestinal systems relevant to skeleton integrity that result in the development of mild normocalcemic hyperparathyroidism. It is important to note that the mild hyperparathyroidism of "normal" aging is probably not a major contributing factor to the development of osteoporosis, since individuals with and without hip fracture have been shown to have similar circulating parathyroid hormone levels, with the exception of those few individuals with significant hyperparathyroidism.

Thyroid Function

Normal aging, in the absence of disease, has no major effect on the function of the thyroid gland and no clinically important influence on the results of diagnostic studies (Livingstone et al. 1987). Thus serum levels of thyroxine, free thyroxine, the 3,5,3'-triiodothyronine (T3) resin uptake test, and a free thyroxine index are not importantly influenced by age. Thyroxine clearance has been shown to decrease with age, but this is coupled with a decrease in the release of thyroxine, resulting in no major overall change in serum levels. While minor age-related declines in T3 have been identified with advancing age, the values remain within the rather broad limits described as "normal" for young populations. It is widely recognized that the most sensitive index of thyroid inadequacy is modest elevation of circulating thyroid-stimulating hormone (TSH) levels and thus there has been substantial interest in the impact of age on TSH secretion. A number of studies have shown that TSH is either unchanged or very slightly increased with age but still within the normal limits. While early studies indicated that the thyrotropin-releasing hormone stimulation of TSH was impaired in elderly men but not in elderly women, more recent evidence suggests that there is no important influence of age on this test (Harman et al. 1984). While thyroid antibodies can be found in higher prevalence in older populations, this does not represent a sensitive or specific screening test for thyroid disease since up to one-third of patients with hypothyroidism have no antithyroid antibodies.

Male Reproductive System

The possible presence of a male climacteric, analogous to the female menopause, has long attracted attention. Early studies suggested a decrease in the level of testosterone and dihydrotestosterone with age. Additional studies on healthy men, who were very carefully screened to exclude underlying disease, are mixed, showing either no effect of age on levels of total testosterone, free testosterone, or the major metabolite, dihydrotestosterone, or a modest decline in levels of these hormones (Harman and Nankin 1985; Harman and Tsitouras 1980). While the majority of current studies show a modest decline in levels, it is clear that this is a variable finding and that many elderly men, even in their 90s, will still have a testosterone level that is not importantly different from that of the average middle-aged man. Normal blood levels reported by some authors may still reflect age-related decreases in secretion of androgens, since androgen clearance falls with advancing age.

Healthy men have shown a modest decrease in luteinizing hormone (LH) levels and a marked increase in follicle-stimulating hormone (FSH) levels and decreases in LH and FSH response to LH-releasing hormone, suggesting a decrease in pituitary gonadotropin reserve or sensitivity. Prolactin levels are either unchanged or increased slightly with age. In healthy men there appears to be no change in testicular size or in sperm number or morphology.

The Duke Longitudinal Study has shown that 75 percent of healthy males over the age of 70 have intercourse at least once a month and over the age of 78, 25 percent are still engaging in regular sexual activity (Pearlman 1972). Martin (1981) found that sexual activity in late life tends to correlate with the degree of sexual activity earlier in life as well as with general health. Sexual response is delayed and greater stimulation is required for a man to obtain an erection, which tends to be less firm in late life. The ejaculatory volume is decreased and men do not appear to have the need to ejaculate with every episode of intercourse. After ejaculation, there is rapid detumescence of the penis and a rather prolonged refractory period before the man is able to have another erection. There is no correlation between levels of serum testosterone and sexual activity in healthy elderly men.

Female Reproductive System

Menopause is one of the most widely recognized age-related biologic changes. While many of the physiologic effects of aging discussed in this chapter are modified strongly by extrinsic factors such as life-style, diet, and habits, this does not appear to be the case with the menopause. The average age of onset of menopause has been remarkably stable at 50 to 51 years for several centuries and appears unrelated to age of menarche, body composition, diet, or socioeconomic status. The only possibly important exception is smoking, which appears to hasten menopause. Though widely considered to be "normal" aging, menopause clearly should not be considered to be harmless, since it is associated with a number of potentially adverse changes including acceleration of age-related bone loss; increase in the risk of coronary heart disease; changes in the female reproductive and urinary tract, particularly thinning and atrophy of the vagina and urethra; and hot flushes, which occur in approximately 50 percent of postmenopausal women and can be very disturbing.

The primary physiologic change underlying the menopause appears to be age-related loss in the number of ova and their associated follicles. The population of ova begins at several million during gestation, falls to 400,000 at menarche and to less than 100 at the menopause. In the years preceding the menopause, the reduction in the number of ova is associated with ovarian resistance to FSH stimulation and reductions in circulating levels of the major estrogen produced by the ovary, 17-beta-estradiol. In the premenopausal period as 17-beta-estradiol levels fall, FSH levels increase with a variable and less pronounced increase in LH levels as well. After age 45 cycle length declines, with the primary reduction being in the follicular phase while the luteal phase remains stable. As menopause nears, the interval between menses lengthens and anovulatory cycles begin prior to the final cessation of bleeding. With the progressive reductions in circulating levels of estradiol, FSH and to a lesser extent LH levels rise. Interestingly, administration of gonadotropin-releasing hormone results in even further increases in FSH and LH in postmenopausal women (Carr and MacDonald 1985).

The menopause is a state of relative rather than absolute estrogen deficiency. Postmenopausally, circulating estrogen levels are maintained at a much lower level than before the menopause. Castration or adrenalectomy does not further reduce estrogen levels in postmenopausal women, since the circulating estrogens, primarily estrone, a physiologically weaker estrogen than estradiol, are produced in extraglandular sites from the metabolism of androstenedione. One of the most important extraglandular sites of estrogen production is adipose tissue. Thus obese elderly postmenopausal women may have substantial circulating estrone levels.

Aging of the Heart

Physiologic age-related changes that occur in the heart are of obvious major clinical importance as a substrate for the development of cardiac disease and as an important predisposing factor in the development of cardiac complications of noncardiac diseases, trauma, or surgery. Perhaps more than most other physiologic areas, elucidation of the relative contributions of intrinsic aging per se and those of extrinsic factors has been very difficult in studies of the heart. This is because of the high prevalence of asymptomatic coronary artery disease in the elderly population and the importance of physical fitness in influencing cardiovascular performance. A number of studies have shown that up to 50 percent of elderly individuals will have severe occlusive disease in at least one coronary artery, although they may not have any symptoms or abnormality in their resting electrocardiogram (White et al. 1950). Investigators now employ exercise tolerance testing and thallium scanning in an effort to identify and exclude individuals with underlying heart disease from the "normal" aged group. The results of such robust studies show much less decline in cardiac function in old age than previous studies, which were undoubtedly contaminated by inclusion of individuals with underlying cardiac disease.

The second major factor, physical fitness, is difficult to quantitate in community-dwelling populations. One must be careful not to exclude all individuals except the very fit, since this would yield a superselect group whose results tell us little about normal aging and have little generalizable clinical relevance. One reasonable approach is to study carefully screened men and women across the adult age range, aggressively trying to exclude underlying heart disease and seeking individuals who are not physically trained but who are fully active in the activities of daily living. In the following discussion the studies cited have generally met these criteria. The literature reviewed deals with the effect of age on cardiac function both under rest and in response to stress in order to provide a broad perspective on the possible clinical implications of the physiologic changes in the aging human heart.

Cardiac function at rest.   The physical examination of the heart is not necessarily altered with age, although nonradiating systolic ejection murmurs, generally attributed to aortic sclerosis, are common over age 75. The electrocardiogram is also generally not importantly changed with age in the absence of disease.

Recent studies of carefully screened individuals from across the adult age range fail to identify an effect of advancing age on cardiac output in the sitting position, but show a modest decline in cardiac output in the supine position. This suggests that older persons do not increase their cardiac output in response to the increased preload associated with the supine position as much as their younger counterparts (Rodeheffer et al. 1984).

Important cardiovascular variables not influenced by age at rest include left ventricular diameter, area and volume, and ejection fraction. There is a very modest decline in basal heart rate with age, which is compensated for by a slight increase in stroke volume to maintain cardiac output. There is no change in peripheral resistance with age, despite a slight increase in systolic blood pressure—which is discussed at length elsewhere in this chapter (Lakatta 1979).

There is a clear increase in left ventricular wall thickness with age. This modest cardiac hypertrophy is probably secondary to the increase in systolic blood pressure. Stroke work, the product of stroke volume and systolic blood pressure, thus increases with age. There is no effect of age on myocardial force production or the extent of shortening under basal conditions.

Early diastolic filling falls with advancing age. This is probably due to age-related prolongation of isometric relaxation time and decreases in cardiac compliance, which are secondary to collagen accumulation in the ventricle. Thus, as the ventricle stiffens with age, relaxation is impaired and filling slows. This may become important when cardiac rate is increased and diastole shortens, leading to inadequate filling, pulmonary venous congestion, and dyspnea.

Taken together, these physiologic studies suggest that there are no inevitable changes with age in cardiac performance, although some modest modifications primarily relating to decreases in left ventricular compliance and subsequent impairment of diastolic function are probably secondary to the hypertrophic response to increases in systolic blood pressure.

Cardiac performance under stress. At various levels of exercise, cardiac output rises in older individuals to similar levels as seen in their younger counterparts. However, maximal heart rate during exercise declines with age, and cardiac output is maintained via an increase in stroke volume and left ventricular end diastolic volume. Although left ventricular ejection fraction declines with age, the absolute amount of blood ejected with each contraction is greater in the elderly, since left ventricular end diastolic volume is clearly increased, and thus an adequate stroke volume can be maintained at a lower ejection fraction (Lakatta 1979).

These changes in cardiac response to stress appear related to the well-documented age-related blunting of the chronotropic and inotropic response of the senescent myocardium to adrenergic stimulation. Since circulating norepinephrine levels are higher in the elderly, both under basal circumstances and in response to graded exercise, inadequate heart rate response clearly cannot be attributed to catecholamine deficiency. Studies of the physiologic mechanisms underlying these findings suggest that they are not related to a decline in adrenergic myocardial receptors but to postreceptor events.

In summary, the senescent human heart is fully capable of maintaining adequate overall function, that is, cardiac output, both under basal circumstances and in response to stress. Specific physiologic effects of aging, primarily related to decreased compliance of the left ventricle and impaired diastolic function as well as impaired chronotropic response to stress, lead to specific adaptations. Thus, adequate cardiac output is maintained during exercise via increases in left ventricular end diastolic volume and stroke volume to compensate for the lack of increase in cardiac output. These physiologic changes are important clinically since they may explain the tendency of older individuals to develop pulmonary venous congestion during uncontrolled atrial fibrillation or other forms of supraventricular tachycardia and also help to explain the blunted response of the elderly to beta-adrenergic agonist and antagonist stimulation.

Isolated systolic hypertension in the elderly. Isolated systolic hypertension is a common entity in the elderly that appears to represent an aggravation of age-dependent processes. The general age-related increase in systolic pressure and fall in diastolic pressure after the middle years results in an increasing prevalence of isolated systolic hypertension (systolic blood pressure, 160 mm Hg; diastolic blood pressure, 90 mm Hg) to 25 percent of men and women over the age of 75 (Tudge 1978). There is general agreement that the major pathophysiologic factor underlying isolated systolic hypertension in the elderly is the age-related decrease in arterial compliance (Rowe 1983). Though some systematic changes in circulating catecholamines and other endocrine factors have been shown to occur with age, to date these have not been shown to contribute importantly to the development of isolated systolic hypertension.

The risk of isolated systolic hypertension. The commonly held view that isolated systolic hypertension should not be treated is based on the misconceptions that since systolic hypertension accompanies "normal" aging it is harmless and that antihypertensive therapy is poorly tolerated by the elderly. Substantial information has now accumulated to indicate that neither of these views is correct.

The 1959 Build and Blood Pressure Study of the Society of Actuaries (Morton 1959) reported on a 19-year follow-up of men and women aged 40 to 69 at entry in the study. For men whose diastolic pressure was 83 to 87 mm Hg, systolic blood pressures in the range of 158 to 167 mm Hg were associated with a 34 percent increase in mortality compared with those with systolic blood pressures in the range of 138 to 147 mm Hg. For women, similar increases in systolic blood pressure were associated with a doubling of mortality rate. The Chicago Stroke Study (Shekelle et al. 1974) followed 2,100 lower socioeconomic class men and women aged 64 to 74 for 3 years. Of the group with diastolic blood pressure less than 95 mm Hg, those with systolic blood pressure greater than 180 mm Hg suffered a mortality rate 59 percent higher than those with systolic blood pressure in the normal range. The Chicago People's Gas Company Study (Dyer et al. 1977) involved a 15-year follow-up of white men aged 40 to 59 at entry. Of the men whose diastolic blood pressure was less than 90 mm Hg, those with systolic blood pressure over 140 mm Hg suffered a 70 percent higher mortality rate than those with lower systolic pressures. In a case-control study, Colandrea et al. (1970) reported the findings on 72 patients with isolated systolic hypertension and 72 age-, sex-, and diastolic-pressure-matched controls. Mean age of entry was 69 years. Over a 4-year follow-up, 10 of the hypertensive patients had fatal cardiovascular events, whereas only 1 member of the control group did.

In addition to the studies cited above reporting increased mortality, data are also available to indicate that substantial morbidity is associated with isolated systolic hypertension. Forette et al. (1982) identified isolated systolic hypertension as a major risk factor for cerebrovascular events and acute myocardial infarction among elderly women (mean age 80 years) followed for 10 years. The Framingham study (Kannel et al. 1981) analyzed the probability of cerebrovascular or cardiovascular disease during prolonged follow-up of low-risk men and women according to their systolic blood pressure and age. This study clearly demonstrated that at any systolic blood pressure level the risk of an adverse cardiovascular or cerebrovascular event increased dramatically with age. In addition, at any age the risk increased substantially with advancing systolic blood pressure. Finally, the relationship between elevated systolic blood pressure and increased risk was modified dramatically with age, with the oldest age groups having the greatest relative risk for any given systolic pressure.

No data are yet available to indicate the benefit or lack of benefit of lowering *systolic* blood pressure to the elderly. However, a recent study, the Systolic Hypertension in the Elderly Program (SHEP), has clearly documented that low doses of thiazide diuretics will substantially lower systolic blood pressure in elderly individuals with isolated systolic hypertension without causing excessive adverse effects (Hulley et al.). This important randomized blinded study included 551 men and women 60 years and older with documented systolic hypertension. Participants received either chlorthalidone (25 to 50 mg/day) or matching placebo. On 1-year followup, 83 percent of the chlorthalidone group and 80 percent of the placebo group were still taking their medications, and of those taking chlorthalidone, 88 percent had reached their goal blood pressure without requiring an additional medication. Analysis of the distribution of individual blood pressure responses to chlorthalidone showed that the response to treatment was rather uniform. Systolic blood pressure in the treatment group fell from 172 mm Hg to 146 mm Hg by the end of the first month of treatment with a slight continued decline through the first year. Diastolic blood pressure did not "bottom out." Compliance with the medication regimen was excellent in both treatment and placebo groups. There was no significant increase in mild or severe side effects in the chlorthalidone group, compared with the placebo group, at 1 month or 1 year. While chlorthalidone is commonly avoided in younger hypertensives because of its tendency to induce potassium depletion, this is not as serious a problem in the elderly, probably because of the lower glomerular filtration rate and renin and aldosterone levels that characterize normal aging. In the SHEP study, the mean decline in serum potassium was limited to 0.5 mEq/l in the treatment group. There was no effect of chlorthalidone treatment on serum cholesterol or glucose levels. There was a very modest, clinically significant increase in serum creatinine levels from 1.05 ± 0.21 to 1.10 ± 0.32 and a modest increase in serum uric acid from 5.7 mg/dl to 6.8 mg/dl.

In summary, this important, large, randomized blinded study indicates that low-dose thiazide diuretic treatment is effective in lowering blood pressure and safe in the management of elderly individuals with isolated systolic hypertension. An even larger multicentered randomized trial is currently underway to determine if lowering systolic blood pressure with antihypertensive medications in elderly individuals with isolated systolic hypertension is associated with significant reduction in the risk of cerebrovascular or cardiovascular disease.

Renal System

Advancing age is associated with progressive loss of renal mass in humans, with renal weight decreasing from 250 to 270 g in young adulthood to 180 to 200 g by the eighth decade. The loss of renal mass is primarily cortical, with relative sparing of the renal medulla. The total number of identifiable glomeruli decreases with age, roughly in accord with the changes in renal weight.

It is generally agreed from histologic studies that normal aging, independent of hypertension or renal disease, is associated with variable sclerotic changes in the walls of the larger renal vessels. These sclerotic changes do not encroach on the lumen and are augmented in the presence of hypertension. Radiographic studies in normotensives demonstrate an increasing prevalence after the seventh decade of abnormalities similar to those seen in hypertension, including abnormal tapering of interlobar arteries, abnormal arcuate arteries, increased tortuosity of intralobular arteries, and a predilection for age-related vascular abnormalities to occur in the polar region. Smaller vessels appear to be spared, with only 15 percent of senescent kidneys from nonhypertensive patients displaying arteriolar changes.

Combined micro-angiographic and histologic studies have identified two very distinctive patterns of change in arteriolar-glomerular units with senescence. In one type, hyalinization and collapse of the glomerular tuft is associated with obliteration of the lumen of the preglomerular arteriole, which results in loss of blood flow. This type of change is seen primarily in the cortical area. The second pattern, seen primarily in the juxtamedullary area, is characterized by the development of anatomic continuity between the afferent and efferent arterioles during glomerular sclerosis. The end point is thus loss of the glomerulus and shunting of blood flow from afferent to efferent arterioles.

Renal blood flow.   Renal plasma flow declines progressively from 600 ml/minute in young adulthood to 300 ml/minute by 80 years of age. The primary factor contributing to this decrease appears to be a reduction in the reno-vascular bed already discussed above. Studies in healthy potential renal donors, ranging in age from 17 to 76 years, indicate that the age-related decrease in flow is not purely a reflection of decreased renal mass, but rather that flow per gram of tissue falls progressively after the fourth decade. There is a highly significant decrease with advancing age in the cortical component of blood flow, with preservation of medullary flow—a finding consistent with the histologic studies reviewed above (Hollenberg et al. 1974). These cortical vascular changes probably account for the patchy cortical defects commonly seen on renal scans in healthy elder adults. Studies employing intravenous administration of vasodilators, including acetylcholine or pyrogen, show similar increases in renal blood flow in all age groups, indicating that the age-related change in renal blood flow is not related to "functional spasm," but appears to be on a fixed or structural basis. Consistent with these findings, vasoconstrictor response to angiotensin is not influenced by age.

Glomerular filtration rate.   The major clinically relevant functional defect arising from the histologic and physiologic changes with aging in the kidney, is a decline in the GFR. Age-adjusted normal standards for creatinine clearance have been established (Rowe et al. 1976). Creatinine clearance is stable until the middle of the fourth decade, when a linear decrease of about 8.0 ml/minute/1.73 m/decade begins. Long-term longitudinal studies indicate substantial variability in the effect of age on creatinine clearance, with as many as one-third of individuals showing no decline in GFR with age. This variability suggests that factors other than aging per se may be responsible for the apparent effect of age on renal function. One important "extrinsic" factor may be blood pressure, since longitudinal studies show that increasing blood pressure levels within the normotensive range are associated with accelerated loss of renal function.

Serum creatinine.   Since muscle mass, from which creatinine is derived, falls with age at roughly the same rate as GFR, the rather drastic age-related loss of GFR is not reflected in an elevation of serum creatinine. Thus, serum creatinine overestimates GFR in the elderly. A healthy 80-year-old man with a creatinine clearance 32 ml/minute less than his 30-year-old counterpart of the same stature and weight will have the same serum creatinine. Depressions of GFR so severe as to result in elevation of serum creatinine above 1.5 mg/dl are rarely due to normal aging, and so indicate the presence of a disease state.

One must consider not only the effects of age but also those of muscle mass on determining the utility of serum creatinine as an estimate of renal function. Elderly debilitated individuals may have a markedly limited muscle mass and glomerular filtration rates as low as 20 to 30 ml/minute with serum creatinine levels of less than 2.0 mg/dl. In these cases, their renal impairment is often overlooked or, at best, underestimated, and these patients are at risk for the development of iatrogenic complications.

In clinical practice, the doses of many drugs excreted primarily by the kidneys are routinely adjusted to compensate for alterations in renal function. This is particularly true of digoxin preparations and aminoglycoside antibiotics. Unfortunately, these adjustments are usually based on serum creatinine values, with the resultant predictable overdose in elderly patients. Dose adjustment should ideally be based on creatinine clearances, even if a timed urine specimen of only a couple of hours is available. If no timed urine specimen can be obtained and only serum creatinine is available, the influence of age must be considered. This can be accomplished by use of the following formula (Cockcroft and Gault 1976):

$$\text{Creatinine clearance (ml/minute)} = \frac{(140 - \text{age}) \times \text{weight (kg)}}{72 \times \text{serum creatinine (mg/dl)}}$$

(15 percent less in females).

Pulmonary System

A central theme of this discussion regarding the physiologic changes with age has been the importance of extrinsic factors, including personal habits, diet, and so forth, as modifiers of the aging process in the absence of disease. Just as increasing levels of blood pressure in the normotensive range influence renal function and physical fitness impacts cardiovascular capacity, cigarette smoking and exposure to hazardous environmental conditions clearly accelerate the progressive changes that occur in pulmonary function in the absence of disease. This section will discuss the changes that occur in the lung, in the absence of obvious extrinsic factors such as cigarette smoking or evidence of pulmonary disease, and will focus on four major areas—pulmonary mechanics, gas exchange, control of respiration, and pulmonary defense mechanisms.

Pulmonary mechanics. Changes with age in the compliance of both the lung and the chest wall account for many of the observed alterations in pulmonary volumes with age. Under normal conditions, the natural tendency of the chest wall to expand is matched by the natural tendency of the lung to collapse so that, under static conditions, lung volume is constant. With advancing age the chest wall becomes stiffer, developing a greater tendency to expand. Simultaneously, the lung becomes stiffer and thus has less of a tendency to collapse. These changes, taken together, explain the finding that functional residual capacity, the volume at which the tendency of the lung to collapse inward is balanced by the tendency of the chest wall to expand outward, increases progressively with advancing age. This increase in functional residual capacity is accompanied by a decrease in vital capacity, or the amount of air exhaled following a maximal inhalation, and an increase in residual volume. Total lung capacity is either constant or declines very slightly with age (Weiss 1980).

Numerous studies have shown that the major flow rates employed in clinical measurements of pulmonary function (i.e., the forced vital capacity and the forced expiratory volume in 1 second) decline with age, although these changes are very variable, with many individuals demonstrating very minor declines.

Gas exchange. The primary determinant of gas exchange is the match of the distribution of blood flow and ventilation in the lung. The decreases in compliance with aging result in closure of airways in the lower portions of the lungs during much of the respiratory cycle and a mismatch of ventilation and perfusion. These changes, along with increases in physiologic dead space, result in progressive declines in arterial oxygen concentration after adulthood. Normal arterial pO_2 for the aged can be estimated by the following formula: $pO_2 = 100 - 0.34 \times$ age. Despite the decline in pO_2 with age there is no change with age in arterial CO_2 content or pH.

Control of respiration. Advancing age is associated with a progressive blunting of both the central and peripheral components of the system that controls respiration. It is unknown whether this decreased respiratory drive is the result of decreased responsiveness to decreases in pO_2 or increases in pCO_2 or whether there is a decreased output from the central respiratory center. Ventilatory drive, as measured by the ventilatory response to hypoxia and hypercapnia, is blunted with normal aging. The magnitude of this effect is slight however, and it generally does not have clinical significance (Kronenberg and Drage 1973).

Pulmonary defense mechanisms. Pulmonary defense mechanisms play a critical role in the prevention of respiratory tract infections. Recognition of the important increase in the prevalence and severity of pneumonia in the elderly has led to substantial study of the influence of normal aging on pulmonary defense mechanisms. In addition to the substantive age-related alterations in systemic immune function, particularly cell-mediated immunity, age-related impairments have been identified in local nonimmune defense mechanisms, including the cough reflex, as well as in laryngeal reflexes and in the rate at which mucus is transported by cilia up the trachea so that it can be expectorated. These changes, when combined with systemic immune changes, place the elderly at enhanced risk for respiratory infection. However, it must be emphasized, as in many other variables, that physiologic changes with age are very variable and that many healthy older persons have respiratory tract defense mechanisms that are within the normal range for younger adult populations.

In summary, there are very substantial reductions in respiratory function with advancing age. Decreases in defense mechanisms make respiratory infection more likely. Decreases in the compliance of the lung and chest wall lead to alterations in gas exchange, which provide older individuals with decreased respiratory reserve. This decreased reserve often becomes critically important in the presence of respiratory infection. In this regard, it is of particular interest to note that longitudinal studies indicate that forced vital capacity is a statistically significant predictor of future mortality in community-based population studies. As such, this measure of respiratory function may begin to approach a useful "biomarker of aging," which provides an index, other than birth date, of the rate of physiologic change in at least one clinically important organ system.

Gastrointestinal System

Esophagus.   Esophageal function is not importantly influenced by normal aging in the absence of disease. While a modest decrease has been found in the amplitude of peristalsis in the esophagus, and older persons are more likely to have other nonspecific motility disturbances, these changes are not generally of clinical relevance. To date, there have been no clear physiologic changes identified as underlying the clearly increased prevalence of hiatus hernia with advancing age.

Stomach and duodenum.   The impaired acid-secreting capacity of the aged stomach is well documented. With advancing age, maximal stimulated gastric acid decreases 10 mEq/hour/decade in men and slightly less in women. The term "gastric atrophy" is generally reserved for individuals with very low or no acid secretion, while "atrophic gastritis" refers to the range of decreased acid production values seen in older persons. An indirect index of gastric acid secretion may be found in the ratio of circulatory pepsinogen I (PI) (which is secreted by mucous and chief cells in the gastric fundus) to pepsinogen II (PII) (secreted by cells in the gastric fundus, cardia, and antrum). Employing a PI/PII ratio less than 2.9 as indicative of gastric atrophy, the prevalence of this disorder increases from 24 percent between ages 60 to 69 years to 37 percent over age 80 years (Krasinski et al. 1986). Impaired gastric acid production has several clinically relevant consequences, including decreased gastric emptying, lowered intrinsic factor levels, enhanced propensity for bacterial overgrowth, and elevated proximal intestinal pH, which influences nutrient and drug absorption. Long-term studies show that atrophic gastritis tends to persist and superficial gastritis progresses slowly to atrophic gastritis.

Other physiologic studies of gastric physiology with advancing age show minor changes. There are no major effects of age on gastric motility, emptying, or the absorption of simple sugars.

Small intestine.   As gastric acid secretion decreases with age, the sterility of the gastrointestinal tract is threatened. Elderly individuals have higher counts of coliform bacteria in the small intestine than their younger counterparts. Blood supply to the intestine is not altered with age.

Absorption of nutrients to the small intestine is, in general, well preserved in the elderly. While occasional deficits do exist, such as in fat absorption, these are minor and have limited, if any, clinical significance.

With regard to vitamins and minerals, there is, as mentioned previously, a progressive reduction in absorption of calcium with advancing age. This is most likely related to decreases in circulating levels of 1,25-dihydroxy-vitamin D_3, rather than structural or primary physiologic changes in the intestine. There is a slight decline in the circulating levels of B_{12} with age, which may be related to B_{12} malabsorption secondary to bacterial overgrowth, but the declines are generally not significant enough to result in clinical evidence of B_{12} deficiency. Absorption of folic acid is adequate in most elderly. This may be due to the fact that the tendency toward decreased absorption induced by higher intestinal pH is compensated by folate production from increased bacterial flora (Russell et al. 1986). Vitamin A absorption increases with age, most likely secondary to age-related declines in the unstirred water layer barrier and increases in pH, thus placing the elderly who ingest large doses of vitamin A supplements at risk for vitamin A toxicity.

Liver, biliary tract, and pancreas.   There are no changes with age in the size or weight of the liver. Standard liver function tests, finding widespread clinical application, are not influenced by age; nor is the bromosulfophthalein retention test. There are, however, important age-related declines in hepatic blood flow and oxidizing systems. The primary clinical impact of these changes is pharmacologic, since they impair the metabolism and increase the half-life of many agents that are modified primarily via hepatic mechanisms. These pharmacologic changes are discussed in detail in Chapter 20. Exocrine pancreatic function is not importantly influenced by age.

Colon.   The high prevalence of constipation or other symptoms of colonic dysfunction has led to the widespread belief that there are major changes with age in the physiology of the colon. On the other hand, a number of studies have shown that the physiology of the large bowel is intact with age in the absence of disease. The reflex responsible for defecation is intact with aging. It has become clear that age-related impairments in large bowel function, which have become so common as to be considered a part of normal aging, are not related to inevitable physiologic changes with age, as much as they are to insufficient dietary fiber, medication use, inadequate food intake, laxative abuse, and inadequate exercise in the elderly.

Importance of Functional Change with Advancing Age

The emphasis in the provision of health care to the elderly should be on maintaining functional capability. Although most older Americans living in the community are cognitively intact and fully independent in their activities of daily living, a substantial number of elderly patients who are not institutionalized report major activity limitations due to chronic conditions. Major functional impairment is clearly age related within the elderly, increasing from approximately 5 percent of individuals age 65 to 74 requiring assistance in basic activities to nearly 35 to 40 percent by age 85. Even if one maintains functional independence into old age, the risk of becoming frail for a long period is still high. For independent persons between the ages of 65 and 70 years, "active life expectancy," that portion of the remaining years characterized by independence, represents about 60 percent, a portion that falls to 40 percent at age 85.

Evaluation of the elderly patient must focus on what the patient can do, relative to what the patient should be able or wishes to do, and on identification of recent functional deficits that may be reversible. Although a complete and precise diagnosis is essential, the functional impact of each diagnosis should be evaluated. Specific diagnoses often have little relation to functional status, and the length of the diagnosis list provides little insight into the specific needs and capabilities of the given elderly patient. Too often a long diagnosis list provides physicians a bias that the patient is multiply impaired and frail although this may not be the case at all. Thus, diagnoses themselves are often a weak criterion for assessing the health care needs of the elderly.

An important component of recognition of the need for data regarding functional status in the elderly is a relationship of functional status to diagnoses and morbidity. As reviewed by Manton (1982), the World Health Organization has proposed a model that describes the linkages among mortality, disability, and morbidity (Figure 2). While it is clear that the overall mortality experience of the elderly population has an underlying curve of morbidity experience in which individuals accumulate diseases and losses in specific capabilities, the specific interactions between the development of diseases and the subsequent development of disability have not been elucidated. It is particularly important to recognize that many different pathologic processes may result in, or contribute to, identical functional impairments. Within a given elderly individual, several coincident pathologic processes interact in a complex fashion to result in disability. This interaction is often strongly influenced by other factors, particularly in the psychosocial sphere.

A major policy issue relates to the importance of clarifying the relationship between changes in the mortality experience of the elderly population and coincident changes in the underlying morbidity and disability experiences. A controversial issue of major importance for health policy is whether future increases in longevity will be associated with prolongation of dependency or whether active life expectancy will increase ("compression of morbidity") as health promotion and disease prevention strategies become increasingly effective. The initial claim that as mortality declines morbidity will also decline has recently been challenged by studies suggesting that the

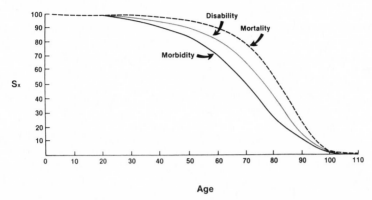

Figure 2. The observed mortality and hypothetical mobidity and disability curves for females in the United States in 1980. (Reproduced with permission from World Health Organization: The uses of epidemiology in the study of the elderly. Technical Report Series 706. Geneva, Switzerland, 1980)

increased life span of the "old old" is not accompanied by decreased morbidity and may actually result in more dramatic increases in the need for health care services.

Approach to Comprehensive Functional Assessment of the Elderly

Evaluation of the elderly patient must focus on what the patient can do, relative to what the patient should be able or wishes to do, and on identification of recent functional deficits that may be reversible. Since elderly persons are especially vulnerable to loss of functional capacity due to interaction of medical problems with adverse economic, psychologic, and social pressures (Habot and Libow 1980), data must be collected in all these domains.

The history taking and physical examination can be difficult in the elderly, as compared with younger patients. Dementia (in 10 percent of the elderly), impaired hearing (in 22 percent), and visual handicaps (in 15 percent) limit communication (Linn and Linn 1980). Effective history taking demands increased skill, time, reliance on significant others, and use of medical records that place the patient's current symptoms in perspective. Physical examination may be time consuming and tedious, especially in the office setting, because of decreased mobility and the length of time required for the patient to disrobe.

One must obtain a thorough medication history and be aware of the special vulnerability of the elderly to the development of adverse effects from medication. Special consideration should be given to the detection of thyroid, rectal, breast, and cervical cancer; occult bleeding; hypertension; postural hypotension; disease in the oral cavity that may impair nutritional status; wax impaction in the ears that may limit hearing; and serious auditory or ophthalmic disorders. Attention should be paid to bowel function and the possible presence of varying degrees of urinary incontinence and sleep disturbance. Specific questions regarding postural stability are mandatory in view of the high prevalence and serious consequences of falls in the elderly.

Reliable, easily administered, brief examinations of mental status, such as the Mini-Mental State Examination (Folstein et al. 1975) and the Blessed Dementia Scale (Blessed et al. 1968), provide valuable data regarding the mental status of elderly persons whose apparently slight cognitive impairment may be incorrectly labeled as "normal" for their age (Kane and Kane 1981). Patients with well-developed social skills who are not subjected to objective mental status testing will often not appear to have as much of a defect in mental function as is actually present. In such cases, the health care provider may not identify mental failure or dementia as a specific problem, and potentially reversible underlying causes, such as drug intoxication, hypothyroidism, azotemia, vitamin B_{12} deficiency, or depression, may not be sought.

A third dimension of functional assessment is evaluation of the patient's social and economic status. The health care of elderly persons, perhaps more than any other age group, is influenced by the social support system available to them. The network of current and potential informal supports, such as family or friends, has an important role in modulating the clinical impact of underlying disease and is often the major determinant in decisions to institutionalize elderly people. For every impaired aged person in a nursing home, there are approximately two, equally impaired elderly people living in the community, who often can remain there by virtue of the critical role of informal support systems, which provide approximately 80 percent of their long-term care.

Illness Behavior in the Elderly

Underreporting of Illness

An important factor underlying functional impairment in the elderly is the failure of many persons to seek assistance. Studies in several countries with varying health care systems indicate that symptoms of serious and treatable diseases often go unreported (Rowe 1983; Anderson 1966). Health problems reported by frail elderly persons are thus frequently only the tip of the iceberg of treatable illness.

This apparently self-destructive behavior springs from the notion on the part of older people that advanced age is necessarily accompanied by illness and functional decline and that many symptoms are thus to be expected rather than treated. Other contributing factors include cognitive impairment; fear of the nature of the underlying illness; and concern about the costs and other negative aspects of hospitalization, diagnostic evaluation, or unpleasant treatment.

As Besdine (1982) has pointed out, nonreporting of symptoms of underlying disease in elderly persons is an especially dangerous phenomenon when coupled with the passive American organizational structure of health care delivery, which lacks prevention-oriented or early detection efforts. He notes that aged persons, burdened by society's and their own ageist views of functional loss with aging, cannot be relied on to initiate appropriate health care for themselves, especially early in the course of an illness.

Multiple Diseases

The coexistence of several diseases has a profoundly negative influence on health and functional independence in the elderly. The number of pathologic conditions in a person is strongly related to age. Elderly persons who live in the community have 3.5 important disabilities per person (Anderson 1966), and the hospitalized elderly have evidence of 6 pathologic conditions per person (Wilson et al. 1962). The entire array of diseases present in an individual patient must be considered as treatment plans are developed.

Atypical or Altered Presentation of Disease in the Elderly

A fundamental principle of geriatric medicine is that many diseases have signs or symptoms in the elderly that differ from those in their younger counterparts. These alterations can take two major forms. First, specific characteristic symptoms of a disease in middle age may be replaced by other symptoms in old age. For instance, in acute myocardial infarction, some studies have suggested that elderly persons are less likely than younger adults to present with chest pain (Pathy 1967). On the other hand, acute myocardial infarction is not "silent" in older persons; instead, they have a variety of other acute signs and symptoms, including syncope, and the sudden onset of left ventricular failure (Besdine 1980). The second difference is that elderly persons may present with nonspecific signs and symptoms (Besdine 1980), such as confusion, weakness, weight loss, or "failure to thrive," instead of specific symptoms indicating the organ or organ system affected.

This chapter has attempted a broad review of current knowledge regarding the physiologic changes with aging and the principles governing thorough evaluation of elderly patients. While these factors are critical to proper care of all elderly patients, they may play especially important and often neglected roles in those individuals in which old age is complicated by psychiatric illness. The emerging data base on the general physiology of aging provides a proper backdrop for detailed discussion of age-related and disease-related alterations in the central nervous system.

References

Abbott RD, Donahue RP, MacMahon SW, et al: Diabetes and the risk of stroke: the Honolulu heart program. JAMA 1987; 257:949

Anderson WF: The prevention of illness in the elderly: the Rutherglen experiment in medicine in old age: proceedings of a conference held at the Royal College of Physicians. London, Pitman, 1966

Besdine RW: Geriatric medicine: an overview, in Annual Review of Gerontology and Geriatrics. Edited by Eisdorfer C. New York, Springer, 1980

Besdine RW: The data base of geriatric medicine, in Health and Disease in Old Age. Edited by Rowe JW, Besdine RW. Boston, Little, Brown, 1982

Blessed G, Tomlinson BE, Roth M: The association between quantitative measures of dementia and of senile changes in the cerebral grey matter of elderly subjects. Br J Psychiatry 1968; 114:797

Bullamore JR, Gallagher JC, Wilkinson R, et al: Effect of age on calcium absorption. Lancet 1970; 2:535

Carr BR, MacDonald PC: The menopause and beyond, in Principles of Geriatric Medicine. Edited by Andrus R, Bierman EL, Hazzard WR. New York, McGraw Hill, 1985

Cockcroft DW, Gault MH: Prediction of creatinine clearance from serum creatinine. Nephron 1976; 16:31

Colandrea MA, Freedman GD, Nichaman MZ, et al: Systolic hypertension in the elderly: an epidemiologic assessment. Circulation 1970; 41:239–245

Davidson MB: The effect of aging on carbohydrate metabolism: a review of the English literature and a practical approach to the diagnosis of diabetes mellitus in the elderly. Metabolism 1979; 28:1095–1101

Dyer AR, Stanler J, Shekille RB, et al: Hypertension in the elderly. Med Clin North Am 1977; 61:513–529

Folstein MF, Folstein S, McHugh PR: Mini-Mental State: a practical method of grading the cognitive state of patients for the clinician. J Psychiatr Res 1975; 12:189

Forette F, de la Fiente X, Golmard JL, et al: The proprostic significance of isolated systolic hypertension in the elderly: results of a ten year longitudinal study. Clin Exp Hypertens 1982; 174:1177–1191

Gillis S, Kozak R, Durante M, et al: Immunological studies of aging: decreased production of and response to t cell growth factor by lymphocytes from aged humans. J Clin Invest 1981; 67:937–942

Gordon T, Shurtleff D: Means at each examination and inter-examination variation of specific characteristics: Framingham study—exams 1–10, in The Framingham Study: An Epidemiological Investigation of Cardiovascular Disease. Edited by Kannel WB. Washington, DC, National Institutes of Health, 1973

Habot B, Libow LS: The inter-relationship of mental and physical status and its assessment in the older adult: mind–body interaction, in Handbook of Mental Health and Aging. Edited by Birren JE, Sloane RB. Englewood Cliffs, NJ, Prentice Hall, 1980

Hannon JH: The Flushings of the Menopause. London, Baillere, Tindall, & Cox, 1927

Harman SM, Nankin HR: Alterations in reproductive and sexual function: male, in Principles of Geriatric Medicine. Edited by Andrus R, Bierman EL, Hazzard WR. New York, McGraw Hill, 1985

Harman SM, Tsitouras PD: Reproductive hormones in aging men: I. Measurement of sex steroids, basal LH and leydig cell response to HCG. J Clin Endocrinol Metab 1980; 51:35

Harman SM, Wehmann RE, Blackman MR: Pituitary-thyroid hormone economy in healthy aging men: basal indices of thyroid function and thyrotropin responses to constant infusions of thyrotropin releasing hormone. J Clin Endocrinol Metab 1984; 58:320

Harris MI, Hadden WC, Knowler WC, et al: Prevalence of diabetes and impaired glucose tolerance and plasma glucose levels in the U.S. population age 20–74 yr. Diabetes 1987; 36:523

Hollenberg NK, Adams DF, Solomon HS, et al: Senescence and the renal vasculature of normal man. Circ Res 1974; 34:309

Hulley SB, Furberg CD, Guyland B, et al: Systolic Hypertension in the Elderly Program (SHEP): antihypertensive efficacy of chlorthalidone. Am J Cardiol 1985; 56:913

Kane RA, Kane RL: Assessing the elderly: a practical guide to measurement. Lexington MA, Lexington Books, 1981

Kannel WB, Wolf PA, McGee DL, et al: Systolic blood pressure, arterial rigidity, and risk of stroke. JAMA 1981; 245:1229

Krasinski SD, Russell RM, Samloff IM, et al: Fundic atrophic gastritis in an elderly population. J Am Geriatr Soc 1986; 34:800

Kronenberg RC, Drage CW: Attenuation of the ventilatory and heart rate responses to hypoxia and hypercapnea with aging in normal men. J Clin Invest 1973; 52:1812

Lakatta EG: Alterations in the cardiovascular system that occur in advanced age. Fed Proc 1979; 38:163

Linn BS, Linn MW: Objective and self-assessed health in the old and very old. Soc Sci Med 1980; 14A:311–315

Livingstone H, Hershman JT, Sawin CT, et al: Prevalence of thyroid disease and abnormal thyroid tests in older hospitalized and ambulatory persons. J Am Geriatr Soc 1987; 35:109

Manton KG: Changing concepts of morbidity and mortality in the elderly population. Milbank Memorial Fund Quarterly 1982; 60:183

Martin CE: Factors affecting sexual functioning in 60–79 year old married males. Arch Sex Behav 1981; 10:399

McKinlay S, Jefferys M: The menopause syndrome. British Journal of Prevent Soc Medicine 1974; 28:108–115

Minaker KL, Meneilly GS, Rowe JW: Endocrinology of aging, in Handbook of the Biology of Aging. Edited by Finch C, Schneider EL. New York, Van Nostrand Reinhold, 1984

Morton PA: Ordinary Insurance! The Build and Blood Pressure Study. Transactions of the Society of Actuaries 1959; 11:987–997

O'Rourke MF: Arterial hemodynamics in hypertension. Circ Res 1970; 6:1234

Pathy MS: Clinical presentation of myocardial infarction in the elderly. Br Heart J 1967; 29:190–199

Pearlman CK: Frequency of intercourse in males at different ages. Medical Aspects of Human Sexuality 1972; 6:92

Rodeheffer RJ, Gerstenblith G, Becker LC, et al: Exercise cardiac output is maintained with advancing age in healthy human subjects: cardiac dilatation and increased stroke volume compensate for diminished heart rate. Circulation 1984; 69:203

Rowe JW: Clinical research in aging strategies and directions. N Engl J Med 1983; 309:1246

Rowe JW: Systolic hypertension in the elderly. N Engl J Med 1983; 309:1246–1247

Rowe JW: Health care of the elderly. N Engl J Med 1985; 312:827

Rowe JW, Andres R, Tobin JD, et al: The effect of age on creatinine clearance in man: a cross-sectional and longitudinal study. J Gerontol 1976; 31:155

Russell RM, Krasinski SD, Samloff IM, et al: Folic acid malabsorption in atrophic gastritis: possible compensation by bacterial folate synthesis. Gastroenterology 1986; 91:1476

Shekelle R, Ostfeld A, Kao A: Hypertension and risk of stroke in an elderly population. Stroke 1974; 5:71

Shock NW, Greulich RC, Anores RA, et al: Normal Human Aging: The Baltimore Longitudinal Study of Aging. Washington, DC, U.S. Department of Health and Human Services, 1984

Tudge C: The biggest risk factor of them all? World Medicine 1978; 13:21

Weale RA: The Aging Eye. New York, Harper & Row, 1963

Weiss ST: Pulmonary system, in Health and Disease in Old Age. Edited by Rowe JW, Besdine RL. Boston, Little, Brown, 1980

White NK, Edwards JE, Dry TJ: The relationship of the degree of coronary atherosclerosis with age in men. Circulation 1950; 1:645

Wilson LA, Lawson IR, Brass W: Multiple disorders in the elderly: a clinical and statistical study. Lancet 1962; 2:841–843

Zavaroni I, Dall'Aglio E, Bruschi F, et al: Effects of age and environmental factors in glucose tolerance and insulin secretion in a worker population. J Am Geriatr Soc 1986; 34:271

Chapter 3

Perceptive Changes with Aging

Ewald W. Busse, M.D.

Pain

Pain is physiologically and psychologically one of the most complex human experiences related to perception. The individual, particularly the very old individual, who is experiencing pain often finds it difficult to describe. It is clear that individual variation increases in late life despite considerable similarity in the stimulus. The sensation of pain is believed to signal current or impending tissue damage. The pain signal is to bring into operation protective measures. There are at least four dimensions of pain protection. They include neurologic, physiologic, behavioral, and affective dimensions. Sternbach (1981) has differentiated, as have other investigators, the difference between acute and chronic pain. He concludes that "an acute pain is a symptom of disease, while chronic pain is a disease within itself" (p. 31). It appears that in order to treat effectively the person with persistent pain, one must have an understanding of the individual's personality, motivation, and emotional factors in the individual's total pain experience, and the role of environment in influencing the patient's behavior and the persistence and exacerbation of pain.

A survey of the prevalence of pain in the United States was undertaken in 1985 (Sternbach 1986). This was a telephone survey of 1,254 persons aged 18 and older believed to represent a cross section of the adult population of the United States and included 48 percent men and 52 percent women. Fourteen percent of those surveyed were 65 years of age and older. The 20-minute interview included questions regarding seven types of pain: headache, backache, muscle pain, joint pain, stomach pain, premenstrual or menstrual pain, and dental pain. They were also questioned about stress reactions and these were called "daily hassles." The survey concluded that young adults aged 18 to 24 were more likely to have all types of pains than any other group; in fact, those aged 65 were found to have a high prevalence of joint pain (71 percent), but for all other pain types reported less than younger adults. These accumulative data may be distorted by the fact that the older woman would not be concerned with menstrual pain and inasmuch as many elderly persons are adentulous, it is unlikely they would have such complaints.

Acute pain promotes survival, while chronic pain is destructive. It disrupts physical, psychologic, and social functions, but it may not impair longevity. Patients with acute pain become less tolerant of exacerbations or the independent appearance of new acute pain. Minor injuries such as stubbing a toe become a major pain experience. The entire organism is hyperalert and often overresponds to a pain signal.

Melzack and Wall (1965) proposed the "gate theory" of pain. It provided an explanation as to how brain activities such as attention, emotion, memories, and so forth can change the gate in various directions—opening or closing it. With the generation of new knowledge, some of the limitations of the gate theory are apparent, but the theory has stimulated research and is useful.

Wall, in 1979, proposed a new approach to the understanding of pain. He delineated three sequential stages of pain: immediate, acute, and chronic. Each of these phases is linked less to injury than to body state. Wall suggests that pain is more of an awareness of a need state than an awareness of an actual event that produces a sensation. This explains why pain can be linked causally to an injury, but it may not be. There are times when injury does not generate pain, and the sensation of pain does not always signal injury. Clearly the behavior associated with internal feelings is powerfully influenced by other events such as emotional responses of fear, anger, anxiety, and concern. All of these emotional responses affect the sensation of pain.

In this approach, pain emerges as a general pattern reaction comprising three distinct and behavioral phases whose intensity and duration determine the final response. Acute pain sets in when one can concentrate on protecting the wound. Acute pain does not set in until attention can be directed wholly or in part to caring for the injury. The acute phase is dominated by pain, but it is also accompanied by anxiety that may be related to past events, the present condition, or future expectations. The first or acute phase changes when the events appear to be under one's control. In fact, the first phase of pain may be skipped and the second phase entered quickly. During this phase steps are taken to reduce the pain and to cope with the injury. The third or chronic phase of pain is marked by a recovery from the injury. Under optimal conditions of healing, the pain gradually declines following the healing process, but in a few patients without permanent injury, the chronic phase drags on far beyond the necessity for recovery. The chronic phase is that of intractable pain. This apparently is the phase associated with the central control trigger of the original theory. Chronic pain is the burden of the numerous pain clinics that have appeared in many medical facilities.

It is of interest to note that there are some structures that have pain fibers only. No other sensations are transmitted from these structures. They are teeth, the middle meningeal artery, arteries at the base of the brain, and at least some scalp arteries. In contrast, there are certain structures that appear to be devoid of pain supply. These include the parenchyma of the brain and the inside of the cheek opposite the lower molar.

Unfortunately, pain research has paid little attention to the influence of age on this important perception. The lack of specificity of acute pain, location, type and intensity, and the increase in chronic pain reduce the reliability of pain as a diagnostic sign or symptom.

Endogenous Pain-Producing Substances

Endogenously occurring chemical substances such as H^+ ions, serotonin, histamine, bradykinin, and prostaglandins have excitatory effects on nociceptors. These substances are designated as endogenous algesics. Some of these substances contribute to the sensation of pain directly by sensitizing the nociceptor or may indirectly influence the nociceptor by their fasoactive effects. Substance P is released from some nociceptive nerve terminals. Substance P has been suggested to be a factor in inflammation and pain, this phenomenon being termed "neurogenic inflammation." A number of substances contribute to the release of Substance P, which results in vasodilatation and local edema caused by increased capillary permeability (Zimmermann 1984).

Neuropeptides and Pain Modulation in the Brain

Accumulated experimental evidence has established that there is a network within the brain that functions to selectively inhibit pain transmission (Fields 1983). This network includes neurons at mid-brain, medullary, and spinal levels. This network is normally activated by endogenous peptides. This analgesic system can be activated by narcotic analgesics, such as morphine, which are believed to mimic the action of the normally occurring endogenous peptides. Some of the endogenous opioid peptides that have been identified include leucine-enkephalin, methionine-enkephalin, alpha-neoendorphin, dynorphin, and the 30 amino acid compound beta-endorphin. Beta-endorphin was first discovered in the pituitary, but has subsequently been shown to be present in the hypothalamus as well. Endogenous opioid peptides are closely associated with the pain-modulating network at diencephalic, mid-brain, medullary, and spinal levels.

Although the opioid network is extremely important, Gebhart (1983) believes that it is likely that pain control involves not only endogenous opioid systems, but nonopioid systems as well.

Hearing

Hearing is a significant loss in later life that can adversely affect social interaction, and is particularly important to the psychiatric physician. A recent study in Britain ("Loss of hearing in the elderly" 1986) supported by the Royal National Institute for the Deaf reports that some 60 percent of people over the age of 70 are thought to be significantly hearing impaired. Only one-sixth of the affected persons are referred to and receive rehabilitation services including hearing aids. In the United States it is estimated that 14.4 to 15.5 million Americans have irreversible hearing loss and only 17 to 27 percent are wearing hearing aids (Rupp and Jackson 1986).

A progressive decline that often appears with advancing age is referred to as presbycusis. Presbycusis is sometimes defined in general terms and often there are specific diagnostic categories. Presbycusis can be defined as the alteration of hearing capacity associated with normal physiologic aging of the auditory system. Presbycusis can be broken into three types. In sensory presbycusis there is a decrement of perception of high frequencies without the loss of speech discrimination. Impairment of speech understanding occurs in neuronal presbycusis. In striatal presbycusis all frequencies show a uniform loss (Busse 1987).

Normal Hearing

The human ear can perceive sounds over a wide range of frequencies from as low as 16 to 20 c/second to as high as 23,000 to 30,000 c/second. There is a great deal of individual variation, and in general, perception of high frequencies is best in early childhood and gradually decreases throughout life. A normal middle-aged adult may have difficulty with anything over 10,000 to 12,000 c/second. In addition to the aging process, there is little doubt that frequent exposure to loud noises contributes to deafness.

The intensity of the sound, that is, the height of the wave, is customarily expressed in decibels. Zero decibels is the intensity that humans can hardly hear. At 10 decibels speech is faintly audible, while quieted speech is approximately 40 decibels. The decibel scale is not one of equalized units. It is a logarithmic scale. Every upward step of 10 decibels represents 100-fold multiplication of sound energy. Thus a sound of 60 decibels is 100 times more powerful than one of 50 decibels.

Unfortunately, a riveter standing approximately 35 feet away from a person produces a sound, the intensity of which is 100 decibels or 10 billion times the intensity that is barely audible. A nearby gunshot blast produces 140 decibels.

The Anatomy and Physiology of the Ear

The outer ear (i.e., the visible, external ear) consists of the pinna, which picks up sound waves, and the external canal, which channels the waves as far as the ear drum. The middle ear is the air-filled cavity containing the ossicles, which conduct sound vibrations from the ear drum to the inner ear. The inner ear is a liquid-filled chamber that contains the cochlea, the vestibule, and the semicircular canals. It is connected to the brain by the auditory nerve.

Over the life span, the pinnacle or external ear grows as much as several millimeters. Atrophy can be seen in the supporting walls of the external auditory meatus. The accumulation of excessive amounts of cerumen within the inner ear is not an uncommon finding in the elderly and can produce a conductive hearing loss. The ear drum separating the middle ear from the external ear often stiffens as a result of aging. The sound is transmitted from the ear drum to three bones. The three bones constitute the ossicular chain—the malleus (hammer), the incus (anvil), and the stapes (stirrup). All of the bones can undergo arthritic changes. Such changes result in a reduction of ability to hear higher frequencies.

The cochlea undergoes at least four major changes. Sensory losses can result from lower elasticity of the basilar membrane that reduces the ampliture and the shearing force on the organ of Corti. This organ includes the receptor cells that are attached to the basilar membrane. The sensory receptors for higher frequencies are located on a thicker, more narrow strip of the basilar membrane; hence, they are more likely to be affected. Neural losses can occur throughout the cochlea and not infrequently are greater at the basal end that mediates high frequencies. Cochlear otosclerosis with or without stapes fixation is a common condition in the elderly.

The stria vascularis, a band of specially differentiated tissues in the cochlea, atrophies with age. This loss apparently interferes with metabolic processes throughout the cochlea, especially of the ionic composition of the endolymph, the fluid within this structure.

Auditory Perception

Auditory perception is affected by several age-related structural and physiologic changes. These declines include alteration and auditory thresholds, pitch discrimination, sound localization, masking, loudness recruitment, and speech comprehension (Schiffman 1985).

At approximately 20 years of age, it is not unusual to observe a beginning loss in sensitivity to pure tones. Most of the losses are at 1,000 Hz and above and frequencies above 4,000 Hz at 30 decibels are especially vulnerable. Males experience greater losses than females. This may be related to exposure to loud noises.

With the passage of time there is a decline in the ability to discriminate among frequencies. These changes are greatest in the higher frequency ranges. The elderly person has greater difficulty localizing sounds, especially those with higher frequencies. With advancing age the presence of background noise frequently masks the reception of important signals.

The condition of loudness recruitment occurs in about 50 percent of the elderly population and makes the use of hearing aids of limited usefulness in situations where high-intensity background noise occurs along with wanted signals of low intensity. Accompanying this condition of loudness recruitment is the possibility that sounds of moderate to high intensities may produce a painful reaction.

The loss of high-frequency sounds that have been previously mentioned results in a decline in ability to identify consonants (particularly *s, z, t, f,* and *g*). Consonants that are said to contribute to "intelligibility" of speech are high-frequency sounds (about 2,000 to 4,000 c/second) while vowels that are the "energy" and "body" of speech are low-frequency sounds (250 to 750 c/second). Consequently, comprehending speech can be a very serious problem. The person may hear the sounds but not understand them.

Speech discrimination, under adverse listening conditions, is seriously affected by age. When test sentences are undistorted or do not compete without stimuli, the effects of age on speech discrimination are relatively small. However, when words overlap or are interrupted, intelligibility scores of older adults, particularly those in the seventh decade or more, are affected. Speech discrimination is disrupted by rapid speech, increased verberation, overlapping of words, and other forms of acoustical distortion (Corso 1986).

Understanding Speech

Many reports on older people emphasize the decline in ability to hear over 3,000 c/second. In a longitudinal study of aging people, it appears that losses of about 4,000 c/second can interfere with understanding speech. This is explained by the fact that speech normally generates many frequencies in the range above 4,000 c/second and these may be critical to understanding the spoken words (Busse and Maddox 1986).

Old people living most of their lives in a quiet, usually rural environment often have better hearing than city persons (Eisdorfer and Wilkie 1972).

Tinnitus

A more or less persistent ringing or buzzing noise in the ears occurs in approximately 80 percent of the population of developed nations at some point during the aging process. It is believed to be the result of the natural degenerative processes of aging and exposure to excessive noise. In some individuals, if the excessive noise can be avoided, the tinnitus will improve or disappear. There are no drugs to cure or eliminate tinnitus. Two devices, hearing aids and so-called masking tapes, sometimes are of use. Tinnitus is an internal noise. If a person can hear what is going around him or her, then the person is less likely to pay attention to the tinnitus. Masking devices work on the premise of counteracting an internal noise with an external noise. Fatigue and stress may add to the appearance of tinnitus. Tinnitus can be attributed to external and middle ear problems, which can be removed by medical or surgical treatment. Tinnitus may be secondary to drugs and can usually be relieved by the elimination or reduction of the causative agent. Tinnitus may be precipitated by exposure to high noises and conservation methods are of use. Tinnitus of sensorineural origin is usually associated with hearing loss and cannot be affected by medical or surgical intervention.

Hearing Aids

The resistance to wearing hearing aids has, in recent years, been changed because of the appearance of in-the-ear aids and the willingness by many prominent people to use hearing aids. President Ronald Reagan acknowledged that he wears an in-the-ear hearing aid in his right ear, and later he began to use a similar device in his left ear. This is consistent with the current recommendation that binaural aids are significantly better than monaural aids. Binaural aids are said to improve the threshold of hearing, increase speech discrimination, generate normal fields of hearing, and provide binaural cues for directional hearing.

Another major advancement has been the approval by the Food and Drug Administration in 1984 of the cochlear implant. This procedure is reserved for adults with profound hearing losses who are unable to be helped by conventional hearing aids. The surgically implanted electrode helps the profoundly deaf person to distinguish various environmental sounds through direct electrical stimulation of the cochlear nerve. The cochlear implant provides the greatest benefit to adults with hearing loss acquired after speech development. Although the cochlear implant is a major advancement, it cannot adequately mimic the large amount of auditory information produced by the cochlea. Patients are often able to perceive some sounds produced in average speech, but speech discrimination is limited (Manning and Meyerhoff 1986).

Vision

There are at least four age-related changes in the structure of the eye that result in significant functional differences. These anatomical changes include (1) flattening of the corneal surface, which reduces refractive power; (2) a clouding of the lens that attenuates available light, especially for short-wave lengths; (3) the loss of the ability of the lens to accommodate; and (4) losses in the efficiency and the number of photoreceptors in the retina (Sekuler et al. 1982). The functions that are particularly affected will be discussed. Pathologic conditions that become more common with advancing age include cataracts, glaucoma, and macular degeneration.

Lens Accommodation and Cataracts

One of the most consistent and perhaps universal manifestations of aging in mammals is the progressive alteration that takes place in the composition of the lens of the eye with advancing age. Criteria have been developed using the lens as a standard to estimate the ages of animals, particularly those captured in the wild. The total protein content of the lens is measured. This protein increases during the entire life span of the animal and after maturity there is primarily an increase in the insoluble protein fraction of the lens. Rearing these animals in a variety of conditions has no appreciable effect on this procedure for estimating age.

The lens throughout the life span increases in both size and thickness because of the continuing proliferation of new cells at the periphery of the lens. As the lens fibers mature they migrate to the central region (the nucleus) where they become compressed and more rigid. Consequently the transparency of the nucleus as well as the overall elasticity of the lens are reduced. In addition, the capsule, the homogeneous acellular structure surrounding the lens, becomes thicker and less permeable. In addition to the lens becoming less transparent for the entire spectrum (white light), the aging lens also becomes markedly less transparent for the blue part of the spectrum. This is due to opacities that accumulate in the lens, usually a yellow-brown substance. For some older people, a true blue appears greenish blue.

Visual impairment due to senile cataract is a very common visual problem in late life. Visual improvement is obtained by cataract surgery and the use of corrective lenses. An artificial lens implant is also possible. Cataract surgery must be decided after evaluation of the presence or absence of coexisting retinal disease. Binocular vision after surgery for a unilateral cataract is possible only if the patient is able to wear a contact lens or if an artificial lens is implanted in the eye.

Cataracts are the result of a gradual loss of lens transparency. There is a painless loss of vision. When opacity is in the central lens nucleus, myopia develops in the early stages so that a presbyopic patient may be able to read without corrective lenses. This is often called second sight.

Macula Degeneration and Glaucoma

Degeneration of the macula is a very serious visual loss. The macula lutea is a small circular area of the retina, about 5 mm in diameter, located at the posterior pole of the eye. Its integrity is essential for good vision, particularly for reading and color perception. The rest of the retina serves the peripheral field with perception of light and gross movement. There are four types of macular degeneration:

1. *Senile pigmentary degeneration* shows irregularities of pigment with areas of pigment loss and pigment clumping.
2. *Disciform degeneration* is characterized early in its clinical course by subretinal neovascularization arising from the choroidal circulation. There is irregular proliferation of the retinal pigment epithelium and overgrowth of glial and connective tissue.
3. *Cystoid degeneration* is the appearance and rupture of large cysts, resulting in a honeycomb appearance. Antiinflammatory therapy may improve some patients.
4. *Primary neuronal degeneration* is characterized histologically as a loss of photoreceptors and their nuclei. This type of degeneration was described in 1980 and it appears to be age related.

In chronic simple or open-angle glaucoma, increased intraoccular pressure leads to optic atrophy. This bilateral, slowly progressive disease causes no symptoms until considerable visual field loss or even blindness has occurred. Early detection is of considerable importance. This can be recognized by measuring the intraoccular pressure and by observation of the optic nerve.

Chronic open angle glaucoma. The cause of this disorder is unknown. It is assumed there are several predisposing factors, especially heredity. The anatomical structures of the eye appear normal, but drainage of the aqueous humor is incomplete. This is the most prevalent form of glaucoma. It is rarely unilateral.

Acute or chronic closed angle glaucoma. This disorder is associated with eyes that have narrow anterior chamber angles. The acute form is usually unilateral and is accompanied by severe head and eye pain, blurred vision, nausea, and vomiting. Chronic angle closure is that of recurrent attacks. It too is accompanied by severe headaches, blurred vision, and halos around lights.

Visual Changes

Presbyopia, which occurs in virtually all aging persons, is a result of the inability of the lens to change its shape. Onset is often around the age of 45, and the common complaint is the inability to see near objects clearly. Fortunately, it is corrected by eye glasses. Presbyopia is thought to have several causes, since the lens becomes more rigid and less amenable to shape change by action of the ciliary muscle. In addition, the ciliary muscles become less effective (Anderson and Palmore 1974).

With aging there is an alteration in light/dark adaptation. The minimal amount of light energy that can be detected by the eye is called the detection level. It is usually measured after the eye has been dark adapted. Detection thresholds increase with age, especially for short wave lengths. Visual threshold alteration is the result of a reduced pupil size, modification in the lens, and altered retinal metabolism. Greater differences in brightness are required by older persons in order to detect a change.

This alteration may be particularly important to those who drive automobiles. Aging increases the susceptibility to glare due to increased dispersion of light that occurs in all of the ocular media. The presence of cataracts greatly increases glare problems.

With aging there is a decline in the ability to read the smallest letters on the Snellen chart. Raising the light intensity and increasing contrast between the object and its background can overcome some of this decrement.

Taste and Smell in Old Age

With advancing age, there is a diminished ability to perceive taste and smell. The changes are the result of the loss of receptors and changes in neuronal pathways. Taste and smell decline with advancing age and alter the ability to distinguish foods and drinks (Schiffman 1978). Some physicians believe that the decline in taste sensitivity is not solely the result of age but is caused by or exacerbated by the use of tobacco, dietary and metabolic deficiencies (B_3 [niacin], B_{12}, zinc), and diseases such as viral and influenza-like infections, multiple sclerosis, hyperthyroidism, diabetes mellitus, and so on. There are many medications commonly used by the elderly that adversely affect taste and smell; these include antirheumatic, antihypertensive, and antiparkinsonism agents, and some psychopharmacologic drugs.

Olfaction

Olfactory receptors cells are specialized bipolar neurons. Their nuclei are located at the base of the epithelium layer. The small receptors are found in the patch of olfactory epithelia that lines the medial and lateral walls of the roof of the nasal cavity. Because of the small size and the inaccessibility of the olfactory cells, the mechanism of odor detection has not been as thoroughly investigated as other sensory mechanisms. Furthermore, the receptors and their cells have not been divided into recognizable groups as is the case with taste receptors and cells. There is evidence that the molecular size, shape, and configuration of the odorant are important elements in olfactory discrimination (Netter 1983).

As to changes of smell with aging, elevated detection and recognition thresholds accompanying the aging process have been reported for coal gas, coffee, menthol, and other substances. Other studies have attempted to determine if perceived intensity proportionate to the stimuli alters with aging (Schemper et al. 1981). It appears that the elderly are less proficient at odor identification. They are less likely to identify four common odors including coffee, peppermint, coal tar, and oil of almonds. Undoubtedly there are individual differences, but living habits as well as the habitual use of olfaction may explain some of these differences.

Gustation

Taste (gustatory) perception is mediated by taste buds, which are pear-shaped organs consisting of approximately 50 cells. Taste cells derive from epithelia surrounding the bud and constantly turn over, with a life span of approximately 10½ days. Taste buds are found on three types of papillae—fungiform, circumvallate, and foliate. These papillae decrease with age. Taste buds are primarily on the tongue; however, a few are on the soft palate and epiglottis.

Different taste sensations are regionally distributed on the tongue. Usually aging is accompanied by a deterioration of taste recognition that progresses from the front to the back of the tongue. Sweet and salt perceptions are particularly vulnerable; hence, many elderly complain that foods taste sour or bitter.

There is evidence that a chronic taste in the mouth, a mild dysgeusia, is present in many elderly people. The persistence of a bad taste makes taste discrimination more difficult. Consequently, improved oral hygiene may improve taste recognition, particularly tastes of lower intensity (Bartoshuk et al. 1986).

Little is known about the gustatory pathways, with the exception of the amygdala, where neurofibrillary tangles (NFTs) are seen. Olfactory pathways are also affected by neuropathologic age changes, particularly senile plaques and NFTs.

Taste changes include alteration of thresholds, changes in perceived intensity, and a decline in ability to identify and discriminate among tastes. Stevens et al. (1984) used a technique of magnitude matching, that is, comparing the relative losses of taste, olfaction, and hearing, to confirm the fact that age reduces the perceived intensity of olfactory sensations to a greater extent than taste. This difference in loss of olfaction as compared to taste was reported by Stevens et al. (1984).

Amplification of Taste and Smell

Recent research (Henki et al. 1976) is attempting to enhance taste and smell perception in the elderly. Direct application of methyl xanthines, including caffeine, to the tongue has been shown to enhance sweet and salty tastes (Schiffman et al. 1985). Zinc sulfate has been found to restore general taste functioning in some people, compensating for a zinc deficiency.

The loss of smell with age is even greater than the loss of taste. The loss of taste and smell affect the elderly person's ability to identify food and discriminate odors.

Tactile Sensation: Vibration

Many studies have reported a loss of tactile sensation with advancing age. Precise quantitative evaluation of the result is often difficult or impossible because modern methods of stimulation were not used and often adequate stimulation control was not possible. However, with modern techniques, vibrotactile methods can be studied and measured on various parts of the body. Vibrotactile thresholds can be measured. The results show a progressive decline in sensitivity at high frequencies over the entire age span—from childhood to late life. The sharpest decrease apparently occurs between 50 and 65 years of age. This is particularly true of the high frequencies. This decreased sensitivity may be attributed to a reduction in the number of Pacinian corpuscles that occurs with aging or to structural changes within the corpuscle (Verrillo 1980).

Nowlin et al. (1985) studied vibratory threshold in relationship to health parameters. Their subjects were 320 white middle-aged and elderly individuals who were studied over a span of 2 years. Within this population, vibratory threshold for both upper and lower extremities increased significantly over the 2-year interval between tests. Alterations in the threshold differences were more marked in the lower extremities than in the upper extremeties. Men showed greater threshold differences than women. Measures of general health demonstrated that those with increased evidence of pathology showed the most alteration in recognition of vibrotactile sensations.

Whanger and Wang (1974) compared control subjects from a longitudinal study of "normal" aging with acute psychiatric patients and chronic psychiatric patients. Although these authors questioned the validity of using vibrotactile measures as an evaluation of the general state of the nervous system, they did confirm that normal elderly subjects show a progressive elevation of the vibratory threshold. The psychiatric patients showed higher levels of virbratory thresholds. The investigators observed that black subjects had significantly lower vibratory thresholds than whites and had significantly higher mean serum B_{12} levels than did their white subjects and patients.

Loss of Teeth

The loss of teeth has been a common feature of aging. It not only has produced inconvenience in eating, but perhaps has contributed to nutritional deficiencies and certainly has altered the appearance of many elderly people. This is particularly true of those who have been unable to wear dentures. In recent years better fitting dentures have become available, and often those that are made with attractive teeth actually improve the appearance of an older person. It is quite possible that in the decades ahead the loss of teeth will not be as common since the use of fluoride in water supplies has effectively reduced the incidence of dental caries. There has also been a reduction in the other factors that contribute to caries. These are a susceptible tooth, a specific bacterium, and a diet rich in sugars. The care of teeth has also improved, and considerable emphasis has been placed on the reduction of dental plaque, which is a soft mass of bacteria on tooth surfaces. Dental plaque often precedes the development of tooth decay. Many scientists believe they are well on their way to developing a vaccine that will protect humans against caries.

In the past, dental decay and tooth loss seemed to be unavoidable facts of aging. Shakespeare and Dickens, as well as other authors, have described unfortunate victims of tooth decay, their smiles revealing pitted, discolored, or altogether missing teeth.

Block (1985) reported a survey of the dental status of the elderly. This survey found that 50 percent of all people over the age of 65 years had lost all of their teeth and that 70 percent of residents of long-term care facilities have no teeth. Approximately one-third of those without teeth have no dentures, have defective dentures, or have partial dentures.

References

Anderson B, Palmore E: Longitudinal evaluation of ocular function, in Normal Aging II—1970–73. Edited by Busse EW, Maddox GL. Durham, NC, Duke University Press, 1974

Bartoshuk LM, Rifkin B, Marks LE, et al: Taste and aging. J Gerontol 1986; 41:51–57

Block M: Dental status of the elderly. Paper presented at the Symposium of the Durham Veterans Administration Geriatric Research, Education, and Clinical Center, August 13, 1985

Busse EW: Clinical characteristics of normal aging, in Teaching and Training in Geriatric Medicine (Volume 1). Edited by Meier-Ruge W. Basel, Switzerland, Karger, 1987

Busse EW, Maddox GL: The Duke Longitudinal Studies of Normal Aging 1955–1980. New York, Springer, 1986

Corso JF: Auditory perception, in Encyclopedia of Aging. Edited by Maddox GL. New York, Springer, 1986

Eisdorfer C, Wilkie F: Auditory changes in the aged: a follow-up study. J Am Geriatr Soc 1972; 20:377–382

Fields L: Recent advances in research on pain and analgesia, in Contemporary Research in Pain and Analgesia (National Institute on Drug Abuse Research Monograph 45). Edited by Brown RM, Pinkert TM, Ludford JP. Washington, DC, U.S. Department of Health and Human Services, 1983

Gebhart GF: Recent developments in the neurochemical bases of pain and analgesia, in Contemporary Research in Pain and Analgesia (National Institute on Drug Abuse Research Monograph 45). Edited by Brown RM, Pinkert TM, Ludford JP. Washington, DC, Department of Health and Human Services, 1983

Henki R, Schechter P, Friedewald W, et al: A double-blind study of the effects of zinc sulfate on taste and smell dysfunction. Am J Med Sci 1976; 272:289–299

Loss of hearing in the elderly. Lancet, February 22, 1986

Manning S, Meyerhoff WL: Bringing hearing to the profoundly deaf: a research report. Geriatrics 1986; 41(3):78–79

Melzack R, Wall PD: Pain mechanisms: a new theory. Science 1965; 150:971–979

Netter FH: The Nervous System: Volume 1. Anatomy and Physiology. West Caldwell, NJ, Ciba, 1983

Nowlin JB, Whanger AD, Cleveland WD Jr: Vibratory threshold and health, in Normal Aging III. Edited by Palmore EB, Busse EW, Maddox GL, et al. Durham, NC, Duke University Press, 1985

Rupp FA, Jackson DD: Primary care for the hearing impaired. Geriatrics 1986; 41(3):75–80

Schemper T, Voss S, Cain S: Odor identification in young and elderly persons. J Gerontol 1981; 36:446–452

Schiffman SS: Changes in taste and smell in older persons. Advances in Research 1978; 2(3):1–7

Schiffman SS: The Salient Sensory Losses with Aging (Aspects of Aging Series No. 3). Philadelphia, Smith Kline & French Laboratories, 1985

Schiffman SS, Gill JM, Diaz C: Methyl xanthines enhanced taste: evidence for modulation of taste by adenosine receptor. Pharmacol Biochem Behav 1985; 22:195–203

Sekuler RD, Kline K, Dismukes: Aging and Human Visual Function. New York, Alan R. Liss, 1982

Sternbach RA: Chronic pain as a disease entity. Triangle 1981; 20(1/2):27–32

Sternbach RA: Survey of pain in the United States: the Nuprin pain report. Clinical Journal of Pain 1986; 2(1):49–53

Stevens JC, Bartoshuk LM, Cain WS: Chemical senses and aging: taste versus smell. Chemical Senses 1984; 9:167–179

Verrillo RT: Age related changes in the sensitivity to vibration. J Gerontol 1980; 35:185–193

Wall PD: The relationship of injury to pain: the John J. Bonica lecture. Pain 1979; 6:253–264

Whanger AD, Wang HS: Clinical correlates of the vibratory sense. J Gerontol 1974; 29:39–45

Zimmermann M: Neurobiological concepts of pain: its assessment and therapy, in Pain Measurement in Man: Neurological Correlates of Pain. Edited by Bromm B. Amsterdam, Elsevier, 1984

Chapter 4

Neuroanatomy and Neuropathology of Aging

F. Stephen Vogel, M.D.

The nervous system evolved phylogenetically over millions of years. Yet only recently in this prolonged interval did the human brain singularly acquire a facility for cognition. Unfortunately, this new attribute is labile. It is transient in each individual brain and its loss is cardinal to senescence.

Highly specialized anatomic and molecular properties were unquestionably prerequisite to the attainment of cognition. Therefore, this chapter will focus initially on the structural attributes of the human brain that seemingly sustain cognitive function. This informational base will then serve in an assessment of the pathogenesis of the intellectual decline that accompanies chronologic age.

Neuroanatomy

The adult human brain weighs approximately 1,350 g. This weight represents glia (astrocytes, oligodendroglia, and ependyma), myelin, blood vessels, and an astronomic number of neurons. The latter has been estimated conservatively at 20 billion. It is an important concept that each neuron is essentially an individual unit of structure while its function is integrated into a consortium with many other nerve cells. The functional capacity of a neuron becomes immutable with anatomic development and cell maturation; however, clearly embryonic neuroblasts have the latitude to evolve functions in accord with the needs of the host, when these needs are expressed early in embryonic development. Thus, a single cerebral hemisphere assumes bilateral motor and sensory functions in the congenital abnormality of hemiatrophy of the brain.

79

The structural character of neurons is also established during embryonic development. Both nerve cells and glia take origin from the germinal mantle, a marginal zone in the subependyma that is densely populated with primitive neuroectodermal cells. Here, and only here, with the rarest exception, do neurons undergo mitotic division, principally in the first trimester of embryonic development. The progeny of these mitoses migrate outwardly into the cerebral cortex, assisted directionally in their migration by slender glial filaments that serve as "guide wires" from the germinal mantle to the cortex. Having gained a permanent cortical position, the neurons differentiate and relinquish their capacity for replication. This acquired inability to divide is nevertheless highly compensated. The neurons attain stability of structure, an attribute that is prerequisite to cognition. Anatomic stability permits the accumulation of information in the present, allows its recall from the past, and facilitates the formulation of concepts for the future. Nevertheless, this property also defines the inescapability of aging, since metabolic errors and metabolic deficiencies now become accumulative. Such metabolic decrements cannot be eliminated by cell division, in a manner that characterizes somatic cells. In summary, the structural stability of the human nervous system is simultaneously the prerequisite to cognition and also the attribute that is cardinal to aging.

Each nerve cell is bounded totally by a three-layered plasma membrane ("unit membrane") that is regionally specialized in structure to form axons, dendrites, and synapses. As with all cells, the plasma membrane controls the molecular flow between the neuron and its environment. As a specialization of neurons, the plasma membrane serves as a site of electrical activity, particularly at synapses, where it facilitates the transfer of signals from neuron to neuron. The nucleus is situated in the perikaryon, that is, the cell body or "soma." The nucleus generally varies proportionally in size to that of the nerve cell, ranging from 5 to 100 mm. Its DNA content controls protein synthesis. However, the production of protein must sustain not only the soma but also the dendrites and axons. This physical relationship is underscored in the "dying back phenomenon" of amyotrophic lateral sclerosis. Herein the distal segments of the motor axons are the initial site of structural degeneration, presumably as a manifestation of a metabolic inadequacy within the perikaryon.

The perikaryon also contains the ribosomes that synthesize proteins. Ribosomes are either free lying, being single or clustered as polyribosomes, or are attached to the endoplasmic reticulum, a structural relationship referred to as "Nissl substance." A neuron may show chromotolysis, characterized structurally as a swelling of the cytoplasmic compartment, a fragmentation of Nissl substance, and a displacement of the nucleus to the plasma membrane. These morphologic alterations signify cell injury and are accompanied by functional compromises.

Mitochondria are largely restricted to the perikaryon. As in most cells, the mitochondria of the nervous system function as a source of energy through glycolysis, a chain reaction that utilizes glucose to produce adenosine triphosphate, with its high-energy bonds. However, nerve cells are distinctive in their obligate need for glucose and also in their inability to store glycogen. These characteristics increase their dependency on circulating glucose and oxygen for uninterrupted aerobic metabolism. Thus, hypoxia and hypoglycemia promptly initiate such pathologic entities as laminar necrosis, a loss of Purkinje cells, and insular sclerosis, among others. Lysosomes also frequent the perikaryon and serve as reservoirs of hydrolytic enzymes. Disturbances in their numbers and presumably in their functional capacities to perform autophagocytosis cause them to accumulate in excessive numbers and to be engorged with lipoprotein waste material. These "lipofuscin granules" are evidence of metabolic wear and tear. They accumulate with age, but their rate of accumulation is also accelerated by metabolic insults, such as hypoxia. The lengthy distance between the perikaryon and the synapse has necessitated a specialization of lysosomes. Nerve transmission across the synapse initiates the production of vesicles; these are modified lysosomes that conduct autophagic activities as pinocytotic or exocytotic vesicles.

Microtubules, neurofilaments, and microfilaments are specialized structures in neurons. Microtubules measure 20 to 30 nm; neurofilaments, 10 nm; and microfilaments, 5 nm. Microtubules are long unbranched cylinders. They are formed principally of the protein tubulin. In nerve cells, microtubules reside predominately in the perikaryon, as individual forms or in small clusters. They are present in lesser numbers in axons. Compounds such as colchicine bind with microtubules and impair their functional participation in axoplasmic transport. Neurofilaments are unique to nerve cells. They are abundant in large axons where they outnumber the microtubules. In small axons and dendrites, microtubules predominate. The ratio of neurofilaments to microtubules is altered moderately as a corollary of age. However, it is modified to an extreme as the result of neurofibrillary tangle formation in Alzheimer's disease.

Microfilaments are abundant in growing nerve processes. They are also present in neuroglia. Compounds such as cytochalasin B greatly interfere with the role of microfilaments in cell motility and presumably also in neuronal axoplasmic transport.

The term "synapse" is derived from the Greek, meaning to connect or to join. It is a locus of specialized anatomy that permits the directional flow of "information" from neuron to neuron. Its directionality is best appreciated in the constancy of the circuitry that defines flow from sensory to motor neurons, and never in the reverse. A synapse is an approximation of the membranes of two neurons, always physically separated by a space approximately 20 nm in width. The contact of an axon to a cell body is termed an axosomatic synapse; between an axon and a dendrite, an axodendritic synapse; between two axons, an axoaxonic synapse; and between two dendrites, a dendrodendritic synapse. At such sites of juxtaposition, neurons release substances that diffuse through the intracellular clefts and serve as neurotransmitters or neuromodulators. The movement of neurotransmitters, ions, or metabolites from one neuron into the synaptic cleft may initiate or modify a function of several contiguous cells, even glia. In addition, the anatomic proximity of juxtaposed membranes permits direct electrical interaction between neighboring nerve cells. The polarity of a synapse is defined by structure; thus the presynaptic terminal is distinguished by the presence of synaptic vesicles, while the postsynaptic processes are marked anatomically by an increased density of the plasma membrane. Functional specialization of synapses is reflected in their shape and size, and also in the number and configuration of synaptic vesicles. For example, small vesicles (20 to 40 nm in diameter), by their size, indicate a content of acetylcholine and characterize the synapse as cholinergic. Medium-sized vesicles (50 to 90 nm) denote the presence of monoamine transmitters, whereas large vesicles (120 to 150 nm) characterize neurosecretory cells, such as those of the hypothalamus, which supply polypeptide hormones to the pituitary. The security of information about the more precisely characterized neurotransmitters, such as acetylcholine, γ-aminobutyric acid, and dopamine, has lent false assurance to our fragmentary knowledge about the numerous, and still putative, neuroactive polypeptides such as somatostatin, vasopressin, endorphin, and so on. This limited knowledge concerning the normal functional roles of these compounds imparts considerable uncertainty to hypotheses that suggest their specific roles in the causation of such disease processes as Alzheimer's disease. Thus, a diminished concentration of acetylcholine in the terminal state of Alzheimer's disease necessitates a clear distinction between causation and an epiphenomenon before its significance assumes meaning.

This brief discussion has focused on the individual neuron and the structural characteristics that evolve through cell differentiation. To a degree, it has also concerned the process of maturation, that is, the evolution of the topography of the nervous system. Ancillary events such as myelinization should not go unnoticed; however, the integrity of myelin seems not to be cardinal to the phenomenon of aging. Its loss seemingly is not a primary event in the aged human nervous system, and therefore our principal concern will remain with the functional unit, the neuron.

The embryonic events of angiogenesis are also important to the functionality of the neural tissues. Abnormal angiogenesis may be responsible for congenital malformations of the nervous system. More important, the continued patency of the cerebral blood vessels is clearly cardinal to aging for it is frequently compromised by atherosclerosis and by hypertensive fibromuscular hyperplasia.

It should be noted that the complex events of embryonic development are accompanied by programmed neuronal cell death. The term "programmed" warrants underscoring because it reflects the purposeful transiency of biologic units within an organism. Thus, defective and superfluous neurons are lost even during this early interval of life. The analogy could be drawn to the "thinning" of a corn field during its most active growth phase. At the point of completed neuronal division, is it then appropriate to character-ize the human nervous system as a "sculptured" entity, cast in stone and incapable of further development or repair, subject only to "aging," to disease, and to degeneration? Ostensibly, this concept has validity, for neurons cannot replicate, oligodendroglial cells cannot remyelinate, and cerebral blood ves-sels are limited in their capacity for structural repair. But even in the human nervous system there is a reparative process termed "plasticity" that suggests that mature neurons have a capacity to sprout and form new synapses. Optimistically, it has been suggested that by the formation of new synaptic circuitry, there is an added ability to learn, an acquired capability to re-member new facts, and a facility to develop new skills. As indicated above, during embryonic development, the migration of neurons, and particularly the development of dendritic processes and the formation of synapses, are dictated largely by the functional needs of the host. Whether plasticity serves a purposeful need in the adult human nervous system, as a reaction to tissue injury or as a response to a neurologic deficit, however, remains beyond current knowledge.

It has been demonstrated that neural tissue can be grafted into an alien nervous system. However, again the capabilities of these cells to perform useful repair of neurologic deficits remains uncertain. In this regard, it must be noted that the "grafting" of embryonic or adult cells selected because of their capability to elaborate substrate, such as dopamine, merely supplies this substrate regionally to metabolically compromised cells. As is true with exogenously administered L-dopa, this substrate temporarily restores a de-gree of functionality to the substantia nigra but does not correct the progres-sive metabolic defect. In time, this intraneuronal metabolic disorder is re-sponsible for neuronal cell death. At this point substitution therapy ceases.

One returns to the question of what then is unique about the human nervous system that "enables" it to acquire a capability for cognition. One can note quantitative differences in the relative mass of the neocortex in humans versus that of lower animals, but these quantitative variables are minor when compared to the grandeur of intellectual function in humans versus its absence (or at least near absence) in lower animals. One is obliged, however, to admit that our own intellectual capacities do not provide us with meaning-ful insight into the origin or the modus operandi of cognition. Being required to acknowledge this major deficit in knowledge, we must still presume to ask, Why does age, or the passage of time, quantitatively modify the cognitive capacities of the human nervous system?

Pathology of Organic Mental Disorders

The concept of aging has been inseparably allied with that of dementia. Thus, the inescapable passage of calendar years has encouraged an acceptance of an age-related cognitive decline. In this context, dementia has been viewed as an unavoidable corollary of "old age." For example, in 1906, Alois Alzheimer described the occurrence of neuritic plaques, excessive intraneuronal fila-ments, and granulovacuolar degeneration in the severely atrophic brain of a 51-year-old woman whose illness was dominated by dementia. Although identical morphologic alterations had been previously observed, generally in lesser degrees, in aged individuals, Alzheimer insisted that this disorder was distinctive because of its relationship to an early decade of life. The entity was termed "presenile dementia" to distinguish it from a disorder that occurred with identical morphology after the age of 65, a disease referred to as "senile dementia." Unfortunately, the rarity of postmortem examinations on patients from mental institutions delayed the realization that the formations of neuritic plaques, neurofibrillary tangles, and granulovacuolar degeneration are mor-phologic expressions of a specific disease process, irrespective of age. For this reason, the terms "presenile" and "senile dementia" have been set aside for the unified designation, "Alzheimer's disease." Clearly, disease states (notably, Alzheimer's disease, cerebrovascular disease, and Pick's disease) occur with increased incidence in the human nervous system with advanced chronologic age. For this reason it is important to examine these entities by seeking ancillary information to the question, Do anatomic and functional alterations occur in the brain as a result of age alone?

A list of known causations of dementia would also include Creutzfeldt-Jakob's disease, as well as Alzheimer's disease, Pick's disease, and cerebrovas-cular disease. However, the transmissibility of Creutzfeldt-Jakob's disease to laboratory animals and also its unfortunate transmission from human to human by corneal transplantation, by pituitary extracts, and by contaminated surgical instruments, clearly characterizes it as an infectious process. This characterization removes Creutzfeldt-Jakob's disease from the "degenerative" or "aging" category and thus from our present consideration.

Alzheimer's Disease

Neurons and neuritic processes are lost during the course of Alzheimer's disease. Gyri narrow, sulci widen, and cortical atrophy becomes apparent both by computerized tomography and at postmortem examination. The atrophic brain of Alzheimer's disease is generally diminished in weight by approximately 200 g. Importantly, however, the histologic features of Alz-heimer's disease can be present in a nervous system unaltered in weight or gross appearance. When atrophy is present, and it usually is, typically it is bilateral and symmetrical and its distribution is predominately frontal and temporal. The degree of atrophy in the parietal–occipital lobes is regularly minimal. The cerebellum is uninvolved and this importantly distinguishes Alzheimer's disease from Creutzfeldt-Jakob's disease. The meninges are not thickened. This feature separates Alzheimer's disease from general paresis or dementia paralytica, with which it shares the characteristics of bilaterality and the frontal symmetry of the atrophy (Figure 1).

Three morphologic alterations serve to individualize Alzheimer's disease: neuritic plaque formation, neurofibrillary degeneration, and granulovacuolar alteration. In view of the chronicity of the disease process, it is remarkable that astrocytes remain so quiescent through the entire course of this prolonged disease process. The minimal extent of astrogliosis contrasts Alzheimer's disease with Pick's disease and Creutzfeldt-Jakob's disease, where astrocytic proliferation adds firmness to the cortical tissues and provides a diagnostic index during histologic examination. Notwithstanding the occasional coexistence of congophilic angiopathy, the cerebral blood vessels ostensibly respond neither in structure nor in patency to the presence of Alzheimer's disease. Interestingly, there is no quantitative variance in the formation of senile plaques or neurofibrillary tangles at the margin of a cortical infarct that might incidentally be present in the cerebrum of a patient with Alzheimer's disease.

Among the cardinal lesions of Alzheimer's disease are the neuritic or Alzheimer plaque, the neurofibrillary tangle, and granulovacuolar degeneration. The latter two are intraneuronal processes, whereas the neuritic plaque is a focal, roughly spheroid area of transformation in the neuropil. Although the two processes, senile plaque formation and the creation of neurofibrillary tangles, are individual and totally distinct in morphology, they conform closely in their geographic distributions. Generally, both predominate in the frontal and temporal cortices and are particularly prominent in the hippocampus. Neurofibrillary degeneration per se is not restricted to Alzheimer's disease but may be observed, for example, in the pigmented neurons of the substantia nigra in postencephalitic parkinsonism.

The senile or neuritic plaque is a focal, rather discrete area of abnormality, globoid in shape, several hundred microns in diameter, and regularly situated in the gray matter. Magnification by electron microscopy discloses the initial alteration to be characterized by segmental enlargement, or aneurysmal dilatation, of each neuritic process that traverses the domain of the plaque. These segmentally enlarged, sausage-shaped neuritites become engorged with degenerated mitochondria and lysosomes, presumably because of stagnation of axoplasmic flow. The globoid lesion curiously remains individual. It attains, and retains, uniformity in size without further enlargement. It may cluster with other plaques, but avoids coalescing. The early lesions have faint argentophilia and thus appear as fine delicate areas of argentophilic, filamentous material. As the senile plaque ages, it acquires density. This composition results from a deposition of native compounds such as acid

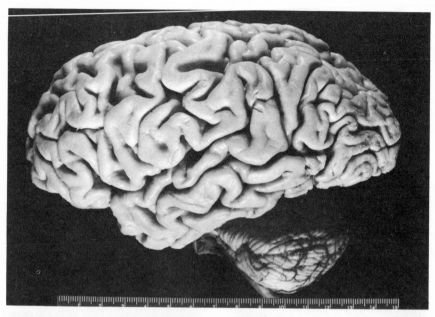

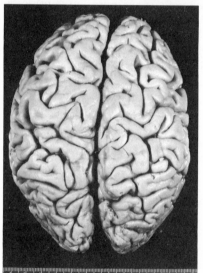
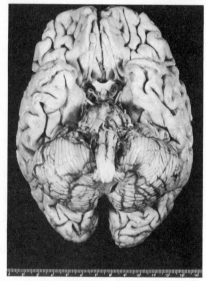

Figure 1. Alzheimer's disease. The brain of a 72-year-old man with a 5-year history of dementia weighed 1,225 g. There is moderate cortical atrophy most marked in the frontal and temporal lobes.

mucopolysaccharides and glycoproteins and, importantly, from the addition of alien substances, notably amyloid. As a result of these accumulations, plaques become stainable by a variety of agents such as Congo red and Alcian blue, among others (Figures 2 and 3).

The senile plaque, in its architectural creation, is totally alien to the cellular and molecular composition of the brain. But this is not the case with neurofibrillary tangle formation, an entity that borrows its structural blueprint, as well as its molecular composition, from the 10-nm neurofilaments that are normally present within neurons and that are sparsely distributed in the perikaryon and axon, for the purpose of propelling axoplasmic flow. The filaments that constitute the fibrillary tangle deviate significantly from normal, both in number and also in their paired, intertwined, helical structure. There remains a degree of order, however, since each individual filament retains an approximate diameter of 10 nm; moreover, the circumferential twist of the two filaments occurs at predictable intervals of 80 nm. Unfortunately, there is a void of knowledge concerning the nature of the stimulus and the molecular events that initiate and conduct the excessive production of neurofilaments and also cause them to wed into helical formations. Although the nature of this stimulus is obscured, the stimulus itself is not seemingly restricted to

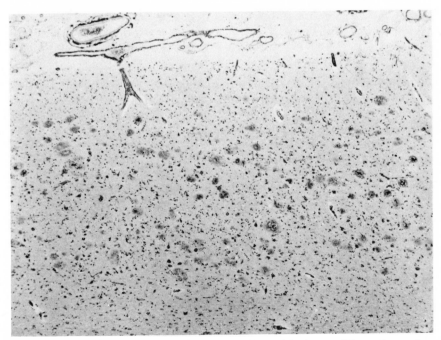

Figure 2. Alzheimer's disease. The entorhinal cortex of the brain of Figure 1 contains numerous neuritic plaques. King stain, 52 ×.

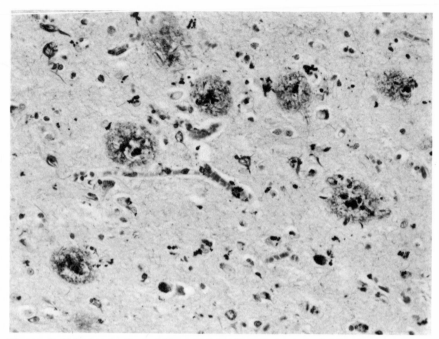

Figure 3. Alzheimer's disease. The neuritic plaques are remarkably discrete, spherical, and of uniform size. Their dense core is amyloid. King stain, 250 ×.

Alzheimer's disease. As has been mentioned, neurofibrillary tangles develop in the pigmented neurons of the substantia nigra in postencephalitic parkinsonism as well as in the Guam-Parkinsonian complex and in the cerebral neurons of pugilists. The helical configuration is unique to the neurons of the human central nervous system and is not a borrowed characteristic from lower members of the phylogenetic scale. Neurons of elderly monkeys and dogs accumulate excessive filaments, but these threads do not become paired or helical in configuration. The phenomenon of helical formation is not necessarily related to overproduction. In progressive supranuclear palsy (Steele-Richardson-Olszewski syndrome) the intraneuronal filaments attain quantitative excess without helical formation. Neurons altered by neurofibrillary degeneration are generally numerous in the entorhinal cortex, among the pyramidal cells of the hippocampus, and in those of the amygdala. They are also encountered without difficulty in the cortex of the frontal and temporal lobes and are generally less numerous in the parietal and occipital areas, with only an occasional example in the brainstem. It is of interest that the neurons that normally accumulate lipofuscin pigment are not prone to develop neurofibrillary tangle formation, even though lipofuscin, termed "wear and tear pigment," is viewed as an expression of "aging." It is also of interest that neurons involved by granulovacuolar degeneration, generally the pyramidal cells of the hippocampus, eschew neurofibrillary degeneration although contiguous neurons may be severely altered by the accumulation of neurofilaments (Figures 4 and 5).

Granulovacuolar degeneration is the least conspicuous member of the triad of lesions in Alzheimer's disease. Involved neurons portray a fine vacuolization of the cytoplasm and each vacuole harbors one or several hyperchromatic granules. The significance of granulovacuolar degeneration is not understood, but it is individual to Alzheimer's disease, and it is not coexistent in the same neuron with the formation of lipofuscin pigment or neurofibrillary degeneration.

There are many hypotheses concerning the pathogenesis of Alzheimer's disease. However, the validity of all remains questionable since none serves to unify the cardinal morphologic expressions of this disordered biologic state. One hypothesis incriminates aluminum as a toxic causation of Alzheimer's disease. The demonstrated tissue levels of aluminum, however, are quantitatively low and elevations are inconsistent. This raises the issue of causation versus a secondary chelating epiphenomenon. Another theory creates an

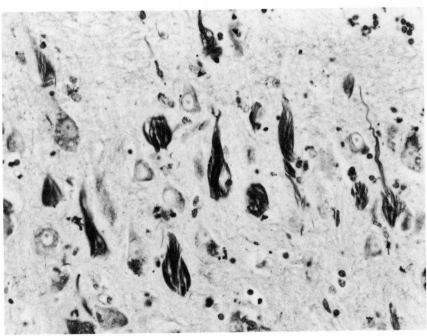

Figure 4. Alzheimer's disease. The pyramidal cell layer (H_2) of the hippocampal cortex of the brain of Figure 1 shows numerous neurons with advanced neurofibrillary degeneration. King stain, 325 ×.

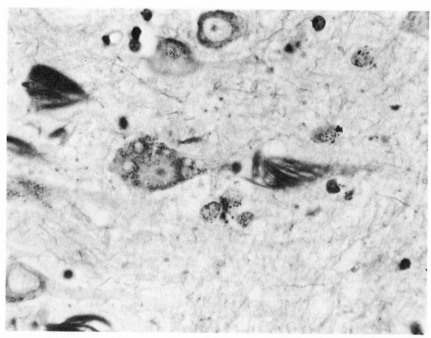

Figure 5. Alzheimer's disease. Neurofibrillary degeneration eschews neurons with granulovacuolar degeneration. King stain, 680 ×.

analogy with parkinsonism wherein Meynert's nucleus serves as the counterpart of the substantia nigra while the purported deficiency of transmitter substance relates to cholinergic compounds rather than those of the dopaminergic system. This theory relies on biochemical determinations performed on tissues altered by a chronic disease state; therein, primary events are obscured by a multiplicity of biochemical epiphenomena. The role of amyloid deposition, as a consequential or coincidental event, keeps open speculation about its possible role in the pathogenesis of Alzheimer's disease. The potential contributions of genes are also under active investigation, but clearly the role of genetics, at worst, is predispositional and should not be exaggerated to imply Mendelian relationships.

Pick's Disease

Classically, Pick's disease, or "lobar sclerosis," features atrophy of a single lobe, notably the frontal or temporal area, wherein the atrophy may attain extreme proportions. An occasional case of Pick's disease is more generalized and may be bilateral and symmetrical. Histologically, the involved cortex is markedly depleted of neurons and their absence is accentuated by marked

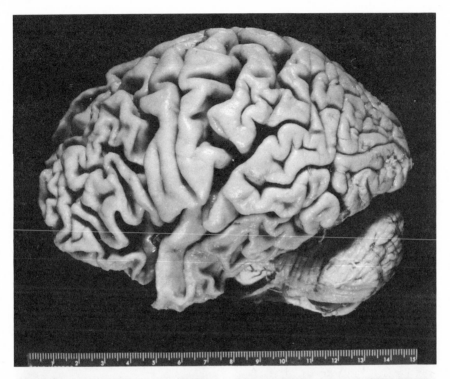

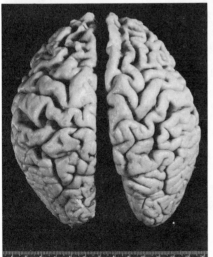
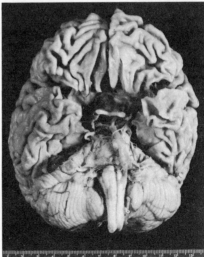

Figure 6. Pick's disease. The brain of a 73-year-old man, institutionalized for dementia of approximately 5 years' duration, weighed 1,075 g. There is severe cortical atrophy in the frontal and temporal lobes.

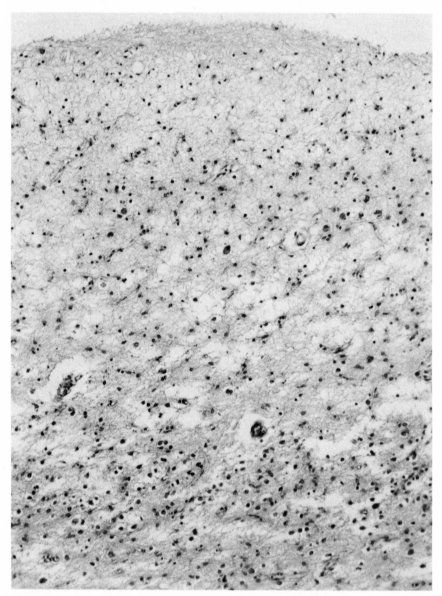

Figure 7. Pick's disease. The entorhinal cortex is almost totally depopulated of neurons and shows marked fibrillary astrogliosis. Luxol fast blue, 100 ×.

astrogliosis. The hallmark of this disease is evidenced in the residual neurons many of which are "ballooned" and within some of which there are one or several faint eosinophilic and argentophilic inclusions, termed "Pick's bodies." Pick's bodies are formed of densely aggregated neurofilaments (Figures 6, 7, and 8).

Thus, the excessive production of neurofilaments characterizes many disease states, notably the following: Pick's disease, by the formation of Pick's bodies; Alzheimer's disease, with the expression of neurofibrillary degeneration; parkinsonism, by the formation of Lewy bodies; and progressive supranuclear palsy. Is the excessive production of neurofilaments a manifestation of age? One would think not and would rather attribute excessive production of neurofilaments to a specific metabolic disturbance rather than a universal event of aging. Even the brain of a centenarian does not always reflect quantitative alterations in neurofibrillary production, and when present, as in Alzheimer's disease or Pick's diesase, the alterations are typically restricted to selected regions or nuclear systems. In summary, both Pick's disease and Alzheimer's disease are more reasonably termed "disease states," rather than aging phenomena.

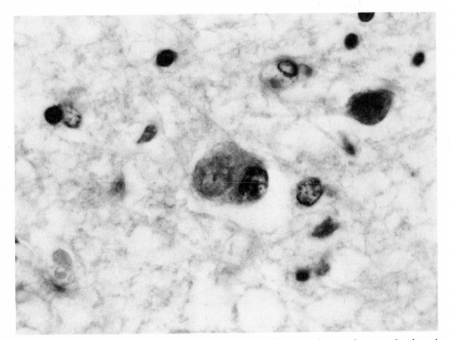

Figure 8. Pick's disease. A residual neuron is ballooned; the nucleus is displaced eccentrically and the cytoplasm contains a Pick body. Luxol fast blue, 1000×.

Multi-infarct Dementia

The stenosis or occlusion of small vessels leads to small infarcts. These are termed "lacunae." The clinical state may be evidenced as dementia; the entity is then referred to as "multi-infarct dementia." Approximately 15 percent of individuals institutionalized because of severe dementia will be found at postmortem examination to have a multiplicity of small cerebral infarcts. These infarcts individually measure less than 1 cm across and although random, are usually most numerous in the basal ganglia, thalamus, and the corona radiata. A loss of cognition generally denotes a global insult to cerebral function. In the situation of multi-infarct dementia, the impairment in integrated neuronal activity denotes interference in the associated pathways in the white matter. The term "Binswanger's disease" has been applied to the morphologic constellation of cerebral arteriosclerosis, multiple microinfarcts, and a diffuse pallor of myelin (Figure 9).

The Brain and Time

The focus is now on that nebulous entity, the aged brain untouched by disease. It is self-evident that with the passage of time, the accumulation of intraneuronal metabolic errors diminishes the ability of neurons to function and, at some interval thereafter, to survive. These events pertain to each nerve cell individually for each is a structural unit of the brain and each is incapable of replication. As evidenced by the rate of neuronal depopulation, the end point of lethal metabolic errors is attained at an earlier chronologic age in cortical neurons than in those of the brainstem or spinal cord.

It is also clear that the biologic or metabolic requirements of individual neurons are further challenged by exogenous toxins and systemic events. For example, unquestionably, the depopulation of neurons is accelerated by impaired vascular integrity, wherein substrates such as oxygen and glucose are diminished and cellular toxic waste materials, such as lactic acid, tend to accumulate. The human being exists in an adverse ecology in which neurons are responsive to exogenous as well as endogenous insults.

The pathogenesis of aging has been thus conceptualized as an exhaustion or depletion of intracellular metabolism occurring insidiously over many years. It is clear that this is a manifestation of the imperfections that characterize all biologic systems. We accept the loss of motor strength that accompanies age, the decrement of visual acuity, and the diminished auditory perception —why do we then question the impairment of cognition that relates to time and not to disease?

The very essence of cognition necessitates stability of structure, but biologic systems, whether they are bacteria, amoebae, or hepatic cells, perpetuate biologic activity only through a capacity for replication. Thus, stability

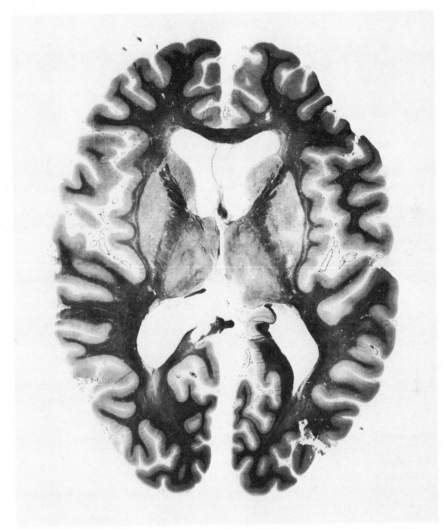

Figure 9. Multi-infarct dementia. A whole mount of a horizontal section shows rarefaction and multiple lacunae, particularly in the right basal ganglia and thalamus. Luxol fast blue.

and longevity are incongruous attributors. Cognition cannot be otherwise than transient in the presence of time. Theologians would suggest that freedom from time is an essence individual to Divinity.

Suggested Readings

Burger PC, Vogel FS: The development of the pathologic changes of Alzheimer's disease and senile dementia in patients with Down's syndrome. Am J Pathol 1973; 73:457–476

Coyle JT, Price DL, Des Long MR: Alzheimer's disease: a disorder of cortical cholinergic innervation. Science 1983; 219:1184–1190

Crapper DR, Krishman SS, Quitkat S: Aluminum neurofibrillary degeneration and Alzheimer's disease. Brain 1976; 99:67–80

Crapper DR, Quitkat S, Krishman SS, et al: Intranuclear aluminum content in Alzheimer's disease, dialysis encephalopathy and experimental aluminum encephalopathy. Acta Neuropathol 1980; 50:19–24

Davies P, Maloney AJR: Selective loss of central cholinergic neurons in Alzheimer's disease. Lancet 1976; 2:1403

Gibson PH: Relationship between numbers of cortical argentophilic and congophilic senile plaques in the brain of elderly people with and without senile dementia of Alzheimer type. Gerontology 1985; 31:321–324

Hooper MW, Vogel FS: The limibic system in Alzheimer's disease. A neuropathologic investigation. Am J Pathol 1975; 85:1–13

Johnston MV, McKinney M, Coyle JT: Evidence for a cholinergic projection to neocortex from neurons in basal forebrain. Proc Natl Acad Sci USA 1979; 76:5392–5396

Khachaturian ZS: Diagnosis of Alzheimer's disease. Arch Neurol 1985; 42:1097–1105

Lloyd B, Brinn N, Burger PC: Silver staining of senile plaques and neurofibrillary change in paraffin-embedded tissues. Journal of Histotechnology 1985; 8:155–156

Munoz-Garcia D, Ludwin SK: Classic and generalized varients of Pick's disease: a clinicopathological, ultrastructural, and immunocytochemical comparative study. Ann Neurol 1984; 16:467–480

Perl DP, Brody AR: Alzheimer's disease: x-ray spectrometric evidence of aluminum accumulation in neurofibrillary tangle-bearing neurons. Science 1980; 208:207

Rogers JD, Brogan D, Mirra SS: The nucleus basalis of Meynert in neurological disease: a quantitative morphological study. Ann Neurol 1985; 17:163–170

Tellez-Nagel I, Wisniewski HM: Ultrastructure of neurofibrillary tangles in Steele-Rchardson-Olszewski syndrome. Arch Neurol 1973; 29:324–327

Terry RD, Peck A, De Teresa R, et al: Some morphometric aspects of the brain in senile dementia of the Alzheimer type. Ann Neurol 1981; 10:184–192

Tomlinson BE, Blessed G, Roth M: Observations on the brains of non-demented old people. J Neurol Sci 1968; 7:331–356

Tomlinson BE, Blessed G, Roth M: Observations on the brains of demented old people. J. Neurol Sci 1970; 11:205–242

Wisniewski K, Jervis GA, Moretz, et al: Alzheimer neurofibrillary tangles in diseases other than senile and presenile dementia. Ann Neurol 1979; 5:288–294

Woodard JS: Clinicopathologic significance of granulovacuolar degeneration in Alzheimer's disease. J Neuropathol Exp Neurol 1962; 21:85–91

Chapter 5

Chemical Messengers of the Brain

Charles B. Nemeroff, M.D., Ph.D.

In the latter part of the 19th century and the beginning of the 20th century, a major controversy occurred in the burgeoning new science of neurobiology. The opposing views in this controversy, which concerned the neuroanatomical basis for communication in the brain, were each championed by a giant in neuroanatomy. Golgi, an Italian neuroanatomist, emphatically believed that nerve cells were connected to each other, forming a nerve net throughout the central nervous system (CNS). In contrast, Ramon y Cajal, the Spanish neuroanatomist, using silver impregnation techniques as well as other methods, concluded that there were gaps (synapses) between adjacent nerve cells. We now know that except for a few well-documented examples in invertebrates, neurons in the mammalian CNS are in fact separated by these synapses and, moreover, that chemical messengers, termed "neurotransmitters" are released from the nerve terminal of one neuron and diffuse in the extracellular fluid across the synapse to act on receptors on adjacent dendrites and cell bodies of neighboring neurons. The chemical nature, biosynthesis, regulation, and mechanism of action of the best studied mammalian CNS neurotransmitters are the subjects of this chapter. In the past 50 years, many neurotransmitters have been identified; below, the criteria for identification of a neurotransmitter are described (Cooper et al. 1986). A discussion of the monoamine, amino acid, and peptide neurotransmitters is then provided. At the end of the chapter, the important roles of particular neurotransmitters in the physiologic changes associated with normal aging and in pathologic states of the aged are briefly described.

This research was supported by National Institute of Mental Health grants MH–39415, MH–42088, MH–40524, and MH–40159 and National Institute of Aging grant AG–05128.

In the peripheral nervous system, it is possible to demonstrate release of a putative neurotransmitter from nerve endings when their nerve fibers are selectively stimulated. This is virtually impossible to demonstrate in the CNS. For this reason, *localization* to presynaptic nerve endings is often substituted as a requisite criterion. This is accomplished by demonstration of a heterogeneous distribution of the putative neurotransmitter in the CNS and by immunocytochemical visualization of the neurotransmitter in nerve terminals, using light and/or electron microscopy and quantitative measurement of the substance in different brain areas by one or another analytic method. Sometimes biochemical measurement and histochemical identification of biosynthetic enzymes responsible for synthesis of the putative neurotransmitter are technically more easily accomplished than directly measuring the candidate transmitter itself. After localization and release, a third criterion that must be fulfilled is synaptic mimicry; that is, exogenous administration of the chemical messenger must mimic the action of the transmitter released by nerve stimulation. This is best accomplished in the CNS by microiontophoretic or pressure ejection of the substance from micropipettes with concomitant electrophysiologic measurements of neuronal activity. A fourth criterion for identification of a novel neurotransmitter is that drugs that augment or antagonize the effects of the released neurotransmitter must exert predictable effects on the action of the administered neurotransmitter. Although certain differences among neurotransmitters exist, the scheme in Figure 1 depicts in general the steps involved in neurotransmission in the mammalian CNS.

Once released, neurotransmitters diffuse across the synaptic cleft where they bind to specific postsynaptic receptor sites, now known to be macromolecular complexes (Figure 2). Neurotransmitter binding sites must exhibit saturability, specificity, reversibility, and biologic activity after reconstitution, to be considered true receptors (Campbell 1984). In many cases, the neurotransmitter receptor is linked to an effector that amplifies the signal by a second messenger system such as cyclic adenosine monophosphate formation or phosphoinositide hydrolysis (Fisher and Agranoff 1987).

Norepinephrine (Noradrenaline)

The norepinephrine-containing neurons are found in the pontine and medullary reticular formation. They typically contain widespread dendritic arborizations and project over long distances to large areas of the brain with extensive collaterals both in ascending projections to the neocortex and hippocampus and in descending brainstem and spinal cord projections. The norepinephrine-containing cell groups in human brain, identified by histofluorescent methods (Dahlstrom and Fuxe 1964; Fuxe 1965), have been termed A_1–A_7 and are shown in Figure 3 (Watson et al. 1986). The A_6 norepinephrine cell group localized in the locus ceruleus, an area of the dorsal pons adjacent to the fourth ventricle, has received considerable attention. This cell

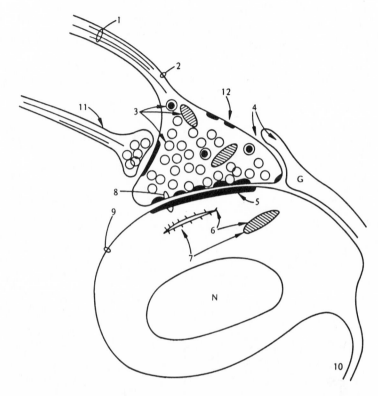

Figure 1. Twelve steps in the synaptic transmission process in an idealized synaptic connection. 1. Transport down the axon. 2. Electrically excitable membrane of the axon. 3. The organelles and enzymes present in the nerve terminal for synthesizing, storing, and releasing the transmitter, as well as for the process of active reuptake. 4. Enzymes present in the extracellular space and within the glia for catabolizing excess transmitter release from nerve terminals. 5. The postsynaptic receptor that triggers the response of the postsynaptic cell to the transmitter. 6. The organelles within the postsynaptic cells that respond to the receptor trigger. 7. Interaction between genetic expression of the postsynaptic nerve cell and its influences on the cytoplasmic organelles that respond to transmitter action. 8. The possible "plastic" steps modifiable by events at the specialized synaptic contact zone. 9. The electrical portion of the nerve cell membrane that, in response to the various transmitters, is able to integrate the postsynaptic potentials and produce an action potential. 10. Continuation of the information transmission by which the postsynaptic cells send an action potential down its axon. 11. Release of transmitter, subjected to modification by a presynaptic (axoaxonic) synapse; in some cases an analogous control can be achieved between dendritic elements. 12. Release of the transmitter from a nerve terminal or secreting dendritic site may be further subject to modulation through autoreceptors that respond to the transmitter that the same secreting structure has released. (Reproduced with permission from Cooper JR, Bloom FE, Roth RH: The Biochemical Basis of Neuropharmacology (fifth edition). New York, Oxford University Press, 1986.)

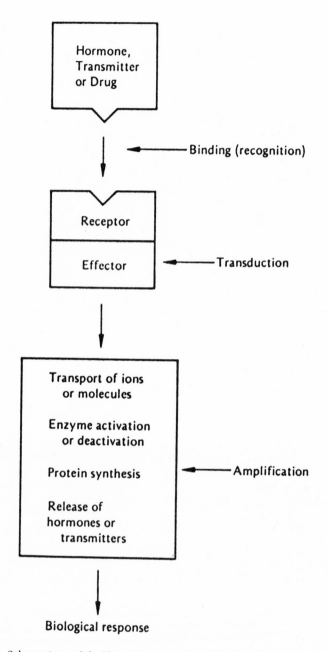

Figure 2. Schematic model of ligand–receptor interaction. (Reproduced with permission from Cooper JR, Bloom FE, Roth RH: The Biochemical Basis of Neuropharmacology. New York, Oxford University Press, 1986.)

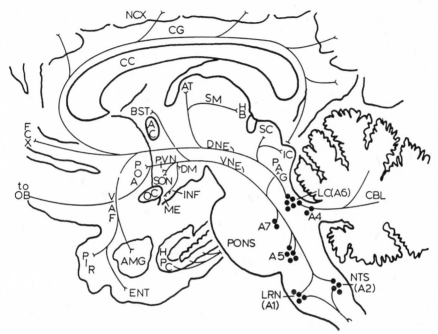

Figure 3. Noradrenergic systems. This schematized parasagittal view of a primate brain shows the location of major norepinephrine-producing cell bodies (solid circles) and their major projections. These cell groups have been designated A_1 to A_7 by Dahlstrom and Fuxe. (Reproduced with permission from Nieuwenhuys R, Voogd J, van Huijzen C: The Human Central Nervous System. New York, Springer-Verlag, 1981.)

group is the source of a dense norepinephrine projection to the hypothalamus, hippocampus, amygdala, and cerebral cortex. Abnormalities in noradrenergic neurotransmission have been postulated to occur in affective disorders, anxiety states, and even schizophrenia (Lake and Ziegler 1985).

The biosynthetic pathways of the major catecholamine neurotransmitters, norepinephrine, dopamine, and epinephrine have been elucidated and their synthesis from the amino acid tyrosine is illustrated in Figure 4. The vast majority of norepinephrine is synthesized within the nerve terminals; a small percentage of the total norepinephrine formed is synthesized within the perikaryon. The rate-limiting step in catecholamine synthesis is the conversion of tyrosine to 3, 4-dihydroxyphenylalanine (DOPA), a reaction catalyzed by tyrosine hydroxylase (TH). This enzyme is a unique constituent of catecholamine neurons, and antisera to TH can be used to visualize catecholamine neurons by immunohistochemistry. Different biochemical methods have now been used in laboratory animals to measure norepinephrine turnover. Turnover is defined as the overall rate at which the amine store is

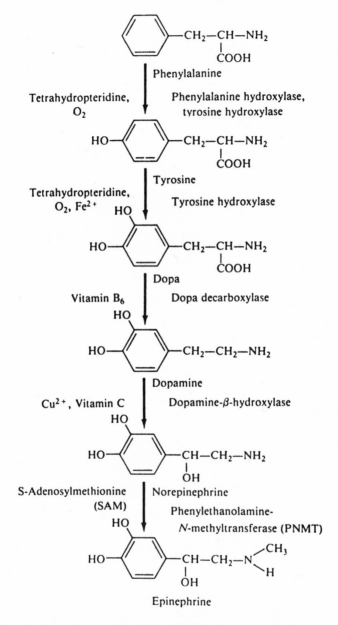

Figure 4. Synthesis of the catecholamine transmitters. The synthesizing enzymes are shown to the right of the arrows; the cofactors and the methyl donor (SAM) are shown on the left. (Reproduced with permission from Reinis S, Goldman JM: The Chemistry of Behavior. New York, Plenum Press, 1982.)

replaced in a given tissue, and it is thought to closely reflect the functional activity of the catecholamine neuron (Cooper et al. 1986). Turnover rates are affected by synthesis, release, and degradation rates. Newly synthesized catecholamines are preferentially released. After release, inactivation of norepinephrine occurs by reuptake into the presynaptic terminal. Within the nerve terminal norepinephrine is degraded by monoamine oxidase; extracellularly, another enzyme, catechol-o-methyltransferase, degrades norepinephrine, though under physiologic conditions this enzymatic inactivation is only a minor component of norepinephrine removal compared to reuptake. The catabolism of catecholamines is shown in Figure 5.

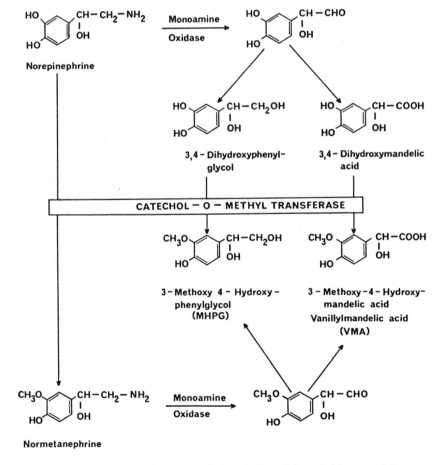

Figure 5. Catabolism of norepinephrine. (Adapted from Feldman and Quenzer [1984].)

As noted above, neurotransmitters such as norepinephrine act on post-synaptic receptors. Adrenergic receptors have been classified on the basis of the affinity of different neurotransmitters and drugs; norepinephrine acts on both α- and β-adrenergic receptors. These have now been subdivided—α_2 receptors are believed to be present on presynaptic norepinephrine terminals and regulate subsequent norepinephrine release. In contrast, α_1 and β receptors are located postsynaptic to norepinephrine terminals.

A variety of pharmacologic agents that act on CNS norepinephrine neurons are now available. These have been used in myriad studies to elucidate the physiologic roles of norepinephrine. Examples of such drugs include α-methyl-p-tyrosine, a TH inhibitor that depletes CNS catecholamines, and 6-hydroxydopamine (6OHDA), which destroys catecholamine neurons. Recently N-(2-chloroethyl)-N-ethyl-2-biomobenzylamine (DSP4) has been used to deplete norepinephrine without altering dopamine availability. It may, however, affect other neurotransmitter systems. Although none of these agents are totally specific in their actions, several different pharmacologic agents have been used to ascertain the role of norepinephrine in physiology and behavior; norepinephrine-containing circuits appear to be involved in learning and memory (Arnsten and Goldman-Rakic 1985), nociception (Kuraishi et al. 1987), sleep (Karacan and Moore 1985), thermoregulation (Milton 1977), and organisms' response to stress (Antelman and Chiodo 1984).

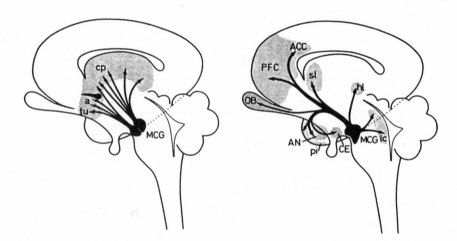

Figure 6.   Dopamine neurons and their pathways in the human brain. (Reproduced with permission from Lindvall O, Bjorklund A: Neuroanatomical localization of dopamine in the brain and spinal cord, in Handbook of Schizophrenia: Volume 2. Neurochemistry and Neuropharmacology of Schizophrenia. Edited by Henn FA, DeLisi LE. Amsterdam, Elsevier, 1987.)

Dopamine

Unlike norepinephrine, which is contained in brainstem neurons that project diffusely to widespread areas of the forebrain, dopamine-containing cells project to more discrete, topographically organized terminal areas. The dopamine neuronal cell groups (termed A_8–A_{15}) are located almost exclusively in the mesencephalon and diencephalon (Dahlstrom and Fuxe 1964). It is of interest that there are many more dopamine neurons in the mammalian brain than norepinephrine neurons; in fact, there are 15,000 to 20,000 dopamine cells per side in the midbrain (Cooper et al. 1986). The distribution and projections of the major dopamine neurons are illustrated in Figure 6. Little is known of the role of the dopaminergic amacrine cells in the retina or the periglomerular cells of the olfactory bulb. The tuberoinfundibular dopamine system with cells in the arcuate and periventricular nuclei of the hypothalamus that project to the median eminence is known to control prolactin secretion; it probably also modulates the secretion of other anterior pituitary hormones (Vance et al. 1987). Little is known about the function of the incertohypothalamic and medullary dopamine systems.

The best studied dopamine circuits are the nigroneostriatal (mesostriatal) system on the one hand, and the mesolimbic and mesocortical dopamine systems on the other (Lindvall and Bjorklund 1987; Wolf et al. 1987). The former arises from cells in the zona compacta of the substantia nigra (A_9) and projects to the neostriatum, including the caudate nucleus, putamen, and globus pallidus. In contrast, the mesolimbic and mesocortical dopamine systems arise in the ventral tegmental area of Tsai (A_{10}), adjacent to the A_9 cell group. The A_{10} cells project to the nucleus accumbens, olfactory tubercle, amygdala, septum, habenula, and locus ceruleus, and to the prefrontal, entorhinal, anterior cingulate, and other cortical areas (Lindvall and Bjorklund 1987). These two major dopamine projections have received considerable attention in psychiatry and neurology. The nigroneostriatal dopamine circuit is known to degenerate in Parkinson's disease. This knowledge formed the basis of L-dopa therapy (Birkemayer and Riederer 1983), the only clinically effective treatment for this disorder. Recently, compelling evidence has appeared indicating that the mesolimbicocortical dopamine system also degenerates in Parkinson's disease (Javoy-Agid and Agid 1980). When patients are administered antipsychotic drugs that block dopamine receptors, they frequently experience extrapyramidal side effects, such as acute dystonias and idiopathic parkinsonism, which are believed to be due to dopamine receptor blockade in the nigroneostriatal system.

The therapeutic effects of antipsychotic drugs are believed to be mediated by dopamine receptor blockade at receptors postsynaptic to mesolimbic and mesocortical dopamine nerve terminals. Compared with the nigroneostriatal dopamine system, relatively little is known about the physiology and pharmacology of the mesolimbicocortical dopamine system. The interested

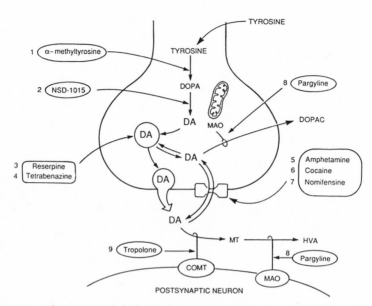

Figure 7. Schematic model of striatal dopaminergic nerve terminal. Drugs that alter dopamine (DA) life cycle include (1) α-methyltyrosine, competitive inhibitor of tyrosine hydroxylase; (2) NSD-1015, inhibitor of DOPA decarboxylase; (3) reserpine, which irreversibly damages DA uptake and storage mechanisms and produces long-lasting depletion of DA; (4) tetrabenazine, which also interferes with DA uptake and storage, but the effects are of shorter duration than reserpine and do not appear to be irreversible; (5) amphetamine, which increases synaptic DA through a number of mechanisms, including induction of release of DA and blockade of DA reuptake; (6) cocaine, which also blocks DA reuptake and induces DA release; (7) nomifensine, also a blocker of DA reuptake, but lacks DA-releasing ability; (8) pargyline, an inhibitor of monoamine oxidase (MAO); and (9) tropolone, an inhibitor of catechol-O-methyltransferase (COMT). HVA = homovanillic acid, 3-MT = 3-methoxytyramine. (Reproduced with permission from Wolf ME, Deutch AY, Roth RH: Pharmacology of central dopaminergic neurons in Handbook of Schizophrenia: Volume 2. Neurochemistry and Neuropharmacology of Schizophrenia. Edited by Henn FA, DeLisi LE. Amsterdam, Elsevier, 1987.)

reader can refer to a recent New York Academy of Sciences monograph on mesolimbic and mesocortical dopamine systems for further information (Kalivas and Nemeroff in press). As with the norepinephrine system, a number of drugs are known to interfere with or augment dopamine neuro-transmission. Their sites of action are schematically illustrated in Figure 7. Subtypes of postsynaptic dopamine receptors have been identified. Although as many as four subtypes have been postulated (D_1, D_2, D_3, and D_4) to exist, most investigators now recognize only two dopamine receptor subtypes, D_1 and D_2.

There is a very strong correlation between the potency of antipsychotic drugs to displace the binding of radiolabeled antipsychotic drugs such as ^{3}H-spiperone or ^{3}H-haloperidol to the D_2 receptor and clinical potency to control psychotic symptoms in neuroleptic-responsive schizophrenic patients (Figure 8). In contrast, blockade of the D_1 receptor inhibits dopamine-stimulated adenylate cyclase activity, and the ability of antipsychotics to block this is not correlated with clinical potency. Thus butyrophenones such as haloperidol are clinically efficacious but do not block dopamine-stimulated adenylate cyclase activity.

The use of drugs that enhance dopamine neurotransmission such as psychostimulants (d-amphetamine, cocaine, and methylphenidate) and drugs that block dopamine receptors such as haloperidol or pimozide, as well as neurotoxins such as 6OHDA, has allowed investigators to study the physiological role of dopamine in the CNS. There is evidence that dopamine neurons

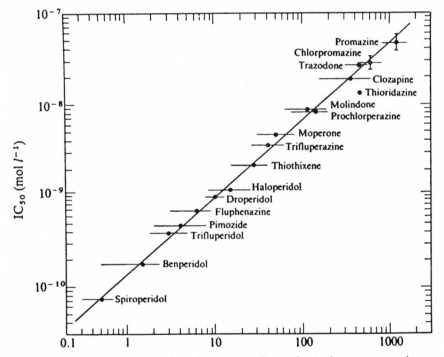

Figure 8. Comparison of the clinical potencies of neuroleptic drugs, measured as average daily dose in treating schizophrenia, with potencies of the same drugs in displacing [^{3}H] haloperidol from dopamine receptor binding sites in vitro (concentration of drug required to displace 50 percent of specific haloperidol binding). (Reproduced with permission from Seeman P, Lee T, Chau-Wong M, et al: Antipsychotic drug doses and neuroleptic/dopamine receptors. Nature 1976;261:717–719.)

serve important reward functions—that dopamine neuronal integrity is essential in order to experience the rewarding effects of food, certain drugs of abuse (opiates, cocaine), and electrical self-stimulation of the brain (Wise 1982). Others have suggested that the interference of reward induced by the disruption of dopamine circuits can be attributed to motor disturbances; that is, the animal is motivated to respond but cannot do so (Koob 1984). There is also evidence that dopamine systems are involved in thermoregulation (Baeyens and Moreno 1983), neuroendocrine homeostasis (Vance et al. 1987), and the pathogenesis of several neuropsychiatric disorders including schizophrenia, Huntington's chorea, and Parkinson's disease.

Epinephrine (Adrenaline)

Until recently it was virtually impossible to unequivocally demonstrate the presence of epinephrine in the CNS. This was because this catecholamine is present in considerably smaller quantities than dopamine and norepinephrine, and in addition, the enzyme that converts norepinephrine to epinephrine and is unique to epinephrine-containing neurons, phenylethanolamine-N-methyltransferase (PNMT), was difficult to assay. The use of sophisticated and sensitive analytic materials and immunocytochemistry with antisera to PNMT has led to the elucidation of two discrete groups of epinephrine-containing perikarya in the CNS: One group (C-1) is located in the lateral tegmentum of the caudal medulla, interspersed with norepinephrine cells. The second group (C-2) is in the dorsal medulla, also interspersed with norepinephrine cells. These two cell groups project to the spinal cord, locus ceruleus, periaqueductal gray, thalamus and hypothalamus, and nuclei of visceral efferent and afferent systems such as the dorsal motor nucleus of the vagus (Foote 1985; Cooper et al. 1986). The biosynthesis of epinephrine is illustrated in Figure 4. Virtually nothing is known of the physiologic role of epinephrine in the mammalian CNS.

Serotonin (5-Hydroxytryptamine)

Serotonin is an indoleamine that was one of the first neurotransmitters identified in the mammalian CNS. The localization of serotonin-containing neurons has been accomplished by the use of histochemical methods. The serotonergic cell groups have been termed B_1–B_9 and are contained within the midline raphe nuclei of the brainstem (Dahlstrom and Fuxe 1964). The more rostral raphe nuclei (e.g., median raphe cells in the midbrain) project to the diencephalon and telencephalon, while the medullary raphe cells send descending projections to the lower brainstem and spinal cord. The ascending serotonin projections are diffuse and widespread, resembling the ascending locus ceruleus noradrenergic projections. A schematic representation of the major serotonergic projections in the mammalian brain is presented in Figure 9.

The biosynthesis of serotonin is illustrated in Figure 10. Unlike catecholamine biosynthesis, in which the rate-limiting step is controlled by the enzyme tyrosine hydroxylase, serotonin biosynthesis is controlled by the availability of the amino acid tryptophan. This is because at normal plasma tryptophan concentrations, brain tryptophan hydroxylase is unsaturated. Thus, CNS concentrations of serotonin can be elevated by loading doses of L-tryptophan. Just as there are pharmacologic tools available to study CNS dopamine and norepinephrine systems, there are also drugs that selectively alter brain serotonin systems. An inhibitor of serotonin synthesis is p-chlorophenylalanine, which competes with tryptophan and binds irreversibly to tryptophan hydroxylase. The neurotoxin 5,7-dihydroxytryptamine, when injected directly into the CNS, selectively destroys serotonin neurons. Figure 11 depicts a nerve terminal with the sites of action of several drugs that affect serotonin neurons. Of particular interest to psychiatrists is the fact that many tricyclic antidepressants such as amitriptyline, chlorimipramine, and imipramine block the

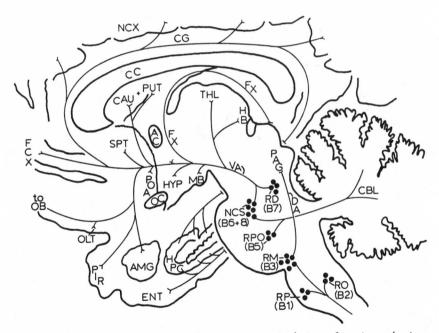

Figure 9. Serotonergic systems. Schematic parasagittal view of a primate brain depicting the serotonin cell groups (solid circles) and their major projections. These groups were designated B_1 to B_9 by Dahlstrom and Fuxe. (Reproduced with permission from Nieuwenhuys R, Voogd J, van Huijzen C: The Human Central Nervous System. New York, Springer-Verlag, 1981.)

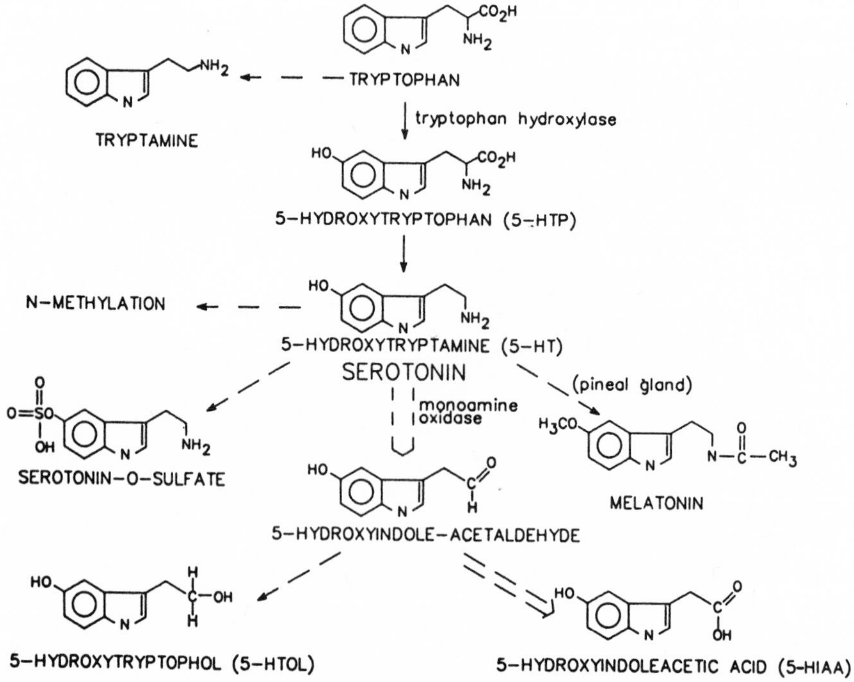

Figure 10. Serotonin metabolism in the central nervous system. (Reproduced with permission from Stahl SM, Wets K: Indoleamines and schizophrenia, in Handbook of Schizophrenia: Volume 2. Neurochemistry and Neuropharmacology of Schizophrenia. Edited by Henn FA, DeLisi L. Amsterdam, Elsevier, 1987.)

reuptake of serotonin into the presynaptic nerve terminal (Baldessarini 1985), which is the primary mode of inactivation of serotonin after its release.

Different serotonin receptor subtypes have been characterized in the mammalian CNS (Hamon et al. 1984); they have been termed $5HT_1$ and $5HT_2$. The $5HT_1$ subtype has now been subdivided into $5HT_{1A}$ and $5HT_{1B}$ subtypes. The serotonin autoreceptor is a $5HT_{1A}$ subtype.

The role of serotonin in the pathogenesis of psychiatric disorders has received considerable attention. Because methylated derivatives of serotonin such as dimethyltryptamine are hallucinogenic and psychotomimetics such as LSD are known to alter serotonergic neurotransmission, a role for serotonin in schizophrenia was postulated many years ago (Jacobs 1987). These data have recently been reviewed (Stahl and Wets 1987). Alterations in serotonin neurotransmission do not seem to be primarily responsible for the signs and symptoms of schizophrenia. In contrast, considerable evidence favors a role for serotonin systems in affective disorders. Measures of serotonin turnover and alterations in presynaptic serotonin nerve terminals have repeatedly been shown to be reduced in depression and suicide (Asberg et al. 1976; Stanley et al. 1982) and certain antidepressants such as fluoxetine, fluvoxamine, and chlorimipramine selectively block serotonin reuptake (Baldessarini 1985). Serotonin has also been postulated to play important roles in aggressive behavior (Brown et al. 1979), sexual behavior (Zemlan 1978), and the modulation of pituitary hormone secretion, particularly adrenocorticotropin (ACTH) (Frohman and Berelowitz 1984).

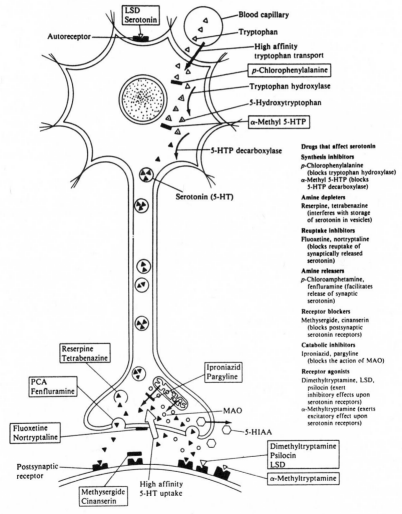

Figure 11. Serotonergic neurons with the sites of action of drugs. (Reproduced with permission from Reinis S, Goldman JM: The Chemistry of Behavior. New York, Plenum Press, 1982.)

Acetylcholine

Acetylcholine is the neurotransmitter contained within the parasympathetic fibers that innervate the heart that Otto Loewi used to unequivocally demonstrate the existence of chemical neurotransmission (Cooper et al. 1986). Elucidation of the neurobiology of cholinergic systems in the mammalian brain has been hampered by the difficulty in measuring acetylcholine, and in visualizing acetylcholine and choline acetyltransferase, the enzyme that synthesizes acetylcholine from acetyl CoA and choline. For these reasons localization of cholinergic pathways in the CNS depended, for many years, on immunohistochemical staining of acetylcholinesterase, the enzyme that degrades acetylcholine (Carson et al. 1978). Unfortunately acetylcholinesterase is contained within both cholinergic and noncholinergic neurons and is therefore not a specific marker. In recent years antisera to choline acetyltransferase have become available and CNS cholinergic circuits have been mapped (Jones and Beaudet 1987).

The distribution of cholinergic neurons and their major projections are shown in Figure 12. In brief, cholinergic neurons are found in the caudate nucleus and putamen as well as in the nucleus accumbens and olfactory tubercle. The caudate–putamen neurons project to the globus pallidus. A very large and important cholinergic cell group is found in the nucleus basalis of Meynert in a region adjacent to the anterior commissure and ventral to the globus pallidus. These cholinergic neurons include those in the substantia innominata, diagonal band of Broca, medial septal nucleus, preoptic area, and globus pallidus that project to the cerebral cortex and hippocampus. These neurons are now known to degenerate in Alzheimer's disease (Coyle et al. 1983). Another group of cholinergic neurons is contained in the pedunculopontine tegmental nucleus within the nucleus cuneiformis. These cells project largely to extrapyramidal structures such as the substantia nigra, subthalamic nucleus, striatum, and globus pallidus (Watson et al. 1986). Other cholinergic neurons include certain brainstem motor nuclei of the cranial nerves.

As briefly noted above, acetylcholine is synthesized by a reaction catalyzed by choline acetyltransferase in which acetyl CoA and choline yield acetylcholine and CoA (Cooper et al. 1986). The rate-limiting step in this reaction is the high affinity uptake of choline, which is blocked by hemicholinium-3. Like the catecholamines, newly synthesized acetylcholine is preferentially released from nerve terminals. Once released, acetylcholine is degraded by acetylcholinesterase.

Considerable information is now available on cholinergic receptors. There are two types—muscarinic and nicotinic. The former have been subdivided into M_1 and M_2 subtypes (Yamanaka et al. 1986). Until recently it was thought that the brain contained only muscarinic cholinergic receptors. It is, however, now evident that nicotinic receptors also exist in the CNS.

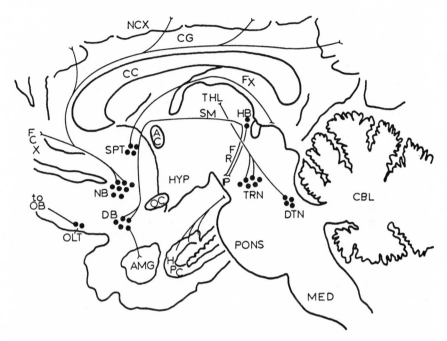

Figure 12. Cholinergic systems. Parasagittal view of a schematized primate brain showing the distribution of cholinergic cell bodies (filled circles) and their projections. Note that while some of these systems have also been confirmed in the human brain, most of our current knowledge of cholinergic systems stems from studies in the rodent brain. (Reproduced with permission from Watson SJ, Khachaturian H, Lewis ME, et al: Chemical neuroanatomy as a basis for biological psychiatry, in American Handbook of Psychiatry. Edited by Berger PA, Brodie HKH. New York, Basic Books, 1986.)

The role of acetylcholine in the CNS remains to be completely elucidated. However, it is likely that it is involved in the central control of neuroendocrine regulation (Frohman and Berelowitz 1984), sleep (Karacan and Moore 1985), and learning and memory (Bartus et al. 1982). Janowsky and Risch (1987) have provided evidence that depression is associated with cholinergic hyperactivity and mania with cholinergic hypoactivity. As noted above, cholinergic neurons in the nucleus basalis degenerate in Alzheimer's disease.

γ-*Aminobutyric Acid*

Considerable evidence has accumulated that supports the hypothesis that γ-aminobutyric acid (GABA) is an inhibitory neurotransmitter in the mammalian CNS (Cooper et al. 1986). It is distributed heterogeneously in the brain and is present in very high (micromolar) concentrations in certain areas including the substantia nigra, globus pallidus, and hypothalamus. γ-Amino-butyric acid containing neurons in the caudate and putamen project to the substantia nigra and globus pallidus. Like acetylcholine, GABA has been difficult to measure, and after death rapid increases in GABA concentration have been noted. The synthesis of GABA has been well characterized—it is formed from glutamate by the enzyme glutamic acid decarboxylase. Antisera to glutamic acid decarboxylase have been used to visualize GABA-containing neurons in the CNS (Figure 13). The catabolism of GABA has also been well characterized; it is degraded by GABA-transaminase to yield glutamate and succinic semialdehyde. After release, GABA acts on postsynaptic receptors resulting in alterations in chloride permeability and membrane hyperpolarization (Enna and Mohler 1987). There is, however, evidence for subtypes of GABA receptors. Moreover, there is considerable evidence that benzodiazepines and certain barbiturates modulate activation of GABA receptors. Many convulsants are GABA antagonists and many anticonvulsants, at least in part, act to facilitate GABA neurotransmission (Lloyd and Morselli 1987).

There is some evidence that GABA is involved in neuroendocrine homeostasis (McCann et al. 1984) and locomotor activity (Mitchell et al. 1985), as well as in the pathogenesis of Huntington's disease, epilepsy, tardive dyskinesia, and even schizophrenia (van Kammen et al. 1982).

Glutamate and Other Excitatory Amino Acids

The concentration of glutamate is higher than any other amino acid in the mammalian CNS. As noted by Engelsen (1986), glutamate and aspartate are considered CNS neurotransmitters on the basis of four salient findings: presynaptic localization in specific neurons, release by physiologic stimuli, identical action to the naturally occurring neurotransmitter, and mechanisms of inactivation. Both glutamate- and aspartate-containing neurons are widely distributed in the CNS and project diffusely throughout the brain. Both amino acids appear to be neurotransmitters in the hippocampus, glutamate in the perforant path, the lateral entorhinal input to the hippocampal molecular layer, and aspartate in the hippocampal input to the dentate gyrus (Watson et al. 1986). Cerebrocortical neurons also apparently use glutamate as a neurotransmitter. Three excitatory amino acid receptors have been identified in the mammalian CNS: N-methyl-D-aspartate, quisqualate, and kainate (Coyle 1987). Glutamate and/or aspartate have been postulated to play a role in epilepsy, cerebral ischemia, Parkinson's disease, and Huntington's disease (Engelsen 1986).

Histamine

Histamine is almost certainly a CNS neurotransmitter. It is found in both mast cells and neurons in the brain. It is formed from histidine by histidine

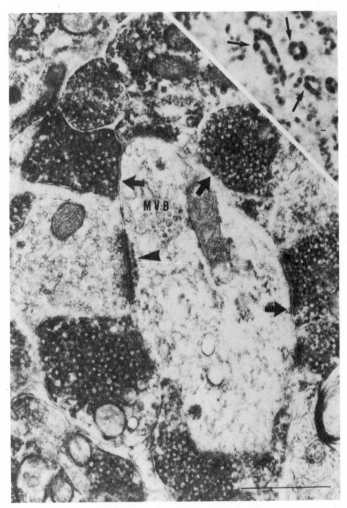

Figure 13. Terminals containing glutamic acid decarboxylase (GAD) in the substantia nigra from speciments incubated in anti-GAD serum. Insert: Semithin (1μm) section of the pars reticulata with obliquely and transversely sectioned dendrites that are encircled by punctate structures containing GAD-positive reaction product (→). Scale bar = 1 μm. The accompanying electron micrograph shows an obliquely sectioned dendrite in the substantia nigra that is surrounded by many axon teminals filled with GAD-positive reaction product that are equivalent to the puncta seen in the insert. Some of the terminals form symmetrical synapses (←), whereas the unstained terminal contains round synaptic vesicles and forms an asymmetrical synapse (◀) with this danditic shaft, multivesicular body (MVB). Scale bar: 1 μm. (Reproduced with permission from Ribak CE, Vaughn JE, Saito K, et al: Immunocytochemical localization of glutamate decarboxylase in rat substantia nigra. Brain Res 1977;116:287-298.)

decarboxylase. It is metabolized by histamine n-methyltransferase. Little is known about the distribution of histamine-containing neurons and histamine receptors in mammals (Cooper et al. 1986).

Neuropeptides

Assessment of the physiologic role and effects of an increasingly large number of peptides in the CNS has become a major focus of scrutiny for many neurobiologists in the last 10 to 15 years. More than 50 neuropeptides have thus far been isolated and sequenced (see Table 1). They range in size from dipeptides (two amino acids joined by a single peptide bond) to large molecules such as ACTH, which is comprised of 39 amino acids. Comprehensive reviews of the neuroanatomical distribution and neurochemical, neurophysiologic, neuropharmacologic, and behavioral effects of a variety of neuropeptides have appeared (Nemeroff and Bissette 1986; Iversen et al. 1983). These data are briefly reviewed with special attention to the literature concerning the human CNS. In particular, the neurobiology of neuropeptides is compared and contrasted with that of the previously described monoamine neurotransmitters.

With little exception, the pattern of peptide discovery has been as follows: First, a crude extract of brain is found to contain one or another biologic activity. This activity is then discovered to be due to the presence of a peptide, and the peptide is eventually purified and sequenced. In 1931, substance P (sub P) was discovered by von Euler and Gaddum, but 40 years passed before its chemical identity was elucidated. Some peptides were discovered in the 1950s, such as insulin, though their presence in the CNS was not recognized until approximately 20 years later. In the 1940s and 1950s, the work of a few pioneering investigators spawned the "new" multidisciplinary field of neuroendocrinology.

For approximately 20 years the greatest impetus for neuropeptide research was the discovery that the various endocrine axes are organized in a hierarchical fashion, with the CNS at the summit; the chemical regulators of adenohypophyseal hormone secretion are now known to be neuropeptides, the hypothalamic hypophysiotropic (release and release-inhibiting) factors. The chemotransmitter–portal vessel hypothesis, expounded by Harris (1955), posited the presence of neurohormones that are released from nerve terminals in the median eminence region of the hypothalamus and are transported from the primary capillary plexus to the anterior pituitary gland by the hypothalamo–hypophyseal venous portal system. Once transported to the anterior pituitary, these releasing factors bind to membrane receptors, which results in the release (or inhibition of release) of one or more pituitary trophic hormones. Millions of sheep and pig hypothalami were processed to eventually yield a few milligrams of the first hypothalamic-releasing hormones to be discovered (Vale and Rivier 1975). These included thyrotropin-

Table 1. Neuropeptides Identified in Mammalian Brain

Thyrotropin-releasing hormone	Cholecystokinin
Gonadotropin-releasing hormone	Secretin
Somatostatin	Gastrin-releasing peptide
Corticotropin-releasing factor	Calcitonin
Growth hormone-releasing factor	Anserine
Thyroid-stimulating hormone	Calcitonin gene-related peptide
Adrenocorticotropin	Carnosine
Luteinizing hormone	Insulin
Prolactin	Glucagon
Growth hormone	Neuromedin N
α-Endorphin	Neuropeptide Y
β-Endorphin	Vasoactive intestinal peptide
γ-Endorphin	Vasopressin
Met-Enkephalin	Oxytocin
Leu-Enkephalin	Vasotocin
Dynorphin	Delta-sleep-inducing peptide
Kytorphin	Melanocyte-stimulating hormone-release
α-Melanocyte-stimulating hormone	inhibiting factor
β-Melanocyte-stimulating hormone	Angiotensin
Neurotensin	Kallikrein
Substance P	Bradykinin
Bombesin	Inhibin
Gastrin	Gallanin
	Motilin

releasing hormone (TRH, a tripeptide), luteinizing-hormone-releasing hormone (LHRH, a decapeptide), and somatostatin (a tetradecapeptide).

These findings have not only resulted in major diagnostic and treatment breakthroughs in clinical endocrinology, but also have had considerable impact in psychiatry as well. It is now becoming more evident that particular psychiatric disorders are often associated with robust and reproducible neuroendocrine abnormalities (Nemeroff and Loosen 1987). Several distinct but related discoveries have led to one inexorable conclusion—that neuropeptides are important neuroregulators in the CNS; they function there as neurotransmitters or neuromodulators and, consequently, also modulate behavior. Moreover, some evidence is concordant with the view that alterations of specific neuropeptide-containing neurons occur in certain neuropsychiatric diseases, especially two common diseases of the elderly, Alzheimer's disease and Parkinson's disease.

Space constraints preclude a detailed discussion of the evidence that supports a neurotransmitter role for each of the neuropeptides (see Table 1) present in the mammalian CNS. As with the monoamines, controversy still exists as to whether these chemical messengers fulfill all of the requisite neurotransmitter criteria.

Neuropeptides are heterogeneously distributed in the CNS. The pattern of distribution of each peptide is relatively unique. Thus in humans and other mammals, neurotensin (NT) is found in high concentrations in the hypothalamus, amygdala, nucleus accumbens, and septum. In contrast, vasoactive intestinal peptide and cholecystokinin are present in high concentrations in the cerebral cortex, as well as in the hippocampus. Other neuropeptides, like LHRH or growth-hormone-releasing factor, have much more restricted patterns of distribution—they are found almost exclusively in the diencephalon.

Because it would be impossible to discuss each of the neuropeptides in detail in this chapter, a single one, NT, is presented as an example. It is hoped that this will serve to acquaint the reader with the experimental approaches used by different investigators to determine whether a candidate neuropeptide fulfills neurotransmitter criteria.

Neurotensin is a peptide composed of 13 amino acids that was discovered by Carraway and Leeman (1973) in extracts of bovine hypothalamus. It was characterized, purified, and finally sequenced by use of several bioassays. The crude extract produced hypotension, hyperglycemia, and vasodilation after intravenous injection in the rat and smooth muscle contraction in vitro. Once sequenced (pGlu-Leu-Tyr-Glu-Asn-Lys-Pro-Arg-Arg-Pro-Tyr-Ile-Leu-OH), the synthetic peptide was synthesized, and antisera were raised against it. Such antisera were subsequently used for both immunohistochemistry and radioimmunoassay experiments, and the results revealed a strikingly heterogeneous CNS distribution of NT.

High concentrations of NT were found in limbic (e.g., nucleus accumbens, amygdala, habenula, and septum) and hypothalamic regions (median eminence, paraventricular nucleus, and preoptic area), whereas low concentrations were found in the hippocampus, cerebral cortex, and cerebellum. Density-gradient centrifugation revealed that most NT is concentrated in the synaptosomal fraction, and further subcellular fractionation localized the peptide to synaptic vesicles. Immunohistochemical studies at the electron microscopic level have confirmed the presence of NT in vesicles contained within nerve terminals.

Neurotensin is released from brain slices by high concentrations of potassium, and this release is calcium dependent. Enzymes (peptidases) that degrade NT have been identified in the mammalian brain. The NT gene has recently been sequenced. Like other neuropeptides, such as the opioid peptides, insulin, and somatostatin, NT is contained within the sequence of a larger prohormone that is synthesized, like most proteins, by deoxyribonucleic acid transcription and subsequent translation. After the prohormone is formed, the active neuropeptide is thought to be liberated by the action of specific peptidase-cleaving enzymes. Once released from the presynaptic terminal, peptides act on specific high-affinity postsynaptic membrane receptors. Indeed, radiolabeled NT has been used in vitro to identify such membrane receptors in the human and rat brain.

Unlike the monoamines, neuropeptides, once released into the synaptic cleft, are inactivated primarily by enzymatic degradation and not by reuptake into the presynaptic terminal. Current knowledge about the transduction of the signal that occurs after neuropeptides bind to their membrane receptor(s) is also quite limited. However, changes in neuronal firing rates have repeatedly been observed after microiontophoretic application of neuropeptides such as NT. Finally, behavioral changes and modifications in response to centrally acting pharmacologic agents have been observed after intracerebroventricular or direct CNS administration of neuropeptides. These latter findings suggest that changes in the extracellular fluid concentration of neuropeptides can produce marked physiologic and pharmacobehavioral alterations.

It is of interest to compare the neurobiology of neuropeptides with that of better studied monoamines. These differences, highlighted by Hughes (1984), are summarized in Table 2. One major difference between these two

Table 2. Comparison of Aminergic and Peptidergic Systems

Amine	Neuropeptides
Biosynthesis Local synthesis in terminals via catabolic enzymes subject to feedback control.	Ribosomal synthesis of protein precursor and enzymatic cleavage to active products in nerve axon. Posttranslational peptide modification occurs (amidation, acetylation, sulfation).
Storage Large and small vesicles, often granulated; specific uptake and storage mechanisms in vesicles.	Large granular vesicles. Protein carriers.
Tissue concentrations vary from 1 to 100 nmol/g.	Tissue concentrations vary from 1 to 1,000 pmol/g.
Release Calcium-dependent exocytosis; quantal.	Calcium dependent.
Inactivation Reuptake into nerve terminal; ester hydrolysis, methylation, and deamination.	Aminopeptidases; endopeptidases; carboxypeptidases.

Source. Hughes J: Strategies for manipulating peptidergic transmission, in Alzheimer's Disease: Advances in Basic Research Therapies. Edited by Wurtman RJ, Corkin SH, Growden JH. Zurich, Proceedings of the Third Meeting of the International Study Group on Treatment of Memory Disorders Associated with Aging, 1984.

classes of neuroregulators is their mode of biosynthesis. As noted earlier, neuropeptides are synthesized by protein synthesis in ribosomes in the perikaryon (usually as a large prohormone) and, after packaging, are transported down the axon to the nerve terminal, where they are subsequently released in active form. In contrast, monoamines are synthesized largely in the nerve terminal region by a series of well-characterized enzymatic steps from an amino acid precursor. The mode of inactivation of these two classes of neuroregulators is also quite different; peptides are inactivated by enzymes (peptidases), whereas monoamines are removed from the synaptic cleft largely by transmitter reuptake into the presynaptic terminal. The physiologic consequences of monoamine release are brief, whereas the action of neuropeptides can be quite sustained.

It is indeed fascinating to consider the recent findings of Hokfelt et al. (1986) and others (Watson et al. 1986) that have convincingly demonstrated colocalization of neuropeptides and monoamines. The colocalization of sub P and serotonin in descending spinal pathways has been the most closely scrutinized example of colocalization. Recently compelling evidence for colocalization of cholecystokinin and dopamine has appeared.

In summary, a large number of neuropeptides are now known to be present in the mammalian CNS. Their unique anatomical localization and the concatenation of behavioral, electrophysiologic, and pharmacologic properties attributed to them make neuropeptides prime candidates for one of the classes of endogenous substances (endocoids) that modulate normal and abnormal behavior. Three types of evidence have been used to evaluate this hypothesis. First, studies in postmortem brain tissue and cerebrospinal fluid (CSF) have been conducted to determine whether the integrity or activity of neuropeptide-containing systems (and their receptors) are altered in neuropsychiatric disorders. Second, peptides have been administered to humans to evaluate their potential therapeutic use. Finally, the effects of peptide receptor antagonists on the behavior and mood of normal volunteers and psychiatric patients have beeen evaluated.

The postmortem tissue and CSF studies have recently been reviewed by Nemeroff and Bissette (1986), Rossor (1988), and Post et al. (1988). In both types of studies, several potentially confounding variables must be carefully evaluated, including patient age and sex, and drug effects. Such considerations increase the likelihood that alterations in peptide concentration (or receptor number) are related to patient diagnosis and not to these "nuisance variables." In postmortem tissue studies, stability of the peptide to be measured must be taken into consideration as well as agonal state, postmortem delay, and cause of death. In CSF and postmortem studies, the time of day (and year) the sample is obtained may be important because of possible circadian and circannual rhythms in the concentrations of certain neurotransmitters and their metabolites (e.g., melatonin and endorphins). In general, neuropeptides have been found to be remarkably stable in postmortem brain tissue and CSF. However, the complexity of neuropeptide neurobiology is demonstrated by the presence of multiple forms of certain neuropeptides that have been found in brain and CSF.

Neurotransmitter Systems in Aging and Alzheimer's Disease

Considerable work has been conducted in determining whether there are age-related alterations in one or another neurotransmitter system in normal aging. Some time ago, I reviewed the salient findings (Lipton and Nemeroff 1978). There is general agreement that a loss of neurons in the CNS occurs in animals and humans with aging. It is evident that this age-related neuronal loss is not anatomically uniform. For example, approximately one-half of the neurons in the superior frontal gyrus are lost in the elderly, whereas the inferior olivary nucleus exhibits virtually no age-related decline. Space constraints preclude a detailed review of age-associated alterations in CNS neurotransmitter systems. There is considerable evidence, however, of age-related alterations in dopamine, norepinephrine, serotonin, acetylcholine, and GABA neural circuits. A particularly impressive example of this is shown in Figure 14 where the number of neurons in the substantia nigra of humans as a function of age is plotted. A clear age-related loss of these neurons, most of which are dopaminergic, is evident. In the remaining portion of this chapter the focus is on alterations in specific chemically defined neurotransmitter systems in Alzheimer's disease, a neurodegenerative disorder that accounts for more than 50 percent of the cases of dementia in the over-50 age group.

Senile dementia of the Alzheimer's type (SDAT) is a debilitating, irreversible disorder characterized by progressive mental impairment. The initial deficit is loss of memory for recent events, but eventually, the patient's cognitive dysfunction is so profound that the capacity for self-care is lost.

The primary histopathologic hallmarks of SDAT in the brain are senile plaques and neurofibrillary tangles (Terry and Katzman 1983). These are primarily localized in the cerebral cortex and hippocampus, and their presence correlates with the degree of cognitive disruption. In addition, certain subcortical structures (e.g., hypothalamus, amygdala, and striatum) also contain neurofibrillary tangles (McDuff and Sumi 1985). The involvement of these structures and the neural pathways emanating from them probably underlie certain of the clinical symptomatology.

Currently, there is no effective therapy to ameliorate the cognitive deterioration characteristic of SDAT. As noted above, the focus of part of this chapter is on the biochemical changes reported to occur in specific neurotransmitter and neuropeptide systems in SDAT. The goals of research in this area are twofold. Most immediately, it is hoped that specific pharmacologic agents can be developed to alleviate some or all of the symptoms of SDAT and/or to retard the progression of the disease. Moreover, this line of research may provide insights into the etiology and pathogenesis of SDAT.

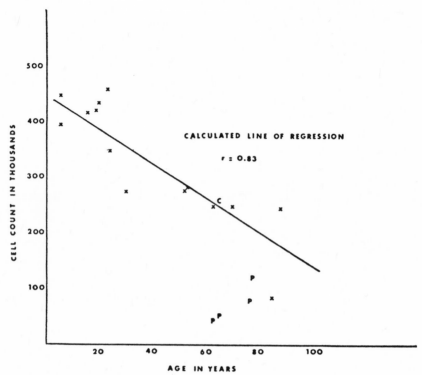

Figure 14. Cell counts in substantia nigra of humans plotted against age. Xs and line represent those dying without neurologic illness; P = Parkinsonian; C = choreic. (Reproduced with permission from McGeer et al. [1977].)

Acetylcholine

There is little question that in SDAT, as noted above, there is a degeneration of the cholinergic pathway that originates in the nucleus basalis of Meynert (NbM) and projects to the neocortex. Virtually every research group that has studied the NbM in SDAT has verified that there is a loss, primarily of the large cells that comprise the primary cholinergic innervation to the cortex (Rossor et al. 1982; Whitehouse et al. 1982; Coyle et al. 1983). It has recently been suggested that rather than a loss of cholinergic cells, the large cells shrink in diameter as a result of retrograde degeneration following cerebrocortical damage (Pearson et al. 1983). Of course, whether the initial damage is at the cortical or NbM levels, it is evident that the NbM–cortical pathway degenerates in SDAT.

In addition to the histochemical studies described above, biochemical indices in neocortex are consistent with a marked reduction of cholinergic neuronal integrity in SDAT. Until recently, because of technical considerations, it was difficult to measure acetylcholine concentrations directly. Thus, the acetylcholine synthetic enzyme, choline acetyltransferase, and the acetylcholine-degrading enzyme, acetylcholinesterase, have been used as markers of the integrity of cholinergic neurons. The former is known to be a more specific marker of cholinergic neurons. Choline acetyltransferase activity is markedly decreased in the cortex and hippocampus of postmortem SDAT tissue (Bowen et al. 1983; Davies 1979). There is a significant negative correlation between measures of cortical cholinergic integrity and measures of neuropathology (e.g., plaques and tangles) in SDAT (Mountjoy et al. 1984). There is also a positive correlation between cholinergic degeneration and tests of mental ability in Alzheimer's disease (Perry et al. 1978). In elderly nonhuman primates, choline acetyltransferase is present in the neurites of some senile plaques, indicating a cholinergic innervation of these plaques (Kitt et al. 1984).

Acetylcholinesterase has been measured largely in CSF to evaluate it as a putative diagnostic tool. Although decreases in CSF acetylcholinesterase content have been observed in some studies (Soininen et al. 1984; Tune et al. 1985), the finding is by no means universal (Davies 1979). Moreover, although the mean acetylcholinesterase activity in the SDAT group is significantly lower than in the controls, considerable overlap between the two groups occurs. The diagnostic utility of CSF acetylcholinesterase concentrations must therefore be considered questionable. However, acetylcholinesterase activity is present in the senile plaques of aged primates, providing further direct evidence for cholinergic involvement in the pathology of SDAT (Struble et al. 1982).

Attempts to demonstrate changes in the number or affinity of acetylcholine receptors in SDAT have mostly been unsuccessful (Davies and Verth 1978). Decreases in muscarinic binding in SDAT have, however, been reported (Reisine et al. 1978). The latter group localized the decreased binding to hippocampus, amygdala, and nucleus accumbens, but not to frontal cortex or striatum. Recently, M_2, but not M_1, muscarinic receptors in cerebral cortex have been reported to be lost in SDAT (Mash et al. 1985). Because the M_2 receptors are hypothesized to be presynaptically located, the accumulated findings have lent credence to the hypothesis that the primary degeneration is within the cholinergic neuron rather than in neurons postsynaptic to the acetylcholine neuron. Consistent with this hypothesis are findings that demonstrate a reduction in choline uptake in hippocampal and cortical synaptosomes prepared from postmortem Alzheimer's tissue (Rylett et al. 1983) and those that show a decrease in acetylcholine synthesis and release in temporal cortex biopsy tissue from patients with SDAT (Sims et al. 1983).

Given the cholinergic degeneration in SDAT and the voluminous evidence supporting a role for acetylcholine in a variety of learning and memory tasks, it is not surprising that much effort has been expended on studying whether pharmacologic enhancement of acetylcholine neurotransmission would ameliorate the symptoms of SDAT. Two main strategies have been employed. In the first, acetylcholine precursors such as choline chloride or lecithin are administered for 2 to 8 weeks and the patients are evaluated on various memory and cognitive tasks. With only a few exceptions, the results have proved disappointing, with little or no improvement seen (Bartus et al. 1982, 1987).

The second major strategy to potentiate cholinergic neurotransmission is by administration of acetylcholinesterase inhibitors such as physostigmine. Modest gains in performance in memory and cognition tests have been reported (Johns et al. 1985). However, the optimal effective dose varies widely, side effects are common, and the improvements are generally transient.

Monoamines

Most evidence supports a decrement in norepinephrine function in Alzheimer's disease. This is primarily reflected in two sets of experimental findings. First, numerous reports have demonstrated that in SDAT, cell loss is observed in the locus ceruleus, which, as noted above, is one of the major groups of norepinephrine perikarya in the CNS (Mann et al. 1984). In addition, the magnitude of the locus ceruleus cell loss is greater in patients who develop Alzheimer's disease at a younger age, formerly referred to as presenile dementia. Second, norepinephrine concentrations are decreased in a variety of postmortem brain regions in SDAT (Adolfsson et al. 1979; Arai et al. 1984a). It is noteworthy, however, that although norepinephrine concentrations have been reported to be decreased in the cerebral cortex, the largest norepinephrine deficit is found in the hypothalamus. This is in contrast to the marked deficits in acetylcholine, somatostatin, and corticotropin-releasing factor (vide infra) that occur primarily in neocortical and hippocampal areas. A significant correlation between clinical symptoms in SDAT and the reduction in hypothalamic norepinephrine has been reported. However, no consistent changes in adrenergic receptors (both α and β) have been found in Alzheimer's tissue (Cross et al. 1984). In one study, norepinephrine uptake was found to be reduced in temporal cortex biopsy tissue from patients with presumed SDAT (Benton et al. 1982). Using data obtained in laboratory animals, it has been suggested that age-related cognitive dysfunction is related to degeneration of norepinephrine pathways (Arnsten et al. 1985). Degeneration of norepinephrine neurons in patients with SDAT may therefore contribute to the cognitive dysfunction observed in this disorder.

The evidence for a dopaminergic involvement in SDAT is, at best, minimal. On the positive side, a number of research groups have found reductions either in dopamine or in the dopamine metabolite, homovanillic acid (HVA), in Alzheimer's tissue. The most consistent reduction in dopamine has been found in the basal ganglia (caudate and putamen) (Gottfries et al. 1983). Concentrations of HVA have been found to be reduced most consistently in CSF (Bareggi et al. 1982; Palmer et al. 1984). However, dopamine in the caudate (Yates et al. 1983b) and HVA in CSF has been reported to be unchanged in Alzheimer's disease (Kay et al. 1984). In contrast to cholinergic and noradrenergic neurons, there is no evidence of cell loss in the midbrain cells of origin of the dopamine pathways in SDAT. One confounding variable in these studies described above (Figure 14) is the reduction in dopamine concentration in the striatum that occurs in normal individuals as they age.

There is clear evidence for Alzhemier's disease-associated degeneration of serotonin neurons. Both serotonergic cell loss and the presence of neurofibrillary tangles have been found in the nucleus raphe dorsalis in SDAT (Yamamoto and Hirano 1985; Ishii 1966). Not surprisingly, reductions in the concentrations of both serotonin and its metabolite 5-hydroxyindoleacetic acid (5-HIAA) have also been observed. Serotonin concentrations are reduced in the hippocampus, hypothalamus, cingulate cortex, and caudate (Gottfries et al. 1983). Reductions in the CSF concentration of 5-HIAA have been reported in CSF of SDAT patients by some (Palmer et al. 1984) and not others (Volicer et al. 1985). Both uptake of serotonin and ^{3}H-imipramine binding, presynaptic serotonin markers, are reduced in the temporal cortex in Alzheimer's disease (Bowen et al. 1983). Serotonin receptor subtypes S_1 and S_2 are reportedly decreased in SDAT, at least in both hippocampal and cortical tissue (Cross et al. 1984; Reynolds et al. 1984).

Neuropeptides

In conjunction with the rapid expansion of research concerning identification of novel neuropeptides, much interest has focused on the potential pathologic involvement of peptidergic neurons in Alzheimer's disease. The concentration of a number of peptides has been measured in postmortem brain tissue and CSF using radioimmunoassay procedures.

Consistent alterations in only two peptides (somatostatin and corticotropin-releasing factor) have been found in Alzheimer's disease. The most widely replicated finding is a reduction in the concentration of somatostatin in several cerebrocortical areas and hippocampus. In a series of pioneering studies, Davies and colleagues found markedly decreased somatostatin concentrations in the hippocampus, mid-frontal cortex, inferior parietal cortex, occipital cortex, superior temporal gyrus, mid-temporal gyrus, and inferior temporal gyrus (Davies et al. 1980; Davies and Terry 1981). Ferrier et al. (1983) also reported a reduction in somatostatin concentration in frontal, temporal, and parietal cortex as well as in the septum of Alzheimer's patients. However, no decrease in hippocampal somatostatin was found. Both my colleagues and I (Nemeroff et al. 1983) and Rossor et al. (1980) have observed reduced somatostatin concentrations in postmortem brain samples from patients with Alzheimer's disease, though the reductions were somewhat more limited than those reported previously. Our group found somatostatin reductions in frontal cortex, temporal cortex, and hypothalamus, but not in parietal cortex, amygdala, caudate nucleus, nucleus accumbens, or posterior hippocampus. In the studies by Rossor et al., decreased concentrations of somatostatin were measured only in temporal cortex. Arai et al. (1984b) reported that the concentration of somatostatin was reduced in the hippocampus, orbital cortex, and putamen. In most studies, Alzheimer's disease-related reductions in somatostatin concentration have not been found in subcortical structures. Both Davies's group and Rossor's group have noted that the reductions in somatostatin concentration are most prominent in patients with early onset of the disease. Recently, somatostatin immunoreactivity has been observed in both the neuritic plaques of primates (Struble et al. 1984) as well as in 30 to 50 percent of cortical plaques in postmortem brain tissue from Alzheimer's disease patients (Armstrong et al. 1985; Morrison et al. 1985).

The CSF studies are largely consistent with the postmortem studies in that somatostatin concentrations are reduced in the CSF of SDAT patients (Bissette et al. 1986). In addition, in a recent pilot study in collaboration with Widerlov and his colleagues, my colleagues and I found that intensive environmental (psychosocial) stimulation of Alzheimer's disease patients results in an increase in CSF concentrations of somatostatin (Karlsson et al. 1985). The use of the reduction of CSF somatostatin as a diagnostic marker for SDAT is of questionable value because of the lack of specificity of this finding. The peptide is also diminished in CSF of patients with major depression, Parkinson's disease with dementia, and multiple sclerosis (Bissette et al. 1986). β-endorphin and ACTH have also been reported to be reduced in the CSF of Alzheimer's patients (Kaiya et al. 1983).

My colleagues and I have recently discovered that corticotropin-releasing factor (CRF) concentrations in the frontal cortex (Brodmann's area 10) and temporal cortex (Brodmann's area 38) are reduced by 50 percent in SDAT (Figure 15); a 70 percent decrease in the CRF concentration was observed in the caudate nucleus of Alzheimer's patients as well (Bissette et al. 1985). These findings have now been confirmed and extended by DeSouza et al (1986); they not only have shown a reduction in CRF concentrations in SDAT, but also have shown a marked increase in the number of CRF receptors.

With the exception of the somatostatin and CRF findings, the majority of the studies that have evaluated the integrity of peptidergic neurons in Alzheimer's disease have proved negative. The following neuropeptides have been scrutinized in some detail: thyrotropin-releasing hormone (Biggins et al. 1983; Nemeroff et al. 1983; Yates et al. 1983a), vasoactive intestinal peptide, cholecystokinin, sub P, and NT. Arai et al. (1984b) reported that vasoactive intestinal peptide concentrations were reduced in insular and cingular cortices in Alzheimer's. Others, however, have been unable to replicate this finding (Ferrier et al. 1983). Discordant findings have also been obtained with

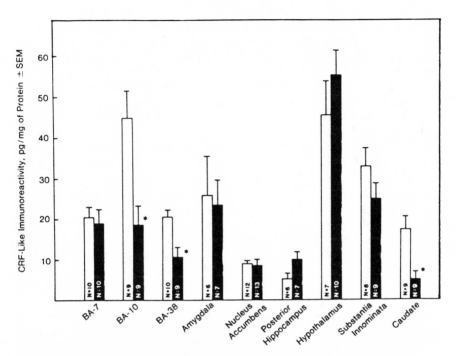

Figure 15.   Regional brain concentration of corticotropin-releasing factor-like immunoreactivity (CRF-LI) in patients with senile dementia of Alzheimer's type and in controls. Graphs represent concentrations of CRF-LI in brain regions from patients dying of senile dementia of Alzheimer's type (solid bars) and controls (open bars). Number of samples from each brain region is shown inside respective bars. Concentration of CRF-LI is shown as mean ± SEM and is reported as picograms per milligram of protein. Statistical significance was sought by Student's t test and is represented by asterisk, which indicates p<.01. (Reproduced with permission from Bissette G, Reynolds GP, Kilts CD, et al: Corticotropin-releasing factor-like immunoreactivity in senile dementia of the Alzheimer type. JAMA 1985; 254:3067–3069.)

sub P. Crystal and Davies (1982) found a slight decrease in cortical sub P, but this was not verified by Ferrier et al. (1983). Cortical cholecystokinin (Ferrier et al. 1983) and NT (Nemeroff et al. 1983) have consistently been found to be unchanged in Alzheimer's disease. We did, however, observe a 30 percent decrease in the NT concentration in the amygdala of Alzheimer's disease patients. Enkephalin and vasoactive intestinal peptide immunoreactive hippocampal pyramidal cells have been reported to contain neurofibrillary tangles in both Alzheimer's disease tissue and aged brain (Kulmala 1985). Neuropeptide-Y-like immunoreactivity is present in 10 to 20 percent of hippocampal neuritic plaques from SDAT tissue (Dawbarn and Emson 1985).

Study of neuropeptide function in Alzheimer's disease is still in its infancy. It is not surprising that the brain regions where somatostatin has been found to be depleted vary slightly across laboratories. In view of the variability in patient populations and the clinical course of the disease, it is, in fact, quite remarkable that such consistent and selective reductions in somatostatin have been found in frontal and temporal cortices. Clearly, much work remains to be done to determine if any relationship exists between the somatostatin deficits and the clinical symptoms of SDAT. Recently, it has been shown that depletion of hippocampal somatostatin induced by cysteamine is associated with deficits in passive avoidance learning (Nemeroff et al. 1987). Studies of somatostatin biosynthesis and receptors are being conducted in several laboratories. Treatment of Alzheimer's disease with neuropeptides including a somatostatin analog, ACTH fragment, vasopressin, as well as the opiate receptor antagonist naltrexone, has been tried without any salutary effect (Nemeroff and Bissette 1986). Problems of limited entry of neuropeptides into brain after parenteral administration and rapid degradation in vivo must be overcome.

Although Alzhemier's disease-associated changes in concentration or receptor binding of the amino acid neurotransmitters, GABA and glutamic acid, are not particularly striking, some differences from control samples have been reported.

Reductions in GABA concentration in the CSF of SDAT patients have been documented (Zimmer et al. 1984). Cortical concentrations of GABA (Mountjoy et al. 1984) and activity of the GABA synthesizing enzyme, GAD (Perry et al. 1978), have been reported to be reduced slightly or not at all (Perry et al. 1984) in Alzheimer's disease. These deficits, however, do not correlate well with estimates of neuron counts, senile plaques, or neurofibrillary tangles. With the exception of Reisine et al. (1978), who found decreased GABA binding in the frontal cortex and caudate nucleus, no changes in GABA receptor binding have been reported in Alzheimer's disease brain tissue.

The material presented in this chapter is a testimony to the advances in neurobiology that have occurred in the last decade. However, we still can account for only 50 percent, at most, of the neurotransmitters in the CNS. Molecular biology has been applied to neuroscience and novel neurotransmitters have been identified. As these advances occur, they can be applied to the neurochemistry of aging and to diseases of the elderly.

References

Adolfsson R, Gottfries CG, Roos BE, et al: Changes in brain catecholamines in patients with dementia of Alzheimer type. Br J Psychiatry 1979; 135:216–223

Antelman SM, Chiodo LA: Stress: its effect on interactions among biogenic amines and role in the induction and treatment of disease, in Handbook of Psychopharmacology (Volume 18). Edited by Iversen LL, Iversen SD, Snyder SH. New York, Plenum Press, 1984

Arai H, Kosaka K, Iizuka R: Changes of biogenic amines and their metabolites in postmortem brains from patients with Alzheimer-type dementia. J Neurochem 1984a; 43:388–393

Arai H, Moroji T,Kosaka K: Somatostatin and vasoactive intestinal polypeptide in post-mortem brains from patients with Alzheimer-type dementia. Neurosci Lett 1984b; 52:73–78

Armstrong DM, LeRoy S, Shields D, et al: Somatostatin-like immunoreactivity within neuritic plaques. Brain Res 1985; 338:71–79

Arnsten AFT, Goldman-Rakic PS: α₂–adrenergic mechanisms in prefrontal cortex associated with cognitive decline in aged nonhuman primates. Science 1985; 230:1273–1276

Asberg M, Traskman, K, Thoren P: 5HIAA in the cerebrospinal fluid. A biochemical suicide predictor. Arch Gen Psychiatry 1976; 33:1193–1197

Baeyens JM, Moreno A: Are two different types of dopaminergic receptors involved in thermoregulation in the rat? in Environment, Drugs and Thermoregulation. Edited by Lomax P, Schonbaum E, Basel, Karger, 1983

Baldessarini RJ: Chemotherapy in Psychiatry (second edition). Cambridge, MA, Harvard University Press, 1985

Bareggi S, Franceshi M, Bonini L, et al: Decreased CSF concentration of homovanillic acid and GABA in Alzheimer's disease. Arch Neurol 1982; 39:709–712

Bartus RT, Dean RL III, Beer B, et al: The cholinergic hypothesis of geriatric memory dysfunction. Science 1982; 217:408–417

Bartus RT, Dean RL, Flicker C: Cholinergic psychopharmacology: an integration of human and animal research on memory, in Psychopharmacology: The Third Generation of Progress. Edited by Meltzer HY. New York, Raven Press, 1987

Benton JJ, et al: Alzheimer's disease as a disorder of isodendritic core. Lancet 1982; 1:456

Biggins J, Perry EK, McDermott JR, et al: Post-mortem levels of thyrotropin-releasing hormone and neurotensin in the amygdala in Alzheimer's disease, schizophrenia and depression. J Neurol Sci 1983; 58:117–122

Birkmayer W, Riederer P: Parkinson's Disease. Vienna, Springer-Verlag, 1983

Bissette G, Reynolds GP, Kilts CD, et al: Corticotropin-releasing factor-like immunoreactivity in senile dementia of the Alzheimer type. JAMA 1985; 254:3067–3069

Bissette G, Walleus A, Widerlov E, et al: Alterations in cerebrospinal fluid concentrations of somatostatin-like immunoreactivity in neuropsychiatric disorders. Arch Gen Psychiatry 1986; 43:1148–1154

Bowen DM, Allen SJ, Benton JS, et al: Biochemical assessment of serotonergic and cholinergic dysfunction and cerebral atrophy in Alzheimer's disease. J Neurochem 1983; 41:266–272

Brown GL, Goodwin FK, Ballenger JC, et al: Aggression in human correlates with cerebrospinal fluid metabolites. Psychiatr Res 1979; 1:131–139

Campbell IC: Receptors: a historical perspective, in Brain Receptor Methodologies. Edited by Marangos PJ, Campbell IC, Cohen RM. New York, Academic Press, 1984

Carraway RE, Leeman SE: The isolation of a new hypotensive peptide, neurotensin, from bovine hypothalami. J Biol Chem 1973; 248:6854–6861

Carson KA, Nemeroff CB, Rone MS, et al: Experimental studies on the ultrastructural localization of acetylcholinesterase in the mediobasal hypothalamus of the rat. J Comp Neurol 1978; 182:201–220

Cooper JR, Bloom FE, Roth RH: The Biochemical Basis of Neuropharmacology (fifth edition). New York, Oxford University Press, 1986

Coyle JT: Excitotoxins, in Psychopharmacology: The Third Generation of Progress. Edited by Meltzer HY. New York, Raven Press, 1987

Coyle JT, Price DL, DeLong MR: Alzheimer's disease: a disorder of cortical cholinergic innervation. Science 1983; 219:1184–1190

Creese I: Biochemical properties of CNS dopamine receptors, in Psychopharmacology: The Third Generation of Progress. Edited by Meltzer HY. New York, Raven Press, 1987

Cross AJ, Crow TJ, Johnson JA, et al: Studies on neurotransmitter receptor systems in neocortex and hippocampus in senile dementia of the Alzheimer type. J Neurol Sci 1984; 64:109–117

Crystal HA, Davies P: Cortical substance P-like immunoreactivity in cases of Alzheimer's disease and senile dementia of the Alzheimer type. J Neurochem 1982; 38:1781–1784

Dahlstrom A, Fuxe K: Evidence for the existence of monoamine-containing neurons in the central nervous system. I. Demonstration of monoamines in the cell bodies of brainstem neurons. Acta Physiol Scand 1964; 62(Suppl 232):1–55

Davies P: Neurotransmitter-related enzymes in senile dementia of the Alzheimer type. Brain Res 1979; 171:319–327

Davies P, Terry RD: Cortical somatostatin-like immunoreactivity in cases of Alzheimer's disease and senile dementia of the Alzheimer type. Neurobiol Aging 1981; 2:9–14

Davies P, Verth AH: Regional distribution of muscarinic acetylcholine receptors in normal and Alzheimer type dementia brains. Brain Res 1978; 138:385–392

Davies P, Katzman R, Terry RD: Reduced somatostatin-like immunoreactivity in cerebral cortex from cases of Alzheimer's disease and Alzheimer senile dementia. Nature 1980; 288:279–280

Dawbarn D, Emson PC: Neuropeptide Y-like immunoreactivity in neuritic plaques of Alzheimer's disease. Biochem Biophys Res Comm 1985; 126:289–294

DeSouza EB, Whitehouse PJ, Kuhar MJ, et al: Reciprocal changes in corticotropin-releasing factor (CRF)-like immunoreactivity and CRF receptors in cerebral cortex of Alzheimer's disease. Nature (London) 1986; 319:593–595

Engelsen B: Neurotransmitter glutamate: its clinical importance. Acta Neurol Scand 1986; 74:337–355

Enna SJ, Mohler H: γ-aminobutyric acid (GABA) receptors and their association with benzodiazepine recognition sites, in Psychopharmacology: The Third Generation of Progress. Edited by Meltzer HY. New York, Raven Press, 1987

Feldman RS, Quenzer LF: Fundamentals of Neurospsychopharmacology. Sunderland, Mass, Sinaver Associates, 1984

Ferrier IN, Cross AJ, Johnson JA, et al: Neuropeptides in Alzheimer's type dementia. J Neurol Sci 1983; 62:159–170

Fisher SK, Agranoff BW: Receptor activation and inositol lipid hydrolysis in neural tissues. J Neurochem 1987; 48:999–1017

Foote SL: Anatomy and physiology of brain monoamine systems, in Psychiatry (Volume 3). Edited by Michaels R, Cavenar JO. Philadelphia, J. B. Lippincott, 1987

Frohman LA, Berelowitz M: The physiological and pharmacological control of anterior pituitary hormone secretions, in Peptides, Hormones and Behavior. Edited by Nemeroff CB, Dunn AJ. New York, Spectrum Publications, 1984

Fuxe K: Evidence for the existence of monoamine neurons in the central nervous system. IV. The distribution of monoamine terminals in the central nervous system. Acta Physiol Scand 1965; 64(Suppl 247): 41–85

Gottfries C-G, Adolfsson R, Aquilonius S-M, et al: Biochemical changes in dementia disorders of Alzheimer type (AD/SDAT). Neurobiol Aging 1983; 4:261–271

Hamon M, Bourgoin S, El Mestikaway S, et al: Central serotonin receptors, in Handbook of Neurochemistry, Receptors in the Nervous System (Volume 6). Edited by Lajtha A. New York, Plenum Press, 1984

Harris GW: Neural Control of the Pituitary Gland. London, Arnold, 1955

Hokfelt T, Fuxe K, Pernow B (eds): Coexistence of Neuronal Messengers: A New Principle in Chemical Transmission (Progress in Brain Research 68). Amsterdam, Elsevier, 1986

Hughes J: Strategies for manipulating peptidergic transmission, in Alzheimer's Disease: Advances in Basic Research Therapies. Edited by Wurtman RJ, Corkin SH, Growden JH. Proceedings of the Third Meeting of the International Study Group on Treatment of Memory Disorders Associated with Aging, 1984

Ishii T: Distribution of Alzheimer's neurofibrillary changes in the brain stem and the hypothalamus of senile dementia. Acta Neuropath 1966; 6:181–187

Iversen LH, Iversen SH, Snyder SH (eds): Neuropeptides. Handbook of Psychopharmacology (Volume 16). New York, Plenum Press, 1983

Jacobs BL: How hallucinogenic drugs work. American Scientist 1987; 75:386–392

Janowsky DS, Risch SC: Role of acetylcholine mechanisms in the affective disorders , in Psychopharmacology: The Third Generation of Progress. Edited by Meltzer HY. New York, Raven Press, 1987

Javoy-Agid F, Agid Y: Is the mesocortical dopaminergic system involved in Parkinson's disease. Neurology 1980; 30:1326–1330

Johns CA, Haroutunian V, Greenwald BS, et al: Development of cholinergic drugs for the treatment of Alzheimer's disease. Drug Development Research 1985; 5:77–96

Jones BE, Beaudet A: Distribution of acetylcholine and catecholamine neurons in the cat brainstem: a choline acetyltransferase and tyrosine hydroxylase immunohistochemical study. J Comp Neurol 1987; 261:15–32

Kaiya H, Tanaka T, Takeuchi K, et al: Decreased level of β-endorphin-like immunoreactivity in cerebrospinal fluid of patients with senile dementia of Alzheimer type. Life Sci 1983; 33:1039–1043

Kalivas PW, Nemeroff CB (eds): The mesolimbicocortical dopamine system. Ann NY Acad Sci, in press

Karacan I, Moore C: Physiology and neurochemistry of sleep, in Psychiatry Update: American Psychiatric Association Annual Review (Volume 4). Edited by Hales RE, Frances AJ. Washington, DC, American Psychiatric Press, 1985

Karlsson I, Widerlov E, Malin E, et al: Changes of CSF neuropeptides after environmental stimulation in dementia. Nordic Psychiatric Journal 1985; 39(Suppl 1):75–81

Kay AD, Milstein S, Kaufman S, et al: 5-HIAA and HVA in the CSF of patients with Alzheimer's disease. Neurology 1984; 34(Suppl 1):161

Kitt CA, Price DL, Struble RG, et al: Evidence for cholinergic neurites in senile plaques. Science 1984; 226:1443–1445

Koob GF: The dopamine anhedonia hypothesis: a pharmacological phrenology. The Behavioral and Brain Sciences 1982; 5:63–64

Kulmala HK: Some enkephalin- or VIP-immunoreactive hippocampal pyramidal cells contain neurofibrillary tangles in the brains of aged humans and persons with Alzheimer's disease. Neurochem Path 1985; 3:41–51

Kuraishi Y, Satoh M, Takagi H: The descending noradrenergic system and analgesia, in Neurotransmitters and Pain Control. Edited by Akil H, Lewis JW. Basel, Switzerland, Karger, 1987

Lake CR, Ziegler MG (eds): The Catecholamines in Psychiatric and Neurologic Disorders. Boston, Butterworth, 1985

Lindvall O, Bjorklund A: Neuroanatomical localization of dopamine in the brain and spinal cord, in Handbook of Schizophrenia: Volume 2. Neurochemistry and Neuropharmacology of Schizophrenia. Edited by Henn FA, DeLisi LE. Amsterdam, Elsevier, 1987

Lipton MA, Nemeroff CB: The biology of aging and its role in depression, in Aging: The Process and the People. Edited by Usdin G, Hofling CJ. New York, Brunner/Mazel, 1978

Lloyd K, Morselli PL: Psychopharmacology of GABAergic drugs, in Psychopharmacology: The Third Generation of Progress. Edited by Meltzer HY. New York, Raven Press, 1987

Mann DMA, Yates PO, Marcyniuk B: Alzheimer's presenile dementia, senile dementia of Alzheimer type and Down's syndrome in middle age from an age related continuum of pathological changes. Neuropathol Appl Neurobiol 1984; 10:185–207

Mash DC, Flynn DD, Potter LT: Loss of M2 muscarine receptors in the cerebral cortex in Alzheimer's disease and experimental cholinergic denervation. Science 1985; 228:1115–1117

McCann SM, Lumpkin MD, Mizunuma H, et al: Recent studies on the role of brain peptides in control of anterior pituitary secretion. Peptides 1984; 5(Suppl 1):3–7

McDuff T, Sumi SM: Subcortical degeneration in Alzheimer's disease. Neurology 1985; 35:123–126 .

McGeer RL, McGeer EG, Suzuki JS: Aging and extrapyramidal function. Arch Neurol 1977; 34:33–35

Milton AS: The hypothalamus and the pharmacology of thermoregulation, in Pharmacology of the Hypothalamus. Edited by Cox B, Morris ID, Weston AH. London, MacMillan Press, 1977

Mitchell IJ, Jackson A, Sambrook MA, et al: Common neural mechanisms in experimental chorea and hemiballismus in the monkey: evidence from 2-deoxy glucose autoradiography. Brain Res 1985; 339:346–350

Morrison JH, Rogers J, Scherr S, et al: Somatostatin immunoreactivity in neuritic plaques of Alzheimer's patients. Nature 1985; 314:90–92

Mountjoy CQ, Rossor MN, Iversen LL, et al: Correlation of cortical cholinergic and GABA deficits with quantitative neuropathological findings in senile dementia. Brain 1984; 107:517–518

Nemeroff CB, Bissette G: Neuropeptides in psychiatric disorders, in American Handbook of Psychiatry. Edited by Berger PA, Brodie HKH. New York, Basic Books, 1986

Nemeroff CB, Loosen PT (eds): Handbook of Clinical Psychoneuroendocrinology. New York, Guilford Press, 1987

Nemeroff CB, Bissette, G, Busby WH Jr, et al: Regional brain concentrations of neurotensin, thyrotropin-releasing hormone and somatostatin in Alzheimer's disease. Society for Neuroscience Abstracts 1983; 9:1052

Nemeroff CB, Walsh TJ, Bissette G: Somatostatin and behavior: preclinical and clinical studies, in Somatostatin. Edited by Reichlin SM. New York, Plenum Press, 1987

Nieuwenhuys R, Voogd J, van Huijzen C: The Human Central Nervous System. New York, Springer-Verlag, 1981

Palmer AM, Sims NS, Bowen DM, et al: Monoamine metabolite concentrations in lumbar cerebrospinal fluid of patients with histology verified Alzheimer's dementia. J Neurol Neurosurg Psychiatry 1984; 47:481–484

Pearson RCA, Sofroniew MV, Cuello AC, et al: Persistence of cholinergic neurons in the basal nucleus in a brain with senile dementia of the Alzheimer's type demonstrated by immunohistochemical staining for choline acetyltransferase. Brain Res 1983; 289:375–379

Perry EK, Tomlinson BE, Blessed G, et al: Correlation of cholinergic abnormalities with senile plaques and mental test scores in senile dementia. Br Med J 1978; 2:1457–1459

Perry EK, Atack JR, Perry RH, et al: Intralaminar neurochemical distributions in human midtemporal cortex: comparison between Alzheimer's disease and the normal. J Neurochem 1984; 42:1402–1410

Post RM, Rubinow DR, Gold PW: Neuropeptides in manic-depressive illness, in Neuropeptides in Psychiatric and Neurological Disorders. Edited by Nemeroff CB. Baltimore, Johns Hopkins University Press, 1988

Reinis S, Goldman JM: The Chemistry of Behavior. New York, Plenum Press, 1982

Reisine TD, Yamamura HI, Bird ED, et al: Pre- and post-synaptic neurochemical alterations in Alzheimer's disease. Brain Res 1978; 159:477–481

Reynolds GP, Arnold L, Rossor MN, et al: Reduced binding of [^{3}H]ketanserin to cortical 5HT2 receptors in senile dementia of the Alzheimer type. Neurosci Lett 1984; 44:47–51

Ribak CE, Vaughn JE, Saito K, et al: Immunocytochemical localization of glutamate decarboxylase in rat substantia nigra. Brain Res 1977; 116:287–298

Rossor MN: Peptides and dementia, in Neuropeptides in Psychiatric and Neurological Disorders. Edited by Nemeroff CB. Baltimore, Johns Hopkins University Press, 1988

Rossor MN, Emson PC, Mountjoy CQ, et al: Reduced amounts of immunoreactive somatostatin in the temporal cortex in senile dementia of Alzheimer type. Neurosci Lett 1980; 20:373–377

Rossor MN, Svendsen C, Hunt SP, et al: The substantia innominata in Alzheimer's disease: an histochemical and biochemical study of cholinergic marker enzymes. Neurosci Lett 1982; 28:217–222

Rylett RT, Ball MJ, Colhoun EH: Evidence for high affinity choline transport in synaptosomes prepared from hippocampus and neocortex of patients with Alzheimer's disease. Brain Res 1983; 289:169–175

Seeman P, Lee T, Chau-Wong M, et al: Antipsychotic drug doses and neuroleptic/dopamine receptors. Nature 1976; 261:717–719

Sims NR, Bowen OM, Allen SJ, et al: Presynaptic cholinergic dysfunction in patients with dementia. J Neurochem 1983; 40:503–509

Soininen H, Pitkanen A, Halonen T, et al: Dopamine-beta-hydroxylase and acetylcholinesterase activities of cerebrospinal fluid in Alzheimer's disease. Acta Neurol Scand 1984; 69:29–34

Stahl SM, Wets K: Indoleamines and schizophrenia, in Handbook of Schizophrenia: Volume 2. Neurochemistry and Neuropharmacology of Schizophrenia. Edited by Henn FA, DeLisi L. Amsterdam, Elsevier, 1987

Stanley M, Virgilio S, Gershon S: Tritiated imipramine binding sites are decreased in the frontal cortex of suicides. Science 1982; 216:1337–1339

Struble RG, Cork LC, Whitehouse PJ, et al: Cholinergic innervation in neuritic plaques. Science 1982; 216:413–415

Struble RG, Kitt CA, Walker LL, et al: Somatostatinergic neurites in senile plaques of aged non-human primates. Brain Res 1984; 324:394–396

Terry RD, Katzman R: Senile dementia of the Alzheimer type. Neurology 1983; 14:497–506

Tune L, Gucker S, Folstein M, et al: Cerebrospinal fluid acetylcholinesterase activity in senile dementia of the Alzheimer type. Ann Neurol 1985; 17:46–48

Vale W, Rivier C: Hypothalamic hypophysiotropic hormones, in Handbook of Psychopharmacology (Vol 5). Edited by Iversen LL, Iversen SD, Snyder SH. New York, Plenum Press, 1975

Vance ML, Kaiser DL, Frohman LA, et al: Role of dopamine in the regulation of growth hormone secretion: dopamine and bromocriptine augment growth hormone (GH)-releasing hormone stimulated GH secretion in normal man. J Clin Endocrinol Metab 1987; 64:1136–1141

van Kamman DP, Sternberg DE, Hare TA, et al: CSF levels of γ-aminobutyric acid in schizophrenia. Arch Gen Psychiatry 1982; 39:91–97

Volicer L, Direnfeld LK, Freedman M, et al: Serotonin and 5-hydroxyindoleacetic acid in CSF. Arch Neurol 1985; 42:127–129

von Euler US, Gaddum J: An unidentified depressor substance in certain tissue extracts. J Physiol (London) 1931; 72:74–87

Watson SJ, Khachaturian H, Lewis ME, et al: Chemical neuroanatomy as a basis for biological psychiatry, in American Handbook of Psychiatry. Edited by Berger PA, Brodie HKH. New York, Basic Books, 1986

Whitehouse PJ, Hedreen JC, White LL, et al: Alzheimer's disease and senile dementia—loss of neurons in the basal forebrain. Science 1982; 215:1237–1239

Wise RA: Neuroleptics and operant behavior: the anhedonia hypothesis. The Behavioral and Brain Sciences 1982; 5:39–87

Wolf ME, Deutch AY, Roth RH: Pharmacology of central dopaminergic neurons, in Handbook of Schizophrenia: Volume 2. Neurochemistry and Neuropharmacology of Schizophrenia. Edited by Henn FA, DeLisi LE. Amsterdam, Elsevier, 1987

Yamamoto T, Hirano A: Nucleus raphe dorsalis in Alzheimer's disease: neurofibrillary tangles and loss of large neurons. Ann Neurol 1985; 17:573–577

Yamanaka K, Kigoshi S, Muramatsu I: Muscarinic receptor subtypes in bovine adrenal medulla. Biochem Pharmacol 1986; 35:3151–3157

Yates CM, Harmar AJ, Rosie R, et al: Thyrotropin-releasing hormone and substance P immunoreactivity in post-mortem brain from cases of Alzheimer-type dementia and Down's syndrome. Brain Res 1983a; 258:45–52

Yates CM, Simpson J, Gordon A, et al: Catecholamines and cholinergic enzymes in pre-senile and senile Alzheimer-type dementia and Down's syndrome. Brain Res 1983b; 280:119–126

Zemlan FP: Influence of p-chloroamphetamine and p-chlorophenylalanine on female mating behavior. Ann NY Acad Sci 1978; 305:621–626

Zimmer R, Teelken AW, Trieling WB, et al: γ-aminobutyric acid and homovanillic acid concentration in the CSF of patients with senile dementia of Alzheimer's type. Arch Neurol 1984; 41:602–604

Chapter 6

Cerebral Metabolism and Electrical Activity

Ewald W. Busse, M.D.

Brain Metabolism

The brain is the most active energy consumer of any organ of the body. The brain represents 2 percent of the total body weight, yet at rest it consumes at least 20 percent of the oxygen used by the entire body. This enormous expenditure of energy appears to be related to maintaining the ionic gradient across the neuronal membrane on which the conduction of impulses depends. There are billions of neurons in the brain demanding this large amount of oxygen. Neurons, under normal conditions, use only glucose and adjust their metabolic rate according to their needs (Dekoninck 1985).

The composition of the human brain in total is approximately 77 to 78 percent water. The distribution of the water content is 83 percent in the gray matter while in the white matter it is 70 percent. The other major components of the brain include 8 percent protein and approximately 10 percent lipids. Both the lipids and protein are higher in white matter (McIlwain and Bacholard 1971). The lipids of the brain are outstanding for their components, which by their amount and nature can be said to characterize the organ. Lipids are two to three times greater in the brain than in muscle. However, in the brain their availability for general metabolism is limited compared to that in most other organs. In contrast, proteins and other simple organic substances make up much of the metabolic and contractile machinery in muscle. Proteins in the brain are approximately half that found in muscle, but they are very important in the brain to carry out of much of its functional activity. Brain cells are bathed in extracellular fluids, and the electrical activity in all neural systems depends on the differential ion concentration between the cellular components and the fluids that surround them. Not only neurons, but glial cells are relatively permeable to ions and so contribute to the electrical conductivity of the brain. It is estimated that extracellular fluid constitutes 21 percent of the volume of the brain. As to cerebral spinal fluid, it is primarily produced by the choroid plexis though some comes from cerebral capillaries. It is assumed that some of this fluid was originally interstitial.

The majority of cerebral organic constituents are synthesized in the brain itself from simpler compounds supplied by the bloodstream. Much of the material that enters the brain from the blood passes through cells that line the capillaries. Eight distinct transport systems have been identified that carry specific substances through this barrier. Each of the transport systems deals with essential substrates that the brain requires to meet its metabolic demands. Since material passes from the blood into the brain, these changes can be measured. The most striking change is that of the absorption of glucose. The brain is unusually dependent on glucose. There are serious limitations as to how far normal glucose can drop before the brain encounters difficulty. If the normal glucose consumption is held to approximately 40 percent, the brain can only continue to work effectively for 10 to 15 minutes with the oxidation of keto acids. However, if the glucose depletion is not of this magnitude, the normal brain has the ability to utilize other metabolites in place of glucose in order to continue its normal function. Measurement of local glucose utilization is possible by positron emission tomography (PET). This is usually accomplished by using fluorodeoxyglucose (see Chapter 11).

Glucose Metabolism and Huntington's Disease

Symptomatic patients with Huntington's disease are known to have reduced glucose metabolism in the caudate nuclei. This reduced metabolism occurs prior to the appearance of any structural changes visible using computed tomography (CT). It now appears possible to predict the subsequent appearance of Huntington's disease by determining the marked reductions in caudate glucose metabolism using PET (Mazziotta et al. 1987).

Cerebral Metabolic Rate

The cerebral metabolism of a substance is expressed as a metabolic rate. The cerebral metabolic rate (CMR) is usually expressed in milliliters or milligrams of the substance that is picked up and used by a measured unit of the brain, often 100 g of brain per minute. To calculate the metabolic rate, one must measure the blood level of a substance before and after it passes through the brain and must determine the rate of blood flow through the brain. Thus, "when arterial blood loses 6.6 ml of oxygen per 100 ml on passing through the brain at the rate of 50 ml per 100 g of brain per minute, the cerebral respiratory rate is 6.6 × 50/100, or 3.3 ml oxygen/100 g/minute" (Dekoninck 1985, p. 154). The rate of blood flow through the brain varies under so-called normal as well as pathologic conditions. Under normal conditions the brain has an effective autoregulation of blood flow. The cerebral metabolic rate tends to remain stable. When comparing different cerebral metabolites, such as oxygen or glucose, quantities of the material are conveniently expressed in molar units (Dekoninck 1985).

In recent years the classical methods of measuring cerebral metabolism in humans by invasive procedures have been replaced by less traumatic procedures, and in addition, regional cerebral blood flow (CBF) and metabolism have been studied.

Cerebral Blood Flow Changes with Age

Freyhan (1951) reported the now generally accepted observation that CBF is significantly reduced in patients with organic dementias and that there is a correlation between intellectual test scores and measurements of global CBF. Seymour (1956) developed an invasive nitrous oxygen technique to study CBF. He concluded that there were progressive blood flow changes with aging. Unfortunately, many of those he studied were hospitalized patients with chronic diseases. Subsequently, Dastur et al. (1963) attempted to rule out the effects of aging by selecting elderly subjects who were in excellent health. His study concluded that age per se cannot account for the decline in CBF. Underlying pathology was the primary culprit.

A few years later, the nitrous oxide technique was replaced by the inhalation method of xenon-133. This nontraumatic, noninvasive method for measuring CBF was particularly welcome since subjects were willing to participate in nonpainful, nonthreatening research. This method permits observation of regional blood flow and of the contrast between blood flow through the gray matter and that through white matter. Blood flow through the gray matter is faster than that through the white matter. A number of the studies that have been reported are concerned primarily with the fast-clearing component of gray matter (Busse and Wang 1985).

In a series of publications (Palmore et al. 1985) from the Duke University longitudinal studies on normal aging, it appears that elderly community residents have a significantly lower blood flow than young controls. These elderly "normal" subjects had a mean age of 80 years. Compared with that of demented patients, CBF of the elderly person is in relatively good condition. This was despite the fact that many of the demented patients were considerably younger (Busse and Wang 1985). The normal subjects were also studied for the relationship of intellectual performance, electroencephalogram (EEG), and CBF. A slower alpha frequency was found in subjects with reduced blood flow, and this in turn paralleled a decline in intellectual performance. The difference in Wechsler Adult Intelligence Scale scores was heavily influenced by a decline in the Performance scale as opposed to the Verbal scale. The deterioration quotient was .30 for the low CBF subjects, compared with 1.9 for the high CBF subjects. A slower alpha frequency was found in subjects with reduced blood flow. The alpha index was .93 for high CBF compared with 8.5 for reduced blood flow (Obrist et al. 1961).

Sex Differences in Cerebral Blood Flow

Mathew et al. (1985) report that age-related reduction in CBF was found to be most marked in the frontal region. Women had higher CBF than men, and the difference was most obvious in the frontal region. It has been observed that women do have a lower hematocrit. Although the authors confirm that women have a lower hematocrit, they do not believe that it is an adequate explanation for the higher CBF in women. In addition to the sex differences, the influence of age was found to be most significant in the frontal area bilaterally.

In an earlier article by Mathew et al. (1985) there is reference to differences in cerebral hemispheres. Unfortunately, they were using handedness as a determinant of dominance when most recent studies use the location of speech to determine which cerebral hemisphere is dominant. They say that other investigators have reported an increase in right hemisphere flow in right-handed people. That seems to be contradictory.

Cerebral Blood Flow and Metabolism Changes in Schizophrenia, Dementia, and Cognition

Mathew et al. (1986) claim that patients with schizophrenia show a lower metabolism in the frontal cortex and this is paralleled by a reduced metabolism of the left cortex. Mathew et al. (1986) they question the validity of these studies as well as other ones suggesting that depressed persons have an alteration in CBF. However, they confirm that most dementias, regardless of their underlying diagnosis, are associated with global reduction in both blood flow and metabolism; also, that the degree of reduction in CBF tends to correlate with impaired performance on psychologic tests.

As for PET, the literature (Mathew et al. 1985) reveals that CBF and oxygen metabolism are reduced in patients with Alzheimer's disease with multi-infarct dementia as compared with normal age matched controls. Again, this physiologic change decreases with losses of mental skills. It is also commented that a study of glucose metabolism is more useful than trying to measure ventricular dilatation by CT as evidence of Alzheimer's disease. This, of course, requires the availability of a PET.

Huntington's disease has also been studied. Kuhl et al. (1981) found a reduction in cerebral metabolism in both the frontal cortex and the corpus striatum.

Ingvar, in a commentary (Mathew et al. 1985), states that the reduction in CBF and metabolic measures in schizophrenia correlate better with so-called negative symptoms—the more negative symptoms, the more pronounced the reduction in blood flow. In contrast, in some patients with schizophrenia hallucinations result in supplemental or increased blood flow to postcentral parts of the cortex as well as in the occipital area.

Buchsbaum (Mathew et al. 1985) states that to adequately study brain function using a PET, a specific sensory condition or task must be given to all subjects since there is considerable variation if the task is not identical or at least similar.

Hoyer (Mathew et al. 1985) states that in Alzheimer's disease variations in CBF, including measures of oxygen and glucose consumption, in all probability reflect states of functional activity rather than indicate primary pathophysiologic abnormalities and differential diagnosis criteria. He also states that there is only a slight reduction in cerebral metabolic rate glucose beyond the age of 70 years in well-documented healthy elderly subjects.

Hoyer also says that the depressive reaction that confuses the possible presence of Alzheimer's disease and results in a type of pseudodementia is accompanied by a reduction in CBF and cerebral metabolism. The glucose metabolism is reduced to around 65 percent and oxygen metabolism to 80 percent.

Magnetic resonance imaging (MRI) permits more accurate definition of small infarcts, cortical atrophy, and ventrical enlargement compared with CT scanning. Magnetic resonance imaging allows better distinction among multi-infarct dementia, Alzheimer's disease, and Pick's disease. This author does not elaborate on how this difference can be observed.

Gur et al., in 1982, reviewed the CBF changes in dementia. Most dementias are associated with global reduction in blood flow and metabolism (Gur et al. 1982; Mathew et al. 1985). In addition, certain focal decreases of CBF are noted in dementias. Alzheimer's disease is associated with more marked decrease in postcentral CBF, while Pick's disease is characterized by a reduction involving the frontotemporal area. Consistent with the diagnosis of multi-infarct dementia is the finding of regional changes in CBF. Maximum CBF reduction is found in the posterior regions of the brain. In general the degree of reduction in regional CBF tends to correlate with impaired performance on psychologic tests; that is, the greater the reduction in CBF, the poorer the performance on psychologic tests.

Utilizing the 133 Xe inhalation technique, Gur et al. (1987) explored the relationship between age and regional CBF and activation by cognitive tasks. The sample consisted of 55 healthy subjects ranging in age from 18 to 72 years. The subjects were studied during rest and during the performance of verbal analysis and spatial orientation tasks. Indices of regional CBF of the gray matter and average regional CBF of both gray and white matter were obtained. They confirmed that with advancing age there is a reduction in blood flow, particularly in the anterior regions of the brain. Interestingly, the extent and pattern of regional CBF changes during cognition were *not* affected by age.

The data suggest that the effects of aging are more pronounced for gray matter profusion and, further, that CBF tends to be higher in women. No significant age and sex interactions were found. An attempt was made to control for hemisphere dominance. It was noted that the increase was relatively greater to the left hemisphere for the verbal tasks and to the right hemisphere for the spatial tasks. Gur et al. (1982) speculated that the differences in hemisphere differences, particularly in the anterior regions, may present some evidence that aging is associated with a reduction in "fluid intelligence." Fluid intelligence is usually associated with memory span, inductive reasoning, mental flexibility, and problem solving. In contrast, "crystallized intelligence" includes verbal comprehension, vocabulary, and fund of knowledge, and seems to be unaffected by aging.

Electroencephalographic Changes with Age

The normal human EEG undergoes progressive changes with age from birth through senescence. There are two distinct components of the normal adult EEG recorded while awake. The alpha rhythm, which is an 8- to 12-per-second rhythmic sine wave, gradually slows with advancing age of both males and females. The second component of normal adult EEG is beta rhythm, or low-voltage fast-activity (LVF) rhythm. Aging does not seem to have a clear impact on this particular rhythm.

Alpha Activity

The slowing of the alpha frequency is the most common change in EEGs recorded after the age of 60. Averaging of a large number of alpha waves is often referred to as the alpha index. This slowing takes place within the alpha range of 8 to 13 c/second. On the basis of results of several investigators, the frequency can be said to decline approximately 0.5 to 0.75 c/second each decade after age 60. Many EEG changes seem to reflect the health status of an individual. Therefore, it is plausible that excessive slowing within the alpha range in elderly adults may not only be the aging problem, but may be related to subclinical pathology. Alpha waves below 8 c/second are often related to demonstrated pathology.

Males in the Duke University longitudinal study were found to have a significantly lower mean alpha frequency than females of comparable age. For blacks and whites living in the United States there does not appear to be any difference in slowing accompanying aging. The alpha slowing within the normal range of 8 to 13 c/second found in elderly community subjects is not paralleled by changes in intellectual performance. In comparison with the young adult average of 10.0 to 10.5 c/second, the mean alpha frequency of mentally normal old subjects is significantly lower, reaching 9.0 to 9.5 c/second around age 70 and 8.5 to 9.0 c/second after age 80. This decline is greater among institutionalized aged patients, particularly those with cerebral vascular disease or neurologic disorders, where the frequency is often 8 c/second or less. Those with obvious dementia usually have frequencies of 7 c/second or less.

Individuals vary widely in the degree to which their EEGs manifest senescent changes. It does appear, however, that vascular disease is an important contributing factor. Patients with arteriosclerotic brain disease show not only a slowing of alpha but also a decline in CBF and cerebral metabolism. In this type of patient, a number of investigators have reported the degree of slowing as quantitatively related to impaired memory and to other aspects of intellectual functioning. This correlation is not nearly as consistent in subjects who remain in the community. It is possible that those who survive in the community are actually adjusting at a borderline level and may be vulnerable to environmental stress that would precipitate the appearance of organic brain disease. There is some evidence that this is true, but the vulnerability of such elderly people deserves greater attention.

A related matter that needs study is the hypothesis that the speed of information processing is dependent on brain wave frequencies. This possibility primarily stems from the work of Surwillo, who found a correlation between the stimulus response interval of a simple auditory reaction time and average duration of alpha waves (Surwillo 1963).

There are other alpha wave changes with aging. In normal young adults the frequency varies about one-tenth of the mean value. If the variation is greater, the rhythm is said to be unstable. If this criterion is applied to older subjects, many of them have unstable EEGs. This apparently has no demonstrated significance.

Several studies indicate that there is a relationship between alpha slowing and decreased longevity. This is not surprising when one recognizes the relationship between vascular disease and alpha slowing. Obrist (1980) showed that over a span of 5 to 7 years the alpha wave slowing in those who died was double that found in survivors. This result has been confirmed by Wang and Busse (1974) and Muller et al. (1975).

An important aspect of the senile EEG is its reaction to sensory stimulation. An alpha-blocking response to light or eye opening has been found to decrease with age in both psychiatric patients and normal subjects. Also, it is claimed that the habituation of the blocking response with repeated stimulation is faster and more complete in elderly community volunteers than in young controls. The magnitude of alpha attenuation, however, is apparently unrelated to motor response speed in normal elderly subjects (Thompson and Botwinick 1968).

Slowing of Theta and Delta Waves

Another common feature of EEG changes in late life, in addition to alpha slowing, is the appearance of scattered slow waves. A slight slowing of the alpha index with scattered 6 to 8 c/second waves is not pathognomonic for any particular disorders. A moderate amount of slowing within the theta range with some delta (i.e., the appearance of delta activity approximately 10 percent or more of the time) is characteristically found in brain disorders whether they are classified as degenerative or vascular in origin. It has been demonstrated that elderly subjects in good health are found to have a mean alpha occipital frequency that is almost a full cycle slower than that found in healthy young adults. Furthermore, about 7 percent of the EEGs in the elderly subjects manifest a dominant frequency of 6 to 8 c/second waves. A good correlation has been demonstrated between EEG frequency and cerebral oxygen consumption and/or CBF (Obrist et al. 1963). Therefore the slowing of the dominant frequency in the majority of elderly people is associated with a decline of cerebral metabolism. Diffuse slow activity, more than any other EEG variable, is related to senile intellectual deterioration. Institutionalized elderly subjects manifest a good correlation between diffuse EEG slowing and tests of cognitive function. This relationship, however, does not hold true in community volunteers, particularly those with borderline or mild slowing, since they do not demonstrate clear intellectual impairment. It is possible that psychologic tests are not sufficiently sensitive to early mental changes (Wang and Busse 1974).

In spite of these unanswered questions, EEG slowing is used to differentiate functional psychiatric disorders from organic mental diseases in old age. This distinction was first emphasized by Luce and Rothschild (1953), by Frey and Sjogren (1959), and by Obrist and Henry (1958). Obrist and Henry found that 70 percent of cases with diffuse slow activity were found to have organic brain syndrome, while 88 percent of those with normal EEGs had functional disorders consisting primarily of depressions and paranoid reactions. These same authors found that a majority of elderly people with diffuse slow activity required hospitalization or died within 1 year after the slow EEG was demonstrated.

Electroencephalogram, Blood Pressure, and Heart Disease

In 1961, a publication appeared linking electroencephalographic changes to blood pressure in elderly persons (Obrist et al. 1961). This study included a total of 233 hospitalized psychiatric patients age 60 or older and 261 of the subjects of the first Duke University longitudinal study. An average blood pressure was obtained by computing the geometric mean of the systolic and diastolic readings as determined by routine physical examination. When several EEG categories were plotted separately against mean blood pressure in the hospitalized group, it was found that the incidence of normal EEGs increased markedly as the blood pressure rose, while the number of diffuse slow and mixed abnormal EEGs was maximum with the lower blood pressure readings.

A similar correlation did not hold for the subjects in the first Duke University longitudinal study. The findings in this study of normal subjects suggested that a mild elevation of blood pressure may tend to preserve a normal EEG by maintaining adequate circulation to the brain, thus compensating for cerebral arteriosclerosis. It was speculated that the diffuse slow activity in many aged psychiatric patients results from the combination of a relatively low blood pressure and cerebral arteriosclerosis (Busse and Wang 1985).

Busse and Wang (1985) divided subjects from the first longitudinal study into four groups: (1) those without heart disease, (2) those who possibly had heart disease, (3) those with definite and compensated heart disease, and (4) those with definite and decomposed heart disease. This study revealed that EEG changes were significantly higher in the subjects with decompensated heart disease compared with those with compensated heart disease and those without heart disease. It was concluded that the brain impairment as evidenced by the EEG changes is probably due to a profound reduction of CBF, which is shown to be proportional to the reduction in cardiac output. Subjects with compensated heart disease also had a mild hypertension. These findings suggest that mild hypertension in some elderly patients may help to maintain the blood flow to the brain and hence to preserve the status of the brain, perhaps at the expense of the heart (Wang and Busse 1974). Sustained severe hypertension, however, is often associated with intellectual decline (Wilkie and Eisdorfer 1961).

Focal Electroencephalographic Abnormalities

The recognition that a relatively high percentage of elderly people had focal EEG abnormalities predominantly over the temporal areas of the brain first occurred in 1949 and 1950. In 1951, with the support of the National Institutes of Health, a research project was undertaken, specifically directed toward EEG changes in late life. This report was published in 1954 (Busse et al. 1954). Since that date, the observation that such foci are common in older people and appear gradually throughout adulthood has been reported by other investigators.

Busse et al. (1954) used three series of community subjects, separated according to socioeconomic criteria. A correlation was found between increased incidence of EEG disturbance and socioeconomic status. This finding is probably influenced by health variables. It has been repeatedly observed that 30 to 40 percent of apparently healthy people have temporal focal abnormalities predominantly on the left side of the brain. In residents of an old-age home, an even higher incidence of focal slowing, 50 percent, was reported by Mundy-Castle in 1962. This report was in agreement with the prior observation, since it indicated that maximum involvement was in the anterior temporal area and 75 percent of these foci were found on the left side. Furthermore, the most prominent foci occurred among normal old people with an adequate social adjustment. A high incidence of temporal lobe EEG alterations has been noted in a number of other studies involved with elderly hospitalized subjects (Harvald 1958; Frey and Sjogren 1959).

Barnes et al. (1956) contrasted community subjects with aged psychiatric patients. Elderly mentally ill patients were found to have a wider distribution of the temporal abnormality extending into the posterior and midtemporal areas. Among patients with organic brain syndrome, the focal changes often took the form of localized accentuated diffuse low activity. Those initial observations and conclusions, that is, that focal slow activity in the anterior temporal area is compatible with a good social adjustment in old age, have not been altered over the years. However, when the focus involves adjacent areas or is associated with a more diffuse disturbance, organic brain syndrome is probable.

In 1982 Kazis et al. also addressed the possible significance of temporal slowing in the EEG in old age. This study involved 2,085 inpatients who were from 60 to 92 years of age. Twenty-seven percent of those studied were found to have temporal abnormalities and 66 percent of these were on the left side. No normal or community living subjects were included. This study concluded that vascular disease contributed to the appearance of temporal focal abnormalities.

Some studies have not observed such a high incidence of temporal foci in elderly people. For example, Obrist, using a midtemporal placement with an ear reference, failed to demonstrate foci in more than a small percentage of aged subjects. Obrist believed that this points to the importance of electrode placement (Obrist 1954).

Temporal focal abnormalities and age of onset. Kooi et al. reported in 1964 similar findings related to EEG patterns of the temporal region in normal adults. These investigators studied 218 neurologically normal subjects who ranged in age from 26 to 81 years. They found an increasing incidence of temporal lobe irregularities with advancing age. In addition, Kooi et al. stated, "Detailed review of the comprehensive clinical data including analysis combining various medical findings reveals no evident medical factors responsible for the common type of temporal transients" (p. 1035). Shortly thereafter, Busse and Obrist made a similar report. Their study was based on 425 normal white volunteer subjects, including those derived from the longitudinal studies, with an age span of 20 to 80 years. It was found that foci occurred in 3.4 percent of subjects 20 to 29 years of age, 8 percent between ages 30 and 39, 20 percent between ages 40 and 49, 22 percent between ages 50 and 59, and 36 percent between ages 60 and 69, with a very gradual increase thereafter (Busse and Obrist 1965).

The dominant background activity and foci.   On the basis of cross-sectional study early in the first Duke University longitudinal study, it was found that an EEG with dominant alpha was found in 61 percent of the subjects. Sixteen percent had LVF activity, 15 percent were diffuse fast, and 7 percent diffuse slow. The average age of these subjects was slightly less than 70 years. As to age distribution and dominant activity, subjects under the age of 70 accounted for 75 percent of the diffuse fast but were not represented in the diffuse slow group. The mean age of subjects in the diffuse fast group was 66.7 years, but in the diffuse slow group it was 77.7 years. Subjects with dominant alpha and LVF activity frequencies were found throughout the age range and were equally divided between those over 70 and those under 70.

As to those with foci, 75 percent of subjects with diffuse slow EEGs had foci, as did 38 percent of those with alpha and 25 percent of the diffuse fast group. Of particular importance is that none of the LVF activity EEGs (normal) contained focal disturbances (Wang and Busse 1969).

Activation of temporal foci.   Hyperventilation tends to exacerbate temporal slowing that is already present, but it does not elicit new unsuspected foci. Passive tilting of the subject, starting from a prone position, does not exacerbate foci or elicit new ones. Electrocardiogram monitoring and blood pressure readings taken during this procedure indicate relatively little hypotensive effect. Five percent inhalation of CO_2 does not eliminate or reduce the severity of a temporal foci. Temporal foci are not reduced or eliminated while the subject is exposed to hyperbaric conditions, and there is no evidence of a change following hyperbaric exposure.

Drowsiness did influence the appearance of foci: 25 percent of foci appeared in a drowsy condition, thus increasing the usual percentage from 30 to 40 percent of subjects. In addition, existing foci became more evident during drowsiness (Busse and Obrist 1963).

The origin of foci.   It has been speculated that temporal foci may originate either from a lesion, possibly in the hippocampal region, or from a remote area outside the temporal lobe. Gershwind and Levitsky reported in 1968 that marked anatomic asymmetries exist between upper surfaces of the left and right temporal lobe in the human brain: The left temporal lobe is usually larger and longer than the right. There is also evidence to suggest that the temporal lobes, particularly the left one, are susceptible to vascular insufficiency.

Clinical implications of temporal foci.   Psychologic deficiencies have been suspected but have not been unequivocally confirmed. In one study involving the longitudinal study subjects, the EEG focus predominantly in the left temporal region was significantly associated with a decline in verbal but not in performance ability. This decline in verbal ability over a span of approximately 2½ years was greater in the focal group than in the nonfocal group (Wang et al. 1970). However, in another study, again involving elderly community subjects, Obrist selected 20 subjects with severe temporal foci and compared them with 20 age-matched cases having normal EEGs. No difference could be found in learning or memory, and survival 12 years later was approximately equal in the two groups (Obrist 1975).

Psychiatric implications of foci. Visser et al. (1987) reported a study correlating temporal lobe abnormalities in EEGs of normal subjects with psychopathologic measures and CT brain scans. Twenty-seven normal individuals between the ages of 65 and 83 years were examined. Fifty-nine percent (16) were found to have focal EEG abnormalities in their left frontal temporal area. Nearly all psychologic test scores were within normal limits for all subjects. However, the scores were lower in the subjects with focal abnormalities compared with those without focal abnormalities. The authors caution that they cannot say that any real deterioration was found in subjects with temporal lobe abnormalities although they were on the low side of the normal range. In a somewhat similar fashion they found "a trend to abnormality" in CT brain scans including a slight dilatation of the third ventricle.

Low-Voltage Fast Activity

Some electroencephalograph researchers do not believe that the beta activity is synonymous with LVF. Chatrian and Lairy (1976) believe that their definition excludes the LVF described by Gibbs and Gibbs (1950), which is characterized by nonrhythmic amorphous fast activity usually not exceeding 10 μv in amplitude. The Duke University longitudinal studies used as the criterion for normal LVF activity all fast waves below 20 μv with no countable frequency. Low-voltage fast activity is considered synonymous with beta activity and is distinguished from F1 and F2 records, which are considered synonymous with gamma activity. Gamma is now considered an obsolete classification; consequently, LVF or beta activity is a type of normal brain wave that includes frequencies above the alpha range usually between 18 and 30 c/second with diminished voltage. Low-voltage fast activity is more often found in the anterior regions of the brain. When it periodically appears in posteriors of the brain, it is disrupting an alpha rhythm and is usually associated with an attention response. The amount of LVF activity appears to be a reflection of the state of arousal in the longitudinal study subjects. It is evident that in the early part of the routine recording in the longitudinal study, LVF is much more in evidence. As the examination progresses, alpha activity not only becomes more prominent in the posterior leads but also spreads anteriorly, replacing varying amounts of LVF.

Complicating the distinction of LVF from beta activity is the separation of beta into two or three types. These types of beta activity are said to occur in some unmedicated, apparently normal adult human subjects. Chatrian and Lairy (1976) separated beta into three types: (1) a central or frontal central rhythm of frequency as high as 30 c/second that is selectively blocked by contralateral movement or touch of moderate intensity, (2) a diffuse beta rhythm frequently between 20 and 25 c/second that is not selectively blocked by any stimulus, and (3) a posterior beta rhythm of 14 to 19 c/second that is selectively blocked by visual stimulus of moderate intensity and mental activity. The diffuse beta potentials can be produced or enhanced by a wide variety of drugs. Chatrian and Lairy (1976) are convinced that none of the three beta rhythms correlates with any psychologic variable or personality traits in normal adults.

Dondey and Gaches (1976) recognized two types of beta activity. The first is referred to as either diffuse or frontal beta activity and is usually under 30 μv in amplitude and between 25 and 40 c/second with a larger amplitude. It is symmetrical although often not synchronous, and it is distinguished from frontal and diffuse beta activity by the fact that it is blocked by voluntary movement or imaginary voluntary movement and also by tactile stimuli. The rolandic beta activities are related to rolandic cortical activities. The frontal and diffuse beta are increased by drugs, as noted by Dondey and Gaches. Cobb (1976) also supported the idea of three types of beta activity. Cobb believed, however, that the occipital beta or fast rhythm is actually a type of fast alpha rhythm since it is usually in the range of 14 to 18 c/second.

Chatrian and Lairy (1976) concluded that there is no adequate evidence of any relationship between normal and excessive beta activity in any psychiatric or neurologic disorder. They speculated that it might be of use when it does not appear in a localized area as the result of a usually drug-induced type of beta activity. Similarly, in another type of drug (for example, Thorazine), the appearance of fast potentials, particularly unilaterally, may give some evidence of a pathological process in the brain. *Mu* is used to designate an apparent subharmonic variant of rolandic beta rhythm. It differs from beta activity in that its frequency is usually between 7 and 11 c/second and it has an arched form (Duterte 1977). Chatrian and Lairy (1976) further concluded that no convincing proof has been conducted so far "suggesting that the presence of 'Mu' waves correlates with psychological variables and personality traits, or normal or mentally ill subjects of psychiatric diagnosis" (p. 30).

Fast Activity—Gamma Waves

Fast waves are above the alpha range and are distinguished from LVF activity on the basis of amplitude and to some degree by regularity. The frequency of fast activity is confined to a relatively narrow spectrum, and its amplitude usually exceeds 25 μv. The original Gibbs EEG adult standards and classification were the initial bases for all interpretations (Gibbs and Gibbs 1950). Hence fast activity included F1 and F2. Evaluations of F1 included determination of amplitude and frequency, the percentage of time it is present, and the number of leads in which it appears. F2 was considered an excessive amount of diffuse fast activity. A greater incidence of fast tracings in females was reported by Mundy-Castle in 1951 and by Vogel in 1965. The amount of fast activity present in normal females increases in young adulthood, reaches a peak at late middle life, and then gradually declines. This fast activity appears predominantly over the precentral areas of both hemispheres and is rarely associated with Mu rhythms (Busse and Obrist 1965). Busse and Obrist (1965) reported that women between the ages of 20 and 39 years have an incidence of 8 percent fast activity. Between the ages of 40 and 59 this increases to 26 percent, and thereafter it does not increase. From age 60 until age 79, there is a decrease to 23 percent. After the age of 80, in females the amount of fast activity appears to begin a gradual decline. That hormonal changes may play a role in the development of fast rhythms in middle-aged females has been suggested by McAdam and Robinson (1956), who observed a significantly greater amount of beta activity in postmenstrual as opposed to premenstrual women. It is evident, however, that the increase in females previously described suggests that if it is hormonally related, it is not directly tied to the menopause.

Thompson and Wilson (1966) suggested that fast activity is associated with superior learning. Obrist (1975) added that the presence of fast activity in the EEGs of elderly persons can probably be regarded as a favorable sign, affecting both longevity and mental capacity. In contrast, fast activity is rarely found in deteriorated senile patients (Obrist 1975).

Roubicek (1977) studied the frequency and amount of fast activity in elderly women. He divided the whole beta band into two parts: 12 to 25 c/second and 25 to 45 c/second. With advancing age, the lower portion of the band, 12 to 25 c/second, continually decreased in abundance, while the percentage of the waves above 25 c/second either did not change or slightly increased. Roubicek believes that the different patterns of change found in these fast waves is probably a sign of diverse physiologic meaning of the waves under and above 25 c/second. He believes that there are at least two unidentified generating sites that influence these different spectra of fast activity.

The Clinical Use of Quantitative Electroencephalographic Techniques

Quantitative EEG techniques include frequency analysis, topographic mapping, statistical comparisons with a normal data base, and other computer-based calculations or displays of EEGs or evoked potential. According

to the American Electroencephalographic Society (1987), "The clinical application of quantitative EEG is considered to be limited and adjunctive" (p. 75).
At the present time these techniques are useful in research, rather than
clinically. Unfortunately, the techniques used in this field vary greatly among
laboratories and so the clinical utility of one technique may not be applicable
in another setting and in another technique. The American Electroencephalographic Society stated, "At present there is no justification for stand-alone
computer-based clinical EEG analysis" (1987, p. 75).

Normal Sleep: Stages and Physiologic Correlates

Sleep patterns change throughout the life span (Kales and Kales 1984).
Normal sleep is usually divided into REM (rapid eye movement) and nonREM
sleep. NonREM sleep has four stages. Stage 1 starts with drowsiness that
moves to light sleep. This stage is a transition stage and is characterized by
slow eye movements and low-amplitude fast waves mixed with scattered slow
waves. Muscle artifact is not unusual during light sleep or drowsiness. Stage 2
is also characterized by mixed frequencies but with increasing amount of
slow waves and the appearance of characteristic sleep spindles, brief runs, or
bursts of 12 to 14 c/second waves. K complexes are a distinctive stimulus
response that can appear during Stage 2. Stages 3 and 4 are periods dominated by slow waves. Stage 3 also is made up of theta waves, usually of 4 to 7
c/second. Stage 4 is characterized by delta waves of 4 or less per second and
often in the range of 1 to 2 per second. Stage 4 is usually considered the
deepest stage of sleep, and the amount of this stage of sleep decreases with
advancing age. It is virtually absent in some elderly subjects.

During the normal nocturnal sleep cycle, brief periods of wakefulness
develop. Children, adolescents, and young adults will have brief periods of
awakening and usually have no recall for the event. Unfortunately, periods of
awakening become very frequent in late life, and many times the elderly
person not only recalls being awake, but experiences varying degrees of
difficulty returning to sleep.

Rapid eye movement sleep occupies 20 to 25 percent of total sleep time.
In adulthood the first REM period of sleep occurs approximately 70 to 100
minutes after the onset of nocturnal sleep. Because normal sleep follows a
definite cycle, periods of REM sleep appear approximately four times per
night. Although the number of REM periods does not appear to change with
advancing age, often one finds that the duration of the REM periods becomes
essentially the same in elderly people. In young adults, the REM portion of
sleep increases in length over the night of sleep. The basic pattern during
REM sleep is not unlike that found in Stage 1.

As to physiologic correlates, temperature regulation appears to be controlled differently during REM sleep than in nonREM sleep (see Chapter 18).
There are also other measurable differences between REM and nonREM

sleep. As one progresses through the stages of nonREM sleep and the slow waves increase in frequency and amplitude, there is a decrease in blood pressure, heart rate, cardiac output, respiratory rate, whole body and brain temperature, total body oxygen consumption, and other changes that affect the excretion of neurotransmitters and neuropeptides. In nonREM sleep, growth hormone is secreted early in the night during Stages 3 and 4. This growth hormone type of secretion is contrasted with corticosteroids that are likely to be excreted during REM sleep late in the night. Rapid eye movement sleep is usually associated with dreaming, and during this period many of the physiologic changes are distinctly different from those that occur during nonREM sleep. When there is an elevation in body and brain temperature there is a faster firing for neurons in the brain and an increase in CBF. There is also an increase in oxygen consumption. Penile erections also occur in conjunction with REM sleep.

As previously mentioned, neurotransmitter secretion and activity alter during stages of sleep. Serotonin has long been believed to have a role in sleep induction and there have been attempts to use the precursor of serotonin, L-tryptophan, which can be given orally to improve sleep and alter the negative impact of so-called jet-lag (Schneider-Helmert and Spinweber 1986). Spinweber et al. (1987) report positive results with sparing of defects of short-term memory, rapid recovery of reaction-time performance, and increased total sleep time on the first night after arrival.

How Much Sleep?

How many hours of sleep are required for an individual to function effectively remains, at last in part, unanswered. It is evident that most elderly people tend to sleep less as they grow older, but often spend more time in bed. Elderly individuals with hypersomnia are often found to have physical disorders that underlie this particular symptom (Kales and Kales 1984). In younger adults, several studies have been carried out to determine differences between long and short sleepers. Such studies would be extremely important to determine the difference between long sleepers and those who spend considerable time in bed. Long sleepers may not be associated with increased psychopathology as reported by at least one study (Hartmann et al. 1972), while it is quite possible that those who spend excessive periods of time in bed are using a method of avoidance of reality problems rather than excessive time in fantasy. Such a debate can only be resolved by all-night polygraphic recordings in a sleep laboratory. To obtain accuracy, Kales and Kales (1984) recommend that several consecutive nights of recordings be conducted. A study reports that Type A behavior is likely to be associated with short sleepers (Hicks et al. 1979). Short sleepers do have a reduction in Stage 2, while they have just as much Stages 3 and 4 as those who sleep 7 to 8 hours per night. Short-term sleepers are usually considered to have 5.5 hours of sleep per night or less. Extremely short-term sleepers spend much of their sleep time in Stages 3 and 4.

The Significance of Changes in Sleep Stages

The importance to psychophysiologic functioning of the various stages of sleep has been given attention and it is evident that certain stages are accompanied by other physiologic changes. Rapid eye movement sleep is often considered to have a critical role in memory and learning. For this reason, the amount of REM sleep has been looked at in elderly people (Prinz 1985). Prinz found that in subjects 70 to 90 years of age greater amounts of REM were associated with stable intellectual functioning, while lower REM sleep levels were related to cognitive decline. Other investigators have advanced the notion that REM sleep activates a reverse learning process (Crick and Mitchison 1983). In short, these investigators say that we gain in order to forget. Other theories hold that REM sleep is accompanied by protein synthesis and adds to the capacity of the brain to function normally. It does appear that the amount and percentage of REM sleep are reduced in mentally retarded people (Feinberg et al. 1969; Petre-Quadens and Jouver 1966).

Sleep Electroencephalogram and Cognition

With the passage of time there are changes in cognitive function and in sleep patterns. Numerous reports have indicated that a correlation exists between certain types of sleep changes and the preservation or the decline in intellectual functioning. For example, Berry and Webb (1985) report a decline in the Ravens score and waking after sleep onset. These authors believe that their work suggests that the variations in cognitive functioning remain independent of somatic functioning as measured by sleep changes until critical thresholds of deterioration in the somatic tissues are reached, either through disease or trauma. When a critical threshold is reached, they believe, there is a stronger relationship between sleep and cognitive variables. The authors, however, state that this hypothesis is not critically tested in their study. They refer to their idea as the discontinuity hypothesis, that is, a lack of relations between cognitive and somatic variables until critical levels of deterioration are exceeded (Roth 1986).

Coherence in Power and Dementia Electroencephalogram

O'Connor et al. (1979) compared power and coherence measures using computer techniques to compare various types of dementia. On the basis of these studies, they believe that these EEG measures reflected a diffuse pathology involved with senile dementia, but identified focal pathology with arteriosclerotic patients.

Kazniak et al. (1979) reported that EEG slowing was the strongest and the most general pathologic influence on cognition in elderly persons without organic brain disease. In those with cerebral atrophy, verbal recall of recent and remote information was the important feature. (No mention is made of the EEG patterns seen in those with cerebral atrophy.)

Minimum Technical Standards for Electroencephalographic Recording and Suspected Cerebral Death

In 1970 the first minimal standard for EEG recording in suspected cerebral deaths was published (International Federation of Electroencephalography 1986a). Subsequently improved EEG instrumentation and the experience of many laboratories have resulted in a revised guideline. This review of the minimal standards for determining brain death is for general information only and is not a complete account. Cerebral death is now designated as electrocerebral inactivity or electrocerebral silence (ECS). ECS is defined as no electrical activity over 2 μV when recording from scalp electrode pairs 10 or more centimeters apart with interelectrode impedances under 10,000 ohms, but over 100 ohms.

Those responsible for recording and judging suspected cerebral death should refer to guideline 3 in the *Journal of Clinical Neurophysiology*. At the present time telephone transmission of EEG cannot be used for determination of ECS in the diagnosis of brain death because of the frequent and unpredictable electrical noise in telephone networks. It is recommended that a minimum of eight scalp electrodes be used; more may be necessary to make certain that the absence of activity is not a focal phenomenon.

As to impedance, it should be remembered that unmatched electrode impedance may distort the EEG. The integrity of the entire recording system must be tested and attention should be given to the filtering systems. Of particular importance is the fact that the international system of electrode placement for ordinary clinical studies is not recommended because the average adult interelectrode distances are between 6 and 6.5 cm. It is to be recalled that longer electrode distances are recommended.

Special attention should be given to the sensitivity of the recording instruments. Much of the contemporary, improved equipment permits extended recording at a sensitivity of 1.5 or 1.0 μV per μV/mm. A single recording should be at least 30 minutes long to be certain that intermittent low-voltage cerebral activity is not missed. In general, it appears to be sensible to do at least two 30-minute recordings. Periods of what appears to be ECS can occur and last up to 20 minutes in low-voltage records (Jorgensen 1974). Unfortunately, there is a wide range of artifacts that can interfere with adequate recording. Electrocardiogram artifact is commonly found in an otherwise ECS record. Ordinarily event-related responses are not a problem, but other types of stimuli can distort the record, such as airway suctioning and other nursing procedures. Patients who have suffered massive overdoses of nervous system depressants may recover from what appeared to be ECS. Obviously the possibility of a drug overdose must be given special attention.

As to the status of evoked potentials in brain-dead patients, median nerve short-latency somatosensory evoked potentials (SSEPs) were studied in patients who met all criteria required for declaring a person brain dead. Certain components of the evoked potential, P13-P14 and N20, were absent in all scalp–scalp channels, although three patients showed P13-P14 in scalp–noncephalic channels. This suggests that this is simply another way of determining the status of any residual brain functioning in patients considered to be brain dead (Belsh and Chokroverty 1987).

Reviewing Electroencephalogram Reports

The practitioner should be aware that guideline 8 of the American Electroencephalograph Society requires that an EEG report consist of three principal parts. The first is an introduction that starts with a statement of the kind of preparation the patient had, if any, for the recording situation. It should note that if the patient has received any medication or any other preparation such as sleep deprivation the state of consciousness and alertness at the time of recording should be documented. The description of the EEG should include all of the characteristics of the recording, both normal and abnormal. This description should be objective, avoiding any judgment. The final component (the interpretation) should include a statement by the interpreter regarding the abnormality or normality of the record followed by a clinical correlation. This correlation should attempt to explain how the EEGs fit or do not fit the total clinical picture.

Summary

Major changes found in the awake EEG of relatively normal elderly persons living in the community are progressive slowing of the alpha rhythm, appearance of fast rhythms in aging females, and development of foci, predominantly in the left anterior temporal region, in approximately one-third of the subjects. Neither the slowing of the alpha frequency within the normal range of 8 to 12 c/second nor the temporal lobe foci can be consistently correlated with intellectual decline, health, or longevity. The increase in fast waves in females, however, may be related to better learning abilities.

Evoked and Event-Related Potentials

The term "evoked potential" is usually used to designate the responses of sensory pathways to sensory or electrical stimuli. "Event-related" potentials are electrical responses to a variety of identifiable events including sensory stimulation, electrical excitation, movement, or other identifiable events. Event-related potentials appear only when the stimulus has meaning for the subject and is alert to the stimulus. The event-related potentials have relatively prolonged latency (see below) and are of largest amplitude overlying the parietal and posterior frontal lobes. In clinical practice, sensory evoked potentials may be used to assess peripheral sensory function, to evaluate the functional integration of sensory projection pathways in the central nervous system, or both (International Federation of Electroencephalography 1986b). The recording of a normal sensory evoked response does not guarantee that the information transmitted is used by the subject. Comatose patients may not respond to an acoustic or visual stimulus but have normal evoked potentials, thus showing that the afferent pathway is intact but is useless for the patient (Goodin et al. 1978).

Evoked potentials are of small amplitude and are usually recorded by noninvasive methods in humans. Computer summation or averaging generally is necessary to resolve them from background "noise" (Stockard et al. 1977). Noise is predominantly the spontaneous electrical activity which is associated with electroencephalography. Signal amplification is a necessity and the customary methods of averaging many trials should be standard practice.

The Characteristics of an Evoked Response

Evoked response is recorded and displayed as a series of electrical waves that, according to the type of evoked potential, vary in form, polarity, frequency, duration, and latency to onset. Further, observations may include interpeak intervals, threshold level, peak amplitude, amplitude ratio, absence of waves, and so on.

Clinical diagnosis frequently requires that measures obtained in individual patients be compared to a population composed of either normals or persons who are carrying a specific clinical diagnosis. The setting of normal limits is usually a decision made by an individual laboratory or investigator.

There are several types of short-latency evoked potentials. Visual system evoked potentials are electrophysiologic responses of the retina and the optic pathways to an appropriate stimulus. Included in visual stimulus evoked potentials are two categories of events: the electroretinogram and cerebral visual evoked potentials. The short-latency auditory evoked potentials are used to detect and approximately locate dysfunctions of the auditory projection pathways. Short-latency auditory evoked potentials are early electrical responses. The auditory pathways that appear in normal subjects are somewhere between 10 and 15 msec of an appropriate acoustic stimulus. Again, there are two categories: (1) the electrocochleogram and (2) the brainstem auditory evoked potentials (BAEPs) or brainstem evoked response (Stockard et al. 1977). The electrocochleogram consists of an electrical response of the cochlea and the auditory nerve to acoustic stimulation. The BAEPs are responses to the auditory nerve, brainstem, and possibly higher subcortical structures to acoustic stimulation. Unfortunately, both these terms are somewhat inappropriate since the primary auditory fibers, rather than the cochlear structure, play a role in the most prominent component of the electrocochleogram and the first component of the BAEP does not develop from the activity in the brainstem, but rather from the auditory nerve. It is the late components of the response that are associated with the brainstem.

All types of responses have certain characteristics; the BAEP that occurs within 10 msec of an appropriate acoustic stimulus consists of up to seven positive waves. The first wave is held by some to arise from the acoustic nerve, the second wave from the cochlear nuclei (medulla), the third from the superior olivary complex (pons), the fourth from the lateral lemniscus (pons), the fifth from the inferior colliculus (mid-brain), the sixth from the medial geniculate (thalamus), and the final (seventh) wave from the thalamocortical auditory radiations (Stockard et al. 1977). The latter waves, which are believed to arise from specific relays in the white matter, are potential points of delay; however, no age-related slowing in central nerve transmission time has been indexed by the BAEP (Harkins 1987). Alterations that do take place in slowing of BAEPs are held to be more health related than attributable to aging.

Another type of evoked potential is the SSEP. These early electrophysiologic responses are the result of appropriate stimulation of somatosensory pathways. A number of body sites can be elected to be used as the site of stimulation for various types of stimuli. Major mixed nerve trunks are easily accessible and therefore are often employed for clinical studies. Short-latency somatosensory evoked potentials occur within 25 to 50 msec of the stimulus.

Clinical Application of Evoked Potentials

The recommended standards for short-latency evoked potentials are limited to their neurologic applications. Sensory evoked potentials may be used to assess peripheral nerve function or to evaluate the functional integrity of sensory projection pathways in the central nervous system. Evoked potentials can play a major role in clinical neurology, allowing identification of local lesions in the central nervous system. Evoked responses are often classified as short latency (occurring within 10 to 15 msec after the stimuli), middle latency (from 15 to 80 msec), or long latency (of approximately 100 msec).

Other classes of sensory evoked potentials, particularly those that occur approximately 30 to 300 msec following an auditory, visual, or somatosensory stimulus, have under certain circumstances been reported to alter with advancing age. A study of the effects on pattern electroretinograms and visual evoked potentials (Celesia et al. 1987) concluded that age changes are found in latency and amplitude. These age-related changes are multifactorial, involving eye optics altered by the aging processes. One important factor is the aging of the retinal neurocircuitry.

Important to cognitive function is one component of an event-related response to a stimulus. This is a positive evoked potential at approximately 30 msec (P300 or P3) that appears following the absence of an expected tone. This occurs when a series of tones is presented in a fixed order and then, after repeated exposure to a series of tones, omission of a tone occurs. If the subject is alert to the absence of this tone, a P300 is likely to occur. The appearance of the P300 is believed to be related to psychologic variables. The P300 in cognitively impaired elderly is reported to be reduced in amplitude with prolonged latency (Harkins 1987).

Negative and Positive Components

The latency of late positive component (LPC), or P300, is thought to mark the completion of the processes of evaluating a stimulus (Busse and Maddox 1985).

A recent report studied the long-latency auditory evoked potential in demented patients with clinically definitive Huntington's disease, Parkinson's disease, and Alzheimer's disease (Goodin and Aminoff 1986). These evoked potential wave forms were in response to frequent and rare tone, not an absent tone. They found significant differences between each of these types of dementia. They were particularly interested in the P300 (P3) component of the longer latency evoked potential. The response to the rare tone was complex. They found, when using normal controls, the components N1, N2, and P3 became progressively longer with increasing age. They believe that their findings suggest a uniform slowing of neuronal transmission with increasing age. In the three patient populations, Alzheimer's disease showed a prolongation of latency of the N2 and P3 components relative to the normal subject but normal N1 and P2 latencies. The patients with Parkinson's and Huntington's diseases showed not only a greater delay in the N2 and P3 but in addition a prolongation of latency of N1 and P2 (Kutas and Hillyard 1984). In addition, 17 percent of the patients lacked N2 and P3 components. Further analysis of the pattern of electrophysiologic response permitted the investigators to correctly identify most of the patients as to type of dementia using a logistic regression model.

Event-related potential associated with the ability to process information appears to be altered by experience and training. Naive subjects respond differently than those with experience and training. The inexperienced group produced a greater amplitude response at the parietal site, while the experienced group showed greater amplitude at the frontal site (N1–P2 and P200). Kobus et al. (1987) suggest that the increased amplitude at the frontal site by the experienced group is related to decision making.

It is obvious that numerous skillful investigators are convinced that evoked potentials will be demonstrated to have great research and expanded clinical value. Recently no major breakthroughs have occurred, but steady progress is being made (Morihisa 1987).

Medications and Evoked Potentials

Bromm (1984) is of the opinion that the evaluation of pain-related evoked potentials holds the best prospects to quantify pain and pain relief in humans. However, he cautions that the distortions common to evoked potential studies must be controlled such as attention, level of arousal, news value of the stimulus, and so forth. Correlation between the late pain evoked potential and verbal reports of pain have been studied in many investigations (Bromm 1984). These amplitudes are obviously diminished under narcotics and even under weak analgesics.

Chapman and Jacobson (1984) express reservations regarding the usefulness of evoked potentials as an approach to assessment of analgesic states. For these investigators, one of the negative features is the lack of understanding of the neurophysiology that underlies evoked poentials. It is extremely difficult to arrive at unequivocal conclusions about generator sites, and there may be multiple generators for the information inherent in a single long-latency wave form. Buchsbaum (1984) found that the somatosensory evoked potential amplitude is diminished with common analgesics such as aspirin and morphine. The amplitude is increased by the opiate antagonist naloxone. He notes that additional information will be generated by studies of simultaneous glucose metabolic rate from PET and evoked potentials.

Deanol is a drug that is believed to be a precursor to acetylcholine. Deanol and a placebo were given over a period of 4 weeks to evaluate the effect of this precursor on cognitive function. No improvements on any of the cognitive tests were shown by subjects receiving the drug. However, the event-related potentials were enhanced in amplitude for subjects receiving the drug in several of the tests. No ready explanation of this dissociation between the lack of any discernible behavioral response or change and the alteration in the event-related potential can be offered (Busse and Maddox 1985).

References

American Electroencephalographic Society: Statement on the clinical use of quantitative EEG. J. Clinical Neurophysiol 1987; 4:75

Barnes RH, Busse EW, Friedman EL: The psychological functioning of aged individuals with normal and abnormal electroencephalograms. II. A study of hospitalized individuals. J Nerv Ment Dis 1956; 124:585–593

Belsh JM, Chokroverty S: Short-latency somatosensory evoked potentials in brain-dead patients. Electroencephalogr Clin Neurophysiol 1987; 68:75–78

Berry DTR, Webb WB: Sleep and cognitive functions in normal older adults. J Gerontol 1985; 40:331–335

Bromm B: Measurement of pain in man, in Pain Measurement in Man: Neurophysiological Correlates of Pain. Edited by Bromm B. Amsterdam, Elsevier, 1984

Buchsbaum MF: Quantification of analgesic effects by evoked potentials, in Pain Measurement in Man: Neurophysiological Correlates of Pain. Edited by Bromm B. Amsterdam, Elsevier, 1984

Busse EW, Barnes RH, Silverman AJ, et al: Studies of the processes of aging: factors that influence the psyche of elderly persons. J Psychiatry 1954; 110:897–903

Busse EW, Maddox GL: The Duke Longitudinal Studies of Normal Aging 1955–1980. New York, Springer, 1985

Busse EW, Obrist WD: Significance of focal electroencephalographic changes in the elderly. Postgrad Med 1963; 34:179–182

Busse EW, Obrist WD: Presenescent electroencephalographic changes in normal subjects. J Gerontol 1965; 20:315–320

Busse EW, Wang HS: Cerebral blood flow changes with age, in Normal Aging III. Edited by Palmore E, Busse EW, Maddox GL, et al. Durham, NC, Duke University Press, 1985.

Busse EW, Wang HS: Electroencephalographic changes in late life, in Normal Aging III. Edited by Palmore E, Busse EW, Maddox GL, et al. Durham, NC, Duke University Press, 1985

Celesia GG, Kaufman D, Cone S: Effects of age and sex on pattern electroretinograms and visual evoked potentials. Electroencephalogr Clin Neurophysiol 1987; 68:161–171

Chapman CR, Jacobson RC: Assessment of analgesic states: can evoked potentials play a role?, in Pain Measurement in Man: Neurophysiological Correlates of Pain. Edited by Bromm B. Amsterdam, Elsevier, 1984

Chatrian GE, Lairy GC: Typical normal rhythms and significant variants, in Handbook of Electroencephalography and Clinical Neurophysiology (Volume 6, Section 1). Edited by Remond A. Amsterdam, Elsevier, 1976

Cobb WA: EEG interpretation in clinical medicine, in Handbook of Electroencephalography and Clinical Neurophysiology (Volume 2, Section 11). Edited by Remond A. Amsterdam, Elsevier, 1976

Crick F, Mitchison G: The function of dream sleep. Nature 1983; 304:111–114

Dastur DK: Effects of aging and cerebral circulation and metabolism in man, in Human Aging: A Biological and Behavioral Study [Public Health Service Publicaton No. 986]. Edited by Birren J. Washington, DC, U.S. Government Printing Office, 1963

Dekoninck WJ: Brain metabolism and aging, in Thresholds in Aging. Edited by Bergener M, Ermini M, Stahelin HB. London, Academic Press, 1985

Dondey M, Gaches J: Semiology in clinical EEG, in Handbook of Electroencephalography and Clinical Neurophysiology (Volume 6, Section 1). Edited by Remond A. Amsterdam, Elsevier, 1976

Duterte F: Catalogue of the main EEG patterns, in Handbook of Electroencephalography and Clinical neurophysiology (Volume 2, Part A). Edited by Remond A. Amsterdam, Elsevier, 1976

Feinberg I, Braun M, Shulman E: EEG sleep patterns in mental retardation. Electroencephalogr Clin Neurophysiol 1969; 27:128–141

Frey TS, Sjogren H: The electroencephalogram in the elderly persons suffering from neuropsychiatric disorders. Acta Psychiatr Scand 1959; 34:438–450

Freyhan FA, Woodford RB, Kety SS: Cerebral blood flow and metabolism in psychoses of senility. J. Nerv Ment Dis 1951; 113:449–496

Gershwind N, Levitsky W: Human brain: left asymmetries in temporal speech region. Science 1968; 161:187–197

Gibbs FA, Gibbs EL: Atlas of Electroencephalography: Volume 1. Methodology and Controls. Cambridge, MA, Addison-Wesley, 1950

Goodin DS, Aminoff MJ: Electrophysiological differences between subtypes of dementia. Brain 1986; 109:1103–1113

Goodin DS, Squires KC, Starr A: Long latency event-related components of the auditory evoked potential in dementia. Brain 1978; 101:635–648

Gur RC, Gur RE, Obrist WD, et al: Sex and handedness differences in cerebral blood flow during rest and cognitive activity. Science 1982; 217:659–661

Gur RC, Gur RE, Obrist WD, et al: Age and regional cerebral blood flow at rest and during cognitive activity. Arch Gen Psychiatry 1987; 44:617–621

Harkins SW: Evoked potentials, in Encyclopedia on Aging. Edited by Maddox GL. New York, Springer 1987

Hartmann E, Baekeland F, Zwilling G: Psychological differences between long and short sleepers. Arch Gen Psychiatry 1972; 26:463–468

Harvald B: EEG in old age. Acta Psychiatr Scand 1958; 33:193–196

Hicks RA, Pellegrini RJ, Martin S, et al: Type A behavior and normal habitual sleep duration. Bulletin of the Psychonomic Society 1979; 14:185–186

Hillyard SA, Kutas M: Electrophysiology of cognitive processing. Annu Rev Psychol 1983; 34:33–61

International Federation of Electroencephalography: Guideline three: minimum technical standards for EEG recording and suspected cerebral death. J Clin Neurophysiol 1986a; 3(Suppl 1):12–17

International Federation of Electroencephalography: Recommended standards for the clinical practice of evoked potential. J Clin Neurophysiol 1986b; 3(Suppl 1):45–49

Jorgensen EO: Requirements for recording the EEG as high sensitivity in suspected brain death. Electroencephalogr Clin Neurophysiol 1974; 36:65–69

Kales A, Kales JD: Evaluation and Treatment of Insomnia. New York, Oxford University Press, 1984

Kazis A, Karlovasitou A, Xafenias D: Temporal slow activity of the EEG in old age. Archiv fuer Psychiatrie und Nervenkrankheiten 1982; 231:547–554

Kazniak AW, Garron DC, Fox JH, et al: Cerebral atrophy, EEG slowing, age, education, and cognitive functioning in suspected dementia. Neurology 1979; 29:1273–1279

Kety SS: Human cerebral blood flow and oxygen consumption as related to aging. Research Publications (Association for Research in Nervous and Mental Disease) 1955; 35:31–45

Kobus DA, Beeler MJ, Strashower K: Electrophysiological Effects of Experience During an Auditory Task. Report No. 87–2. Washington, DC, Naval Health Research Center, 1987

Kooi DA, Güvener AM, Tupper CJ, et al: Electroencephalographic patterns of the temporal region in normal adults. Neurology 1964; 14:1029–1035

Kutas M, Hillyard SA: Event-related potentials in cognitive sciences, in Handbook of Cognitive Neurosciences. Edited by Gaxzangia. New York, Plenum Press, 1984

Luce RA, Rothschild D: The correlation of electroencephalographic and clinical observations in psychiatric patients over 65. J Gerontol 1953; 8:167–172

Mathew RJ, Margolin RA, Kessler RM: Cerebral function, blood flow, and metabolism: a new vista in psychiatric research. Integr Psychiatry 1985; 3:214–225

Mathew R, Wilson W, Tant R: Determinants of resting regional CBF in normal subjects. Biological Psychiatry 1986; 21:907–914

Mazziotta JC, Phelps ME, Pahl JJ, et al: Reduced cerebral glucose metabolism in asymptomatic subjects at risk for Huntington's disease. N Engl J Med 1987; 316(7):357–362

McAdam W, Robinson R: Senile intellectual deterioration and the electroencephalogram. J Ment Sci 1956; 102:819–825

McIlwain H, Bacholard HS: The chemical composition of the brain, in Biochemistry and the Central Nervous System, (fourth edition). London, Churchill Livingstone, 1971

Morihisa JM: Functional brain imaging techniques, in Psychiatry Update: American Psychiatric Association Annual Review (Volume 6). Edited by Hales RE, France AJ. Washington, DC American Psychiatric Press, 1987

Muller HF, Grad B, Engelsmann F: Biological and psychological predictors of survival in a psychogeriatric population. J Gerontol 1975; 30:45–52

Mundy-Castle AC: Theta and beta rhythm in the electroencephalograms of normal adults. Electroencephalogr Clin Neurophysiol 1951; 3:477–486

Mundy-Castle AC: Central excitability in the aged, in Medical and Clinical Aspects of Aging. Edited by Blumenthal HT. New York, Columbia University Press, 1962

Obrist WD: The electroencephalogram of normal aged adults. Electroencephalogr Clin Neurophysiol 1954; 6:235–244

Obrist WD: Cerebral physiology of the aged: relation to psychological function, in Behavior and Brain Electrical Activity. Edited by Burch N, Altshuler HL. New York, Plenum Press 1975

Obrist WD: Cerebral blood flow and EEG changes associated with aging and dementia, in Handbook of Geriatric Psychiatry. Edited by Busse EW, Blazer DG. New York, Van Nostrand Reinhold 1980

Obrist WD, Henry C: Electroencephalographic findings in aged psychiatric patients. J Nerv Ment Dis 1958; 126:254–267

Obrist WD, Busse EW, Henry CE: Relation of electroencephalograms to blood pressure in elderly persons. Neurology 1961; 2:151–158

Obrist WD, Sokoloff L, Lassen NA, et al: Relationship of EEG to cerebral blood flow and metabolism in old age. Electroencephalogr Clin Neurophysiol 1963; 15:610–619

O'Connor KP, Chichester W, Shaw JC, et al: The EEG and differential diagnosis in psychogeriatrics. Br J Psychiatry 1979; 135:156–162

Palmore E, Busse EW, Maddox GL, et al (eds): Normal Aging III. Durham, NC, Duke University Press, 1985

Petre-Quadens O, Jouver M: Paradoxical sleep and dreaming in the mentally retarded. J Neurol Sci 1966; 3:608–612

Prinz PN: Sleep patterns in the aged, in Normal Aging III. Edited by Palmore E, Busse EW, Maddox GL, et al. Durham, NC, Duke University Press, 1985

Roubicek J: The electroencephalogram in the middle-aged and the elderly. J Am Geriatr Soc 1977; 25:145–152

Roth M: Implications and outlook: neurobiological aspects, in Dimensions in Aging. Edited by Bergener M, Ermini M, Stahelin HB. New York, Academic Press, 1986

Schneider-Helmert D, Spinweber C: Evaluation of L-tryptophan for treatment of insomnia: a review. Psychopharmacology 1986; 89:1–7

Spinweber C, Webb S, Gillin J: Field Trial of L-tryptophan in reducing sleep-loss effects (Report No. 86–15). Washington, DC, Naval Health Research Center, 1987

Stockard JJ, Stockard JE, Sharbrough FW: Detection and localization of occult lesions with brain-stem auditory responses. Mayo Clin Proc 1977; 52(12):761–769

Surwillo WW: The relation of simple response time to brain wave frequency and the effects of aging. Electroencephalogr Clin Neurophysiol 1963; 15:105–111

Thompson L, Wilson S: Electrocardial reactivity and learning in the elderly. J Gerontol 1966; 21:45–51

Thompson LW, Botwinick J: Age differences in the relationship between EEG arousal and reaction time. J Psychol 1968; 68:167–172

Visser SL, Hooijer C, Jonker C, et al: Anterior temporal focal abnormalities in EEG in normal aged subjects: correlations with psychopathological and CT brain scan findings. Electroencephalogr Clin Neurophysiol 1987; 66:1–7

Vogel FS: Genetic aspects of the EEG. Electroencephalogr Clin Neurophysiol 1965; 19:196–197

Wang HS, Busse EW: EEG of healthy old persons: a longitudinal study, dominant background activity and occipital rhythm. J Gerontol 1969; 24:419–426

Wang HS, Busse EW: Brain impairment and longevity, in Normal Aging II. Edited by Palmore EB. Durham, NC, Duke University Press, 1974

Wang HS, Busse EW: Correlates of regional cerebral blood flow in elderly community residents, in Blood Flow and Metabolism in the Brain. Edited by Harper M, Jennett B, Miller D, et al. Edinburgh, Churchill Livingstone, 1975

Wang HS, Obrist WD, Busse EW: Neurophysiological correlates of the intellectual function of elderly persons living in the community. Am J Psychiatry 1970; 126:39–46

Wilkie FL, Eisdorfer C: Intelligence and blood pressure in the aged. Science 1961; 172:959–962

Chapter 7

The Psychology of Aging

Ilene C. Siegler, Ph.D., M.P.H.
Leonard W. Poon, Ph.D.

In the 1980s, the field of the psychology of aging has consolidated and deepened in traditional research areas such as memory and personality and exploded in other new areas of particular relevance to geriatric psychiatry—namely, neuropsychology and health psychology. The growth of literature in geriatric psychiatry is extraordinary and is estimated to double every 10 years (Birren and Cunningham 1985). Alzheimer's disease has emerged as a scientific, social, and political force (see Heckler 1985). Research opportunities for behavioral scientists have been increased as well (Khachaturian 1985). The explosion of research in psychopharmacology and psychophysiology as well as the revolution of interest in cognitive sciences have all had an impact on changes in the knowledge base of the psychology of aging. Training of clinically oriented psychologists to work with the aged has been formalized, including curriculum and research recommendations (Santos and VandenBos 1982). Complex multivariate data analyses are now typical in the psychology of aging and new methods of analysis are becoming widespread (Schaie and Hertzog 1985).

This chapter was written under the assumption that the reader has access to a previous review chapter (Siegler 1980) for an overview of the organization of theory and data in the psychology of adult development and aging through 1980. In this chapter we concentrate on updating the literature relevant to geriatric psychiatry, paying careful attention to the clinical rele-

Dr. Siegler's work is supported in part by grants AG03188 and AG05128 from the National Institute on Aging and grant HL36587 from the National Heart, Lung and Blood Institute.

163

vance of research findings. The chapter is organized into three substantive areas: (1) experimental and cognitive psychology, (2) personality and social psychology, and (3) health and behavior.

Review of Available Handbooks

Many of the recent developments in the psychology of adult development and aging can be found in a set of volumes that have appeared in the past 6 years. Most notable are the second editions of the first three volumes in this set—*Handbook of the Biology of Aging* (Finch and Schneider 1985), *Handbook of the Psychology of Aging* (Birren and Schaie 1985), and *Handbook of Aging and the Social Sciences* (Binstock and Shanas 1985)—and the aging chapters in the *Handbook of Developmental Psychology* (Wolman 1982). Each of the three volumes was designed to supplement its earlier edition, and the present chapter will provide a key as to which chapters in those books have data of relevance to our concerns. In particular, the *Psychology of Aging* handbook serves not only to update the literature but also to provide the space for some theoretical formulations to guide future research. In addition, a new series of edited volumes, the *Annual Review of Gerontology and Geriatrics* (Maddox and Lawton 1988), provides another source of material. Journals have also been important sources of progress. For psychology, the new journal *Psychology and Aging* and the edited volumes *Aging in the 1980s* (Poon 1980) and *Handbook of Clinical Memory Assessment of Older Adults* (Poon et al. 1986), published by the American Psychological Association, are evidence of a growing maturity of interest in geropsychology within the official psychology community. The *Encyclopedia of Aging* (Maddox et al. 1987) provides short, efficient reviews on many topics in the psychology and psychiatry of aging. Some of the groups conducting major longitudinal studies of aging have published volumes that summarize their findings. These include studies primarily of psychologic content, such as the Berkeley studies (Eichorn et al. 1981) and the Harvard Studies of Adult Development (Vaillant 1983), as well as multidisciplinary studies such as the Baltimore Longitudinal Studies of Aging (Shock et al. 1984), the Duke Longitudinal Studies (Busse et al. 1985; Palmore et al. 1985), and a review of the psychologic aspects of seven major studies (Iowa, Aging Twins, Seattle, Duke, Bonn, Baltimore, and AT&T Managers) in the volume edited by Schaie (1983). Mednick et al. (1984) provide a *Handbook of Longitudinal Research* that reviews 31 studies of adolescents and adults in normal and clinical populations. This is an excellent catalogue of the special populations that have been studied in addition to the more familiar studies of normal aging. The chapters are organized by study and give the major variables, hypotheses tested, and major references for each study. The emphases in these studies with traditional longitudinal designs are on the processes of aging with groups of subjects defined by disease status or social role and followed for almost a generation in many cases.

The Multiple Uses of Age as a Variable in Aging Research

There are two approaches in the developmental psychology of aging: (1) experimental aging research versus developmental research and (2) a psychology of aging versus a psychology of the aged. In experimental aging research, older persons are used as the subjects in research designs. The intent of the research is to illustrate the processes under study (e.g., memory) by comparing the performances of younger versus older persons. There is no intent to infer the developmental processes that would explain the observed differences. Typically, experimental studies are cross-sectional and have strong implicit assumptions. Those assumptions are that (1) the processes inferred in explaining the differences between the age groups represent the change that must occur and (2) the younger group will, with time, become like the older group and the older group used to be like the younger group (see Siegler et al. 1980; McCrae and Costa 1984). Botwinick (1973) indicated the potential fallacy in such assumptions by quoting a talk by Robert Kastenbaum who set the scene in the northeastern United States with a large older immigrant population. He noted that all of the older persons spoke with an accent, while none of the younger persons did. He concluded that surely the development of a foreign accent must be one of the prime manifestations of aging on the psychologic level. It is clear in this example that cultural, rather than developmental, factors account for the observed age differences. Relatively few cross-sectional studies of age differences take the charge of explaining intervening processes seriously. Longitudinal studies assume that the birth cohorts of the individuals and the actual times of measurement do not influence the processes observed. In times of social and cultural change, such assumptions are not always valid. In studies of clinical populations, changes in models of diagnosis and modes of treatment are likely to make longitudinal findings harder to interpret.

Another clash of views in the psychology of aging is whether aging is seen as a continuation of the life span, where attention is paid to the developmental processes or whether elderly persons themselves are the only object of study, which is in essence a psychology of the aged rather than of aging. Geriatric psychiatry is by definition more concerned with the psychology of the aged. The psychology of aging or the life span view emphasizes the continuity of patterns of behavior across the life cycle and is consistent with the case history approach in psychiatry. In areas where cohort variation is important (social and historical trends) the best predictors of the behavior of a group of older persons may well be their own behaviors measured at an earlier point in time. To the extent that future generations of elderly are influenced by social change, a psychology of the aged will become increasingly dated. However, both aspects—psychology of aging and psychology of the aged—have generated important data to be considered, and findings from both areas are reviewed below.

Cognitive Psychology: Basic Research Findings

The term "cognition" subsumes the range of human intellectual functioning. Cognition is, for example, to perceive, to remember, to reason, to make decisions, to solve problems, and to form complex structures of world knowledge. The application of our knowledge of the capacities and limitations of these cognitive processes with normal and abnormal aging can have profound impact on the quality of the daily life of older persons. For example, the knowledge can be used to improve human factor and environmental design, policies on work and retirement, accuracy of clinical assessment, and effectiveness of remediation and rehabilitation when they are warranted.

Although all cognitive processes are intimately interrelated, age-related changes in memory functioning have received by far the largest share of research effort. Two reasons could account for its large share of attention. First, memory decline is one of two major concerns articulated by community-dwelling elderly adults, the other being loss of energy (Lowenthal et al. 1967). Second, memory dysfunction is a major behavioral benchmark in neuropsychopathology, for example, dementia of the Alzheimer's type (Kaszniak et al. 1986). To demonstrate the prolific growth of memory and aging research, there are at least 20 reviews of research findings on various aspects of memory and aging since 1980 (Kaszniak et al. 1986).

Because so much has been written about memory function and aging, this section will first highlight findings in four relatively new cognitive research areas that have practical implications on everyday functioning as well as providing insight toward common memory complaints by geriatric patients. These areas are text processing, speech comprehension, spatial cognition, and problem solving. Second, research findings on memory functioning will be updated from the perspectives of normative changes and Alzheimer's disease. For recent comprehensive reviews see Salthouse (1982a, 1985) and Poon (1985, 1986; Poon et al. in press).

Individual Differences in Cognitive Functions

In examining the literature comparing cognitive performances among age groups, it is useful to keep in mind that the level of cognition can be affected by a number of individual, environmental, and task characteristics in addition to chronologic age (Poon 1985). Depending on the task and the situation, some individuals tend to excel in certain types of performance and not in others. For example, in some cognitive tasks, some adults with high intelligence and education will show minimal decline in their performances with increasing age, while significant decline is observed with adults with lower intelligence and education (e.g., Bowles and Poon 1982; Poon and Fozard 1980). For those tasks, intelligence and education, rather than chronologic age, are the important determinants of performance. In some cognitive tasks that are well practiced the amount of age decline tends to be small or nonexistent (Salthouse 1982a). On the other hand, older persons tend to perform less well in new or novel situations (Poon 1985). These effects will be evident in the following summary of findings across a number of cognitive tasks.

Cognition and aging research thus far has concentrated on differences between age groups in cognitive performance; however, more attention is being placed on identifying the effects of the individual, the environment, and the task characteristics in addition to chronologic age to better understand the obtained cognitive differences among age groups.

Text processing. Earlier studies of verbal memory and aging employing serial or paired-associate learning procedures found substantial age deficits (see Siegler 1980 for a review). A number of investigators have asked how accurately these findings could predict the processing of written or spoken information in everyday life. These questions initiated a number of recent research programs investigating age differences in "discourse" or "prose" processing—the acquisition of spoken or written communications.

The first generation of research on text processing presented contradictory and conflicting findings. Some studies found clear-cut age deficits (e.g., Gordon and Clark 1974; Cohen 1979; Zelinski et al. 1980), while others found no age difference (e.g., Taub 1979; Meyer and Rice 1981; Harker et al. 1982). These conflicting findings apparently were a blessing in disguise, for they provided the impetus for the second generation of research to examine in detail the possible contributions of individual difference, the properties of the text to be processed, and the task demand on the observed processing performance (for detailed reviews see Meyer and Rice in press; Hartley in press).

From the individual difference perspective, the level of education and verbal intelligence seems to account for a portion of the age effects on performance (Meyer and Rice in press). Age deficits in prose recall appear to be significant for average and low-verbal-ability adults with mainly high school education. However, mixed results also come from studies in which adults have high vocabulary scores and a college education. From the task perspective, faster presentation rates tend to compromise the elderly more than the young adults (Hartley in press). This set of results seems to support the finding of cognitive slowing with increasing age.

The organization of the text was found to be a meaningful variable that could also explain some of the conflicting results in the literature. Older adults with high verbal ability appear to utilize text structure as well as young adults (Meyer and Rice in press). They could take advantage of organized structures to facilitate their processing. On the other hand, low-verbal-ability older adults show less sensitivity to text structures that could assist them in the processing task.

These second- and third-generation research programs are seeking answers to questions that could help us understand the impact of everyday processing demands on the older learners as well as insights on how to facilitate better acquisition and retention of prose information. A bottom line of this type of research on the acquisition of more meaningful information is that age-related differences are not as large as indicated by earlier studies of age differences in serial or paired associate learning.

Speech comprehension. Another type of discourse processing is the processing of spoken speech. Whereas written material can be scanned and reviewed during processing, spoken speech can be processed only in a serial manner. While older adults have been shown to suffer from auditory processing deficits (see Olsho et al. 1985 for a review) and in speed of processing (Poon 1985), it is surprising that older adults have not been noticed to have a disproportionate amount of problems in processing everyday conversations or spoken input from television or radio.

There is overwhelming evidence why older persons should have difficulty in processing spoken discourse. One of the major contributors is peripheral hearing decline, presbycusis, which includes the loss of sensitivity in the higher frequency range of hearing, an increased probability of recruitment, and an increased probability of phonemic regression or decreased intelligibility.

Indeed, a number of studies have found clear deficits in the ability of older adults to process spoken speech (Cohen 1979, 1981; Cohen and Faulkner 1982; for a review see Stine et al. 1986). How peripheral hearing deficits interact with available central processing resources is an important question for both the understanding of speech comprehension for older individuals and the design of methods to compensate for the deficit.

Several groups of investigators are attempting to find answers to the above questions. In an experiment in which subjects must detect predictable or not predictable target words presented in varying levels of noise, Cohen and Faulkner (1983) found that elderly listeners were making greater use of the context as the noise level increased. Similar findings were reported by Nickerson et al. (1981) in that elderly subjects actually detected more target words imbedded in cocktail-party noise than did younger subjects. The finding suggested that older adults use the word-sentence context to compensate for their peripheral hearing deficits.

In another experiment reported by Wingfield et al. (1985), young and elderly subjects processed word strings that varied in syntactic constraints and were presented at varying speeds. While the performance of all subjects was affected by speech rate and the degree of linguistic constraint, the performance of the elderly group was differentially depressed by increasing speech rate and by decreasing linguistic constraints. In other words, the results suggested that the older listeners do rely on both the redundancy of language and linguistic constraints to maintain an acceptable level of performance. Together, these preliminary results suggest that peripheral hearing decline is being compensated for by the experience of the older listener and that therapeutic procedures may do well to take into account the individual's cognitive strengths and experiences in remediating peripheral hearing losses.

Spatial cognition. Spatial, in contrast to verbal, cognition refers to a set of processing abilities that some investigators describe as right hemisphere functions. To translate this sort of functioning to everyday demands, spatial cognition describes our ability to recognize faces, pictures, and symbols; find our way around the store or neighborhood; locate or find an object; and so on. In clinical settings, clinicians are confronted with the problem that some older adults are particularly disoriented spatially and sometimes cannot find their way, even in familiar surroundings.

Are older adults particularly compromised in spatial compared with verbal functioning? This is a question that is drawing increasing research attention, but relatively few data are available at present. Two sets of issues are germane to this question. First, are older adults indeed more compromised in spatial compared with verbal processing? The limited research to date has produced conflicting results. Reviews of psychometric and neuropsychologic literature (Klisz 1978; Albert and Kaplan 1980) support the notion that there is differential neurologic decline in right hemisphere functions. On the other hand, controlled laboratory experiments examining the processing of spatial stimuli (e.g., Park et al. 1983) found minimal or no age difference. Research programs are needed to reconcile the differences between the psychometric and information-processing results.

Second, if there is a differential decline in spatial processing, the origin of this differential decline must be traced. Is the observed deficit a result of biologically determined differential decline in the right hemisphere, or is the right hemisphere decline due to differential disuse of the right compared with left hemisphere functioning over the life span? Although the two questions seem circular, modes of remediation would be different depending on the answers.

Current research addressing the common problems of spatial orientation (navigation around stores and neighborhoods), memory for spatial location, and spatial problem solving has begun to examine the relationships among individual spatial abilities, adaptive processes, and situational demands (for a review of the research, see Kirasic, in press). Although the research is pretty much in its infancy, this direction of research could point to the common and unique contributions of spatial and verbal abilities to different sets of everyday spatial demands. For example, Walsh et al. (1981) reported that spatial abilities were significant predictors of neighborhood knowledge, and in turn, neighborhood knowledge was a significant predictor of the use of goods and services in the neighborhood. However, spatial abilities had negligible impact on the individual's neighborhood use. In another study examining the efficiency of shopping routes in supermarkets, Kirasic (1981) reported that individuals' psychometric spatial abilities seemed to be poor predictors of shopping efficiency for any age group. From a clinical evaluation perspective, tests of right hemisphere functioning do not always predict everyday spatially related problems. It is clear that more than spatial ability is involved in planning one's shopping route within a store, and it would be important to pursue how spatial and other cognitive abilities interact in various situational demands for successful adaptation for the community-dwelling aged.

Problem solving. A series of recent discussions (Denney in press; Hartley in press) addressed the study of age-related changes in problem solving from both the standard psychometric intelligence tradition and tests imitating problems encountered in everyday situations. These interchanges differentiated between the goals of *predicting* problem-solving abilities in everyday life and *understanding* the individualized problem-solving mechanisms, strategies, or antecedents of performance. The result of this discussion will increase our knowledge of the roles of individual abilities, experience and expertise, and situational demands in problem-solving performances in adulthood.

An often discussed question is whether traditional problem-solving tasks are relevant or predictive of everyday problem-solving situations for older adults. In making predictions, a test must have predictive validity and correlate well with measures of everyday performances. The answer to this question seems to be yes, in that performance in laboratory problem-solving tasks that were developed for use with children and young adults decreases in a linear fashion after early adulthood (for reviews see Botwinick 1984; Denney 1982; Giambra and Arenberg 1980; Salthouse 1982b). The results hold for both cross-sectional and longitudinal comparisons. At the same time, performance in everyday problem-solving tasks tends to show somewhat similar age trends in that middle-aged adults can in some situations perform better than the young adults; however, performance decline is still evident for the aged adults (Denney in press). From this perspective, traditional psychometric tests can predict in a reasonable fashion everyday problem-solving performances.

From the perspective of understanding the mechanisms of everyday problem solving, the use of traditional ability tasks has limited value. A lesson to learn from the problem-solving research is that if we want to understand basic mechanisms, the chosen tests or tasks must be representative of the actual situation, must have external validity, and must be able to identify or test factors that contribute to performance variability. Although there is limited current research in this area, the studies of Hartley (in press) and Denney (in press) are noteworthy. Both investigators set out to examine problem-solving skills, frequency, and styles of the various age cohorts to define the environment of the problem solver and the complex behavior of problem solving, individual differences, and aging.

Memory Functioning: Normative Changes and Alzheimer's Disease

As stated earlier, investigations of memory functioning in both normal and abnormal aging have garnered a significant amount of research resources over the years. Poon (1985) lists 20 reviews on memory and normative aging that have been published since 1980. He demonstrates the prevalence of the information-processing approach in examining age-related differences in memory components, stages, and processes. This approach postulates that information flows from input to output through a series of stages. At the early stage of information, registration is sensory (iconic and echoic) memory, a preattentive and highly unstable system. Primary (short-term) and secondary (long-term) memory (Waugh and Norman 1965) are responsible for the acquisition and retention of new information. Primary memory is conceptualized as a limited-capacity store in which information is still "in mind" as it is being used. If the information is not rehearsed instantaneously so that it can be stored in secondary memory, the information will be lost. Secondary memory is a repository of newly acquired information. Finally, tertiary memory is a repository for well-learned and personal information.

It is important to note that this "linear" model is one of several theoretical models of memory functioning; however, its prevalence in the study of normal aging and in abnormal memory functioning makes it easy to compare findings on the functioning of the theoretical memory stages in normal and abnormal processes.

Normative aging. Siegler (1980) provided an in-depth description of age-related differences in memory functioning. The results have been robust, and only a cursory review will be attempted here.

A global summary of normal age-related changes in memory is presented in Table 1 and 2. Table 1 shows that there is a general age-related decline in speed of retrieval from the various theoretical memory stores, and Table 2 shows that the locus of the age-related decline in memory capacity is found primarily in secondary memory (Fozard 1980). Thus, although sensorimotor slowing is inevitable with aging, this slowing apparently does not appreciably affect the capacities of sensory, primary, or tertiary memory. Aging, however, exerts a profound effect in the acquisition and retrieval of new information in secondary memory.

As described in the previous sections, a significant amount of recent research effort has been vested in examining the effects of individual, situational, and task differences on age differences in acquisition and retrieval of

Table 1. Cross-Sectional Experimental Evidence for Age-Related Slowing of Memory Processes

Component Affected	Memory Store				
	Sensory	Primary	Secondary	Working	Tertiary
Perceptual motor	Positive	Positive	Positive	—	Positive
Decision making	—	Positive	Positive	Positive	Negative

Note. Reprinted with permission from Fozard (1980).

Table 2. Evidence for Age-Related Declines in Memory Capacity

Type of Study and Type of Evidence	Memory Store				
	Sensory	Primary	Secondary	Working	Tertiary
Cross-sectional studies					
Anecdotal	—	Positive	Positive	Positive	Positive
Psychometric	—	Negative	Positive	—	Negative
Experimental	Positive	Negative	Positive	Positive	Negative
Longitudinal studies					
Anecdotal	—	—	—	—	—
Psychometric	—	Negative	Positive	—	Negative
Experimental	—	—	Positive	—	—

Note. Reprinted with permission from Fozard (1980).

information. The exploration of memory functioning in naturalistic as opposed to laboratory settings, the use of world knowledge, and the use of training strategies, memory mnemonics (memory aids), and practice all contribute to a more comprehensive view of memory and aging.

Alzheimer's disease. In contrast to the prolific number of reviews on research in memory and normative aging, there are relatively fewer studies evaluating changes of memory functions in Alzheimer's disease employing the information-processing procedures. The essential feature of the syndrome of dementia is a loss of intellectual ability of sufficient severity to interfere with social or occupational functioning (American Psychiatric Association 1987). Additional diagnostic criteria include the presence of memory impairment and disturbance in at least one of the following: abstract thinking, judgment, higher cortical function, and personality. Exclusionary criteria include evidence of clouded consciousness and conditions other than organic mental disorders. Memory dysfunction is one of the earliest signs of dementia of the Alzheimer's type, and memory is perhaps the most severely affected function as the disease progresses.

Research to date shows that patterns of memory functioning are distinctly different between normative aging and Alzheimer's disease. In normal aging, memory deficit is focused on secondary memory, the acquisition and retrieval of new information. In contrast, Alzheimer's disease exerts profound effects on all memory stages and stores.

It is noted that some information-processing tasks may be too complex for patients with a moderate level of disease severity. Although this criticism should be seriously considered, the difficulty of the information-processing task can be adjusted so that mildly to moderately impaired patients could perform the tasks adequately. In the studies reviewed in the following sections, results are based on studies of only those patients who could clearly comprehend the instructions and perform the task appropriately.

Table 3 reviews a number of studies evaluating the effects of Alzheimer's disease on primary memory. Five different paradigms are employed. The results are unanimous that primary memory is impaired and that the magnitude of impairment is related to the severity of the disease.

Table 4 presents a review of 32 studies clustered into eight different secondary memory paradigms. Secondary memory impairments have been noted in all the studies. Alzheimer's patients, in comparison to normal aged controls, are impaired in learning, delayed recall, and recognition memory for both verbal and nonverbal stimuli. Again, the degree of dysfunction is related to the severity of the disease. Two studies have noted that signal detection analysis of the performances showed that the deficit was in memory deficiency and not in a change in criterion employed by the patient.

Although there are a limited number of studies that examined the effects of Alzheimer's disease on tertiary and remote memory, Wilson et al. (1981)

Table 3. Investigations of Primary Memory in Patients with Alzheimer's Disease

Task	Measure	Results	Authors
Digit span	Accuracy	Patients impaired; impairment related to behavioral indices of dementia severity and physiologic (EEG) index of cerebral dysfunction; increased impairment seen after 1 year for some patients	Larner (1977) Kaszniak et al. (1979a) Kaszniak et al. (1979b) Crook et al. (1980) Corkin (1982) Danziger and Storandt (1982)
Word span	Accuracy	Patients impaired	Miller (1973)
Block span	Accuracy	Patients impaired; degree of impairment related to severity of impairment in ADL	Corkin (1982)
Brown-Peterson distractor task (consonant trigrams)	Accuracy of recall after various retention intervals	Patients impaired for all but O-S delay; impairment related to severity of impairment in ADL	Corkin (1982)
Immediate verbal free-recall task	Number of words recalled in each serial position of presentation	Patients impaired in recall of words at end of list; validated procedure for scoring primary memory confirms deficit; patients show deterioration in primary memory over 3 years	Miller (1971) Kaszniak et al. (1981) Wilson et al. (1983a) Wilson and Kaszniak (1986)

Note. EEG = electroencephalogram; ADL = activities of daily living. Reprinted with permission from Kaszniak et al. (1986).

reported that memory for colloquial events and famous persons is severely compromised in the patient group.

Intellectual Functioning

Research on intellectual functioning has one of the longest and most productive records in the psychology of aging (see Siegler 1980; Birren et al. 1983). Manton et al. (1986), employing a fuzzy clustering paradigm (grade of membership analysis: Woodbury and Clive 1974; Woodburry and Manton 1982), evaluated cognitive and intellectual performance in the full Duke Longitudinal Study data population. Results indicated that measures of memory, reaction time, and intelligence in the entire population over 21 years of data collection and 30 years of mortality follow-up described five patterns among the participants. The patterns were generally ordered from below average to superior intelligence. The mean ages of the patterns were 78.5, 79.1, 73.7, 79.3, and 74.4. The data also indicated clear relationships between poorer physical health (from heart disease or dementia) and declining cognitive performance, but not mental health as measured by depression ratings.

Hertzog and Schaie (1986) report a new analysis of data from the Seattle Longitudinal Studies with two longitudinal sequences of 162 persons tested in 1956, 1963, and 1970; the second sample was tested in 1963, 1970, and 1977. Data were analyzed with LISREL IV to evaluate the stability of individual differences in intellectual functioning as assessed by the Primary Mental Abilities Test. These techniques speak not only to assessment of stability or change in individual differences in performance (Do individuals maintain their same place relative to each other?), but to the underlying organizational components of intelligence measured by the test and their intercorrelations. The analyses are complex, but the results were relatively clear, indicating a high degree of stability in intellectual functioning across the adult age span with support for factorial invariance.

Patterns of stability and change across the life cycle vary according to the ability that is measured. McCrae et al. (1987) reported declines in divergent thinking (a component of creativity) consistently with cross-sectional, longitudinal, and cross-sequential analyses, although the declines with the longitudinal sequences were the smallest. Steuer et al. (1981) reported on the ability of the critical loss ratio to predict survivorship in the remaining participants of the New York State Psychiatric Institute study of senescent twins who were retested in 1973 (14 women and 8 men ages 83 to 99). By 1978, 12 had died, making it possible to evaluate 5-year survival. Critical loss was not able to distinguish between groups. However, a diagnosis of organic brain syndrome in 1973 was related to death by 1978. In a similar reanalysis of the Duke Longitudinal Study survivors, changes in scores on the full-scale Wechsler Adult Intelligence Scale no longer predicted mortality with the same degree of efficiency as before (Siegler 1985). Longitudinal data sets provide measures

Table 4. Investigations of Secondary Memory in Patients With Alzheimer's Disease

Task	Measure	Results	Authors
Verbal shopping list task (10 words)	Trials to accurate recall; delayed recall; recognition	Patients impaired in learning, delayed recall, and recognition	McCarthy et al. (1981)
Learning progressively longer lists above word span	Accuracy of recall; trials to criterion	Patients impaired	Miller (1973)
Verbal paired-associate learning	Accuracy; trials to criterion	Patients appear consistently impaired, with some evidence of longitudinal deterioration; impairment correlated with severity of EEG slowing and cerebral atrophy seen on CT scan	Inglis (1959); Caird et al. (1962); Inglis and Caird (1963); Barbizet and Cany (1969); Kaszniak et al. (1979a); Kaszniak et al. (1979b); de Leon et al. (1980); Corkin (1982); Danziger and Storandt (1982); Rosen and Mohs (1982); Wilson et al. (1982a)
Nonverbal paired-associate learning (geometric forms)	Trials to criterion for recognition	Moderately and severely demented patients impaired	Corkin (1982)
Story recall test	Accuracy of immediate recall; percentage accuracy of retention after delay	Patients impaired in immediate and delayed recall and percentage of retention	Logue and Wyrick (1979); Brinkman et al. (1983); Danziger and Storandt (1982); Osborne et al. (1982)

Task	Measure	Findings	References
Verbal free-recall task (lists of 7 to 32 words)	Accuracy of recall	Patients impaired in recall, particularly in primacy component of serial position curve; severity of impairment increases over time; stimulus manipulations suggest patients are deficient in encoding semantic and organizational features; recent studies indicate scores for primary and secondary memory are correlated for patients with Alzheimer's disease but not for the normal elderly.	Miller (1971, 1975, 1978) Diesfeldt (1978) Kaszniak et al. (1981) Wilson et al. (1983a) Wilson and Kaszniak (1986)
Verbal recognition memory task	Accuracy of forced-choice recognition	Patients impaired, with evidence for relative inability to make use of semantic cues; signal detection analysis reveals the deficit to be in memory efficiency and not in decision criteria; two studies show, at least for moderately demented patients, an absence of the normal low-frequency word advantage in hit rate	Miller (1975) Miller and Lewis (1977) Kaszniak et al. (1981) Corkin (1982) Wilson et al. (1982b) Wilson et al. (1983b)
Facial recognition memory task	Accuracy of forced-choice recognition	Patients impaired; signal detection analysis indicates the impairment is due to memory inefficiency and not altered decision criterion	Wilson et al. (1982b)

Note. CT = computed tomography; EEG = electroencephalogram. Reprinted with permission from Kaszniak et al. (1986).

of functioning in the old-old who are surviving members of longitudinal populations. Many of these studies started in the mid-1950s. Long-term participants in these studies are reaching the century mark, providing new opportunities to understand the oldest old.

Applications of Cognitive Changes

Important application of the data in cognitive psychology is in how middle-aged and older adults perform in situations in which learning of new information is required and in the workplace (see Cross 1981; Stagner 1985).

The action in learning has switched from the question "Can older persons learn?" to "What is the most effective way to teach older persons the things they want to learn?". Willis (1985) reviewed the major findings and concluded that older persons' learning capacities are greater and more plastic than had been realized. Baltes et al. (1986) replicated and extended earlier work done by Baltes and Willis (1982) at Pennsylvania State University. Older subjects (ages 60 to 86) participated in a short-term (10 sessions) longitudinal training session on measures of fluid intelligence. A pretest and each of three posttests were composed of a 3.5-hour battery of intelligence tests. Gains of those older persons who had practice training were highly significant and related to the degree of similarity of the abilities practiced in the training program to the abilities required to do well on the intelligence tests. Transfer of training was found to be relatively specific, indicating that training programs should be guided toward the specific skills that older persons need to learn. Baltes et al. (1986) interpret their findings as suggesting a higher degree of reserve in fluid intellectual capacity for the elderly than had been shown previously. Older persons after training were able to solve more difficult problems and were more accurate at all levels of performance.

Willis and Schaie (1986) evaluated the effects of cognitive training in panel members of Schaie's Seattle Longitudinal Study. Individuals with a mean age of 72.8 (range, 64 to 95) were classified as stable versus decliners over a 14-year period on inductive reasoning and spatial orientation. Of the 107 subjects, 46.7 percent were stable, 15 to 16 percent had declined on one measure, and 21.8 percent had declined on both measures. A training program was devised to provide training on the ability that had declined. Both stable and decline groups benefited significantly from training, about the same amount; that is, decliners performed at their previous levels and stables increased above previous levels of performance. These results are quite convincing in indicating that target training can be expected to be effective for older persons on complex tasks at very old ages.

Issues of productivity and age remain important. Horner et al. (1986) studied age and research productivity of male academic psychologists in four cohort groups: 1909–1914, 1919–1924, 1929–1934, and 1939–1944. A cross-sequential design that evaluated age and cohort was employed. Cross-sectionally, the publication rate peaked at ages 35 to 44 (1.2 publications per year), was similar at ages 25 to 34 and 45 to 54, and declined thereafter. This pattern was repeated in analysis of each longitudinal cohort. Individual differences were evaluated by looking at three rates of publication. Medium- and low-frequency publishers followed the overall trend. High-frequency publishers showed a linear decline after ages 25 to 34. Stability within category was high. Forty-three percent of the sample remained within the same category throughout their life cycle. While overall level of productivity declines with age, the stability of individual levels of performance is also seen, replicating a pattern seen in many ability measures assessed over the life cycle.

Sterns (1986) has reviewed the literature on training and retraining of older workers with an emphasis on practical applications about what is known about adult development and how it can be applied. The role of worker for an older person remains an option in a very real sense. Sterns and Alexander (1987) present a state-of-the-art review of industrial gerontology and point out that plant closings, reductions in force, and the introduction of new technologies will continue to confront the role of age in the workplace. While the Age Discrimination in Employment Act of 1967 offers individuals protection, the individuals must be willing to file suit to ensure their rights, and/or employers must either agree with the law or be afraid of enforcement to act in a nondiscriminatory manner (see Edelman and Siegler 1978 for a history of the act). Older persons appear less likely to be willing to make discriminatory attributions (Siegler 1979).

Personality and Social Psychology

The dynamics of normal personality across the adult life cycle have continued to be a productive area of research, while a social psychology of adult development and aging, from a psychologic perspective, has emerged in the past 6 years. This social psychology includes studies of interpersonal behaviors (Lachman 1986a, 1986b), social support (Cohen and Syme 1985), attribution paradigms (Lachman and McArthur 1986), and health psychology (Siegler and Costa 1985). Research on the stress/illness paradigm, life events, and models of coping continue to be major contributors to understanding developmental patterns in middle and later life. Whitbourne (1985) analyzes three major models of coping and adaptation: life events, cognitive appraisal, and subjective well-being.

Patterns of Personality Functioning

Bengtson et al. (1985) present a creative approach to a review of the personality literature with a focus on self and self-concept. In a series of excellent tables they review the studies on self-concept with cognitive components; personality scales and self-esteem as an evaluative component; and conative (self-management) components of self-conceptions with behavior–observer ratings. Their analysis of the literature suggests the following trends: greater stability in objective (e.g., self-report paper-and-pencil tests) than in subjective measures of personality (e.g., ratings from interviews); maintenance of levels of self-esteem in later life; different adaptations and responses by different personality typologies to life events; consistent sex differences are found; however, relationships with age are less clear. Not all personality patterns have the same consequences. Better adjusted patterns earlier in life may well lead to more positive outcomes later in life.

There have been important new reports from major studies of adult personality. Kelly and Conley (1987) reported new analyses from Kelly's longitudinal study of 300 engaged couples. They were recruited in 1935–1938 and were followed for the next 45 years to look at the relationship between couples' personality and their marital compatibility. Data on the couples' personality come from peer ratings made by five acquaintances who rated the couples in 1935–1938 on the Personality Rating Scale, which has scores on four traits: neuroticism, social extraversion, impulse control, and agreeableness. Additional data were collected in 1954–1955 and 1980–1981. Marital stability and marital satisfaction, the two criterion variables, were assessed in 1980–1981. Data were available on 199 couples who remained married and 50 divorces (39 between 1935 and 1954 and 11 between 1955 and 1980). A joint criterion was developed (divorced versus stable, but unhappy marriage versus happy marriage). Results of a regression analysis indicated that husband's neuroticism, wife's neuroticism, and husband's impulse control accounted for 14.78 percent of the variance in outcome. An additional 10 percent of the variance was accounted for by 14 marriage attitude variables. While age was not a variable in the analyses presented, the subjects were aged 20 to 30 at entry into the study in the middle 1930s and thus members of the 1905–1915 birth cohorts who are today's elderly.

Vaillant (1983, 1984) describes the Study of Adult Development at Harvard Medical School. Two very different samples, undergraduates from Harvard College and adolescent boys from Boston (selected as nondelinquent controls), have been followed for 40 years in two prospective studies. The differences in socioeconomic status of the two samples, but the general similarity of design, make them excellent companion studies. Vaillant and Milofsky (1980) evaluated Erikson's theory of adult development by categorizing each man's developmental stage at age 47. They formulate Erikson's model as a spiral with periods of stability alternating with periods of change. They relegate transitions to the realm of individual psychopathology and/or cultural anthropology. They test their model by evaluating three propositions: (1) Different stages will be reached at different ages; (2) the model should be independent of social class and education; and (3) the stages should be sequential. Their conclusions were most interesting. There were no specific age linkages to achievement of the stages, development was relatively independent of social status, and the developmental tasks that Erikson suggested were observed in an ordered sequence. The warning that development is a process and not a series of tasks to be completed is a useful one. Long and Vaillant (1984) looked at the adult outcomes at age 47 of 456 inner city Boston adolescents in 1940. Ratings of the childhood families of the men (from chronically dependent to nonproblem but poor) served as the major predictor variable. The results indicated that by middle age, these childhood variables did not differentiate in terms of adult social class, income, employment record, number of sociopathic symptoms, and health/mental health rating scale. Only time in jail was more frequent for those from multiproblem families as children. An analysis of the individual differences in the sample, those who had the best and worst outcomes, suggested that childhood IQ and childhood coping skills were correlated with upward mobility while those who remained in low socioeconomic status or drifted down were as adults alcoholic or mentally ill. These prospective data underscore the importance of prospective data in making causal attributions about development. Long and Vaillant point out that all subjects were white, male, and selected for nondelinquency and that the time period from 1940 to 1975 provided an opportunity structure different from both earlier and later periods.

Caspi and Elder (1986) view successful aging as expressed by high life satisfaction. Using data on 79 women from the Berkeley Guidance Study, they examined the impact of adaptive resources in young adulthood (intellectual ability and emotional health) in interaction with social class (middle versus working class) during the Great Depression. Those who lost more than 35 percent of 1929 assets and income were viewed as deprived, while those who lost less than 35 percent of assets and income were viewed as nondeprived in order to predict life satisfaction in 1970. Their results indicated different relationships for different social classes. For women in the middle class, emotional health in early adulthood was related to life satisfaction in old age. For working class women, the relationships were more complex: Intellectual ability in young adulthood, mediated through social involvement, was related to life satisfaction for the working class women. The impact of deprivation was also opposite. Middle-class women who were deprived during the Depression had higher levels of life satisfaction in old age, whereas for the working class, deprivation during the Depression led to lower life satisfaction in old age. Caspi and Elder stated the real meaning of their research question: "Why do similar misfortunes lead one person toward bitterness and another toward satisfaction?" (1986, p. 22). Their answer involves the interaction of personal resources, historical factors, and social conditions. This thoughtful study suggests a beginning maturity in sociopsychologic research that can begin to deal with the complexities of human development in an appropriate way.

Levinson (1986) summarizes his view of the life cycle and provides a nice conceptualization of his thoughts on adult development. His work on the seasons of a woman's life is not yet available for perusal; however, his discussion in this article (1986) does not suggest that it will be very different from men's lives. After reviewing the key constructs of his view of adult development—the conceptualization of a life structure with alternating periods of structure building and structure changing (transitions)—he argues that the biographic model of data collection is an important way to understand the content of adult lives. The most controversial aspect of his work to others in adult development has been the finding of relatively tight age linkages to the stages of adulthood, which he says replicate on empirical evidence. Roberts and Newton (1987) reported the findings of four doctoral dissertations on 39 women aged 28 to 53 who were interviewed with a biographic interview similar to Levinson's study of 40 men to evaluate his findings on adult development. Support was found in that similar age ranges and themes were evident. However, the content was different and all in all provided replication of the major themes of Levinson's work.

Haan et al. (1986) report on stability and change in Q-sort descriptions of personality from data collected over a 50-year period in the Institute of Human Development Studies at Berkeley. No evidence was found for stage theories of development. There was a high degree of variability in developmental pattern as a function of the sex of the person, the time interval, and the characteristic. Six major dimensions of personality were studied: self-confident/victimized; assertive/submissive; cognitively committed; outgoing/aloof; dependable; warm/hostile. There were measures from age 6 to ages 54 to 61. The findings were extremely complex and interesting. Among the important general observations were (1) developmental trends were most evident in age-adjusted analysis; (2) childhood and adolescence were times of stability and individual predictability; and (3) the transition from adolescent to adult was the most unstable. Females changed more dramatically than males and sex differences were large and striking.

Cooper and Gutmann (1987) compared the ego mastery styles of 50 middle-aged (ages 43 to 51) women in two groups: 25 who had children living at home (at least one child under age 18 who was financially dependent) and 25 whose children were independent and expected to remain so. All 50 women were currently employed teachers. They evaluated differences in Thematic Apperception Test (TAT) measures of ego mastery, a paper-and-pencil measure of androgyny, and interview measures of gender identity. There were differences in mastery on four of the five TAT cards in the direction of more "masculine" responses on behalf of the women no longer parenting, even though there were no between-group differences on the paper-and-pencil measure of androgyny. These results are interpreted as supporting Gutmann's view of a decline in sex role differences after the needs of parenting are taken care of.

Costa et al. (1986) report data from the National Health and Nutrition Examination Survey (NHANES) I Follow-up in order to evaluate stability and change in normal personality. The original survey was conducted from 1971 to 1975 and was a stratified probability sample of the noninstitutionalized civilian population aged 1 to 74. The first follow-up was conducted in 1981 to 1984 on 14,407 adults aged 32 to 88 years old at follow-up (Costa and McCrae 1986). Essentially, the findings indicate an extraordinary degree of stability in these data, replicating other longitudinal findings (see McCrae and Costa 1984) as well as their own findings from the Baltimore Longitudinal Study population (Costa and McCrae 1980).

Caspi and Elder (1986) suggest that stability of personal dispositions such as those studied by Costa and McCrae may partly depend on stability of social conditions—life in the middle class may lead to greater stability by providing more stable conditions for behavioral continuity. The replication of the stability with the national data argues against the class interpretation, as do the prospective findings of Long and Vaillant (1984). Individual life histories studied by Levinson (and those who use a retrospective biographic method) may provide a picture of change because they have been studies of the role of the self in various contexts. Bengtson et al.'s (1985) review finds less consistency vis-à-vis self than in terms of personality traits and characteristics. Furthermore, retrospective studies are able to cover the full time span of the subjects' memories and thus may cover a greater time span (and greater variance due to memory processes), accounting for part of the discrepancy that has appeared to be method variance. What is clear from this review is that overall summary statements about personality and age are likely to be over-simplifications.

Social Interactions and Attributions

Social interactions may be influenced by stereotypes. Research by Schmidt and Boland (1986) indicates that both positive and negative stereotypes of older persons are much more complex than had been thought. The myth of the generalized "older adult" is no longer a societal stereotype, at least among educated university students ages 18 to 33. Lachman and McArthur (1986) studied causal attributions of young (mean age 19.3) versus old (mean age 74.9) men and women made for their own and another's (both same age and opposite age group) performance on cognitive (memory and problem solving), social (independence and nurturance), and physical (strength and speed) domains. Three causes were rated: internal stable (ability), internal unstable (effort), and external. Lachman and McArthur interpret their complex findings as more positive than previous studies and as extremely realistic views of elderly by themselves as well as by younger persons.

There has been a developing interest in the role of social support as a moderating variable in the lives of middle-aged and older persons. Brodhead et al. (1983) reviewed the evidence relating social support to health and concluded that there is a strong relationship. Schulz and Rau (1985) reviewed the evidence on social support across the adult life course. They evaluated support in coping with a variety of normative and nonnormative life events; Their conclusions were that the size of the network remains relatively constant (8 to 15 persons); in nonnormative events, a larger network is helpful; diverse networks are helpful in coping with normative but off-time events; and the stability in the network can mean that negative as well as positive effects persist. Minkler (1985) reviewed the evidence on social support of the elderly. She noted that after the age of 70 networks tend to be smaller, most of the elderly have the basic support network, and relationships between social support and other variables appear to be similar for the elderly and for younger age groups. The elderly are more unique in their problems than in the way constructs operate.

Pilisuk et al. (1987) evaluated medical care utilization in older (ages 40 to 72, mean age 49) members of a health maintenance organization for a 5-year period. Social support was measured by a 65-item schedule of social functioning yielding three factors: spouse/family support, friend support, and positive network orientation (nonparanoid/trustful). Results indicated increased utilization as a function of older age, higher stress, and lower social support. Rook (1987b) reviewed five studies that compared the role of social support versus companionship. The effects were mediated by stress such that in conditions of high stress, support was helpful, but in low stress support had negative effects. Companionship, independent of stress, was generally positive. Krause (1987) found that older persons who were higher in giving and receiving social support had fewer depressive symptoms under conditions of financial strain, arguing for the role of social support as a buffer between depression and financial strain. The buffering effect of social support was also reported by Cutrana et al. (1986) in a group of community elderly measured at 6-month intervals. Rook (1987a, 1987b) evaluated the reciprocity of social exchange in a group of 120 older women. Loneliness was associated with unbalanced reciprocity in both giving more and receiving less. Results differed between friends and children, with well-being highest when the women received more from their children.

Social support is not always positive. It implies a reciprocal relationship, and the provider of the support may experience extreme stress and depression. Gallagher et al. (in press) review the set of negative emotions experienced by caregivers of Alzheimer's disease patients (depression, anger, and anxiety). Scharlach (1987) evaluated two interventions to relieve strain between elderly mothers and their daughters. A cognitive–behavioral presentation designed to reduce the daughters' feelings of responsibility to more realistic levels was more effective than an educational presentation designed to increase the daughters' awareness of their mother's needs.

Larson et al. (1986) compared family and friends as sources of psychological well-being. Ninety-two retired adults carried pagers for one week and filled out self-reports when signaled. They were randomly signaled once per 2-hour time block between 8 A.M. and 10 P.M. As a group, 76 percent of the pages were responded to, providing data on 3,412 self-reports of activity and affect. Married and unmarried were analyzed separately. The married spent their time with their spouse (41.6 percent) or alone (38.9 percent). The unmarried spent 65.8 percent of their time alone. Children occupied 6.8 percent of the unmarried subjects' time and 2 percent of the married subjects' time (plus 4 percent with children and spouse together). Friends occupied 14.2 percent of the time of the unmarried and 5.2 percent of the married subjects' time (plus an additional 2.8 percent for spouse and friends). There were substantial differences in subjective state that varied as a function of the companion. Being with friends was consistently reported to have a higher positive affect than being with family for both the married and the unmarried. For the married, spouse and friends had a higher affect than friends alone. While the authors do not suggest the following as an interpretation, there are two variables they did not measure: (1) the arena of choice that is present with friends and not with family, and (2) that social support is reciprocal and family members often demand more than do friends.

Social changes and their impact on older persons as members of families have been significant. The psychologic impact of divorce and stepparenting on the grandparent generation is beginning to become the subject of research (Datan et al. 1987). Issues of reduced fertility suggest that the next generation of elders will need to find nonfamilial arrangements (Aizenberg and Treas 1985) and speaks to the importance of research on friendship networks among the elderly.

Schlossberg (1987) introduced the concept of mattering (Rosenberg and McCullough 1981) to audiences in adult development. Mattering is the degree to which we feel we matter to others. For many adults and older persons, much of the stress in middle and later life that requires coping can be usefully conceptualized as searches for environments in which mattering needs are successfully fulfilled. The literature on social support and its health and coping effects continues to grow. There is little reason to believe that once the mechanisms of action of social support are understood they will be different for persons of different ages, holding important life situations constant.

Health and Behavior

As the capacity for increased length of life expands decade by decade it becomes clear that we have very different subgroups among the elderly (Siegler 1985). Variations in health, rather than age, are responsible for the age differences that are seen (Siegler and Costa 1985). The frail, impaired elderly appear to have very little in common with their more robust age peers. Similarly, the data are beginning to show that even in the middle years, premature morbidity and mortality may be lessened by attention to modification of risk factors (see Schoenbach 1985). Thus attention to behavioral factors and their relationship to health is important for practical as well as theoretical reasons. The real issues for geropsychology are the contributions of our research to improved diagnosis and treatment of middle-aged and older persons and the extent to which our research efforts can help reduce risk factor profiles and disability during middle and later life. In this section we will review research findings on clinical assessment, risk factors, health behaviors, and interventions with older patient populations.

Assessment of Cognitive Function

Clinical psychologists and neuropsychologists are often confronted with cognitive complaints from older clients. It has been noted that about 80 percent of the cognitive complaints are memory related (Kaszniak et al. 1986). Are these complaints indicative of "malignant memory loss" or just "benign senescent forgetfulness"? Although there are numerous standardized memory and cognitive assessment batteries, there is no general agreement among clinicians about which battery provides the appropriate sensitivity and specificity in diagnosing memory dysfunction in older adults (Erickson et al. 1980). For example, the Wechsler Memory Scale was found to have limited power for detecting specific deficits (Erickson and Howieson 1986), the Guild Memory Test was found to be too complex for some patients (Gilbert et al. 1968), and the Randt Memory Test (Randt et al. 1980) was found lacking in the measurement of nonverbal memory. The clinician's dilemma in test selection is further illustrated by the common complaint among clinicians that some tests bear no resemblance to the everyday cognitive functioning of the patient.

There are three major reasons for the difficulty in cognitive assessment. First, memory and cognition consist of many subsystems and are multidimensional in nature. Second, many individual, environmental, and situational characteristics can influence these cognitive functions. Third, there are wide and variable ranges of responses that can be considered normal functioning. The multivariate nature of cognition makes it clear why the level of functioning is fluid and subject to intra- and interpersonal variability.

When dysfunction is in the early stages, the fluid nature of cognition makes it a challenge to estimate the probability of dysfunction and to isolate the locus of the dysfunction. The uncertainty of isolating early cognitive dysfunction could have contributed to an estimated high percentage of misdiagnosis (10 to 50 percent) in diagnosing cases of possible Alzheimer's disease by clinicians (Gurland and Cross 1986).

For recent reviews on clinical assessment see Poon et al. (1986), Gurland and Cross (1986), Eisdorfer (1986), Crook (1986), Thompson (1986), Kaszniak and Davis (1986), and Zarit et al. (1985).

Informed Decision Making in Differential Diagnosis

It is fair to state that every clinician has his or her favorite tests and modes of hypothesis testing in making differential diagnoses, and there is no one correct approach in test selection to confirm hypotheses. It is important, however, to know precisely the goal of the evaluation, because some tests are designed to predict, others to understand, and some to do both. The selection for a test or a set of tests should, therefore, be guided by the prototypical behavioral symptoms of the disease, the hypotheses of the clinician, and the previously demonstrated sensitivity and specificity of a test, as well as by psychometric properties of the test. This process necessitates informed decision making on the part of the clinician.

Recent development in tests for intake of signs and symptoms, classification of severity of symptoms, and in-depth reviews of psychometric, neuropsychologic, and information-processing approaches for the analysis of underlying cognitive mechanisms can provide a sound initial basis to make informed judgments in differential diagnosis.

Three clusters of instruments are available to assist the clinician to systematically outline the nature of memory and cognitive complaints. The first cluster comes from questionnaire or interview studies that were designed to study metamemory (the effects of the feeling of knowing). A number of memory complaint questionnaires are available and could be adopted for clinical use (see review by Gilewski and Zelinski 1986). The second cluster of instruments comes from rating scales designed for drug studies and minimental status examinations that are employed to provide a cursory survey of cognitive and noncognitive factors (for reviews see McDonald 1986; Reisberg et al. 1986; Ferris et al. 1986). Finally, the third cluster of instruments that could assist in the evaluation of complaints comes from depression assessment inventories. These instruments can help the clinician differentiate and relate complaint symptoms with depression and performance (for reviews see Yesavage 1986; Gallagher 1986).

The classification of symptom severity is a difficult task at best, owing to individual differences and variability in responses. The efforts of two investigative teams to define stages of cognitive impairment in Alzheimer's disease could provide some insight for individual clinicians. They are the work of Reisberg et al. (1986) and Rosen et al. (1986).

Finally, several recent summaries provide information that would be useful for informed decision making in test selection: For rationale for the neuropsychologic approach, see Corkin et al. (1986) and Goldberg and Bilder (1986); for the diagnostic link between brain–behavior dysfunctions, see Riege et al. (1986); for the information-processing approach, see Kaszniak et al. (1986); and for the psychometric approach, see Ferris et al. (1986).

Another interesting question concerns the changes in cognitive functioning seen in psychiatric disorders aside from Alzheimer's disease. Niederehe

and Rusin (in press) review the evidence about changes in cognitive functioning across the life span in chronic schizophrenia. They argue that information-processing deficits have been reported as a function of both schizophrenia and normal aging and speculate on their interactions. Comparisons of
younger versus older patient groups have yet to provide any important
insights, and the authors argue for more longitudinal research.

Behavioral medicine.   Behavioral medicine is the study of the role that
behavioral factors can play in our understanding of the causes and consequences of disease (Rodin 1987). The area of behavioral medicine is an
outgrowth of the traditional area of psychosomatic medicine. It is particularly
useful in the study of aging because so many diseases of the elderly have
behavioral components and because the elderly respond to behavioral treatment approaches. Similarly, there has been an increase of attention to the
elderly in public health (see Phillips and Gaylord 1985).

Risk factors.   Behavioral factors have been shown to be important in the
prediction of coronary heart disease (Williams et al. 1980, 1985; Friedman and
Booth-Kewley 1987) and in the treatment of arthritis (Verbrugge 1987) as well
as diabetes (Surwit et al. 1982). Little is known about the role of behavioral
factors in the etiology of stroke, dementia (see Mortimer and Schumann
1981), or cancer (see Fox 1978), but behavioral treatments have proved to be
of use.
     The Type A behavior pattern appears to be an independent risk factor for
coronary heart disease. However, recent studies have reported that this is
more likely to be true as a predictor of premature mortality and morbidity—
that is, under age 50 to 55 for coronary heart disease (see Anderson 1987;
Williams et al. 1986; Siegler et al. 1985). The strongest arguments to date are
for selection bias: that is, those who are high on the Type A behavior pattern
are those who are selected out by death or disease. Those who survive are
therefore, as a group, more likely to be Type B. It is interesting that in their
generally excellent meta-analysis of psychological predictors of coronary
heart disease, Booth-Kewley and Friedman (1987) pay little attention to age as
a mediator except to report that in prospective studies controlled for other
risk factors (smoking, serum cholesterol, blood pressure, or education) none
of the risk factors—including age—were important mediators between Type
A and coronary heart disease.

Health behaviors.   Leventhal et al. (1985) review the evidence of preventive health behaviors across the life cycle. They focus on specific health
and risk behaviors. Prohaska et al. (cited in Leventhal 1985) asked 390 adults
ages 20 to 34, 35 to 49, and over 50 about the practice of 20 health habits.
Respondents over 50 years old were significantly more likely to report
avoiding harmful health habits. They were less likely to engage in strenuous

exercise and more likely to get medical check-ups. Prohaska et al. also asked subjects to rate the efficacy of the health behaviors. There were no age differences in perceived effectiveness of the health behaviors. Older people were more likely to believe that specific modifications were effective for particular diseases. Leventhal et al. (in press) argue that a major mechanism of older persons for engaging in health preventive behaviors and in coping with illness is in shifting affective appraisal. This mechanism is similar to the coping view of Lazarus and his colleagues (Lazarus and Folkman 1984) of problem-focused versus emotion-focused coping strategies. Our own findings on coping with stressful life events support the view that emotion-focused coping is particularly effective for coping with health events that cannot be modified (George and Siegler 1985). Felton and Revenson (1987) studied middle-aged and older persons with hypertension, rheumatoid arthritis, diabetes, and cancer. Coping was measured by six factor analytically derived scales from Lazarus's Ways of Coping Scale. The results indicated that there were complex interactions of age, coping strategy, and the measure of illness tested, which suggested that any simplistic findings about age relationships are unlikely to be true.

Folkman et al. (1987) evaluated age differences in stress and coping processes in two samples, married couples in which the wife was age 35 to 45 ($n = 150$), and retired men and women ages 65 to 74 ($n = 141$). Individuals were interviewed in their homes once per month for 6 months. Daily hassles were measured with 46 items that were factored into eight scales: household responsibilities, finances, work, environmental/social issues, home mainte-nance, health, personal life, and family and friends. Cognitive appraisal and coping were assessed by interview in which a stressful event was recalled. Coping was measured with a 31-item version of the Ways of Coping Scale that had scales measuring confrontive coping, distancing, self-control, seeking social support, escape–avoidance, planful problem solving, and positive reap-praisal. Age, gender, and age × gender interactions were tested with a multivariate analysis variance, and all were significant. Patterns depended on the particular hassle, although an inspection of results presented in a table suggests that younger people had more hassles. Hassles were evaluated in terms of frequency and relative frequency. Coping scales and situations were also evaluated. Across all types of encounters, middle-aged persons were more likely to use active strategies and older persons more likely to use more passive strategies. While attempts were made to control for situation used to assess coping, the severity of situations for young and old may have varied such that health meant something different for each. There was relatively little evidence for sex differences.

Students of health behaviors are often oriented toward intervention strategies. Leventhal et al. (in press) argue that more primary prevention efforts should be made with the elderly. But a major barrier to their success is that elderly persons are quite adept at accepting the distress of daily life as normal and coping by psychologic reorganizations. Thus a shift to a preventive strategy may be done at significant emotional cost.

Rodin (1986) reviewed the evidence relating health, locus of control, and aging. She argues that the elderly are particularly vulnerable to health-control issues because the role of stress is increased both by experiencing more stress-inducing events and/or environmental challenges and by having an increased physiological vulnerability to the effects of stress. She reports on some exciting preliminary data from a community sample of older persons (aged 62 to 91). Baseline measures of immunocompetence were taken from 24-hour urine samples, and indices of B, T4, and T8 cell function were correlated with age, health, life satisfaction, major life events, expectation of stressors, and sense of control. Recency of life events and effects of these events on the respondents', sense of control were the major psychosocial predictors of immune function. These data begin to present the outlines for potential mechanisms whereby stress can be seen to influence health in the elderly.

Cicirelli (1987) studied health locus of control in elderly patients in a general hospital setting. He found that those who were highly external in their beliefs (believed that outcomes were controlled by powerful others) were better adjusted to the inpatient hospital setting, which was a setting of high constraint.

Woodward and Wallston (1987) evaluated the relationship between older persons' desire for control of their health, age, and self-efficacy. Subjects were 119 adults aged 20 to 99. They measured desire for control of health care specific to situation, desire for information, and general desire for control. Self-efficacy was measured by presenting situations; if the situation was a true one, then they were asked their degree of confidence in their ability to handle the situation. A health care self-efficacy scale was designed to measure the individual's level of self-confidence to each of the items in the health locus of control and health information scales. Three age groups were 20 to 39, 40 to 59, and 60 to 99. While the young and middle-aged groups were generally similar, together they were different from the older group on all health locus of control and self-efficacy measures. Individuals over age 60 had a lower desire for control over their health and for control in general, as well as lowered self-efficacy.

These results may also be seen as realistic. Siegler and Gatz (1985) evaluated older persons' locus of control for causing an event to happen versus their locus of control for the handling of an event. These had quite different patterns. Since health events are generally uncontrollable, the findings of Woodward and Wallston may be seen as in the realistic direction. Lachman (1986b) has reviewed the evidence for stability and change in locus of control. The literature is contradictory. Nonetheless, Lachman makes a cogent point, which is that elderly persons acknowledge the increasing importance of external sources of control in their lives while simultaneously maintaining their own sense of internality. Baltes and Reisenzein (1986) review evidence from Baltes's research program on dependency in the elderly. Behaviors were observed of both elderly persons and children in institutional settings. Their results indicate that dependent behaviors of elder persons are often followed by complementary social consequences and are thereby reinforced. Thus, dependency seems to allow the older persons to attain passive control in a highly constrained setting. The theme of realism about control appears to be the most parsimonious explanation for the varied findings about control and aging.

Behavioral treatments are beginning to be applied to nursing home populations as well. Moran and Gatz (1987) reported increases in psychosocial competence among nursing home residents after short-term group therapy. As more and more older persons survive with disabilities, the role of rehabilitation becomes more critical and a greater part of the rehabilitation literature becomes concerned with geriatrics (Kemp 1985). Stephens et al. 1987) evaluated psychosocial factors in the rehabilitation of 48 elderly stroke patients with moderate levels of expressive and receptive speech who were randomly selected from a year's worth of discharges from a rehabilitation hospital. Subjects were interviewed about positive and negative interactions with members of their social networks in their homes (12.5 percent were discharged to nursing homes) and their overall adjustment. Those who reported higher positive social interactions had higher cognitive scores, and those with higher negative social interactions had poorer morale and fewer symptoms. These results are interesting, but the directionality cannot be evaluated properly in the cross-sectional design. Similarly, as the data base develops on the effect of psychotherapeutic interventions with a wide variety of older patients in a wide variety of clinical settings, the efficacy of treatment is seen to follow successful treatment principles that are generalizable across the life span and provide an optimistic view of the role of therapeutic interventions in enhancing the quality of life of older persons (Gatz et al. 1985).

Longevity, Successful Aging, and Thoughts for the Future

Longevity and successful aging are two distinct constructs. They are not always found together; one might even argue that they are seldom found together. However, later life is often measured with one of these common yardsticks. They are convenient positive end points for aging research. In evaluating factor analytic studies of psychologic well-being, Okun and Stock (1987) conclude that three factors are adequate to describe the phenomenon of well-being: positive affect, negative affect, and cognition. Older persons cognitively manipulate their perceptions to maintain appropriate psychologic well-being in the face of imperfect circumstances. Often correlations between objective circumstances and psychologic well-being are weak (as evidenced by the generally high levels of well-being in institutions). Costa et al. (1987) report on a longitudinal analysis of psychological well-being in the National Health and Nutrition Examination Survey Follow-up Study. Neither the sample nor the analysis can be faulted; thus the conclusions for stability of mean levels in psychologic well-being from ages 25 to 74 and a 9-year time period are impressive indeed.

The purpose of this chapter has been to give an overview of the theory and data in the psychology of aging and the aged in order to provide a set of benchmarks to the question "What is normal aging?" and to review the recent additions to the psychologic literature. Processes of normal aging are being described in ever greater detail. In addition, we are developing data on persons who are aging and survive with nonlethal disorders. Is this normal or abnormal aging? The field of the psychology of aging is no longer as isolated as it once was. There has been an increase of activity in research on public health and behavioral medicine that has been reflected in the number of papers dealing with behavioral factors in middle-aged and older persons (see Maddox et al. 1987; Siegler in press). Research focusing on the behavior of middle-aged and older persons and the contributions of behavioral modes of therapy in the treatment of older persons have made this a particularly interesting time to review the literature in the psychology of adult development and aging.

References

Aizenberg R, Treas J: The family in late life: psychosocial and demographic considerations, in Handbook of the Psychology of Aging, Second Edition. Edited by Birren JE, Schaie KW. New York, Van Nostrand Reinhold, 1985

Albert MS, Kaplan E: Organic implications of neuropsychological deficits in the elderly, in New Directions in Memory and Aging: Proceeding of the George Talland Memorial Conference. Edited by Poon LW, Fozard JL, Cermak LS, et al. Hillsdale, NJ, Erlbaum, 1980

American Psychiatric Association. Diagnostic and Statistical Manual of Mental Disorders (Third Edition, Revised). Washington, DC, American Psychiatric Association, 1987

Anderson, NB: Coronary prone behavior, in Encyclopedia of Aging. Edited by Maddox, GL, Atchley RC, Poon LW, et al. New York, Springer, 1987

Baltes MM, Reisenzein R: The social world in long-term care institutions: psychosocial control toward dependency, in The Psychology of Control and Aging. Edited by Baltes, MM, Baltes PB. Hillsdale, NJ, Erlbaum, 1986

Baltes PB, Willis SL: Enhancement (plasticity) of intellectual functioning in old age: Penn State's adult development and enrichment project (ADEPT), in Aging and Cognitive Process. Edited by Craik FIM, Trehub SE. New York, Plenum Press, 1982

Baltes PB, Dittman-Kohli F, Kliegl R: Reserve capacity of the elderly in aging-sensitive tests of fluid intelligence: replication and extension. Psychology and Aging 1986; 1:172–177

Barbizet J, Cany E: A psychometric study of various memory deficits associated with cerebral lesions, in The Pathology of Memory. Edited by Talland GA, Waugh NC. New York, Academic Press, 1969

Bengtson VL, Reedy MN, Gordon C: Aging and self-conceptions: personality processes and social contexts, in Handbook of the Psychology of Aging. Edited by Birren JE, Schaie KW. New York, Van Nostrand Reinhold, 1985

Binstock RH, Shanas E (eds): Handbook of Aging and the Social Sciences (second edition). New York, Van Nostrand Reinhold, 1985

Birren JE, Cunningham W: Research on the psychology of aging: principles, concepts, and theory, in Handbook of the Psychology of Aging (second edition). Edited by Birren JE, Schaie KW. New York, Van Nostrand Reinhold 1985

Birren JE, Schaie KW (eds): Handbook of the Psychology of Aging (second edition). New York, Van Nostrand Reinhold, 1985

Birren JE, Cunningham WR, Yamamoto K: Psychology of adult development and aging, in Annual Review of Psychology. Edited by Rosenzweig MR, Porter LW. Palo Alto, CA, Annual Reviews, 1983

Booth-Kewley S, Friedman HS: Psychological predictors of heart disease: a quantitative review. Psychol Bull 1987; 101:343–362

Botwinick J: Aging and Behavior. New York, Springer, 1973

Botwinick J: Problem solving: forming concepts, in Aging and Behavior. Edited by Botwinick J. New York, Springer, 1984

Bowles NL, Poon LW: An analysis of the effect of aging on recognition memory. J Gerontol 1982; 37:212–219

Brinkman, SD, Largen JW, Gerganoff S, et al: Russell's revised Wechsler memory scale in the evaluation of dementia. J Clin Psychol 1983; 39:989–993

Brodhead E, Kaplan BH, James SA, et al: The epidemiologic evidence for a relationship between social support and health. Am J Epidemiol 1983; 117:521–537

Busse EW, Maddox GL: The Duke Longitudinal Studies of Normal Aging 1955–1980. New York, Springer, 1985

Caird WK, Sanderson RE, Inglis J: Cross validation of a learning test for use with elderly psychiatric patients. Ment Sci 1962; 108:368–370

Caspi A, Elder GH: Life satisfaction in old age: linking social psychology and history. Psychology and Aging 1986; 1:18–26

Cicirelli VG: Locus of control and patient role adjustment of the elderly in acute-care hospitals. Psychology and Aging 1987; 2:138–143

Cohen G: Language comprehension in old age. Cognitive Psychology 1979; 11:412–429

Cohen G: Inferential reasoning in old age. Cognition 1981; 9:59–72

Cohen G, Faulkner D: Memory for discourse in old age. Discourse Processes 1982; 4:253–265

Cohen G, Faulkner D: Word recognition: age differences in contextual facilitation effects. Br J Psychol 1983; 74:239–251

Cohen S, Syme SL (eds): Social Support and Health. Orlando, FL, Academic Press, 1985

Cooper KL, Gutmann DL: Gender identity and ego mastery style in middle-aged, pre- and post-empty nest women. Gerontologist 1987; 27:347–352

Corkin S: Some relationships between global amnesias and the memory impairments in Alzheimer's disease, in Alzheimer's Disease: A Report of Progress in Research. Edited by Corkin S, Davis KL, Growdon JH, et al. New York, Raven Press, 1982

Corkin S, Growdon JH, Sullivan EV, et al: Assessing treatment effects: a neuropsychological battery, in Handbook for Clinical Memory Assessment of Older Adults. Edited by Poon LW. Washington, DC, American Psychological Association, 1986

Costa PT Jr, McCrae RR: Still stable after all these years: personality as a key to some issues in adulthood and old age, in Life Span Development and Behavior. Edited by Baltes P, Brim O. New York, Academic Press, 1980

Costa PT Jr, McCrae RR: Cross-sectional studies of personality in a national sample: 1. Development and validation of survey measures. Psychology and Aging 1986; 1:140–143

Costa PR Jr, McCrae RR, Zonderman AB: Cross-sectional studies of personality in a national sample: 2. Stability in neuroticism, extraversion, and openness. Psychology and Aging 1986; 1:144–149

Costa PR Jr, Zonderman AB, McCrae RR, et al: Longitudinal analyses of psychological well-being in a national sample: stability of mean levels. J Gerontol 1987; 42:50–55

Crook T: Overview of Memory Assessment Instruments, in Handbook for Clinical Memory Assessment of Older Adults. Edited by Poon LW. Washington, DC, American Psychological Association, 1986

Crook T, Ferris S, McCarthy M, et al: Utility of digit recall tasks for assessing memory in the aged. J Consult Clin Psychol 1980; 48:228–233

Cross KP: Adults as Learners. San Francisco, Jossey-Bass, 1981

Cutrona C, Russell D, Rose J: Social support and adaptation to stress by the elderly. Psychology and Aging 1986; 1:47–54

Danziger WL, Storandt M: Psychometric performance of healthy and demented older adults: a one-year follow-up. Paper presented at the annual meeting of the Gerontological Society of America, Boston, 1982

Datan N, Rodeheaver D, Hughes F: Adult development and aging, in Annual Review of Psychology. Edited by Rosenwig MR, Porter HW. Palo Alto, CA, Annual Reviews, 1987

de Leon MJ, Ferris SH, George AE, et al: Computed tomography evaluations of brain–behavior relationships in senile dementia of the Alzheimer's type. Neurobiol Aging 1980; 1:69–79

Denney NW: Cognitive change, in Handbook of Developmental Psychology. Edited by Wolman BB, Stricker G. Englewood Cliffs, NJ, Prentice Hall, 1982

Denney NW: Everyday problem solving: Methodological issues, research findings, and a model in Cognition in Everyday Life. Edited by Poon LW. New York, Cambridge University Press, in press

Diesfeldt HFA: The distinction between long-term and short-term memory in senile dementia: an analysis of free recall and delayed recognition. Neuropsychologia 1978; 16:115–119

Edelman CD, Siegler IC: Federal Age Discrimination in Employment Law: Slowing Down the Gold Watch. Charlottesville, VA, The Michie Company, 1978

Eichorn DH, Clausen JA, Haan N, et al. (eds): Present and Past in Middle Life. New York, Academic Press, 1981

Eisdorfer C: Conceptual approaches to the clinical testing of memory in the aged: an introduction to the issues, in Handbook for Clinical Memory Assessment of Older Adults. Edited by Poon LW. Washington, DC, American Psychological Association, 1986

Erickson RC, Howieson D: The clinician's perspective: measuring change and treatment effectiveness, in Handbook for Clinical Memory Assessment of Older Adults. Edited by Poon LW. Washington, DC, American Psychological Association, 1986

Erickson RC, Poon LW, Walsh-Sweeney L: Clinical memory testing of the elderly, in New Directions in Memory and Aging: Proceedings of the George A Talland Memorial Conference. Edited by Poon LW, Fozard JL, Cermak LS, et al. Hillsdale, NJ, Erlbaum, 1980

Felton BJ, Revenson TA: Age differences in coping with chronic illness. Psychology and Aging 1987; 2:164–170

Ferris SH, Crook T, Flicker C, et al: Assessing changes in Alzheimer's disease: memory and language, in Handbook for Clinical Memory Assessment of Older Adults. Edited by Poon LW. Washington, DC, American Psychological Association, 1986

Finch CE, Schneider EL (eds): Handbook of the Biology of Aging. New York, Van Nostrand Reinhold, 1985

Folkman S, Lazarus RS, Pimley S, et al: Age differences in stress and coping processes. Psychology and Aging 1987; 2:171–184

Fox BH: Premorbid psychological factors related to cancer incidence. J Behav Med 1978; 1:45–133

Fozard JL: The time for remembering, in Aging in the 1980s: Psychological Issues. Edited by Poon LW. Washington, DC, American Psychological Association, 1980

Friedman, HS, Booth-Kewley S: The "disease-prone personality": a meta-analytic view of the construct. Am Psychol 1987; 42:539–555

Gallagher D: Assessment of depression by interview methods and psychiatric rating scale, in Handbook for Clinical Memory Assessment of Older Adults. Edited by Poon LW. Washington, DC, American Psychological Association, 1986

Gallagher D, Wrabetz A, Lovett S, et al: Depression and other negative affects in family caregivers, in Alzheimer's Disease Treatment and Family Stress: Directions for Research. Edited by Light E, Lebowitz B. Washington, DC, U.S. Government Printing Office

Gatz M, Popkin SJ, Pino CD, et al: Psychological interventions with older adults, in Handbook of the Psychology of Aging (second edition). Edited by Birren JE, Schaie KW. New York, Van Nostrand Reinhold, 1985

George LK, Siegler IC: Stress and coping in later life, in Normal Aging III. Edited by Palmore E, Busse EW, Maddox GL, et al. Durham, NC, Duke University Press, 1985

Giambra LM, Arenberg D: Problem solving, concept learning, and aging, in Aging in the 80s: Psychological Issues. Edited by Poon LW. Washington, DC, American Psychological Association, 1980

Gilbert HG, Levee RF, Catalano FL: A preliminary report on a new memory scale. Percept Mot Skills 1968; 27:277–278

Gilewski MJ, Zelinski EM: Questionnaire assessment of memory complaints, in Handbook for Clinical Memory Assessment of Older Adults. Edited by Poon LW. Washington, DC, American Psychological Association, 1986

Goldbert E, Bilder RM: Neuropsychological perspectives: retrograde amnesia and executive deficits, in Handbook for Clinical Memory Assessment of Older Adults. Edited by Poon LW. Washington, DC, American Psychological Association, 1986

Gordon SK, Clark WC: Application of signal detection theory to prose recall and recognition in elderly and young adults. J Gerontol 1974; 29:64–72

Gurland BJ, Cross PS: Public health perspectives on clinical memory testing of Alzheimer's disease and related disorders, in Handbook for Clinical Memory Assessment of Older Adults. Edited by Poon LW. Washington, DC, American Psychological Association, 1986

Haan N, Millsap, R, Hartka E: As time goes by: change and stability in personality over fifty years. Psychology and Aging 1986; 1:220–232

Harker JO, Hartley JT, Walsh DA: Understanding discourse—a life-span approach, in Advances in Reading/Language Research (Volume 1). Edited by Hutson BA. Greenwich, CT, JAI Press, 1982

Hartley JT: Memory for prose: perspectives on the reader, in Cognition in Everyday Life. Edited by Poon LW. New York, Cambridge University Press, in press

Heckler MM: The fight against Alzheimer's disease. Am Psychol 1985; 40:1240–1244

Hertzog C, Schaie KW: Stability and change in adult intelligence: 1. Analysis of longitudinal covariance structures. Psychology and Aging 1986; 1:159–171

Horner KL, Rushton JP, Vernon PA: Relation between aging and research productivity of academic psychologists. Psychology and Aging 1986; 1:319–324

Inglis J: A paired associate learning test for use with elderly psychiatric patients. Ment Sci 1959; 105:440–448

Inglis J, Caird WK: Modified digit spans and memory disorder. Diseases of the Nervous System 1963; 24:46–50

Kaszniak AW, Davis KL: Instrument and data review: the quest for external validators, in Handbook for Clinical Memory Assessment of Older Adults. Edited by Poon LW. Washington, DC, American Psychological Association, 1986

Kaszniak AW, Garron DC, Fox JH: Differential effects of age and cerebral atrophy upon span of immediate recall and paired-associate learning in older patients suspected of dementia. Cortex 1979a; 15:285–295

Kaszniak AW, Garron DC, Fox JH, et al: Cerebral atrophy, EEG slowing, age, education, and cognitive functioning in suspected dementia. Neurology 1979b; 29:1273–1279

Kaszniak AW, Poon LW, Riege W: Assessing memory deficits: an information-processing approach, in Handbook for Clinical Memory Assessment of Older Adults. Edited by Poon LW. Washington, DC, American Psychological Association, 1986

Kelly, EL, Conley JJ: Personality and compatibility: a prospective analysis of marital stability and marital satisfaction. J Pers Soc Psychol 1987; 52:27–40

Kemp B: Rehabilitation and the older adult, in Handbook of the Psychology of Aging (second edition). Edited by Birren JE, Schaie KW. New York, Van Nostrand Reinhold 1985

Khachaturian ZS: Progress of research on Alzheimer's disease: opportunities for behavioral scientists. Am Psychol 1985; 40:1251–1255

Kirasic KC: Study the "hometown advantage" in elderly adults' spatial cognition and spatial behavior. Paper presented as part of the symposium "Spatial Cognition in Older Adults: From Lab to Life" at the meetings of the Society for Research in Child Development, Boston, 1981

Kirasic KC: Acquisition and utilization of spatial information by elderly adults: implications for day-to-day situations, in Cognition in Everyday Life. Edited by Poon LW. New York, Cambridge University Press, in press

Klisz D: Neuropsychological evaluation in older persons, in The Clinical Psychology of Aging. Edited by Storandt M, Siegler IC, Elias MF. New York, Plenum Press, 1978

Krause N: Chronic financial strain, social support, and depressive symptoms among older adults. Psychology and Aging 1987; 2:185–192

Lachman ME: Locus of control in aging research: a case for multidimensional and domain-specific assessment. Psychology and Aging 1986a; 1:34–40

Lachman ME: Control: change and cognitive correlates, in The Psychology of Control and Aging. Edited by Baltes MM, Baltes PB. Hillsdale, NJ, Erlbaum, 1986b

Lachman ME, McArthur LZ: Adult age differences in the ability to cope with situations. Psychology and Aging 1986; 1:117–126

Larner S: Encoding in senile dementia and elderly depressives: a preliminary study. British Journal of Social and Clinical Psychology 1977; 16:379–390

Larson R, Mannell R, Zyzanek J: Daily well-being of older adults with friends and family. Psychology and Aging 1986; 1:117–126

Lazarus RS, Folkman S: Stress, Appraisal, and Coping. New York, Springer, 1984

Leventhal H, Prohaska TR, Hirschman RS: Preventive health behavior across the life-span, in Prevention in Health Psychology. Edited by Rosen JC, Solomon LJ. Hanover, NH, University Press of New England, 1985

Levinson DJ: A conception of adult development. Am Psychol 1986; 41:3–13

Logue P, Wyrick L: Initial validation of Russell's revised Wechsler memory scale: a comparison of normal aging versus dementia. J Consult Clin Psychol 1979; 47:176–178

Long, JVF, Vaillant GE: Natural history of male psychological health, X1: escape from the underclass. Am J Psychiatry 1984; 141:341–346

Lowenthal MF, Berkman PL, Beuler JA, et al: Aging and Mental Disorder in San Francisco. San Francisco, Jossey-Bass, 1967

Maddox GL, Lawton MP (eds): Annual Review of Gerontology and Geriatrics, Volume 8. New York, Springer, 1988

Maddox GL, Atchley RC, Poon LW, et al. (eds): Encyclopedia of Aging, New York, Springer, 1987

Manton, KG, Siegler IC, Woodbury MA: Patterns of intellectual development in later life. J Gerontol 1986; 41:486–489

McCarthy M, Ferris SH, Clark E, et al: Acquisition and retention of categorized material in normal aging and senile dementia. Exp Aging Res 1981; 7:127–135

McCrae RR, Costa PT: Emerging Lives, Enduring Dispositions. Boston, Little, Brown, 1984

McCrae RR, Arenberg D, Costa PT Jr: Declines in divergent thinking with age: cross-sectional, longitudinal, and cross-sequential analyses. Psychology and Aging 1987; 2:130–137

McDonald RS: Assessing treatment effects: behavior rating scales, in Handbook for Clinical Memory Assessment of Older Adults. Edited by Poon LW. Washington, DC, American Psychological Association, 1986

Mednick S, Harway M, Finello K: Handbook of Longitudinal Research. New York, Praeger, 1984

Meyer BJF, Rice GE: Information recalled from prose by young, middle, and old adults. Exp Aging Res 1981; 7:253–268

Meyer BJF, Rice GE: Prose processing in adulthood: the text, the learner, and the task, in Cognition in Everyday Life. Edited by Poon LW. New York, Cambridge University Press, in press

Miller E: On the nature of the memory disorder in presenile dementia. Neuropsychologia 1971; 9:75–78

Miller E: Short- and long-term memory in presenile dementia (Alzheimer's disease). Psychol Med 1973; 3:221–224

Miller E: Impaired recall and the memory disturbance in presenile dementia. British Journal of Social and Clinical Psychology 1975; 14:73–79

Miller E: Retrieval from long-term memory in presenile dementia: two tests of an hypothesis. British Journal of Social and Clinical Psychology 1978; 17:143–148

Miller E, Lewis P: Recognition memory in elderly patients with depression and dementia: a signal detection analysis. J Abnorm Psychol 1977; 86:84–86

Minkler M: Social support and health of the elderly, in Social Support and Health. Edited by Cohen S, Syme SL. Orlando, FL, Academic Press, 1985

Moran JA, Gatz M: Group therapies for nursing home adults: an evaluation of two treatment approaches. Gerontologist 1987; 27:588–591

Mortimer JA, Schumann LM (eds): The Epidemiology of Dementia. New York, Oxford University Press, 1981

Nickerson RS, Green DM, Stevens KN, et al: Some experimental tasks for the study of the effects of aging on cognition, in Design Conference on Decision Making and Aging JSAS: Selected Documents in Psychology. Edited by Poon LW, Fozard JL. Washington, DC, American Psychological Association, 1981

Niederehe G, Rusin MJ: Schizophrenia and aging: information processing patterns, in Schizophrenia, Paranoia and Schizopheniform Disorders in Late Life. Edited by Miller NE, Cohen GD. New York, Pergamon Press, in press

Okun MA, Stock WA: Correlates and components of subjective well-being in the elderly. Journal of Applied Gerontology 1987; 6:95–112

Olsho LW, Harkins SW, Lenhardt ML: Aging and the auditory system, in Handbook of the Psychology of Aging (second edition). Edited by Birren JE, Schaie KW. New York, Van Nostrand Reinhold, 1985

Osborne DP, Brown ER, Randt CT: Qualitative changes in memory function: aging and dementia, in Alzheimer's Disease: A Report of Progress in Research. Edited by Corkin S, Davis KL, Growdon E, et al. New York, Raven Press, 1982

Palmore E, Busse EW, Maddox GL, et al (eds): Normal Aging III. Reports from the Duke Longitudinal Studies, 1975–1984. Durham, NC, Duke University Press, 1985

Park DC, Puglisi JT, Sovacool M: Memory for pictures and spatial location in older adults: evidence for pictorial superiority. J Gerontol 1983; 38:582-588

Phillips HT, Gaylord SA (eds): Aging and Public Health. New York, Springer, 1985

Pilisuk M, Boylan K, Acredolo C: Social support life stress, and subsequent medical care utilization. Health Psychol 1987; 6:273–288

Poon LW (ed): Aging in the 1980s: Psychological Issues. Washington, DC, American Psychological Association, 1980

Poon LW: Differences in human memory with aging: nature, causes and clinical implications, in Handbook of the Psychology of Aging. Edited by Birren JE, Schaie KW. New York, Van Nostrand Reinhold, 1985

Poon LW (ed): Handbook for Clinical Memory Assessment of Older Adults. Washington, DC, American Psychological Association, 1986

Poon LW, Fozard JL: Age and word frequency effects in continuous recognition memory. J Gerontol 1980; 35:77–86

Poon LW, Gurland BJ, Eisdorfer C, et al: Integration of experimental and clinical precepts in memory assessment: a tribute to George Talland, in Handbook for Clinical Memory Assessment of Older Adults. Edited by Poon LW. Washington, DC, American Psychological Association, 1986

Poon LW, Rubin D, Wilson B (eds): Cognition in Everyday Life. New York, Cambridge University Press, (in press)

Randt CT, Brown ER, Osborne DP Jr: A memory test for longitudinal measurement of mild to moderate deficits. Clinical Neuropsychology 1980; 2:184–194

Reisberg B, Ferris SH, Borenstein J, et al: Assessment of Presenting Symptoms, in Handbook for Clinical Memory Assessment of Older Adults. Edited by Poon LW. Washington, DC, American Psychological Association, 1986

Riege WH, Harker JO, Metter EJ: Clinical validators: brain lesions and brain imaging, in Handbook for Clinical Memory Assessment of Older Adults. Edited by Poon LW. Washington, DC, American Psychological Association, 1986

Roberts P, Newton PM: Levinsonian studies of women's adult development. Psychology and Aging 1987; 2:154–163

Rodin J: Health: control and aging, in The Psychology of Control and Aging. Edited by Baltes MM, Baltes PB. Hillsdale, NJ, Erlbaum, 1986

Rodin J: Behavioral medicine, in Encyclopedia of Aging. Edited by Maddox GL, Atchley RC, Poon LW (eds): New York, Springer, 1987

Rook KS: Social support versus companionship: effects on life stress, loneliness, and evaluations by others. J Pers Soc Psychol 1987a; 52:1132–1147

Rook KS: Reciprocity of social exchange and social satisfaction among older women. J Pers Soc Psychol 1987b; 52:145–154

Rosen WG, Mohs RC: Evolution of cognitive decline in dementia, in Alzheimer's Disease: A Report of Progress in Research. Edited by Corkin S, Davis KL, Growdon, et al. New York, Raven Press, 1982

Rosen WG, Mohs RC, Davis KL: Longitudinal changes: cognitive, behavioral, and affective patterns in Alzheimer's disease, in Handbook for Clinical Memory Assessment of Older Adults. Edited by Poon LW. Washington, DC, American Psychological Association, 1986

Rosenberg M, McCullough BC: Mattering: inferred significance to parents and mental health among adolescents. Research in Community and Mental Health 1981; 2:163–182

Salthouse TA (ed): Adult Cognition: An Experimental Psychology of Human Aging. New York, Springer-Verlag, 1982a

Salthouse TA: Decision making and problem solving, in Adult Cognition: An Experimental Psychology of Human Aging. Edited by Salthouse TA. New York, Springer-Verlag, 1982b

Salthouse TA: A Theory of Cognitive Aging. Amsterdam, North-Holland, 1985

Santos JF, VandenBos GR (eds): Psychology and the Older Adult: Challenges for Training in the 1980s. Washington, DC, American Psychological Association, 1981

Schaie KW (ed): Longitudinal Studies of Adult Psychological Development. New York, Guilford Press, 1983

Schaie KW, Hertzog C: Measurement in the psychology of adulthood and aging, in Handbook of the Psychology of Aging (second edition). Edited by Birren JE, Schaie KW. New York, Van Nostrand Reinhold, 1985

Scharlach AE: Relieving feelings of strain among women with elderly mothers. Psychology and Aging 1987; 2:9–13

Schlossberg, NK: Understanding and reaching adult learners. McGill Journal of Education 1987; 22:5–14

Schmidt DF, Boland SM: Structure of perceptions of older adults: evidence for multiple stereotypes. Psychology and Aging 1986; 1:255–260

Schoenbach VJ: Behavior and life style as determinants of health and well-being in the elderly, in Aging and Public Health. Edited by Phillips HT, Gaylord SA. New York, Springer, 1985

Schulz R, Rau MT: Social support through the life course, in Social Support and Health. Edited by Cohen S, Syme SL. Orlando, FL, Academic Press, 1985

Shock NW, Greulich RC, Costa, PT Jr, et al. (eds): Normal Human Aging: The Baltimore Longitudinal Study of Aging. Washington, DC, National Institutes of Health, 1984

Siegler IC: Attitudes about age discrimination. Paper presented at Gerontological Society of America, San Diego, 1979

Siegler IC: The psychology of adult development and aging, in Handbook of Geriatric Psychiatry. Edited by Busse EW, Blazer DG. New York, Van Nostrand Reinhold, 1980

Siegler IC: Toward a developmental health psychology. Division 20 Presidential Address. Presented at the annual meeting of the American Psychological Association, Los Angeles, 1985

Siegler IC: Developmental health psychology, in The Adult Years: Continuity and Change. Edited by Storandt M, VandenBos GR. Washington, DC, American Psychological Association, in press

Siegler IC, Costa PT Jr: Health behavior relationships, in Handbook of the Psychology of Aging (second edition). Edited by Birren JE, Schaie KW. New York, Van Nostrand Reinhold, 1985

Siegler IC, Gatz M: Age patterns in locus of control, in Normal Aging III. Reports from the Duke Longitudinal Studies, 1975–1984. Edited by Palmore E, Busse EW, Maddox GL, et al. Durham, NC, Duke University Press, 1985

Siegler IC, Nowlin JB, Blumenthal JA: Health and behavior: methodological considerations for adult development and aging, in Aging in the 1980s: Selected Contemporary Issues. Edited by Poon LW. Washington, DC, American Psychological Association, 1980

Siegler IC, Nowlin JB, Blumenthal JA, et al: Type A behavior pattern in later life. Paper presented at the meeting of the International Association of Gerontology, New York, 1985

Stagner R: Aging and industry, in Handbook of the Psychology of Aging (second edition). Edited by Birren JE, Schaie KW. New York, Van Nostrand Reinhold, 1985

Stephens MAP, Kinney JM, Norris VK, et al: Social networks as assets and liabilities in recovering from stroke in geriatric patients. Psychology and Aging 1987; 2:125–129

Sterns HL: Training and retraining adult and older adult workers, in Age, Health and Employment. Edited by Birren JE, Robinson PK, Livingston JE. Englewood Cliffs, NJ, Prentice-Hall, 1986

Sterns HL, Alexander RA: Industrial gerontology, in Annual Review of Gerontology and Geriatrics (Volume 7). Edited by Schaie KW. New York, Springer, 1987

Steuer J, LaRue A, Blum JE, et al: Critical loss in the eighth and ninth decades. J Gerontol 1981; 36:211–213

Stine EL, Wingfield A, Poon LW: How much and how fast: rapid processing of spoken language in later adulthood. Psychology and Aging 1986; 1:303–311

Surwit RS, Scovern AW, Feinglos MN: The role of behavior in diabetes care. Diabetes Care 1982; 5:337–342

Taub HA: Comprehension and memory of prose materials by young and old adults. Exp Aging Res 1979; 5:3–13

Thompson LW: Measurement of Depression: Implications for assessment of cognitive function in the elderly, in Handbook for Clinical Memory Assessment of Older Adults. Edited by Poon LW. Washington, DC, American Psychological Association, 1986

Vaillant GE: The Natural History of Alcoholism: Causes, Patterns, and Paths to Recovery. Cambridge, MA, Harvard University Press, 1983

Vaillant GE: The study of adult development at Harvard Medical School, in Handbook of Longitudinal Research. New York, Praeger, 1984

Vaillant GE, Milofsky E: Natural history of male psychological health: IX. Empirical evidence for Erikson's, model of the life cycle. Am J Psychiatry 1980; 137:1348–1359

Verbrugge LM: Sex differences in health, in Encyclopedia of Aging. Edited by Maddox GL, Atchley RC, Poon LW, et al. New York, Springer, 1987

Walsh DA, Krauss IK, Regnier VA: Spatial ability, environmental knowledge, and environmental use: the elderly, in Spatial Representation and Behavior Across the Life Span. Edited by Liben L, Patterson A, Newcomb N. New York, Academic Press, 1981

Waugh NC, Norman DA: Primary memory. Psychol Rev 1965; 72:89–104

Whitbourne SK: The psychological construction of the life span, in Handbook of the

Psychology of Aging (second edition). Edited by Birren JE, Schaie KW. New York, Van Nostrand Reinhold, 1985

Williams RB, Haney TL, Lee KL, et al: Type A behavior, hostility and coronary atherosclerosis. Psychosom Med 1980; 42:539–549

Williams RB, Barefoot JC, Shekelle RB: The health consequences of hostility, in Anger, Hostility and Behavioral Medicine. Edited by Chesney MA, Rosenman RH. New York, Hemisphere/McGraw-Hill, 1985

Williams RB, Barefoot JC, Haney TL, et al: Type A behavior and agiographically documented coronary atherosclerosis in a sample of 2,289 patients. Paper presented at the American Psychosomatic Society Meetings, Baltimore, 1986

Willis SL: Towards an educational psychology of the older adult learner: intellectual and cognitive bases, in Handbook of the Psychology of Aging (second edition). Edited by Birren JE, Schaie KW. New York, Van Nostrand Reinhold, 1985

Willis SL, Schaie KW: Training the elderly on ability factors of spatial orientation and inductive reasoning. Psychology and Aging 1986; 1:239–247

Wilson RS, Kaszniak AW: Longitudinal changes: progressive idiopathic dementia, in Handbook for Clinical Memory Assessment of Older Adults. Edited by Poon LW. Washington, DC, American Psychological Association, 1986

Wilson RS, Kaszniak AW, Fox JH: Remote memory in senile dementia. Cortex, 1981; 17:41–48

Wilson RS, Bacon LD, Kaszniak AW, et al: The episodic–semantic memory distinction and paired associate learning. J Consult Clin Psychol 1982a; 50:154–155

Wilson RS, Kaszniak AW, Bacon LD, et al: Facial recognition memory in dementia. Cortex 1982b; 18:329–336

Wilson RS, Bacon LD, Fox JH, et al: Primary memory and secondary memory in dementia of the Alzheimer Type. Journal of Clinical Neuropsychology 1983a; 5:337–344

Wilson RS, Bacon LD, Kramer RL, et al: Word frequency effect and recognition memory in dementia of the Alzheimer type. Journal of Clinical Neuropsychology 1983b; 5:97–104

Wingfield A, Poon LW, Lombardi L, et al: Speed of processing in normal aging: effects of speech rate, linguistic structure, and processing time: J Gerontol 1985; 40:579–585

Wolman BB (ed): Handbook of Developmental Psychology. Englewood Cliffs, NJ, Prentice Hall, 1982

Woodbury MA, Clive J: Clinical pure types as a fuzzy partition. Journal of Cybernetics 1974; 4:111–121

Woodbury MA, Manton KG: A new procedure for analysis of medical classification. Methods of Information in Medicine 1982; 21:210–220

Woodward NJ, Wallston BS: Age and health care beliefs: self-efficacy as a mediator of low desire for control. Psychology and Aging 1987; 2:3–8

Yesavage JA: The use of self-rating depression scales in the elderly, in Handbook for Clinical Memory Assessment of Older Adults. Edited by Poon LW. Washington, DC, American Psychological Association, 1986

Zarit SH, Eiler J, Hassinger M: Clinical assessment, in Handbook of the Psychology of Aging (second edition). Edited by Birren JE, Schaie KW. New York, Van Nostrand Reinhold, 1985

Zelinski EM, Gilewski MJ, Thompson LW: Do laboratory tests relate to self-assessment of memory ability in the young and old?, in New Directions in Memory and Aging: Proceedings of the George Talland Memorial Conference. Edited by Poon LW, Fozard JL, Cermak LS, et al. Hillsdale, NJ, L. Erlbaum, 1980

Chapter 8

Social and Economic Factors

Linda K. George, Ph.D.

The experience of psychiatric disorders in later life is related to a variety of biologic, psychologic, and social/economic factors. Similarly, a broad range of factors affect the likelihood and timing of recovery from mental illness and the probability that appropriate treatment will be sought and obtained. Consequently, a comprehensive examination of geriatric psychiatry must include the contributions of multiple disciplines. Previous chapters have emphasized the physiologic, neurologic, sensory, and psychologic changes that accompany the aging process. In this chapter, the social and economic conditions of later life are examined. (For the sake of convenience, henceforth the shorter term "social factors" will be used, though economic factors also are included in the chapter.) Particular attention is paid to the ways that social conditions serve as risk factors for psychiatric disorders, as contingencies that affect the course of recovery from mental illness, and as determinants of mental health service utilization.

An adequate depiction of psychiatric disorders must include a process or dynamic perspective. The experience of psychiatric disorder varies over time as psychiatric symptoms onset and remit. Help seeking and the course of care for psychiatric disorders also are longitudinal phenomena. Consequently, the most useful studies of psychiatric disorders empirically examine the course of illness and use of mental health services. The distinctive facets of geriatric psychiatry are affected by additional dynamic processes. The aging process

This work was supported by grant P50 MH40149 from the National Institute of Mental Health to the Department of Psychiatry, Duke University.

itself leads to intraindividual changes that can alter the likelihood of experiencing psychiatric disorders and/or using mental health services. Age changes in social factors are of interest in this chapter. However, in the social and economic arenas, the effects of *social* change, generating cohort differences, also must be examined. As documented later, social and economic factors have changed substantially across cohorts of older adults, and these cohort differences have important implications for understanding the impact of social factors on psychiatric disorders and mental health service utilization during later life.

Given the importance of age changes versus cohort differences in reaching conclusions about the role of social factors in geriatric psychiatry, these terms will be examined in more detail. "Age changes" refer to the changes in organisms that occur simply as a function of age. True age changes will be observed with considerable regularity across time and place because they are developmental in nature. Most biologic phenomena that change with age, as well as some psychologic and social attributes, appear to be driven by this type of internal, species-specific developmental agenda. Other differences observed between older and younger adults represent the effects of social change that is external to the individual. The term "cohort" is used to refer to groups of people born at particular times (e.g., the 1920 cohort consists of all persons born in 1920). Cohorts that experience different historical and environmental conditions often differ from each other in ways that reflect these external conditions rather than developmental phenomena. As numerous authors have noted (Mason et al. 1973; George et al. 1981; Riley 1985), in the absence of specific kinds of longitudinal data, it is difficult to empirically distinguish between age changes and cohort differences. Moreover, some phenomena clearly are affected by both age changes and cohort differences (George et al. 1981).

Although it is empirically difficult to determine whether a given age difference represents an age change or a cohort difference, it is important to keep this distinction in mind for three reasons. First, this distinction is critical to attributions of etiology or causality. In their pure forms, age changes reflect developmental phenomena and cohort effects reflect the effects of social or environmental conditions. Second, this distinction is relevant to generalization of research findings. If a risk factor for psychiatric disorder changes with age, the observed pattern will be broadly applicable (i.e., across cohorts). If a risk factor for psychiatric disorder differs across age groups because of differences in environmental exposure, the effects of that risk factor—or at least its distribution in the older population—may be cohort specific. Third, the distinction is important for purposes of intervention. If levels of a given risk factor differ substantially across cohorts, it may be possible to target interventions to the environmental conditions that place certain cohorts at greatest risk. If, instead, a given risk factor alters with age, intervention must be targeted toward alteration of a developmental trajectory.

In this chapter, then, two process phenomena will be examined simultaneously. First, the processes underlying the experience of psychiatric disorders and mental health service utilization will be examined from a social perspective. Second, the degree to which the social factors associated with psychiatric disorders and/or mental health service utilization change with age or differ across cohorts also will be considered.

This chapter is organized in five sections. The first section examines social characteristics as risk factors for psychiatric disorders in later life. The social risk factors examined include demographic factors (e.g., race and sex), indicators of social integration (e.g., social roles and availability of social support), socioeconomic conditions (primarily income), and the experience of stressful life events. The second section examines the degree to which exposure to social risk factors for psychiatric disorders changes with age and varies across cohorts. A central issue of concern here is whether current cohorts of younger and middle-aged adults have experienced or will confront environmental conditions that will make them more or less at risk for psychiatric disorders during later life than current cohorts of older adults. The third section of the chapter focuses on the impact of social factors on recovery from psychiatric disorders during later life. The central question of interest is whether social factors alter the probability or timing of recovery. The fourth section examines social factors as determinants of mental health service utilization among older adults. An important distinction is made between help seeking (which reflects the decisions and behaviors of individuals needing mental health services) and provider behavior (i.e., how providers respond to persons presenting psychiatric problems). The final section of the chapter examines the impact of social and economic policies on older adults. These policies and programs have impact directly, by affecting the likelihood of help seeking for psychiatric problems, and indirectly, by affecting some of the social risk factors for mental illness in later life, and thereby influencing the psychiatric status of older adults.

Social Risk Factors for Psychiatric Disorders

Theoretical Model

Slowly but surely a consensual conceptual model of the social precursors of psychiatric disorders is emerging in the social science, epidemiologic, and social psychiatry literatures. The model remains vague in terms of specific operationalizations and statistical estimation; nonetheless, an overarching theoretical orientation has been forged. Table 1 presents our view of the general conceptual model that emerges from previous research. It is a stage model in the sense that each higher stage represents what are hypothesized to be increasingly proximate precursors of psychiatric disorders.

There are six stages of social risk factors. The first stage consists of

Table 1. Stage Model of the Social Precursors of Psychiatric Disorders

Stage Number	Stage Name	Illustrative Indicators
I.	Demographic variable	Age, sex, race/ethnicity
II.	Early events and achievements	Education, childhood traumas
III.	Later events and achievements	Occupation, income, marital status, fertility
IV.	Social integration	Personal Attachments to social structure (e.g., religious affiliation, community roles), environmental context (e.g., neighborhood stability, economic climate)
V.	Vulnerability and protective factors	Social support versus isolation, chronic stressors
VI.	Provoking agents and coping efforts	Life events, coping strategies

demographic variables that are associated with differential risk of psychiatric disorders. Virtually all studies of social risk factors for psychiatric disorders include demographic variables, particularly age, race, and sex. In spite of consensus concerning the importance of demographic variables, the causal mechanisms that underlie the relationships between demographic factors and psychiatric disorders remain unclear. One type of explanation suggests that demographic factors serve as proxies for more mechanistic social factors. For example, the greater prevalence of depressive symptoms among women than men may be accounted for by sex differences in other risk factors such as marital status, income, and exposure to social stress. It also is possible, however, that demographic variables serve as proxies for biologic mechanisms. In this review, the social meanings of demographic factors are emphasized; nonetheless, the possible biologic mechanisms should not be overlooked. Indeed, most recent research on the etiology of mental illness emphasizes the multiple types of risk factors that are implicated in psychiatric morbidity.

Stages II and III of the generic model represent events and achievements relevant to mental health outcomes that are distinguished primarily on the basis of their timing and recency. Stage II consists of relatively early experiences that are hypothesized to have persisting effects on individuals' vulnerability to psychiatric disorders. Examples of such experiences include childhood traumas (e.g., early death or marital disruption of parents) and level of educational attainment. Stage III consists of later events and experiences, including family relationships and socioeconomic achievements. In most studies, Stage III indicators are based on individuals' *current* statuses, reinforcing the temporal distinction between Stage II and Stage III risk factors. It should be noted that Stage II risk factors need not be experiences that occurred during childhood or early adulthood; rather, any experiences that occurred prior to the current time may be relevant. Again, causal interpretation of relationships between risk factors and psychiatric outcomes is problematic. For example, some investigators view higher levels of education and income primarily as resources that facilitate effective coping; others view them as resulting in exposure to environments that directly affect psychiatric status. Future research will need to address the specific mechanisms by which these factors affect mental health outcomes. Current efforts are focused on generating accurate estimates of the magnitude of the relationships between these risk factors and psychiatric disorders.

Stage IV consists of potential risk factors that have been less consistently examined in studies of psychiatric disorders but that receive considerable support from some prevous research. The term "social integration" has been used in two ways in previous research. Some investigators define social integration at the individual level, referring to individuals' attachments to formal aspects of the social structure (e.g., religious affiliations or participation in voluntary organizations). Others define social integration at the aggregate level, referring to levels of stability and organization in the broader environments within which individuals function. This review will examine social integration at both the individual and aggregate levels. The rationale for examining social integration as a risk factor for psychiatric disorders is that individuals who are exposed to social disorganization and/or lack meaningful attachments to community structures are more vulnerable to psychiatric morbidity, because lack of social integration is psychologically stressful, because social integration facilitates effective coping, or both.

Finally, Stages V and VI represent the classes of social risk factors that have received greatest empirical attention in recent research. Vulnerability and protective factors refer to personal assets and liabilities that alter the probabilities of psychiatric problems. Chronic stressors are primary examples of vulnerability factors and social support is a major illustration of a hypothesized protective factor. Provoking agents and coping efforts are more specific and proximate than vulnerability and protective factors. Life events are the primary provoking agents examined in previous research and are viewed as sudden sources of stress that may be sufficiently severe to trigger the onset of psychiatric morbidity, especially in the presence of other risk factors. Coping efforts refer to the specific actions taken to confront a particular source of stress; effective coping may either prevent stresses from generating negative mental health outcomes or minimize their effects on psychiatric status. Stages V and VI are distinguished primarily on the basis of specificity and immediacy. For example, although life events and chronic stressors are both important because of the stresses they generate, life events are more discrete and bounded. Similarly, social support is viewed as a generalized resource for defusing stress whereas coping efforts are specific to particular stresses.

The model in Table 1 must be taken as a heuristic abstraction—as a useful way of summarizing trends in the literature on social risk factors for psychiatric disorders rather than as a conceptual model that has received consensual approval. Undoubtedly some investigators would classify the social precursors of psychiatric disorders in somewhat different categories. Moreover, most available studies do not include all the categories of risk factors included in Table 1. Nonetheless, most studies implicitly or explicitly adopt both the basic categories of risk factors and their ordering.

Thus far, the conceptual framework depicted in Table 1 has been described in terms of direct effects (i.e., the relationships, either bivariate or multivariate, between risk factors and psychiatric outcomes). An additional complexity is the possibility of interaction effects (i.e., that the effects of one risk factor are contingent on the presence or level of another risk factor). In theory, any combination of risk factors may interact to alter the risk of psychiatric disorders. Evidence of such interactions will be included in this review. One illustration will be used at this point to describe the potential importance of risk factor interactions. Because of the theoretical and empirical attention it has received, we will use the interaction between life events and social support as the illustration. Some investigators propose that life events and social support exert independent effects on mental health outcomes, with life events increasing the risk of psychiatric disorders and social support reducing the risk. This is a hypothesis of direct effects. Other investigators suggest that social support buffers the effects of life events on psychiatric outcomes, maintaining that life events increase the risk of psychiatric disorders only (or primarily) among persons who lack adequate social support. This is an interaction hypothesis. Direct versus interaction effects are not mutually exclusive. It is possible, for example, that life events and social support directly affect mental health and that life events are especially damaging in the absence of social support. The important point is that examination of the social risk factors for psychiatric disorders includes not only consideration of multiple risk factors, but also their interrelationships.

As presented, there is nothing distinctively age related about the conceptual framework in Table 1—and this is a purposeful and appropriate decision. Extant literature does not indicate that the social risk factors that place older adults at increased risk for psychiatric disorders are substantially different from those that place younger and middle-aged adults at increased risk. Instead, the social risk factors for psychiatric disorders are distributed differentially across life stages and, perhaps, across cohorts. Thus, as documented below, the major age-related pattern with regard to the social risk factors for psychiatric disorders appears to be varying exposure across age groups.

Methodologic Issues

Although the model is heuristic, review of previous research permits a preliminary assessment of its utility. Prior to reviewing the evidence, however, four methodological issues must be briefly noted.

Measuring psychiatric disorders. Psychiatric disorders have been operationalized in a variety of ways in previous studies. Conceptually, two dimensions underlie most of this variability: (1) diagnostic versus symptom measures and (2) the degree to which the measures tap general psychopathology versus specific diagnostic categories. With regard to the first dimension, some instruments are designed to measure psychiatric disorders using formal diagnostic criteria, typically the *Diagnostic and Statistical Manual of Mental Disorders (Third Edition-Revised)* (DSM-III-R; American Psychiatric Association 1987), the Feighner (Feighner et al. 1972), or the Research Diagnostic Criteria (Spitzer et al. 1978) nosologic systems. Other measures are simple symptom scales in which higher numbers of symptoms are assumed to represent more severe psychiatric morbidity.

The second dimension applies primarily to symptom measures. Some scales include symptoms from a spectrum of disorders and generate measures of global psychopathology. Others measure symptoms within a single diagnostic category (e.g., depression or anxiety). Some of the inconsistencies observed across studies with regard to the effects of specific risk factors undoubtedly reflect the use of different methods of measuring psychiatric disorders. For example, several studies suggest that older people report more depressive symptoms, on average, than do middle-aged and younger adults, but that the prevalence of major depression (as a diagnosis) is lower among older than younger persons (cf. Blazer et al. 1987a; Gurland et al. 1980). Moreover, some risk factors may be important for certain psychiatric disorders but irrelevant to others. For example, there are substantial sex differences in the prevalence of alcohol abuse/dependence and depression, whereas they are minimal for many other disorders (cf. Meyers et al. 1984). These kinds of inconsistencies cannot be dismissed as simple measurement effects, but must be carefully examined from both scientific and clinical perspectives. Until such examinations are conducted, however, variability in the ways psychiatric disorders are measured will continue to complicate conclusions about the importance of various risk factors for mental health outcomes.

A final measurement issue should be noted. Virtually all extant research focuses on the social risk factors associated with functional rather than organic psychiatric disorders. Consequently, this review is restricted to the social risk factors for functional psychiatric disorders.

Sample composition. Variations in samples also account for some of the inconsistencies observed across studies. Not surprisingly, samples vary widely in size and composition, which in turn affects distributions of social risk factors. Consequently, sample composition must be taken into account when synthesizing the research findings across studies.

The age compositions of the samples used in previous research are especially relevant to this review. Some previous studies of the relationships between social risk factors and psychiatric outcomes relied exclusively on data from older adults. More frequently, however, previous studies used data from samples covering much broader age ranges (i.e., age 18 and older). These two types of sample design generate different, but valuable kinds of information. Investigations based on samples of older adults provide in-depth views of how social risk factors operate during later life. Such designs cannot identify risk factor efforts that are distinctive to old age, however. In contrast, data from age-heterogeneous samples can be used to determine (1) the role of age itself as a risk factor for psychiatric disorders and (2) whether other risk factors vary in direction or magnitude across age groups.

Complexity of analyses. Differences in the types and complexity of the statistical techniques used across studies also complicate the task of synthesizing findings from previous research. Some studies provide only bivariate estimates of the relationships between risk factors and psychiatric disorders. Though often tantalizing, such studies are ultimately unsatisfying because it is not clear whether the observed relationships are meaningful or spurious (i.e., disappear in the face of statistical controls). Investigators increasingly recognize the importance of multivariate analyses in which the relationships between risk factors and psychiatric outcomes are examined with potentially confounding and/or interrelated risk factors statistically controlled. Thus, findings from multivariate analyses will receive special attention in this review.

Cross-sectional versus longitudinal studies. The present theoretical model of the social precursors of psychiatric disorders is explicitly dynamic: Categories of risk factors are ordered in terms of their presumed temporal and causal proximity to the onset of psychiatric morbidity. Unfortunately, most available studies are based on cross-sectional data. Such studies can be used to suggest the existence of hypothesized effects, but they cannot provide evidence of temporal order. Nor can cross-sectional data provide information about the lag between exposure to a risk factor and the onset of mental illness. Evidence of temporal order and lagged effects can be obtained only from longitudinal data.

For the purposes of this chapter, other kinds of longitudinal data also are needed. More specifically, information is needed about the extent to which exposure to social risk factors for psychiatric disorders changes with age and varies across cohorts (i.e., across historical time). Fortunately, longitudinal data concerning changes in the hypothesized social risk factors for psychiatric disorders are more plentiful.

Evidence Bearing on the Theoretical Model

Evidence bearing on the theoretical model now can be extracted from previous research. As just noted, methodologic differences across studies render this task difficult and imprecise. Overall, however, the model receives considerable support from previous research. Of particular interest is the fact that few risk factors appear to operate differently across age groups—though, as noted later, the distributions of risk factors often are related to age or cohort.

Demographic variables. Age is related to the risk of psychiatric disorders, but the associations are complex. Some studies based on symptom scales report increased psychiatric disorder among older than younger adults (cf. Warheit et al. 1975), although most report no meaningful age differences (cf. Veroff et al. 1981). A different pattern emerges with respect to diagnoses of specific psychiatric disorders. Most of these studies report lower prevalence of psychiatric disorders among older than younger adults (with the obvious exception of organic mental disorders). These age differences are observed for estimates of both current and lifetime prevalence (cf. Meyers et al. 1984; Robins et al. 1984). The degree to which these age differences in the prevalence of both current and lifetime disorders reflect cohort differences remains unclear, but it is a critical issue for future research.

Sex differences in the prevalence of psychiatric morbidity are consistently reported across studies. Women report increased levels of psychiatric disorders when symptom scales are used (Gore and Mangione 1983; Thoits 1987; Kessler 1979). Studies based on diagnoses, however, suggest that symptom scales mask considerable variation across specific disorders: Affective and somatic disorders are more prevalent among women, alcohol and substance abuse disorders are more common among men, and schizophrenia and most anxiety disorders are unrelated to gender (cf. Myers et al. 1984; Blazer et al. 1985). Interestingly, a limited research base suggests an interaction between sex and age, such that sex differences in the prevalence of psychiatric disorders narrow during old age.

Race and ethnic differences in the prevalence of psychiatric disorders are observed less consistently across studies. Most studies based on symptom measures report higher rates of disorder among nonwhites, especially blacks (Dohrewend and Dohrenwend 1969; Warheit et al. 1975). Race differences typically are not observed, however, in studies based on diagnostic measures, with an important exception being increased rates of alcohol and drug abuse among nonwhites (cf. Myers et al. 1984; Blazer et al. 1985). Moreover, most race and ethnic differences in the prevalence of psychiatric disorders can be accounted for by differences in socioeconomic status (Warheit et al. 1975; Dohrenwend 1975), though some recent research questions these findings (Kessler and Neighbors 1986).

Early events and achievements. There is considerable evidence that early events and achievements have persisting effects on psychiatric status throughout adulthood. Along with other indicators of socioeconomic status, education is associated with the prevalence of psychiatric disorders. In general, low education increases the risk of psychiatric disorder (Holzer et al. 1986; Dohrenwend and Dohrenwend 1969). This is certainly the case for symptom measures, but it also largely holds true for diagnostic measures. There is limited evidence, however, that some psychiatric disorders may be more prevalent among the highly educated or may exhibit a curvilinear relationship with education. Some studies, for example, report a positive relationship between education and major depression (Blazer et al. 1985). Other studies suggest that the relationship between education and major depression is curvilinear, with persons of both very low and very high levels of education exhibiting higher prevalence of the disorder (Holzer et al. 1986).

Although there is a common assumption that early childhood traumas place individuals at increased risk of psychiatric morbidity, solid evidence supporting that assumption has been relatively rare. Several studies, however, support this assumption for psychiatric symptoms and certain specific psychiatric disorders (Langner and Michael 1963; Brown and Harris 1978; Crowell et al. 1987). Although these studies did not focus specifically on late life, older adults were included in the samples. These data are complemented by findings from clinical studies, some of which focused specifically on older persons (cf. Kaminsky 1978; McMordie and Blom 1979).

Later events and achievements. Not surprisingly, current life conditions also are significantly related to the prevalence of psychiatric disorders. Low socioeconomic status, usually indexed by occupation and income (as well as education), is strongly related to levels of psychiatric symptoms and typically is associated with increased risk of specific psychiatric diagnoses (Holzer et al. 1986; Blazer et al. 1985; Dohrenwend and Dohrenwend 1969).

Retirement is obviously a major transition of later life—a transition that removes individuals from the occupational structure and results in significant income loss. Though direct evidence is scarce, it does not appear that retirement increases the risk of psychiatric disorders (cf. Maddox 1970; Atchley 1976). Thus, socioeconomic background appears to be a stronger predictor of psychiatric morbidity during late life than retirement-related changes in economic status.

The relationship between marital status and psychiatric disorders remains ambiguous despite considerable research. In general, marital status appears to be weakly associated with psychiatric morbidity, regardless of whether symptom scales or diagnostic measures are used (Thoits 1987; Gove 1972; Blazer et al. 1985). Two caveats must be added to this conclusion, however. First, undesirable changes in marital status appear to have negative effects on mental health, especially in the few months immediately subsequent to marital disruption (Glick et al. 1974; Brown and Harris 1978). For young and middle-aged adults, marital disruption typically takes the form of separation or divorce; for older adults, marital disruption typically results from widowhood. These relatively bounded changes in marital status are usually viewed as life events, however. Second, to the extent that marital disruption (especially divorce or separation) is related to psychiatric disorders, the causal order of that relationship remains problematic. That is, it is not clear whether marital disruption leads to psychiatric disorder or whether preexisting psychiatric disorder precipitates marital dissolution.

Evidence linking fertility to psychiatric disorders is very limited. The few data available suggest that the presence of minor-age children may increase the risk of psychiatric illness among women, especially employed women; however, this conclusion remains controversial (Kandel et al. 1985; Aneshensel et al. 1981; Ross and Huber 1985). Certainly there is no evidence that fertility history is related to psychiatric status during later life.

Social integration. Although it has received limited attention in previous research, available evidence suggests that social integration may be an important buffer against psychiatric morbidity. At the individual level, religious affiliations and participation in voluntary organizations have received most attention. A growing body of literature suggests that church attendance and participation in other religious activities is associated with decreased risk of psychiatric disorders (Neff and Husaini 1985; Wheaton 1983; Veroff et al. 1981). Similar benefits are reported for participation in voluntary organizations, though the research base is smaller (Veroff et al. 1981; Grusky et al. 1985). All previous studies in this area are based on cross-sectional data; consequently, causal order remains problematic. Moreover, to my knowledge, no studies have examined this issue specifically in the context of later life.

At the aggregate level, most studies have focused on two dimensions of the social environment: (1) its degree of stability and organization and (2) economic conditions, especially levels of unemployment. In both areas, research results have been mixed, with some studies finding significant relationships between disruptive environmental conditions and the prevalence of psychiatric disorders and other studies failing to do so (cf. Dooley et al. 1981; Kasl and Harburg 1975; Leighton 1974). Again, this writer is not aware of any studies that have focused on the impact of macroenvironmental conditions on the psychiatric status of older adults.

One additional indicator of social integration that has received attention in previous research is urban versus rural residence. Studies based on measures of psychiatric symptoms typically find elevated levels of psychopathology among urban residents (Dohrenwend and Dohrenwend 1974; Schwab et al. 1974; Mueller 1981; Brown and Prudo 1981; Comstock and Helsing 1976). Studies based on specific diagnoses suggest a more complex pattern in which place of residence has different effects for particular disorders. A recent study of urban and rural residents of the southeast United States, for example, found that (1) place of residence was unrelated to most psychiatric disorders; (2) a few disorders, particularly major depression, were more prevalent among urban residents; and (3) one disorder, alcohol abuse/dependence, was significantly more prevalent among rural residents (Blazer et al. 1985). Data from that same study indicated that the urban-rural differences observed were greatest among young adults and were minimal among older persons (Crowell et al. 1986).

Vulnerability and protective factors.   Though they have received less attention than life events, chronic stressors are the vulnerability factors most frequently examined in previous research. The specific chronic stressors that have received most empirical scrutiny are job stress, chronic financial strain, and chronic physical illnesses—and all three have been related to increased risk of psychiatric morbidity (cf. House 1981; Ross and Huber 1985; George et al. in press). Because retirement is a normative, usually voluntary, and nearly universal transition during later life, occupational conditions are unlikely to be a significant risk factor for psychiatric disorders among older adults. Both chronic financial problems and chronic physical conditions have been linked to increased psychiatric problems among older and younger adults (Ross and Huber 1985; Krause 1987; George et al. in press-b; Aneshensel et al. 1984). Interestingly, a recent body of literature suggests another chronic stressor that is especially (though not exclusively) prevalent among older adults: caregiving responsibility for an impaired older adult, a responsibility typically shouldered by family members, especially spouses. Like other chronic stressors, caregiving has been documented to increase the risk of psychiatric morbidity (George and Gwyther 1986; Fengler and Goodrich 1979). Most studies of chronic stressors have measured psychiatric disorders using symptom scales rather than diagnostic tools.

The primary protective factor examined in previous research is social support. There is consensus that social support is a multidimensional phenomenon; there is much less agreement, however, concerning the number and nature of its dimensions. Increasingly, however, investigators recognize at least three major dimensions: (1) social network—the number and structure of the network of persons available to provide support, (2) tangible support—the specific instrumental and emotional services provided to individuals by their families and friends, and (3) perceptions of social support—subjective evaluations of satisfaction with the adequacy of available support. Most studies suggest that high levels of social support are associated with decreased risk of psychiatric morbidity and that perceived support is the dimension most strongly related to mental health outcomes (Cohen and Wills 1985; Dean et al. 1981; Cutrona et al. 1986; Kessler and McLeod 1985). In addition, however, limited but tantalizing evidence suggests that tangible support may be especially important for older adults.

Provoking agents and coping efforts. Life events may be the social risk factors for psychiatric disorders that have received greatest attention. Life event studies are based on two major research strategies: (1) studies of aggregated life events (i.e., summing all the events that individuals experienced in a given time period) and (2) studies of specific life events (e.g., widowhood or retirement). Research based on both strategies suggests that life events—especially those that are perceived as negative—are robustly related to increased risk of both psychiatric symptoms and specific psychiatric disorders, especially depression, alcohol abuse, and generalized anxiety (cf. Brown and Harris 1978; Neff and Husaini 1985; Cronkite and Moos 1984; Blazer et al. 1987b). Moreover, these relationships have been observed in both age-heterogeneous samples and samples of older adults.

Findings with regard to the stress-buffering hypothesis (i.e., that life events have stronger negative effects on psychiatric outcomes in the absence of adequate social support) are less consistent. The majority of evidence appears to support the stress-buffering hypothesis—a conclusion also reached in two recent reviews (Cohen and Wills 1985; Kessler and McLeod 1985). Two caveats should be appended to this conclusion. First, evidence favoring the stress-buffering hypothesis is largely restricted to studies employing psychiatric symptom scales or measures of depression and in which perceptions of social support are examined (Kessler and McLeod 1985). Second, relatively few studies of stress buffering have been based on older samples.

Both common sense and social science theory suggest that adequate coping will partially determine whether stress has negative effects on mental health outcomes. Scientific efforts to delineate the nature of coping are just beginning to make headway; assessment of coping effectiveness remains primitive. Studying the effects of coping is particularly problematic because different stressors elicit, permit, and require different coping strategies. In spite of these problems, there is limited evidence that coping methods alter the probabilities that stress has negative impact on mental health outcomes— and some of that evidence is based on data from older samples (cf. Pearlin and Schooler 1978; Folkman and Lazarus 1980; Felton et al. 1980).

Age Changes and Cohort Differences in Social Risk Factors

Thus far, we have considered one set of dynamics affecting psychiatric disorders in later life: the impact of social factors on the risk of mental illness. A second set of dynamics also must be considered: age changes and cohort differences that affect exposure to social risk factors for psychiatric disorders. To the extent that exposure to risk factors varies with age or differs across cohorts, the proportion of the older population at risk of psychiatric morbidity also varies. Thus, the six categories of social risk factors for psychiatric disorders will be reexamined with a focus on age changes and cohort differences that affect the prevalence and distribution of those risk factors during later life.

Demographic variables. Age and sex are largely irrelevant in this context because sex is a fixed characteristic of organisms and age changes are the focus of this examination. Cohort differences in the age structure of society merit brief note, however. As is well documented, industrialized societies have been aging throughout this century because of increasing life expectancy and decreasing fertility—and this trend will continue well into the next century (Myers 1985; Uhlenberg 1977).

As a result of this trend, a larger proportion of the population of persons with psychiatric disorders will consist of older adults. This does not necessarily mean that a larger proportion of the older population will experience mental illness, though it is possible that increased life expectancy will have this effect. For example, several authors have suggested that recent increases in the prevalence of organic mental disorders, especially Alzheimer's disease, are a direct result of increased life expectancy (Mortimer et al. 1981). There is no evidence that changes in life expectancy will result in increased incidence of functional psychiatric disorders during later life, but that possibility cannot be ruled out.

Race/ethnicity is a fixed characteristic that does not change with age. Again, however, there are cohort differences in the ethnic compositions of societies. In the United States, for example, current cohorts of older adults include substantial proportions of persons who migrated to the United States from Europe and Russia. Migration from these countries declined precipitously after World War II, however, and future cohorts of elderly will differ in this regard. Currently, there is relatively little migration to the United States, with the majority of that migration flowing from Central America, South

America, and the Far East. It is not clear how the size or composition of the migrant population affects the prevalence of psychiatric disorders in later life.

Early events and achievements. Education typically is completed during early adulthood and does not change thereafter. There are substantial cohort differences in average levels of education, however. Compared with their middle-aged and younger peers, current cohorts of older adults average relatively low levels of education (Streib 1985). Given evidence (noted above) that education is negatively related to the prevalence of most psychiatric disorders, increasing levels of education may bode well for the mental health of future cohorts of older adults.

Childhood traumas become fixed experiences for individuals and do not change over time. Again, however, cohort differences are possible. Though there are few solid data on historical trends, it is likely that there are cohort differences in the experience of particular kinds of childhood traumas. Compared with their younger peers, current cohorts of older adults are more likely to have experienced parental death at an early age and severe poverty during childhood (because of the Great Depression) (Elder 1974, 1979). Conversely, current cohorts of young adults are substantially more likely to have experienced parental separation or divorce during childhood (cf. Cogswell and Sussman 1972; Furstenberg 1979). The implications of these cohort differences for mental health during later life remain unclear.

Later events and achievements. As noted for education, occupational attainment and income are higher among younger than older cohorts (Streib 1985). Unlike education, however, occupation and income are strongly affected by retirement during later life. Nonetheless, in light of evidence documenting the mental health benefits of higher socioeconomic status, future cohorts of older adults may be at less risk of psychiatric disorders than current cohorts.

Family formation factors also differ substantially across cohorts. Compared with current cohorts of older adults, younger adults now are less likely to marry, are more likely to marry for the first time at later ages, are more likely to divorce, are less likely to have children, and have fewer children (Treas 1977; Bengtson and Treas 1980). These patterns generate major cohort differences in family size and structure. It is not clear whether or how these family changes will affect psychiatric outcomes during adulthood and old age.

Social integration. In American society, personal attachments to community structures tend to change with age. Participation in religious, civic, and other organizations tends to peak during late middle age and decline thereafter as a result of health and mobility problems. Consequently, lack of formal social attachments is more common in later life than at younger ages.

Data concerning possible cohort differences in personal attachments to social structure are very rare. Some authors suggest that there has been a trend away from community participation (Bellah et al. 1985). Data supporting this conclusion, however, are scant and of questionable quality. Moreover, even if this trend exists, its meaning remains ambiguous. It may be, for example, that recent cohorts invest greater personal commitment in fewer community structures.

Conclusions about exposure to social disorganization at the aggregate level also are difficult because of the absence of data. Many would argue that increased rates of crime, technologic change, and residential mobility signal increasing social disorganization (Bellah et al. 1985; Bender 1978), affecting both current cohorts of older adults and the developmental histories of future cohorts of the elderly. On the other hand, levels of financial security have increased steadily over this century, resulting in a more materially secure population. Whatever the actual balance of these trends, substantial numbers of older adults are exposed to sources of social disorganization, including economic dislocations, residential mobility, and even "aging in place" in deteriorating neighborhoods (George 1987).

Vulnerability and protective factors. As noted previously, some chronic stressors, including financial problems and physical illnesses, are age related. That is, financial resources decrease (U.S. Senate Special Committee on Aging 1982; Palmore et al. 1985) and physical health problems increase (U.S. Department of Health and Human Services 1981) during later life. Cohort differences also may operate. The socioeconomic achievements of particular cohorts, the economic climate of the larger society, and the availability of income maintenance policies differ across time and can make financial strain more or less common during later life for particular cohorts. Similarly, medical advances affect both the health status of cohorts prior to old age and the ability to cure or manage chronic illnesses during later life. Policies that facilitate access to health care services also have impact on the likelihood of impaired physical functioning during old age. The majority of available evidence suggests that future cohorts will enter old age with better physical health and greater financial resources than current cohorts. These trends should bode well for decreasing the risk of psychiatric disorders during later life.

Social networks tend to decrease in size and change in composition during later life (Antonucci 1985; Kahn and Antonucci 1980). These changes result primarily from the death or impairment of significant others. In spite of these changes, the vast majority of older adults are not socially isolated and report highly adequate levels of emotional and instrumental assistance from friends and families (Shanas 1979a, 1979b). Cohort differences in the size and structure of support networks are likely. Social trends in family formation patterns strongly suggest that older persons in the future will be less likely to have spouses, children, siblings, and extended kin (Bengtson and Treas 1980;

Treas 1977). It is possible, however, that nonfamilial relationships will compensate for these changes.

Provoking agents and coping efforts. There is considerable evidence that age is related to the occurrence of life events. Compared with their younger peers, older adults average fewer life events overall, but are more likely to experience specific types of events (e.g. widowhood and other deaths, health events, and retirement) (Lowenthal et al. 1975; Hughes et al. 1988). From a mental health perspective, these patterns have mixed implications. On the one hand, fewer life events should decrease the risk of psychiatric disorders. On the other hand, some events that are more common during later life also are associated with increased risk of psychiatric morbidity, particularly depression. Neither empirical evidence nor theoretical speculation suggests major cohort differences in the frequency or timing of life events during old age.

Information about the relationship between age and coping efforts is slim and ambiguous. This reflects both the limited research base and the difficulties inherent in studying coping. To the extent that older adults experience age-related life events, age-related coping efforts also can be expected (George and Siegler 1982). At this point, there is no evidence of age-related declines in coping effectiveness. Nor is there good reason to expect major cohort differences in coping styles or effectiveness. These conclusions, however, are based on an absence of data rather than empirical evidence.

Social Factors Affecting Recovery from Psychiatric Disorders

Given that social factors are substantially implicated in the onset and prevalence of psychiatric disorders, it is plausible to expect that social factors also may influence the course of and the timing of recovery from psychiatric morbidity. For example, we might expect that life events and/or chronic stressors would exacerbate psychiatric problems and impede recovery from them. Similarly, social support and effective coping might be hypothesized to truncate the natural course of mental illness and facilitate recovery.

Unfortunately, very little previous research has examined the role of social factors in the course and timing of recovery from psychiatric illness. In large part this is because of limited information about the natural history of psychiatric disorders. Longitudinal studies are badly needed to delineate the course and natural history of the major psychiatric disorders. (There has been, of course, substantial research examining treatment efficacy. Clinical trials, however, are not adequate for describing the natural history of psychiatric disorders.) Given information about the longitudinal course of psychiatric morbidity, a variety of more specific research questions could be addressed. In essence, multiple courses or trajectories of symptom onset and remission are to be expected for any psychiatric disorder. An initial task is the identification and description of these trajectories. Subsequently, research should focus on identification of the factors that are related to different illness trajectories. For example, one factor that should alter the trajectory of symptom onset and remission is mental health treatment. That is, effective psychiatric treatment should be associated with a more benign illness course and, ideally, a shorter interval between illness onset and recovery. Moreover, different treatment modalities may be related to different illness trajectories, permitting evaluation of therapeutic efficacy in a context that is broader than the usual clinical trial.

Two potential sources of variation in the trajectories of psychiatric disorders are especially relevant to this review. First, since the focus is on geropsychiatry, it is important to determine whether age itself is related to illness course and duration. The second relevant issue is the role of social factors in altering the trajectory of psychiatric morbidity. Extant data about both of these issues are scant in volume and largely restricted to two psychiatric disorders: major depression and alcohol abuse/dependence. Of particular interest is the fact that these two disorders exhibit very different patterns of symptom onset and remission.

A few studies have compared the course of major depression in older adults versus younger and middle-aged adults. The data used in these studies are based on follow-up assessments of clinical samples, with the follow-up intervals ranging from 1 to 3 years after the index episode of major depression. In general, most of these studies suggest that (1) between one-third and one-fourth of the older adults will recover from the index episode and remain relatively symptom free throughout the follow-up interval (with the remainder either exhibiting no recovery or reporting a pattern of recovery and subsequent relapse), and (2) the prognosis for recovery is somewhat poorer among older than among young or middle-aged adults (Cole 1983; Murphy 1983; Post 1972). A more recent study, however, reported minimal differences between middle-aged and older adults in the likelihood of recovery from an episode of major depression over a 1- to 2-year follow-up interval (George et al., in press-a). In addition, in the absence of sustained recovery, older adults were more likely to report no recovery whereas middle-aged participants were more likely to report recovery with subsequent relapse. Clearly, these studies provide only an initial effort to trace the natural history of depressive disorder during later life. Longitudinal studies that include multiple assessments of psychiatric status over a lengthy follow-up interval (e.g., 3 to 5 years) are especially needed. The possibility that age of onset of first episode of major depression affects illness course and duration also merits attention in that one study (Cole 1983) suggests that late onset of first episode is associated with better prognosis.

Available evidence suggests that alcoholism exhibits a natural history considerably different from that for depression. Using the most extensive longitudinal data available to date, Vaillant (1983) describes three major patterns of alcohol-related disorders: (1) a consistent pattern of occasional abuse that does not lead to dependence, (2) an atypical pattern of early and massive alcohol misuse that leads to dependence during early adulthood, and (3) the major pattern, in which "social drinking" on a regular basis leads to persistent heavy drinking and eventual dependence. Unfortunately, however, Vaillant's rich descriptions of alcoholism trajectories are based on data that do not extend to later life. There is general recognition that the population of older alcoholics contains two groups: (1) persons who developed alcoholism earlier in life and persist in abusive or dependent alcohol consumption during old age and (2) late-onset alcoholics, for whom problem drinking emerges for the first time during late life. There also is considerable evidence that late-onset alcohol problems are more strongly related to social risk factors than early-onset alcoholism. It remains unclear, however, whether age of onset is related to prognosis of recovery. Again, further effort is needed.

Information on the effects of social factors other than age on the course and duration of psychiatric disorders also is very limited. With regard to depression during later life, results are inconsistent across studies. Several social factors have been associated with poorer outcome of late life depression in one or more longitudinal studies: severe life events (Murphy 1983), poor physical health (Baldwin and Jolley 1986), and inadequate social support (Holahan and Moos 1981; Pattison et al. 1979; George et al. in press-a). On the other hand, some studies fail to replicate these findings, especially those for social support (cf. Henderson 1981).

A somewhat richer but still incomplete knowledge base is available concerning the role of social factors in the course and duration of alcohol problems. Vaillant (1983) reports that social support and religious participation increase the probability of recovery from alcoholism, though these factors explain only a small proportion of the variation in illness duration. Similarly, Helzer et al. (1984) report that social isolation (primarily absence of a spouse or confidant) predicts longer duration of acute episodes of alcoholism and, interestingly, that social isolation is more important for older than younger alcoholics. These authors also report that more favorable outcome is associated with female gender, white race, and higher socioeconomic status among older alcoholics. Other studies support the conclusion that life events are related to poorer prognosis during later life (Finney et al. 1980; Wells-Parker et al. 1983) and that marriage increases the likelihood of recovery, especially among older men (Bailey et al. 1965). Some investigators also suggest that these social factors are more potent predictors of outcome for late-onset than for early-onset alcoholism (Abrahams and Patterson 1978-1979; Rosin and Glatt 1971; Schuckit et al. 1980).

In summary, available data suggest that both age and other social factors may be significantly related to the course and duation of psychiatric disorders in general and among older adults in particular. Extant evidence is largely restricted to only two psychiatric disorders: major depression and alcohol abuse/dependence. Additional effort clearly is needed to firmly identify the role of social factors in the process of symptom onset and remission. Especially worthy of exploration are social risk factors and psychiatric disorders that have not been examined previously.

Before leaving this topic, a final issue merits brief mention. The limitations of cross-sectional data for reaching conclusions about the dynamics of psychiatric illness were previously noted. Earlier comments focused specifically on problems of causal order between social risk factors and psychiatric outcomes (e.g., are life events risk factors for the onset of psychiatric disorders, or does psychiatric morbidity increase the risk of negative life experiences?). Another limitation of cross-sectional data is especially relevant to the issue of illness course and recovery. Using cross-sectional data, it is impossible to disentangle the role of social factors as predictors of illness onset from their role as predictors of illness course and duration. Consequently, although observed relationships between social factors and psychiatric disorders in cross-sectional studies are typically interpreted as evidence of the importance of social factors for illness onset, we may instead be observing correlates of illness duration.

Help Seeking for Psychiatric Disorders

Social factors have been demonstrated to play a meaningful, though not fully understood, role in the onset and course of psychiatric disorders. They also are related to the likelihood that individuals will seek help for psychiatric problems and the source from which help is sought. In this section, the roles of social and economic factors in seeking help for psychiatric disorders are examined. We begin with summaries of the two major theoretical perspectives that social scientists have used to understand help seeking for physical and mental illness. Subsequently, evidence supporting these perspectives is presented, with special attention to help seeking during later life.

Social Determinants of Help Seeking: The Andersen Model

For the past two decades, the central sociologic question in health services research has been equality of access. The major theory guiding most of this research was developed by Ronald Andersen and his colleagues at the University of Chicago (Andersen 1968; Aday and Andersen 1975; Andersen et al. 1975, 1976; Andersen and Newman 1973). This simple, but elegant theory posits that health service use is a function of three generic classes of variables: predisposing characteristics, enabling factors, and need factors. Predisposing characteristics refer to social and attitudinal variables that predispose certain individuals to seek help from medical providers. Sex, age, education, and attitudes about the efficacy of the medical profession are examples of predisposing characteristics. Enabling factors refer to resources that facilitate health service use, including income, health insurance, and structural factors such as the availability of physicians. Thus, both predisposing characteristics and enabling factors are largely social or economic variables. Need factors are the signs and symptoms of disease that can trigger the decision to seek health services. Andersen and his colleagues argued that in an equitable health care system, need should be the determining factor in health service use and that predisposing and enabling factors should be irrelevant. Conversely, to the extent that predisposing and enabling factors are significant predictors of health service use, there is evidence of inequality.

Initial analyses based on this model, conducted in the 1960s and early 1970s, documented substantial inequity in health service utilization, although need factors were the most powerful predictors of service use (cf. Andersen 1968; Herman 1972; Hyman 1970). Persons with low incomes and who lacked health insurance were less likely to use services in the presence of need than their more advantaged peers. Similarly, certain demographic groups—primarily elderly, unmarried women, and the children of unmarried women— were less likely to use health services in the presence of need. In the late 1960s, Medicare and Medicaid were enacted, with the explicit goal of improving access to medical care for the poor and elderly. By the mid and late 1970s there was clear evidence that these programs had been effective in equalizing access to health services. Since the mid-1970s, analyses based on the Andersen model have repeatedly indicated that the effects of income and demographic characteristics on health service use have weakened substantially, and the influence of need has become even stronger (cf. Cleary et al. 1982; Kessler et al. 1981; Kulka et al. 1979; Wolinsky 1978). Evidence concerning the Andersen model as applied specifically to mental health service utilization is presented below.

One further conceptual issue needs to be addressed concerning the Andersen model. As applied in previous research, the Andersen model has been used to predict both receipt of any services and volume of service use. But recent thinking suggests that these measures of health service use are not substitutable—the model is suitable for examining one issue but not the other (George 1986). The decision to seek or not seek health care is largely in the hands of the individual. Thus, receipt of any service is a measure of help seeking. In contrast, volume of health service use is in large part the decision of the health care provider (i.e., the provider determines the need for return visits and on what schedule). (Considerable research suggests that social factors influence provider behavior as well as help seeking. Space limitations preclude review of these relationships here.) Previous research indicates that model fit and explained variance are substantially stronger for predicting who does and who does not seek help than in identifying those persons who obtain a little versus a lot of services (George 1986). Thus, the Andersen model can be more appropriately viewed as a model of help seeking rather than as a model of service utilization more broadly.

Health Belief Models

The term "health belief model" is used to subsume a variety of specific theories of the decision to seek help for medical or psychiatric problems. In the interest of brevity, this review will focus on the substantial congruence among the models encompassed by this conceptual schema, but the plural form (i.e., health belief models) will be used as a consistent reminder of the underlying diversity of detail.

Health belief models rest on the assumption that beliefs and attitudes are the primary determinants of behavior. The basic tenets of health belief models were best delineated by Rosenstock (1966, 1974) and Becker (1974). In brief, health belief models posit that the decision to seek help for medical or psychiatric problems is a function of four key beliefs, each of which must be present for help seeking to occur: (1) belief that one is susceptible to disease, (2) belief that one's symptoms are sufficiently severe to merit attention, (3) belief in the efficacy of medical treatment, and (4) belief that the costs of treatment are reasonable in relation to the probability of relief from pain or restoration of functioning.

Some investigators have ordered this configuration of beliefs into a process framework, usually proposing four stages in the decision to seek help (cf. Robinson 1971; Anderson and Bartkus 1973; Horwitz 1977; Kirscht 1974). First the individual must recognize that he or she is experiencing pain or departure from normal functioning—a self-attribution referred to as symptom recognition (cf. Anderson and Bartkus 1973; Banks and Keller 1971). The second step is symptom attribution: Once a symptom is recognized, the individual must assess its severity and make an attribution about its probable cause (Banks and Keller 1971; Anderson and Bartkus 1973). If a symptom is not perceived as being relatively severe, further attention (including help seeking) in unlikely. Given that the symptom is perceived as sufficiently severe to merit attention, the individual still must make an attribution concerning its probable cause. In general, available research suggests that help seeking from medical and psychiatric professionals occurs when symptoms are attributed to physical or mental conditions, are viewed as requiring immediate attention or are on a course of escalating impairment, and can be relieved only by professional treatment. The third stage in the help-seeking process is the decision to seek help. It is at this stage that beliefs about the efficacy of health care providers and about the equity of health care costs become especially salient. Even if symptoms are recognized and attributed to medical causes, help seeking will not occur unless the individual believes that the health care system offers efficacious treatments and that the costs of those treatments are commensurate with the benefits to be obtained (Horwitz 1977; Kirscht 1974). The final stage of the process is selection of a specific health care provider or setting. Such choices are made at two levels: at the generic level, resulting in the choice of a certain type of provider and setting, and at the specific level, resulting in the choice of a particular provider or setting (Anderson and Bartkus 1973; Houpt et al. 1979).

In general, research results have supported the importance of health beliefs for help seeking (cf. Kasl 1974; Langlie 1977; Radalet 1981; Hallauer 1972), although few available studies have traced the decision-making process longitudinally. A very important pattern revealed by these studies is the existence of large individual differences in the extent to which individuals recognize symptoms, make accurate attributions concerning their severity and etiology, evaluate the costs and benefits of medical treatments, and select health care providers. The accuracy with which individuals make these attributions and assessments is of considerable importance. One type of inaccuracy results in failure to obtain needed health services and can lead to unnecessary (and sometimes serious or irreversible) losses of functioning. On the other hand, unwarranted concern about transitory or trivial symptoms can lead to excess service use, elevated health care costs, inappropriate use of the sick role (with the accompanying loss of productivity, burden on family members, and so forth), and increased risk of iatrogenic disease.

Evidence for Mental Health Services

Although both the Andersen model and health belief models have been applied primarily to help seeking for physical illnesses, they also have proved useful for understanding help seeking for psychiatric disorders. In addition, help seeking among the elderly has been examined from both perspectives.

Applications of the Andersen model to mental health service use suggests that psychiatric services are viewed both by the public and by reimbursement programs as more discretionary and less important than services for physical health problems. Recent analyses suggest that the Andersen model differs somewhat depending on whether one is predicting use of general health services or predicting visits to specialty mental health providers (cf. George 1986; Kessler et al. 1981; Kulka et al. 1979). Need factors remain the strongest single predictor of health service use for both physical and mental health problems. Nonetheless, predisposing and enabling factors are stronger predictors of mental health service use than of general health service use. Lower income and education, lack of insurance or limited insurance coverage, being male, being a member of a racial or ethnic minority, and being old are all associated with lower likelihood of using specialty mental health services in the presence of need for such services. Consequently, but not surprisingly, public and private health care financing programs have not been as successful in equalizing access to mental health services as for general health services.

Interestingly, research on help seeking among older adults has identified an enabling factor that was omitted from the original Andersen model: social support. Controlling for level of need and other relevant predictors, older persons embedded in active and supportive social networks are more likely to receive both general medical care and specialty mental health services than are their more socially isolated age peers (cf. Murdock and Schwartz 1978; Smith 1985). Limited evidence suggests that social support may operate as an enabling factor for younger and middle-aged adults also (Salloway and Dillon 1973).

Health belief models also have contributed to our understanding of help seeking for psychiatric disorders. In particular, these models provide information about the reasons that people are less likely to seek help for psychiatric problems than for physical symptoms and why persons with psychiatric disorders often seek help from primary care physicians rather than mental health specialists. Symptom recognition is less likely for mental health problems than for psychiatric symptoms, symptom attribution is less likely to lead to the decision to seek help for psychiatric symptoms than for physical illnesses, projected cost/benefit ratios often are viewed as less attractive for mental health service use (in part because a greater proportion of those costs must be paid out of pocket), and many persons with psychiatric disorders prefer to seek help from their usual sources of care (i.e., primary care physicians) than from mental health professionals.

There also is some evidence that social factors are related to the health beliefs relevant to help seeking. Most important, for our purposes, is the considerable evidence that older adults are less likely than their younger peers to (1) recognize psychiatric symptoms, (2) make accurate attributions about their severity and etiology (the tendency of older adults to somatize psychiatric symptoms is especially relevant here), (3) view mental health services as efficacious, and (4) seek help from specialty mental health providers (Greenley and Mechanic 1976; George et al. 1987). In this regard, however, it is interesting to note that older adults with psychiatric disorders are as likely to seek help for them as are younger adults, but the elderly are more likely than their younger peers to seek services from a primary care physician rather than a mental health specialist (George et al. 1987). Other social characteristics also are associated with health beliefs. For example, some investigators suggest that women are more likely than men to recognize symptoms, to view them as severe and medically relevant, and to believe that the benefits of medical care outweigh their costs (cf. Nathanson 1975; Cleary et al. 1982). Similarly, persons of lower socioeconomic status and members of racial or ethnic minorities have been reported to be less accurate in recognizing symptoms and making accurate attributions about their etiology and significance (cf. Hetherington and Hopkins 1969; Kulka et al. 1979). These demographic groups also have been reported to be especially likely to present psychiatric symptoms in somatic terms.

In summary, research based on both the Andersen model and health belief models documents the substantial role that social and economic factors play in help seeking for psychiatric disorders. Findings from applications of the Andersen model demonstrate that need factors are the strongest predictors of health service use, but that social and economic factors explain additional variation in help seeking. Moreover, social and economic factors are especially important for help seeking from the specialty mental health sector. Health belief models elucidate the process by which and conditions under which symptoms (or need factors) result in help seeking. In addition, health beliefs are significantly related to several social characteristics, including age.

The Relevance of Public Policies and Programs

In order to complete this overview of the role of social and economic factors in psychiatric disorders, it is necessary to examine the impact of public policies and programs. Evidence has already been reviewed that social factors (1) are implicated in the onset and risk of psychiatric disorders during later life, (2) probably alter the trajectory of illness course and duration, and (3) play a substantial role in both the decision to seek help for psychiatric morbidity and the choice of a provider from whom to seek help. Public policies also are relevant because they alter the distributions of social and economic factors within the older population and among age groups in society and because they can be targeted directly at the precursors of psychiatric disorders.

It should be noted that public policies and programs are methods of intervention. Not all policies are intended to affect the prevalence of psychiatric morbidity in later life. Indeed, most current policies are intended to achieve very different goals. Nonetheless, because public policies and programs alter the distributions of social and economic characteristics of the elderly, they frequently affect—directly or indirectly—the prevalence and distribution of psychiatric disorders during later life.

At the federal level in the United States, programs for the elderly are concentrated in two areas: income maintenance and health care financing. Social Security is the major income program used by older Americans, but it is augmented by Supplemental Security Insurance, food stamps, and other policies that transfer economic assets to older adults. In addition, a variety of policies ensure that older adults are taxed at lower rates than other Americans, thus permitting the elderly to retain a larger proportion of their incomes. As noted in earlier sections, income adequacy and financial resources are related to both the risk of psychiatric disorders in later life and the likelihood that mental health services will be obtained. Thus, these income maintenance policies undoubtedly affect the prevalence and distribution of psychiatric disorders in later life.

As previously noted, Medicare and Medicaid are the major public health care financing programs in the United States and were designed to serve the elderly and the poor, respectively. Medicare coverage is nearly universal among current cohorts of older adults, and a sizeable minority of older

Americans is covered by Medicaid. Evidence already presented documents the fact that Medicare and Medicaid greatly increased accessibility to health services for older adults and the socioeconomically disadvantaged. Thus, although these health care financing programs probably have had little effect on the risk of psychiatric disorders in later life, they clearly have had a beneficial impact on help seeking and health service utilization by older adults. Though the beneficial impact of Medicare and Medicaid cannot be questioned, the mental health benefits provided by these programs, especially Medicare, are much more restricted than those provided for physical illness and are inadequate for many older persons with psychiatric disorders.

Space limitations preclude a review of other, less universal policies and programs targeted in whole or in part to older adults—programs ranging from veterans' benefits (e.g., at age 65, all veterans become eligible for health care in Veterans Administration facilities) to senior centers to subsidized housing. It is important to realize, however, that all of these programs have the potential to favorably affect the risk factors for psychiatric disorders during later life and/or on patterns of help seeking for psychiatric disorders. Moreover, additional programs, some yet to be designed and some that have been tested on a demonstration basis, could be implemented that would alter the risk of psychiatric morbidity during later life either directly or indirectly. As one illustration, health education programs hold considerable promise as a method for increasing the accuracy of symptom recognition and attribution during later life (Hallauer 1972; Carnahan and Nugent 1975).

One issue emphasized throughout this chapter has been the degree to which risk factors for psychiatric disorders vary across cohorts. Awareness of cohort differences is especially relevant to generalizing over time and anticipating future trends. The policy arena is one area, however, in which speculation is very difficult. Policy changes can alter and have altered the distributions of social risk factors for psychiatric disorders and, especially, access to and quantity of mental health service use during later life. But policy changes are the result of shifting political climates that are difficult to anticipate with any degree of accuracy. Anticipation of the future is further complicated by the fact that the psychiatric status of future cohorts of older adults will be affected by policies and programs to which they are exposed during earlier stages of the life course. Thus, we will have to be content to note that major policy changes have the potential to generate cohort differences in the prevalence and distribution of psychiatric disorders and in patterns of help seeking for mental health problems during later life.

Summary

Social and economic factors play complex roles in the prevalence and distribution of psychiatric disorders in later life. In some cases, the links between social characteristics and psychiatric morbidity are direct and clear-cut. Examples of such relationships include the link between life events and increased risk of psychiatric disorders and the association between financial resources and help seeking for psychiatric problems. In other areas, however, the links between social factors and psychiatric morbidity are indirect and ubiquitous, affecting the social environments within which individuals develop and function. Clearly there is more to be learned about these complex relationships than we know now. Nonetheless, there is striking evidence that psychiatric status during later life is related in strong and complex ways to social and economic factors.

References

Abrahams R, Paterson P: Psychological distress among the community elderly: prevalence, characteristics, and implications for service. International Journal of Aging and Human Development 1978–1979; 9:1–19

Aday LA, Andersen R: Access to Medical Care. Ann Arbor, MI Health Administration Press, 1975

American Psychiatric Association: Diagnostic and Statistical Manual of Mental Disorders (Third Edition-Revised). Washington, DC, American Psychiatric Association, 1987

Andersen R: A Behavioral Model of Families' Use of Health Services. Chicago, University of Chicago Center for Health Administration, 1968

Andersen R, Newman JF: Societal and individual determinants of medical care utilization in the United States. Milbank Q 1973; 51:95–124

Andersen R, Kravits J, Anderson O: Equity in Health Services. Cambridge, MA, Ballinger, 1975

Andersen R, Lion J, Anderson O: Two Decades of Health Services: Social Survey Trends in Use and Expenditures. Cambridge, MA, Ballinger, 1976

Anderson JR, Bartkus D: Choice of medical care: a behavioral model of health and illness behavior. J Health Soc Behav 1973; 14:348–362

Aneshensel CS, Frerichs RR, Clark VA: Family roles and sex differences in depression. J Health Soc Behav 1981; 22:379–393

Aneshensel CS, Frerichs RR, Huba GJ: Depression and physical illness: a multiwave, nonrecursive causal model. J Health Soc Behav 1984; 25:350–371

Antonucci TC: Personal characteristics, social support and social behavior, in Handbook of Aging and the Social Sciences. Edited by Binstock RH, Shanas E. New York, Van Nostrand Reinhold, 1985

Atchley RC: The Sociology of Retirement. Cambridge, MA, Schenkman, 1976

Bailey M, Haberman P, Alksne H: The epidemiology of alcoholism in an urban residential area. Quarterly Journal of Studies on Alcohol 1965; 26:19–40

Baldwin RC, Jolley DJ: The prognosis of depression in old age. Br J Psychiatry 1986; 149:574–583

Banks F, Keller M: Symptom experience and health action. Med Care 1971; 9:498–502

Becker MH: The health belief model and sick role behavior. Health Education Monographs 1974; 2:409–419

Bellah RN, Madsen R, Sullivan WM, et al: Habits of the Heart. Berkeley, University of California Press, 1985

Bender T: Community and Social Change. New Brunswick, Rutgers University Press, 1978

Bengtson VL, Treas J: The changing family context of mental health and aging, in Handbook of Mental Health and Aging. Edited by Sloane RB, Birren JE. Englewood Cliffs, NJ, Prentice-Hall, 1980

Blazer D, George LK, Landerman R, et al: Psychiatric disorders: a rural/urban comparison. Arch Gen Psychiatry 1985; 42:651–656

Blazer D, Hughes DC, George LK: The epidemiology of depression in an elderly community population. Gerontologist 1987a; 27:281–287

Blazer D, Hughes D, George LK: Stressful life events and the onset of a generalized anxiety syndrome. Am J Psychiatry 1987b; 144:1178–1183

Brown GW, Harris T: Social Origins of Depression: A Study of Psychiatric Disorder in Women. London, Tavistock, 1978

Brown GW, Prudo R: Psychiatric disorder in a rural and an urban population: I. Aetiology of depression. Psychol Med 1981; 11:581–599

Carnahan J, Nugent C: The effects of self-monitoring by patients on the control of hypertension. Am J Med Sci 1975; 269:69–73

Cleary PD, Mechanic D, Greenley JR: Sex differences in medical care utilization: an empirical investigation. J Health Soc Behav 1982; 23:106–119

Cogswell BE, Sussman MB: Changing family and marriage forms: complications for human service systems. Family Coordinator 1972; 21:505–516

Cohen S, Wills TA: Stress, social support and the buffering hypothesis. Psychol Bull 1985; 98:310–357

Cole MG: Age, age of onset and course of primary depressive illness in the elderly. Can J Psychiatry 1983; 28:102–104

Comstock G, Helsing K: Symptoms of depression in two communities. Psychol Med 1976; 6:551–563

Cronkite RC, Moos RH: The role of predisposing and moderating factors in the stress-illness relationship. J Health Soc Behav 1984; 25:372–393

Crowell BA Jr, George LK, Blazer D, et al: Psychosocial risk factors and urban/rural differences in the prevalence of major depression. Br J Psychiatry 1986; 149:307–314

Crowell BA Jr, George LK, Blazer DG: Psychiatric and social outcomes of child abuse. Arch Gen Psychiatry (1987, under review)

Cutrona C, Russell D, Rose J: Social support and adaptation to stress by the elderly. Psychology and Aging 1986; 1:47–54

Dean A, Lin N, Ensel WM: The epidemiological significance of social support systems in depression, in Research in Community and Mental Health (Volume 2). Edited by Simmons RG. Greenwich, CT, JAI Press, 1981

Dohrenwend BP: Sociocultural and social-psychological factors in the genesis of mental disorders. J Health Soc Behav 1975; 16:365–392

Dohrenwend BP, Dohrenwend BS: Social Status and Psychological Disorder. New York, Wiley, 1969

Dohrenwend BP, Dohrenwend BS: Psychiatric disorders in urban settings, in American Handbook of Psychiatry (second edition): Volume 2. Child and Adolescent Psychiatry, Sociocultural and Community Psychiatry. Edited by Caplan G. New York, Basic Books, 1974

Dooley D, Catalano R, Jackson R, et al: Economic, life, and symptom changes in a nonmetropolitan community. J Health Soc Behav 1981; 22:144–154

Elder GH Jr: Children of the Great Depression. Chicago, University of Chicago Press, 1974

Elder GH Jr: Historical change in life patterns and personality, in Life-Span Development and Behavior (Volume 2). Edited by Baltes PB, Brim OG. New York, Academic Press, 1979

Feighner JP, Robins E, Guze SB, et al: Diagnostic criteria for use in psychiatric research. Arch Gen Psychiatry 1972; 26:57–63

Felton BJ, Brown P, Lehmann S, et al: The coping function of sex-role attitudes during marital disruption. J Health Soc Behav 1980; 21:240–247

Fengler AP, Goodrich N: Wives of elderly disabled men: the hidden patients. Gerontologist 1979; 19:175–183

Finney J, Moos R, Mewborn CR: Posttreatment experiences and treatment outcome of alcoholic patients six months and two years after hospitalization. J Consult Clin Psychol 1980; 48:17–29

Folkman S, Lazarus RS: An analysis of coping in a middle-aged community sample. J Health Soc Behav 1980; 21:219–239

Furstenberg FF: Recycling the family: perspectives for a neglected family form. Marriage and Family Review 1979; 3:12–22

George LK: Psychological and social determinants of help-seeking. Position paper, National Institute of Mental Health, Depression Awareness, Recognition, and Treatment Program, 1986

George LK: Non-familial support for older persons: who is out there and how can they be reached?, in Handbook of Applied Gerontology. Edited by Lesnoff-Caravaglia G. New York, Human Sciences Press, 1987

George LK, Gwyther LP: Caregiver well-being: a multidimensional examination of family caregivers of demented adults. Gerontologist 1986; 26:253–259

George LK, Siegler IC: Stress and coping in later Life. Educational Horizons 1982; 60:147–154

George LK, Siegler IC, Okun MA: Separating age, cohort, and time of measurement: analysis of variance or multiple regression. Exp Aging Res 1981; 7:297–314

George LK, Blazer DG, Winfield-Laird I, et al: Psychiatric disorders and mental health service use in later life: evidence from the Epidemiologic Catchment Area Program, in Epidemiology and Aging. Edited by Brody J, Maddox GL. New York, Springer, 1987

George LK, Blazer DG, Hughes DC, et al: Social support and the outcome of major depression. Br J. Psychiatry, in press-a

George LK, Landerman R, Blazer D, et al: Concurrent morbidity between physical and mental illness: an epidemiological examination, in Mechanisms of Psychological Influences on Physical Health, with Special Attention to the Elderly. Edited by Carstensen LL, Neale J. New York, Plenum Press, in press-b

Glick IO, Weiss RD, Parkes CM: The First Year of Bereavement. New York, Wiley, 1974

Gore SE, Mangione TW: Social roles, sex roles and psychological distress: additive and interactive models of sex differences. J Health Soc Behav 1983; 24:300–312

Gove WR: The relationship between sex roles, marital status, and mental illness. Social Forces 1972; 51:34–45

Greenley JR, Mechanic D: Social selection in seeking help for psychological problems. J Health Soc Behav 1976; 17:249–262

Grusky O, Tierney K, Manderscheid RW, et al: Social bonding and community adjustment of chronically mentally ill adults. J Health Soc Behav 1985; 26:49–63

Gurland BJ, Dean L, Cross P, et al: The epidemiology of depression and dementia in the elderly: the use of multiple indicators of these conditions, in Psychopathology of the Aged. Edited by Cole JO, Barrett JE. New York, Raven Press, 1980

Hallauer D: Illness behavior—an experimental investigation. J Chronic Dis 1972; 25:599–610

Helzer JE, Carey KE, Miller RH: Predictors and correlates of recovery in older versus younger alcoholics, in Nature and Extent of Alcohol Problems Among the Elderly. Edited by Maddox G, Robins LN, Rosenberg N. Rockville, MD, National Institute on Alcohol Abuse and Alcoholism, 1984

Henderson S: Social relationships, adversity and neurosis: an analysis of prospective observations. Br J Psychiatry 1981; 138:391–398

Herman M: The poor: their medical needs and the health services available to them. Annals of the American Academy of Political and Social Sciences 1972; 399:12–21

Hetherington R, Hopkins C: Symptom sensitivity: its social and cultural correlates. Health Serv Res 1969; 4:63–70

Holahan CJ, Moos RH: Social support and psychological distress: a longitudinal analysis. J Abnorm Psychol 1981; 90:365–370

Holzer CE, Sheal BM, Swanson JS, et al: The increased risk for specific psychiatric disorders among persons of low socioeconomic status. Am J Soc Psychiatry 1986; 6:259–271

Horwitz A: The pathways to psychiatric treatment: some differences between men and women. J Health Soc Behav 1977; 18:169–178

Houpt JL, Orleans CS, George LK, et al: The Importance of Mental Health Services for General Health Care. Cambridge, MA, Lexington, 1979

House JS: Work Stress and Social Support. Reading, MA, Addison-Wesley, 1981

Hughes DC, Blazer DG, George LK: Age differences in life events: a multivariate controlled analysis. International Journal of Aging and Human Development 1988; 27:207–220

Hyman M: Some links between economic status and untreated illness. Soc Sci Med 1970; 4:387–399

Kahn RL, Antonucci TC: Convoys over the life course: attachment, roles and social support, in Life-Span Development and Behavior (Volume 3). Edited by Baltes PB, Brim OG. New York, Academic Press, 1980

Kaminsky M: Pictures from the past: the uses of reminiscence in case work with the elderly. Journal of Gerontological Social Work 1978; 1:19–31

Kandel DB, Davies M, Ravers VH: The stressfulness of daily social roles for women: marital, occupational, and household roles. J Health Soc Behav 1985; 26:64–78

Kasl SV: The health belief model and behavior related to chronic illness. Health Education Monographs 1974; 2:433–454

Kasl SV, Harburg E: Mental health and the urban environment: some doubts and second thoughts. J Health Soc Behav 1975; 16:268–282

Kessler RC: Stress, social status, and psychological distress. J Health Soc Behav 1979; 20:259–272

Kessler RC, Neighbors HW: A new perspective on the relationships among race, social class, and psychological distress. J Health Soc Behav 1986; 27:107–115

Kessler RC, Brow RL, Broman CL: Sex differences in psychiatric help-seeking: evidence from four large-scale surveys. J Health Soc Behav 1981; 22:49–64

Kessler RC, McLeod JD: Social support and mental health in community samples, in Social Support and Health. Edited by Cohen S, Syme SL. New York, Academic Press, 1985

Kirscht JP: The health belief model and illness behavior. Health Education Monographs 1974; 2:387–408

Krause N: Chronic financial strain, social support, and depressive symptoms among older adults. Psychology and Aging 1987; 2:185–192

Kulka RA, Veroff J, Douvan E: Social class and the use of professional help for personal problems: 1957 and 1976. J Health Soc Behav 1979; 20:2–16

Langlie JR: Social networks, health beliefs, and preventive health behavior. J Health Soc Behav 1977; 18:244–260

Langner TS, Michael ST: Life Stress and Mental Health. London, Collier-Macmillan, 1963

Leighton AH: Social disintegration and mental disorder, in American Handbook of Psychiatry (second edition): Volume 2. Child and Adolescent Psychiatry, Sociocultural and Community Psychiatry. Edited by Caplan G. New York, Basic Books, 1974

Lowenthal MF, Thurnher M, Chiriboga D: Four Stages of Life. San Francisco, Jossey-Bass, 1975

Maddox GL: Adaptation to retirement. Gerontologist 1970; 10:14–18

Mason KO, Mason WM, Winsborough HH, et al: Some methodological issues in cohort analysis of archival data. American Sociological Review 1973; 38:242–258

McMordie WR, Blom S: Life review therapy: psychotherapy for the elderly. Perspect Psychiatr Care 1979; 4:162–166

Mortimer JA, Schuman LM, French LR: Epidemiology of dementia: overview and prospectives, in The Epidemiology of Dementia. Edited by Mortimer JA, Schuman LM. New York, Oxford University Press, 1981

Murdock SH, Schwartz DF: Family structure and the use of agency services: an examination of patterns among elderly native Americans. Gerontologist 1978; 18:475–481

Mueller D: The current status of urban-rural differences in psychological disorder: an emerging trend for depression. J Nerv Ment Dis 1981; 169:18–27

Murphy E: The prognosis of depression in old age. Br J Psychiatry 1983; 142:111–119

Myers GC: Aging and worldwide population change, in Handbook of Aging and the Social Sciences. Edited by Binstock RH, Shanas E. New York, Van Nostrand Reinhold, 1985

Myers JK, Weissman MM, Tischler GL, et al: Six-month prevalence of psychiatric disorders in three communities. Arch Gen Psychiatry 1984; 41:959–970

Nathanson C: Illness and the feminine role: a theoretical review. Soc Sci Med 1975; 9:57–62

Neff JA, Husaini BA: Stress-buffer properties of alcohol consumption: the role of urbanicity and religious identification. J Health Soc Behav 1985; 26:207–221

Palmore E, Burchett B, Fillenbaum GG, et al: Retirement: Causes and Consequences. New York, Springer, 1985

Pattison EM, Lleamas R, Hurd G: Social network mediation of anxiety. Psychiatric Annals 1979; 9:56–67

Pearlin LI, Schooler C: The structure of coping. J Health Soc Behav 1978; 19:2–21

Post F: The management and nature of depressive illness in late life: a follow-through study. Br J Psychiatry 1972; 121:393–404

Radalet ML: Health beliefs, social networks, and tranquilizer use. J Health Soc Behav 1981; 22:165–173

Riley MW: Age strata in social systems, in Handbook of Aging and the Social Sciences. Edited by Binstock RH, Shanas E. New York, Van Nostrand Reinhold, 1985

Robins LN, Helzer JE, Weissman MM, et al: Lifetime prevalence of specific psychiatric disorders in three sites. Arch Gen Psychiatry 1984; 41:949–958

Robinson D: The Process of Becoming Ill. London, Routledge and Kegan Paul, 1971

Rosenstock IM: Why people use health services. Milbank Q 1966; 44:94–127

Rosenstock IM: The health belief model and preventive health behavior. Health Education Monographs 1974; 2:354–386

Rosin A, Glatt M: Alcohol excess in the elderly. Quarterly Journal of Studies on Alcohol 1971; 32:53–59

Ross CE, Huber J: Hardship and depression. J Health Soc Behav 1985; 26:312–327

Salloway JC, Dillon PB: A comparison of family networks and friend networks in health care utilization. Journal of Comparative Family Studies 1973; 4:140–147

Schuckit M, Atkinson J, Miller P, et al: A three-year followup of elderly alcoholics. J Clin Psychiatry 1980; 41:412–416

Schwab J, Warheit G, Holzer C: Mental health: rural-urban comparisons. Ment Health Soc 1974; 1:265–274

Shanas E: The family as a social support in old age. Gerontologist 1979a; 19:169–174

Shanas E: Social myth as hypothesis: the case of family relations of old people. Gerontologist 1979b; 19:3–9

Smith K: Sex differences in benzodiazepine use among the elderly: effects of social support. Doctoral dissertation, Duke University, Durham, NC, 1985

Spitzer RL, Endicott J, Robins E: Research Diagnostic Criteria (RDC) for a Selected Group of Functional Disorders (third edition). New York, New York State Psychiatric Institute, 1978

Streib GF: Social stratification and aging, in Handbook of Aging and the Social Sciences. Edited by Binstock RH, Shanas E. New York, Van Nostrand Reinhold, 1985

Thoits PA: Gender and marital status differences in control and distress: common stress versus unique stress explanations. J Health Soc Behav 1987; 28:7–22

Treas J: Family support systems for the aged: some social and demographic considerations. Gerontologist 1977; 17:486–491

Uhlenberg P: Changing structure of the older population of the USA during the twentieth century. Gerontologist 1977; 17:197–202

U.S. Department of Health and Human Services: Health in the United States 1981. Washington, DC, U.S. Government Printing Office, 1981

U.S. Senate Special Committee on Aging: Aging and the Work Force: Human Resources Strategies. Washington, DC, U.S. Government Printing Office, 1982

Vaillant GE: The Natural History of Alcoholism. Cambridge, MA, Harvard University Press, 1983

Veroff J, Douvan E, Kulka RA: The Inner American. New York, Basic Books, 1981

Warheit GL, Holzer CE, Arey SA: Race and mental illness: an epidemiologic update. J Health Soc Behav 1975; 16:243–256

Wells-Parker E, Miles S, Spencer B: Stress experiences and drinking histories of elderly drunken driving offenders. J Stud Alcohol 1983; 44:429–437

Wheaton B: Stress, personal coping resources, and psychiatric symptoms: an investigation of interactive models. J Health Soc Behav 1983; 24:208–229

Wolinsky FD: Assessing the effects of predisposing, enabling, and illness-morbidity characteristics on health service utilization. J Health Soc Behav 1978; 19:384–396

Chapter 9

The Epidemiology of Psychiatric Disorders in Late Life

Dan G. Blazer, M.D., Ph.D.

The epidemiology of psychiatric disorders in late life is the study of the distribution of psychiatric disorders among the elderly and those factors that influence this distribution (MacMahon and Pugh 1970). As applied scientists, epidemiologists devote their inquiries to the identification, treatment, and prevention of disorders within the population. Though psychiatric investigators have taken advantage of many advances in scientific technology, there is, in contrast, little use of the methods of science in shaping the clinical care of older persons. Geriatricians and geriatric psychiatrists bridge an uncomfortable gap between the science and the art of medicine. Roberts (1977) suggested that epidemiology is not only the basic science of preventive and community medicine but also may serve as the basic science of clinical practice. In this chapter, the goals of epidemiology will be reviewed as they relate to the care of the psychiatrically impaired older adult.

In contrast to the substantive sciences, epidemiology is primarily a way of thinking about health and disease beyond the traditional clinical approach (Morris 1975). Platt (1952) described the need for the epidemiologic method as follows:

> Wherein then lies the need for training physicians in science . . . ?
> First, . . . the training is needed because scientific discipline is the anti-

This research was supported in part by Clinical Research Center for the Study of Psychopathology in the Elderly grant MH-40159.

dote to a surfeit of the art of medicine, which, carried too far, degenerates into medical lifemanship. . . . [T]he clinician who knows only the art . . . may end by deceiving not only his patients but himself. . . . Self-deception is the sin against which scientific discipline protects. (p. 978)

The care of the impaired older adult is fraught with pitfalls that lead to uncertainty in clinical decision making (Weinstein and Feinberg 1980). Uncertainty can arise from errors in collecting clinical data; for example, the patient may report one complaint but the physician records another. Problems in case identification are especially prevalent in late life, for the older adult may not express those symptoms traditionally associated with psychiatric diagnoses derived from the *Diagnostic and Statistical Manual of Mental Disorders (Third Edition-Revised) (DSM-III-R)*. (American Psychiatric Association 1987). Other data may be ambiguous, for observers may differ in their ability to detect symptoms and signs of a disorder. For example, laboratories may vary in the assay of cortisol, thus complicating the interpretation of the dexamethasone suppression test (DST). Still further uncertainty may surround the relation between clinical information and the presence of a disease. How are clinicians to distinguish the ubiquitous problems of the worried well from serious and treatable psychiatric disorders? Finally, uncertainty about the effects of treatment may derive from a lack of knowledge of the outcome of disorders in their natural state.

The beginning of the study of psychiatric disorders in the elderly is an understanding of the population at risk, i.e., that group of individuals from which psychiatric disorders may arise. The increasing percentages of older adults in developed countries is a poignant testimony to the need for increased study of psychiatric disorders and mobilization of services for older adults. A demographic profile and projection of the aging U.S. population is presented in Table 1.

Although both the number and percentage of older adults have increased progressively throughout the 20th century, a dramatic increase will occur in the first half of the 21st century, primarily because of the aging of the "baby boom" generation. In other words, between 1995 and 2030, the number of persons age 65 and older in the United States will double (as it doubled from 1950 to 1985). If the average retirement age remains the same and persons continue the trend to enter the work force in their early 20s, the impact of an aging population upon the economy of the country, not to mention the need for health care, will be dramatic. This can be seen by the profound increase in the age/dependency ratio. Flexibility in retirement and other social and economic changes will help modify the impact of this "squaring" of the population pyramid. Nevertheless, this demographic revolution will affect every individual and every institution in our society (Pifer and Bronte 1986).

Although changes in the total number and percentage distribution of the population across the life span are affected primarily by changes in fertility,

Table 1.   Demographic Profile and Projection of the Aging U.S. Population, Showing the Population 65 Years of Age and Older and the Annual Average Increases for 1950–2050

Year	U.S. Population 65 and Older	% of Total Population 65 and Older	Age Dependency Ratio[a]
1950	12,397,000	8.1	14
1965	18,451,000	9.5	18
1984	28,040,000	11.8	20
1995	33,887,000	13.1	22
2010	39,196,000	13.8	23
2030	64,580,000	21.2	39
2050	67,412,000	21.8	40

Note. Adapted from Siegel JS, Taeuber CM: Demographic perspectives on the long-lived society. Daedalus 1986;115(1):77–117. Based on *Current Population Reports* of the U.S. Census Bureau, Series P-25, Nos. 311, 519, 917, 952, and 965. The projections are presented in Spender G: Projections of the population of the United States, by age, sex, and race: 1983 to 2080. *Current Population Reports,* Series P-25, No. 952, May 1984. Projections are from the middle series.

[a]Age dependency ratio $= \dfrac{\text{Population 65 years and over}}{\text{Population 20–64 years}} \times 100.$

changes in mortality within the aging population have affected the demographics of late life as well. The life expectancies for males and females in 1983 were 71 and 78 years, respectively (Siegel and Taeuber 1986). Much of the difference between the sexes in life expectancy at birth can be accounted for by differences in mortality after the age of 65. For example, on the basis of data available in 1983, a female who had lived to age 65 could expect to live an additional 18.6 years, whereas a male could expect to live an additional 14.2 years. The relative contributions of genetic and environmental factors to this difference in longevity have been debated extensively. Cigarette smoking, more prevalent in males, has certainly contributed to the difference. Nevertheless, the more stressful and physically demanding occupations that males engaged in through much of the 20th century may explain the difference as well. These potential mortality risks are dynamic across the sexes, for more women are entering the work place at all levels and more women are smoking. Females may have a genetic advantage in life expectancy, however.

As much as the overall changes in the demographics of the 65+ have commanded the attention of health care planners, perhaps an even more dramatic revolution has occurred among the oldest old. Persons 85 and older currently are the most rapidly growing age group in the American population (Rosenwaike 1985). Though they constituted less than 1 million persons in 1960, by the year 2000 nearly 5 million persons will be 85 years of age and older and will constitute nearly 15 percent of the 65+ age group. These oldest old will require increased medical and psychiatric services, for at the age of 85, they enter a time of life characterized by a high prevalence and incidence of dementia and possibly other psychiatric disorders (such as depression). Given the frailty of the oldest old, medical care must be attended judiciously and therefore will require even greater resources.

Given the magnitude of the task facing geriatricians and geriatric psychiatrists, what can epidemiologic studies contribute to the mental health care of these older adults? Morris (1975) has suggested the following uses of epidemiology:

1. The identification of cases (e.g., can the symptom pattern of depression in the elderly be readily identified in community as well as clinical populations of older adults?)
2. The distribution of psychiatric disorders in the population (e.g., what is the prevalence and/or incidence of dementia?)
3. The historical trends of mental illness among the elderly (e.g., has the incidence of suicide increased, decreased, or remained the same among the elderly over the past 50 years?)
4. The etiology of psychiatric disorders in late life (e.g., are social factors more prevalent in the etiology of late-life psychiatric disorders, given less potential for genetic influence?)
5. The use of psychiatric and other mental health services by the elderly (e.g., do psychiatrically impaired older adults in the community use psychiatric services?).

Each of these uses will be reviewed in this chapter.

Case Identification

Clinicians constantly face the task of distinguishing abnormality from normality. Though most epidemiologists and clinicians agree on the core symptoms of psychiatric disorders throughout the life cycle, the absolute distinction between a case and a noncase is not easily established. Many of the symptoms and signs of a psychiatric disorder in late life may be ubiquitous with the aging process, thus blurring the distinction between cases (i.e., persons requiring medical attention) and noncases. Epidemiologists can assist the clinician in developing meaningful clusters of persons with varying degrees of morbidity. Case identification is also the foundation of descriptive epidemiology; that is, it is the numerator of the equation from which prevalence and incidence proportions are derived.

What is a case? Copeland (1981) suggests that the question be turned by epidemiologists, with advantage, to "A case for what?" The choice of a construct for a case depends on the particular scientific or clinical inquiry of the investigator. If the clinician wishes to identify a group of older adults suffering from initial insomnia (in order to determine the value of a new short-acting sedative–hypnotic agent), the prevalence and severity of a target symptom—initial insomnia—defines the case. The sleep difficulty may result from a number of different underlying disorders, but this is irrelevant to the purpose of the study.

For most clinicians, however, the goal of case identification in psychiatry is to develop a process of diagnosis that reflects an underlying reality (Blazer 1982). According to Goodwin and Guze (1979), diagnosis is prognosis. Diagnostic categories that approximate true disease processes have a number of characteristics, including the following:

1. A category should be distinguished on the basis of patterns of symptomatology;
2. A category should predict the outcome of a disorder;
3. The category should reflect underlying biologic reality, confirmed by family and genetic studies;
4. Laboratory studies should eventually validate a diagnostic category (e.g., the use of rapid eye movement latency or the DST in delineating melancholic depression);
5. The classificatory scheme should identify persons who may respond to a specific therapeutic intervention, such as a particular form of psychotherapy or a specific group of medications (Weissman and Klerman 1978).

Still others may define a case on the basis of severity of symptoms or social and interpersonal impairment secondary to the symptoms. This approach to case identification is less popular among clinicians, who are more inclined to "treat a disease" than to "improve function." Improved function should derive from remission of the disease. Nevertheless, function may have special relevance to the care of older adults. When managing chronic illnesses, such as primary degenerative dementia of senile onset (senile dementia of the Alzheimer's type), the improvement or maintenance of functioning is the primary goal of the clinician. In addition, family members and even patients may be more concerned with improved functioning than symptom alleviation. Improved sleep and appetite and a decline in suicidal ideation in a depressed older adult may not translate into a perceived recovery from a depressive episode by the family. Rather, they may focus on the quality of interpersonal interactions and social functioning.

Regardless of the approach taken to identify cases, most clinicians and clinical investigators maintain an inappropriate desire to achieve perfection in the separation of cases from noncases. The epidemiologic method, for the most part, depends on a clear distinction between cases and noncases (Kleinbaum et al. 1982), yet most older adults do not ideally fit their psychiatric diagnosis (Strauss et al. 1979). Regardless of the diagnostic system, unusual or borderline cases that cannot be clearly placed in a single category always exist. This has led some investigators to consider the possibility of "fuzzy sets" as a means by which cases can be more realistically distinguished (Clive et al. 1983; Swartz et al. 1986). Not only can older adults manifest more than one disease simultaneously, for example, major depression and primary degenerative dementia, they do not fit easily into the prescribed categories of *DSM-III-R* (generalized anxiety is not easily disentangled from a major depressive episode in an agitated older adult). Most natural clustering of older adults into categories is perceptually "fuzzy" (Rosch 1978), for natural categories rarely possess necessary and sufficient properties of criteria. Boundaries between closely related categories are ill defined. The use of fuzzy-set theory, however, is in its infancy in psychiatric epidemiology of the elderly. Nevertheless, some of the methods of case identification, such as the symptom checklist and standardized interview approaches that archive symptoms, are adaptive to the development of fuzzy sets.

Regardless of the approach taken to case identification, for a diagnosis to be a useful means of communicating clinical information, it must be reliable and valid. To pass the test of reliability, a diagnosis must be consistent and repeatable. Standardized or operational methods for identifying psychiatric symptoms and the availability of specific criteria for psychiatric diagnoses have greatly improved the reliability of case identification between psychiatrists and psychiatric epidemiologists. Reliability, however, does not ensure validity, that is, the test of whether a case identified by a particular method reflects underlying reality. Unlike other medical specialties, clinicians who work with the psychiatrically ill focus their skills, for the most part, on thoughts, feelings, and actions. No standard exists for testing the truth of a particular syndrome identified in a particular manner.

Once the criteria are set for case identification, a number of approaches to identifying cases have been used in psychiatric epidemiologic studies of the elderly. Though each contributes to our understanding of psychopathology in late life, each presents unique problems. Historically, the most frequently used method of case identification in epidemiologic surveys has been chart reviews or the establishment of case registries (New York State Department of Mental Hygiene 1960; Farris and Dunham 1939; Pasamanick et al. 1959). Diagnoses in these studies rely totally on a clinician's evaluation of the patient. Variability in criteria used by clinicians, variability in the socioeconomic status of the patient, and variability of criteria for disorders across the life cycle may each contribute to a bias in these studies (Clausen and Kohn 1959).

A second approach to case identification is the use of self-administered symptom scales and personality inventories. Frequently used scales in epidemiologic surveys include the Center for Epidemiology Studies Depression Scale (CES-D) (a scale that screens for depressive symptoms), the Short Portable Mental Status Questionnaire (SPMSQ), and the Folstein Mini-Mental State Exam (MMSE) (Radloff 1977; Pfeiffer 1975; Folstein et al. 1975). These scales are advantageous in that they do not subjectively assign patients to a particular diagnostic category (unlike case registries), yet they suffer from a lack of diagnostic specificity and occasionally clinical relevance. For example, the severity of depressive symptoms following the loss of a loved one may be similar to those of a major depressive episode with melancholia. Though the diagnosis of, and intervention for, these two disorders would be very different, a symptom checklist could distinguish the two.

In recent years, a commonly used means of case identification in both clinical and community studies has been the standardized interview. The Present State Examination (PSE), the Schedule for Affective Disorders and Schizophrenia (SADS), and the Diagnostic Interview Schedule (DIS) are examples of the most frequently used interview schedules (Wing et al. 1974; Spitzer and Endicott 1978; Robins et al. 1981). These instruments are generally based on diagnostic systems, such as *DSM-III-R*, that identify specific criteria for a particular diagnostic category. They tend to be reliable and generally are valid. Nevertheless, the standardized interviews tend to rely on a particular diagnostic system from which they were developed. In addition, there are "trade-offs." The more clinical judgment contributes to the identification of a case, the less reliable cases tend to be (though cases identified by a less structured schedule may reflect clinical judgment better than a highly structured interview that eliminates clinical judgment).

Finally, one of the more frequently used epidemiologic methods in community studies relies on the judgment of a clinician to assess the probability that a psychiatric disorder is present on the basis of data from a survey questionnaire. Clinicians are asked to estimate the chances that a particular individual in the community would be given a psychiatric diagnosis if interviewed clinically. This approach tends to maximize the clinical adjustment in evaluating a forced-response questionnaire. The method suffers, however, because it cannot distinguish between different types of psychiatric impairment and therefore is less clinically relevant. For example, the distinction between major depression and dementia may be blurred, despite the relatively distinct approaches to therapy that are implied in the specific diagnoses. The Midtown Manhattan Study, from which interesting data have been published relevant to cohort phenomena, utilized this approach (Srole and Fischer 1981).

The Distribution of Psychiatric Disorders

Descriptive studies of the epidemiology of psychiatric impairment have concentrated on either overall mental health functioning or the distribution of specific psychiatric disorders in the population. Reports from these studies usually begin as general observations of the relationship of impairment or specific disorders to such characteristics as age, sex, race, occupation, and social class. These trends provide the template for more in-depth studies of the genetic and psychosocial contributors to the etiology of disorders and the

Table 2. Prevalence of Cognitive Impairment in Community and Institutional Populations

Site	Sample	n	Age	Assessment Strategy	Prevalence (%)
Epidemiologic Catchment Area (Robins et al. 1984)					
New Haven	Community	607	65+	MMSE	5 (severe impairment)
Baltimore	Community	923	65+	MMSE	5.1 (severe impairment)
St. Louis	Community	576	65+	MMSE	4.0 (severe impairment)
EPESE (Huntley et al. 1986)					
New Haven	Community	2,811	65+	SPMSQ (nine items)	5.3 (moderate to severe impairment)
Iowa	Community (entire population of two rural counties)	3,673	65+	SPMSQ (nine items)	1.3 (severe impairment)
East Boston	Community	3,812	65+	SPMSQ (nine items)	6.0 (severe impairment)
New York (Goldfarb 1962)	Institution	451	65+	MSQ	87 (moderate or severe)
Durham County (Blazer 1978)	Institution	100	65+	SPMSQ	47 (severe impairment)
Minnesota (Teeter et al. 1976)	Institutionalized Medicaid Patients	74	96% were ≥ 65	SPMSQ	59.4 (moderate or severe)

Note. MMSE = Mini-Mental Status Exam; SPMSQ = Short Portable Mental Status Questionnaire; MSQ = Mental Status Questionnaire.

Table 3. Prevalence of Dementia in Community and Institutional Populations

Site	Sample	n	Age	Assessment Strategy	Prevalence (%)
Sweden (Essen-Möller et al. 1956)	Rural community	443	65+	Psychiatric interviews	10.8 mild and 5.0 severe organic brain syndrome
Sweden (Persson 1980)	Community and institution	460	70+	Psychiatric interviews	1.3 severe organic brain syndrome
England (Kay et al. 1970)	Community	758	65+	Psychiatric interviews	6.2 severe organic brain syndrome
Minnesota (Teeter et al. 1976)	Institution	74	96% were ≥ 65	Psychiatric interviews	45.9 chronic brain syndrome
Baltimore (Folstein et al. 1985)	Community	923	65+	Psychiatric interviews and laboratory studies	2.0 Alzheimer's disease; 2.8 multi-infarct dementia; 1.3 mixed or unspecified dementia
Maryland (Rovner et al. 1986)	Institution	50	96% were ≥ 66	Standardized interview	56 primary degenerative dementia; 22 multi-infarct dementia; 4 Parkinson's dementia

epidemiology of mental health care utilization. Frequencies of disorders within the population are usually presented in terms of a proportion, that is, the percentage of persons suffering from a defined impairment or specific disorder within the population. Almost all such studies are estimates based on community samples of larger populations.

The prevalences of cognitive impairment and dementia in selected community and institutional populations, as determined in selected studies, are presented in Tables 2 and 3. The prevalence of severe cognitive impairment usually reported within community populations is approximately 4 to 6 percent, as illustrated by the data presented. This prevalence of cognitive impairment must not be mistakenly assumed to be the prevalence of Alzheimer's disease or actual cerebral impairment (since such studies measure nothing more than cognitive functioning). For example, the prevalence of cognitive "impairment" is affected by the educational level of the population being studied and other sociocultural factors that may affect performance of cognitive tasks. When institutional populations are studied, the range of severe cognitive impairment clusters around 50 percent in most studies. Though the prevalence of dementia in institutional populations is undoubtedly much higher than in the community, once again these prevalence figures must not be misinterpreted as representing the prevalence of actual dementia in institutions.

Even in community studies performed by clinicians, the prevalence of subtypes of dementia, such as multi-infarct dementia or primary degenerative dementia of senile onset, is not usually reported. Rather, investigators will report the level of severity of generalized organic brain syndromes. Within community populations, these prevalences vary, but most reports hover around 5 percent for severe organic brain syndrome. One exception was the two-stage approach to the identification of dementia in a study reported by Folstein et al. (1985). First, the investigators screened the population using the MMSE. Next, they evaluated in detail those persons who demonstrated impairment on the MMSE. Results from this evaluation were surprising. Though the overall prevalence of dementia was 6.1 percent, the relative distribution between multi-infarct dementia and Alzheimer's disease was different from that usually reported: 2.8 percent multi-infarct dementia versus 2.0 percent Alzheimer's disease (primary degenerative dementia). One explanation for these findings is the relatively high proportion of blacks in the community sample studied (unlike most clinical samples of dementia).

In Tables 4 and 5, the prevalence of selected psychiatric symptoms and disorders in community populations is presented. If the entire adult life cycle were included, then many of the symptoms reported would find their highest frequency among the elderly, especially symptoms of hypochondriasis and sleep difficulties. Most studies of depressive symptoms across the life cycle in the past have documented a higher prevalence in late life (Warheit et al. 1973). A relatively higher frequency of certain symptoms in elderly popula-

Table 4. Prevalence of Psychiatric Symptoms in Community Populations of Older Adults

Site	n	Age	Assessment Strategy	Symptoms/ Disorder	Prevalence (%)
Durham County (Blazer & Williams 1980)	997	65+	OARS Depression Scale	Depression	15
New Haven (Huntley et al. 1986)	2,811	65+	CES-D ($\geq$16)	Depression	15
Durham County (Blazer and Houpt 1979)	997	65+	Selected questions	Hypochondriasis	14
San Francisco (Lowenthal and Berkmen 1967)	589	60+	Selected questions	Suspicious	17
Durham County (Christenson and Blazer 1984)	997	65+	MMPI	Persecutory ideation	4
Iowa (Huntley et al.1986)	3,217	65+	Selected questions	Trouble falling asleep Awakes during the night Sleepy during the day	14 34 31

Table 5. Prevalence of Selected Psychiatric Disorders in Community Populations of Older Adults

Site	n	Age	Assessment Strategy	Disorder	Prevalence (%)
New Haven Epidemiologic Catchment Area (Myers et al. 1984)	3,058	65+	Diagnostic Interview Schedule	Major depression Dysthymia Alcohol abuse Schizophrenic/ schizophreniform disorder	M = 0.5; F = 1.6 M = 1.8; F = 3.1 M = 3.0; F = 0.0 M = 0.0; F = 0.9
England (Kay et al. 1964)	297	65+	Psychiatric interviews	Anxiety and dysthymic disorder	5–10
North Carolina (George et al. 1986)	1,297	65+	Diagnostic Interview Schedule	Generalized anxiety disorder	5.5

tions, however, does not necessarily signify an increased frequency of specific psychiatric disorders. The paradox of relatively high reports of depressive symptoms and relatively low reports of the prevalence of major depressive episodes illustrates this point (Blazer 1982b). Diagnostic categories, as are found in *DSM-III-R*, are clusters of symptoms and signs that derive their validity, not from the overall weight of symptomatology, but rather from regularities in the clustering of history, the persistence of symptoms over time, a predictable outcome, a common pathophysiology, and possibly common biochemical disturbances. As biologic markers of psychiatric disorders are identified, laboratory diagnostic techniques will be complements to the symptoms reported. As our knowledge progresses in the area of nomenclature, new categories of symptoms may be lumped together to define a particular syndrome. As Morris (1975) noted, each succeeding generation will split and lump groups of symptoms and signs to suit its own purposes, given the current biomedical and clinical understanding of disease entities.

Symptoms, the most objective clinical indicators of psychopathology, may reflect more than one diagnostic entity. On the other hand, symptoms may not be associated with any disorder of interest to the clinician. For example, decreased appetite can result from a number of sources. At a given time, grief reactions, more frequent in late life than at other stages of the life cycle, may be virtually indistinguishable from major depressive episodes, based on loss of appetite alone. As allowed in *DMS-III-R*, grief may be distinguished from major depression only when a loss of significance is identified. Loss of appetite also accompanies major life adjustments such as a forced change of residence or a decline in economic resources. Most commonly, loss of appetite in late life is a result of poor physical health.

Further review of Table 5 indicates that psychiatric disorders other than depression are also found in a lower prevalence among the elderly than at other stages of the life cycle. The relatively decreased prevalence of alcohol abuse has been well documented in the literature, as has been the decreased prevalence of schizophrenia and schizophreniform disorders. The virtual absence of these disorders in the Epidemiologic Catchment Area data (Myers et al. 1984) may reflect selective mortality. On the other hand, it may also reflect the case-finding techniques used (for the investigators did not attempt to identify the homeless). The community data do not include individuals in institutions, and many chronic schizophrenics in late life may be institutionalized. In addition, late-life schizophrenics may have a "burned-out" symptom picture and, coupled with poor reporting, may not meet the criteria for schizophrenia. By far the most frequent of the psychiatric disorders to be found in the elderly are the anxiety disorders. These disorders have received relatively little attention in the literature but should be considered in more detail.

A further question derives from these data. Do unique late-life symptom presentations render the RDC and *DSM-III-R* inadequate as a nomenclature?

Table 6. Prevalence of Selected Psychiatric Disorders among Older Adults in Selected Treatment Facilities

Site	n	Age	Assessment Strategy	Disorder	Prevalence (%)
Inpatient geriatric evaluation unit (Cheah and Beard 1980)	262	45+ but primarily 55+	Psychiatric interviews	Dysphoria/depression	31.3
Medical surgical inpatient facility (Folks and Ford 1985)	195	60+	Psychiatric interviews	Major depression Paranoid disorder/Schizophrenia	26.0 4.6
Intermediate care facility (Rovner et al. 1986)	50	96% were ≥ 66	Psychiatric interviews	Major depression Paraphrenia	6 2
Skilled nursing facilities (Teeter et al. 1976)	74	96% were ≥ 65	Semistructured psychiatric interviews	Schizophrenia Depressive neurosis Psychotic depression	6.7 21.6 4.0

The *DSM-III-R* provides age-specific categories for children, but not for the elderly. Clinicians who work with the elderly, however, have often commented that depression may be masked in late life through presentation of symptoms of poor physical health or pseudodementia. Yet there is no compelling evidence for developing a new diagnostic classification specific to older adults. Though *DSM-III-R* may not identify all older persons with significant psychiatric symptoms, those persons who do qualify for a *DSM-III-R* diagnosis are not unlike persons at other stages of the life cycle (Blazer 1980a; Blazer et al. in press).

The prevalence of psychiatric disorders (other than dementia) in treatment facilities is presented in Table 6. As can be seen, the prevalence of dysphoria and major depression in treatment facilities is much higher than that found in community populations. Many depressed older adults may be selectively admitted to medical inpatient units or long-term care facilities (since older adults are less likely to use specialty psychiatric care). The lower prevalence of these disorders in the community, therefore, should not lull the clinician into believing that psychiatric problems are of little consequence for older adults.

Historical Studies

Psychiatrists follow patients for relatively short periods of time during the course of their illnesses. In addition, they practice within a relatively brief window of historical time. Epidemiologic studies add a perspective to current cross-sectional findings in population and clinical surveys. Some disorders, such as tuberculosis, are known to wax and wane; new disorders may emerge, such as acquired immune deficiency syndrome dementia; and old ones, such as smallpox, are eradicated or disappear naturally (Morris 1975). Historical studies in psychiatric epidemiology are rare, especially of the elderly. Temporal changes of most behaviors of psychiatric interest, unlike infectious diseases, must be determined over years rather than months, an exception being the clustering of psychiatric emergencies after the Christmas season or the increase in suicide during the spring of the year (Hillard et al. 1981; Lester 1979). Constructs of case identification have changed over the years, and therefore it is rare to find a study in which similar methods of case identification were applied at two points distant enough in time to establish historical trends. Longitudinal studies are also fraught with methodologic problems, especially problems with follow-up.

The study of changes in suicide frequency among older adults during the 20th century illustrates the value of longitudinal studies, despite the methodologic problems associated with such studies. Suicide rates in 1980 were positively correlated with age, although the correlation was not as dramatic as it was in the year 1970. As can be seen in Figure 1, the correlation is almost totally explained by the dramatic increase in frequency of suicide after the age

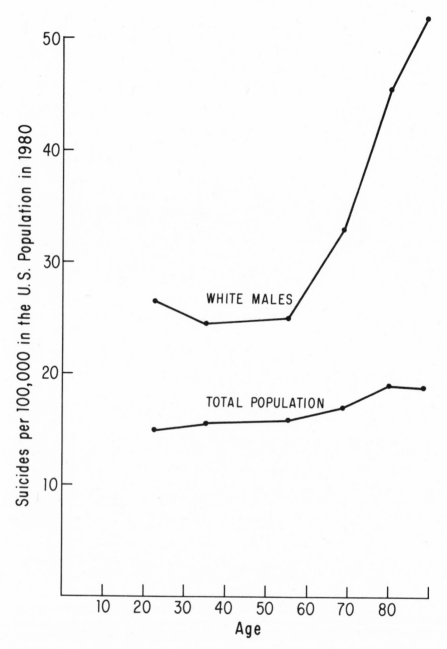

Figure 1. U.S. suicide rates in 1980. (Reproduced with permission from Blazer DG, Bachar JR, Manton KG: Suicide in late life: review and commentary. J Am Geriatr Soc 1986; 34:519–525.)

of 60 years in white males.

Why has there been a flattening of the century-long trend for suicide rates to increase with age? Suicide rates at any point in time are determined by at least three factors: age, generational or cohort effects, and unique stressors for a particular age group at a particular point in time (i.e., period effects). Both age and generational effects were demonstrated to predict suicide in the United States since 1900 in a study by Murphy and Wetzel (1980). This generational effect was illustrated in a study by Haas and Hendin (1983). Age groups were studied at four points in time from 1908 to 1970. Cohorts entering the 15- to 24-year-old age group showed significantly different suicide rates. The 15- to 24-year-olds in 1908 had a suicide rate of 13.5 per 100,000, in contrast to the rate of the same age group in 1923 of 6.3 per 100,000. The 1908 cohort has continued to have relatively higher rates of suicide at every age through life, though both cohorts showed increases in suicide rates with age. In other words, a cohort is presently passing through the 65 to 80 years age window, which has always had lower rates of suicide than the cohort passing through the 80 to 95 years age window. When examined cross-sectionally, the curve is flattened. Younger cohorts (such as the 1946, or baby-boom, cohort) have increased rates of suicide. If their trend follows previous trends in the 20th century and they are followed by cohorts with lower suicide rates, the slope of the curve will change once again.

Murphy et al. (1986), in a study of suicides in England and Wales, were able to demonstrate a marked period effect. In a cohort analysis of recorded suicides from 1921 to 1980, a fall in suicide rates of successively older cohorts was identified (in contrast to figures in the United States). Murphy postulated the impact of period events, specifically, World War II and the detoxification of domestic gas. The last hypothesis is especially intriguing. Before the early 1960s, domestic gas in England and Wales contained large amounts of carbon monoxide. One of the more popular means of suicide was putting one's head in a gas oven, particularly among the middle aged and the elderly. As domestic gas was converted to a methane-based product in the 1960s, the rate of gas poisoning decreased dramatically in the more elderly age groups. This was not offset by increasing rates of suicide by other means, suggesting that withdrawal of a method of suicide could result in a net saving of life.

Observing these historical studies, one can observe that many factors contribute to changing rates in at least one indicant of psychiatric disorder, that is, suicide. Concomitant changes in other factors are less well understood, but may be especially relevant to the study of psychiatric disorders in the elderly. Klerman et al. (1985) suggest that the relatively low prevalence of depression in late life, compared with that of other age groups in the 1980s, may be a result of cohort phenomenon. Current cohorts of older adults appear remarkably protected against severe or clinically diagnosed depressive disorders. Younger cohorts, in contrast, have exhibited higher rates of major depression throughout the life cycle. Since there is no reason to expect the rates for younger cohorts to decrease as they enter late life (i.e., there is no evidence of a period effect), the relatively low prevalence of major depression in late life will be a transient phenomenon.

An additional historical consideration in the study of psychiatric disorders is the study of incidence and duration of disorders. Cumulative incidence, the probability of developing a disorder over a specified period of time (usually 1 year), is less important to the health care provider at a given point in time but very relevant to the planning for services in the future. The duration of a psychiatric disorder in late life, such as senile dementia, interacts with both incidence and prevalence. For example, the incidence of primary degenerative dementia or senile dementia of the Alzheimer's type appears relatively unchanged over the past 15 to 20 years (though accurate studies are still lacking). Nevertheless, dementia patients receive better health care and appear to follow the general trend of the aging population—an increased life expectancy. Therefore the prevalence of the disorder over time (in addition to a higher number of cases because of more older adults at risk) is increasing, leading to a greater burden of dementia within the community (Gruenberg 1980).

Etiologic Studies

One of the more important tasks of epidemiology is to identify factors that can either predispose individuals to developing psychiatric disorders or precipitate such disorders (Blazer and Jordan 1985). Both genetic and environmental causative agents can be identified in population studies. Yet the significance of this research has only recently achieved some status in psychiatry and has rarely been applied to geriatric psychiatry.

The contribution of epidemiology to uncovering hereditary trends in mental disorder is best illustrated by the work in senile dementia. Heston et al. (1981) studied the relatives of 125 probands who suffered from dementia of the Alzheimer's type as identified at autopsy. The risk of dementia in first-degree relatives varied with the age of the person at the onset of dementia. Those persons who were first-degree relatives of someone with Alzheimer's disease were more likely to develop the disease earlier in life, suggesting that the inherited form of Alzheimer's disease accelerates the onset of the disease. In a more recent study by Barclay et al. (1986), a family history for dementia was positive in 35.9 percent of Alzheimer's patients, compared with 5.6 percent of individuals who were cognitively intact.

Other investigators have suggested an association between early-onset Alzheimer's disease and Down's syndrome. Heyman et al. (1983) studied 68 Alzheimer's disease patients with clinical onset before the age of 70. Secondary cases of dementia were found in 17 (25 percent) of the families, affecting 22 of the probands' siblings and parents. An increased frequency of Down's syndrome was observed among relatives of the probands, a rate of 3.6 per

1,000, compared with the expected rate of 1.3 per 1,000. Heston et al. (1981) not only found an excess of Down's syndrome in the families of Alzheimer's patients but also identified an increased frequency of lymphoma and immune diatheses among family members, suggesting that immune system disorders are associated with an increased risk for Alzheimer's disease. Another finding that has been shown to be increasingly frequent among Alzheimer's patients is a history of head trauma (Heyman et al. 1983).

Among the more intriguing genetic studies, however, are those of Folstein and Breitner (1981). These investigators suggest that a subtype of primary degenerative dementia (PDD) may be transmitted as an autosomal dominant trait with complete penetrance (Folstein and Breitner 1981; Chase et al. 1983). In the original Folstein and Breitner investigation, they found the presence of aphasia and apraxia distinguished patients suffering from primary degenerative dementia who had a family history of the disease from those who did not have a history. In a study of 39 cases of PDD, patients with relatives suffering from the disease were less often able to complete a sentence on the MMSE than those who did not have afflicted relatives ($p <$ .05). Among those individuals who were unable to write a sentence, the investigators found a fourfold increased risk of dementia than in the general population. In a follow-up study, Folstein and colleagues found that among 54 nursing home patients diagnosed with PDD, 40 were considered aphasic and agraphic and 14 were not. Among the first-degree relatives of the aphasic/ agraphic PDD patients, there was a 44 percent risk of senile dementia by age 90, approaching the 50 percent rate for a genetic disorder that is autosomal dominant with complete penetrance.

Physical agents in the environment, such as the bacterium syphilis and the ingestion or absorption of certain chemicals, have long been known to cause cognitive problems. Some of these agents may lead to other psychiatric symptoms as well. Two illustrative studies demonstrate the effect of such agents on the brain.

Goodwin et al. (1983) studied 260 noninstitutionalized men and women between the ages of 60 and 94. These individuals were not found to have serious illnesses or to be clinically malnourished or vitamin deficient on clinical examination. Dietary intake for these subjects was calculated. The nutrients measured included protein, vitamin C, vitamin B_{12}, folic acid, riboflavin, thiamine, niacin, and pyridoxine. Blood samples were obtained to determine the blood levels of these specific nutrients. The investigators discovered a significant relationship between scores on memory tests and blood levels of vitamin C and folic acid in these generally well-functioning older adults. These results suggest that there may be variables, such as nutrient levels, that provide an opportunity for intervention in the relationship between primary (innate) and secondary (environmentally induced) changes with aging and cognitive functioning. Gerontologists have long sought such intervening variables that may allow clinical intervention to prevent or mitigate deficits that were previously ascribed to primary aging.

Parker et al. (1983) investigated the relationship between alcohol use and cognitive functioning. They studied 1,937 employed men and women who were asked about their alcohol consumption during the previous month. In addition, their vocabulary skills and abstraction abilities were investigated. Results from the study suggested a linear relationship between the amount of alcohol consumption during the previous month and cognitive impairment. The relationship held for the men and those women whose drinking patterns resembled the men's. This model suggests that cognitive performance may be decreased by alcohol consumption prior to the postintoxication period, and since this relationship is linear, even moderate alcohol intake may lead to impairment in congitive functioning. The implications of these findings for the elderly are evident.

By far the most frequently investigated environmental factor associated with psychiatric disorders are social factors. The changing roles and circumstances of older adults are considered by many investigators to stress older adults and therefore contribute to the onset of psychiatric disorders and cognitive difficulties. Blazer (1980b), in a study of 986 community-based older adults, found the crude estimate of relative risk for mental health impairment, given a life event score greater than or equal to 150 on the Schedule of Recent Events, to be 2.14. A relative risk of 1.73 ($p < .01$) was estimated when a binary regression procedure was used, controlling for physical health, economic status, social support, and age. In a study of individuals 55 years of age and older by Murrell et al. (1983), social factors, including widowhood, divorce, separation, and decreased income, were related to depressive symptomatology in the community.

Nevertheless, the study of social factors in relation to psychiatric disorders must not be viewed simplistically. The mitigating effect of social support, the perception of the event (as well as the occurrence of the event), the expectancy of the event, and the perceived importance of the event may all contribute to the impact of environmental stress upon the older adult. In a previous study (Blazer 1982b), I have suggested a number of possible mechanisms by which environmental stress and social support may interact with psychiatric disorders:

1. Environmental stressors, including stressful life events, may cause or contribute to the development of a psychiatric disorder. The bulk of the literature on stressful life events as precipitants of depressive disorders is based on this hypothesis.
2. Environmental stressors may decrease physical health status, and the older adult thus reacts to the decline in physical health with the development of a reactive psychiatric disorder, such as an adjustment disorder with depressed mood.
3. Environmental stressors an individual experienced in the remote past

may contribute to physical and psychologic changes that predispose the older adult to develop a psychiatric disorder in late life. Studies of early deprivation (such as the death of a parent in childhood) exemplify this hypothesis.

4. Social isolation may contribute to the onset of a psychiatric disorder. For example, lack of social stimuli may contribute to increased paranoid ideation in an older adult.

5. Environmental stressors may be buffered by the perceived or actual social support to an individual. In other words, when social support is decreased, the causal relationship between environmental stress and psychiatric disorder is enhanced.

6. The lack of important specific social relations, such as the absence of a spouse or confidant, may predispose to the development of a psychiatric disorder. Studies of the increased risk for depression in the year following the loss of a spouse or confidant derive not only from the stress of the loss but also from the absence of the relationship in the succeeding year.

7. The absence of a satisfactory social network may lead to decreased frequency of social interaction, which in turn leads to an increased likelihood of the development of certain psychiatric disorders. For example, lack of social relations may increase the prevalence of hypochondriacal symptoms and the use of health services (thus increasing social contact).

Health Service Utilization

Epidemiologic studies provide a disturbing profile of the use of mental health services by the elderly. Though older adults are less likely to use community-based psychiatric services than any other age group, they are more likely to use psychotropic medication. Shapiro et al. (1984), in a study of three communities (New Haven, Baltimore, and St. Louis), found that 6 to 7 percent of the adults had made a visit during the 6 months prior to evaluation to a health care provider for mental health reasons. The 65 + group infrequently received care from mental health specialists, even if they were identified in the community as suffering from a *DSM-III* psychiatric disorder or severe cognitive impairment. German et al. (1985) analyzed data from Baltimore in greater detail. Of those persons under the age of 65, during the 6 months prior to the evaluation, 8.7 percent had made a visit to a specialty or primary care provider for mental health care. For those aged 65 to 74, the rate was 4.2 percent; and of those 75 and older, only 1.4 percent received such care. In the 75 + age group, not one person among the 292 individuals interviewed saw a specialty mental health provider. The investigators concluded that the likeliest source of care for older individuals suffering from emotional or psychiatric problems is their primary care provider within the context of a visit made for physical medical problems.

In contrast, the use of psychotropic drugs has increased among older adults. In a nationwide survey, Mellinger et al. (1978) found that 40 percent of the men over age 60 and 44 percent of women over age 60 who suffered from psychiatric distress had used a psychotherapeutic drug during the preceding year, while 17 percent and 20 percent, respectively, were regular users. In a study by Rossiter (1983) from another national survey, 23.4 percent of persons 65 and older were using some central nervous system agent at the time of the survey, higher than any other age group (for example, only 14.4 percent of the 25- to 54-year-old age group used these agents). Ray et al. (1980), in a review of prescriptions for Medicaid patients residing for at least 1 year in nursing homes in the state of Tennessee, found that 43 percent of these individuals had received antipsychotic drugs during the preceding year and 9 percent were chronic recipients.

Yet the value of community surveys does not end with a description of patterns of health services use. Such investigations are especially useful for determining the needs of services for the noninstitutionalized and institutionalized elderly. By sampling elderly community populations, researchers can collect data on rates of impairment, need for services, perceived needs or demands for services, and the current use of services. This information can be used by government and private agencies to chart effective evaluative, treatment, and preventive programs. This development is especially relevant to the care of older adults, as they tend to be isolated, their psychiatric impairment may be masked, and they are less active advocates for their mental health needs.

Such an approach is illustrated by a study from North Carolina (Blazer 1978). In a statewide survey, 8 percent of the elderly in the community suffering from functional mental impairment were receiving mental health services at the time of the survey. The problem was compounded by the fact that for the elderly, mental health services were not integrated with other services available. The overlap of impairments was documented in this study as well. Blazer and Maddox (1982) reviewed a seven-step model, modified from Wing (1968), to use these data for the development of a new service for older adults. First, a target population was identified through an epidemiologic survey of Durham County. Next, the appropriate types of services for this population were determined through a needs assessment of the population. Because cognitive impairment was highly correlated with impairment in other areas, it was decided that an integrated program of psychotherapy, psychotropic medication management, medical evaluation, and social interaction would be the most appropriate way to develop the necessary services. The third step was to assess the perception of need for services, since this would affect the level of use. Ten percent of the sample expressed some need for counseling, while 31 percent of the cognitively impaired stated they experienced such a need. Fourth, current use was assessed. Only 10 of the 997 subjects (1 percent) were receiving any kind of counseling or psychotherapy, although 20 percent were taking some type of psychotropic medication, almost always prescribed by a primary care physician.

The fifth step, closely tied to the fourth, was to assess the impact of other factors on service utilization. One factor was economic resources. The assumption that those with adequate financial resources would seek private care rather than use a public clinic, as was planned, had to be considered. Since 40 percent of those who were impaired had inadequate finances, these were identified as those persons who would potentially use such a clinic. The sixth step addressed the need for personnel to represent the interdisciplinary needs described above. It was decided that a part-time staff, including a psychiatrist, a social worker, a physician with experience in geriatric medicine, and a registered nurse with experience in geriatric nursing, as well as a receptionist/secretary, would meet the needs. In addition, the staff would make efforts to integrate their services with existing service providers such as primary care physicians and social service agencies. The final step was to assess the accuracy of planning efforts after the clinic was established. Four years after the inception of the clinic, the plans suggested that the flow of patients was about as expected and the mix of staff was appropriate to delivering the care conceived initially. As predicted, most of those seen were individuals with multiple impairments who could not afford usual medical and psychiatric care.

References

American Psychiatric Association: Diagnostic and Statistical Manual of Mental Disorders (Third Edition-Revised). Washington, DC, American Psychiatric Association, 1980

Barclay LL, Kheyfets S, Zemcov A, et al: Risk factors in Alzheimer's disease, in Alzheimer's Disease and Parkinson's Disease: Strategies for Research and Development. Edited by Fisher A, Hanin I, Lachman C. New York, Plenum Press, 1986

Blazer D: The OARS Durham surveys: description and application, in Multidimensional Functional Assessment: The OARS Methodology (Second Edition). Durham, NC, Center for the Study of Aging and Human Development, Duke University, 1978

Blazer D: The diagnosis of depression in the elderly. J Am Geriatr Soc 1980a; 28:52–58

Blazer D: Life Events, mental health functioning and the use of health care services by the elderly. Am J Public Health 1980b; 70:1174–1179

Blazer DG: Depression in Late Life. St. Louis, C. V. Mosby, 1982a

Blazer D: The epidemiology of late life depression. J Am Geriatr Soc 1982b; 30:587–592

Blazer D, Houpt JL: Perception of poor health in the healthy older adult. J Am Geriatr Soc 1979; 27:330–334

Blazer DG, Jordan K: Epidemiology of psychiatric disorders and cognitive problems in the elderly, in Psychiatry (Volume 3). Edited by Michels R, Cavenar JO. Philadelphia, J.B. Lippincott, 1985

Blazer DG, Maddox G: Using epidemiology survey data to plan geriatric mental health services. Hosp Community Psychiatry 1982; 33:42–45

Blazer, D, William CD: The epidemiology of dysphoria and depression in an elderly population. Am J Psychiatry 1980; 137:439–444

Blazer DG, Bachar JR, Manton KG: Suicide in late life: review and commentary. J Am Geriatr Soc 1986; 34:519–525

Blazer DG, Bachar JR, Hughes DC: Major depression with melancholia: a comparison of middle-aged and elderly adults. J Am Geriatr Soc, in press

Chase GA, Folstein MF, Breitner JCS, et al: The use of life tables and survival analyses in testing genetic hypotheses with an application to Alzheimer's disease. Am J Epidemiol 1983; 7:590–597

Cheah KC, Beard OW: Psychiatric findings in the population of a geriatric evaluation unit: implications. J Am Geriatr Soc 1980; 28:153–156

Christenson RM, Blazer DG: Epidemiology of persecutory ideation in an elderly population in the community. Am J Psychiatry 1984; 141:1088–1091

Clausen JA, Kohn ML: Relation of schizophrenia to the social structure of a small city, in Epidemiology of Mental Disorder. Edited by Pasamanick B. Washington, DC, American Association for the Advancement of Science, 1959

Clive J, Woodbury MA, Siegler IC: Fuzzy and crisp set theoretic-based classification of health and disease: a qualitative and quantitative comparison. J Med Syst 1983; 7:317–332

Copeland J: What is a "case"? A case for what?, in What Is a Case? The Problem of Definition in Psychiatric Community Surveys. Edited by Wing JK, Bebbington P, Robins LN. London, Grant McIntyre, 1981

Essen-Möller E, Larsson H, Uddenberg CE, et al: Individual traits and morbidity in a Swedish rural population. Acta Psychiatr Neurol Scand [Suppl] 1956; 100

Farris RE, Dunham HW: Mental Disorders in Urban Areas. Chicago, University of Chicago Press, 1939

Folks DG, Ford CV: Psychiatric disorders in geriatric medical/surgical patients. South Med J 1985; 78:239–241

Folstein MF, Breitner JCS: Language disorder predicts familial Alzheimer's disease. Johns Hopkins Medical Journal 1981; 149:145–147

Folstein MF, Folstein SE, McHugh PR: "Mini-Mental State": a practical method for grading the cognitive state of patients for the clinician. J Psychiatr Res 1975; 12:189–198

Folstein M, Anthony JC, Parhad I, et al: The meaning of cognitive impairment in the elderly. J Am Geriatr Soc 1985; 33:228–235

George LK, Hughes DC, Blazer DG: Urban/rural differences in the prevalence of anxiety disorders. American Journal of Social Psychiatry 1986; 6:249–258

German PS, Shapiro S, Skinner EA: Mental health of the elderly: use of health and mental health services. J Am Geriatr Soc 1985; 33:246–252

Goldfarb AI: Prevalence of psychiatric disorders in metropolitan old age and nursing homes. J Am Geriatr Soc 1962; 10:77–84

Goodwin DW, Guze SB: Psychiatric Diagnosis (Second Edition). New York, Oxford University Press, 1979

Goodwin JS, Goodwin JM, Garry PJ: Association between nutritional status and cognitive functioning in a healthy elderly population. JAMA 1983; 249:1917–1921

Gruenberg EM: Epidemiology of senile dementia, in Epidemiology of Aging. Edited by Haynes SG, Feinleib M. Washington, DC, U.S. Department of Health and Human Services, 1980

Haas AP, Hendin H: Suicide among older people: projections for the future. Suicide Life Threat Behav 1983; 13:147–154

Heston LL, Mastri AR, Anderson E, et al: Dementia of the Alzheimer's type: clinical genetics, natural history, and associated conditions. Arch Gen Psychiatry 1981; 38:1085–1090

Heyman A, Wilkinson WE, Hurwitz BJ, et al: Alzheimer's disease: genetic aspects and associated clinical disorders. Ann Neurol 1983; 14:507–515

Hillard JR, Holland JM, Ramm D: Christmas and psychopathology: data from a psychiatric emergency room population. Arch Gen Psychiatry 1981; 38:377–381

Huntley J, Brock DB, Ostfeld AM, et al: Established Populations for Epidemiologic Studies of the Elderly: Resource Data Book (NIH Publication No. 86-2443). Washington, DC, National Institute on Aging, 1986

Kay DWK, Beamish P, Roth M: Old age mental disorders in Newcastle upon Tyne: I. A study of prevalence. Br J Psychiatry 1964; 110:146–158

Kay DWK, Bergmann K, Foster EM, et al: Mental illness and hospital usage in the elderly: a random sample followed up. Compr Psychiatry 1970; 11:26–35

Klerman GL, Lavori PW, Rice J, et al: Birth-cohort trends in rates of major depression among relatives of patients with affective disorder. Arch Gen Psychiatry 1985; 42:689–694

Lester D: Temporal variation in suicide and homicide. Am J Epidemiol 1979; 109:517–520

Lowenthal MF, Berkman PL: Aging and Mental Disorders in San Francisco: A Social Psychiatric Study. San Francisco, Jossey-Bass, 1967

MacMahon B, Pugh TF: Epidemiology: Principles and Methods. Boston, Little, Brown, 1970

Mellinger GD, Balter MB, Manheimer DI, et al: Psychic distress, life crisis, and use of psychotherapeutic medications: national household survey data. Arch Gen Psychiatry 1978; 35:1045–1052

Morris JN: Uses of Epidemiology (Third Edition). Edinburgh, Churchill Livingstone, 1975

Murphy E. Lindesay J, Grundy E: Sixty years of suicide in England and Wales. Arch Gen Psychiatry 1986; 43:969–977

Murphy GE, Wetzel RD: Suicide risk by birth cohort in the United States, 1949 to 1974. Arch Gen Psychiatry 1980; 37:519–523

Murrell SA, Himmelfarb S, Wright K: Prevalence of depression and its correlates in older adults. Am J Epidemiol 1983; 117:173–185

Myers JK, Weissman MM, Tischler GL, et al: Six-month prevalence of psychiatric disorders in three communities. Arch Gen Psychiatry 1984; 41:959–969

New York State Department of Mental Hygiene, Mental Health Research Unit: Mental Health Survey of Older People. Utica, NY, State Hospital Press, 1960

Parker DA, Parker ES, Brody JA, et al: Alcohol use and cognitive loss among employed men and women. Am J Public Health 1983; 73:521–526

Pasamanick B, Roberts DW, Lemkau PW, et al: A survey of mental disease in an urban population: prevalence by race and income, in Epidemiology of Mental Disorder. Edited by Pasamanick B. Washington, DC, American Association for the Advancement of Science, 1959

Persson G: Prevalence of mental disorders in a 70-year-old urban population. Acta Psychiatr Scand 1980; 62:119–139

Pfeiffer E: A Short Portable Mental Status Questionnaire for the assessment of organic brain deficit in elderly patients. J Am Geriatr Soc 1975; 23:433–441

Pifer A, Bronte DL: Introduction: squaring the pyramid. Daedalus 1986; 115(1):1–12

Platt R: Wisdom is not enough: reflections on the art and science of medicine. Lancet 1952; 2:977–980

Radloff LS: The CES-D scale: a self-report depression scale for research in the general population. Applied Psychological Measurement 1977; 1:385–401

Ray WA, Federspiel CF, Schaffner W: The study of antipsychotic drug use in nursing homes: epidemiologic evidence suggesting misuse. Am J Public Health 1980; 70:485–491

Roberts CJ: Epidemiology for Clinicians. London, Pitman Medical Publishing, 1977

Robins LN, Helzer JE, Croughan J, et al: The National Institute of Mental Health Diagnostic Interview Schedule: its history, characteristics, and validity. Arch Gen Psychiatry 1981; 38:381–389

Robins LN, Helzer JE, Weissman MM, et al: Lifetime prevalence of specific psychiatric disorders in three sites. Arch Gen Psychiatry 1984; 41:949–958

Rosch E: Principles of categorization, in Cognition and Categorization. Edited by Rosch E, Lloyd BB. Hillsdale, NJ, Erlbaum, 1978

Rosenwaike I: A demographic portrait of the oldest old. Milbank Mem Fund Q 1985; 63:187–205

Rossiter LF: Prescribed medicines: findings from the National Medical Care Expenditure Survey. Am J Public Health 1983; 73:1312–1315

Rovner BW, Kafonek S, Fillipp L, et al: Prevalence of mental illness in a community nursing home. Am J Psychiatry 1986; 143:1446–1449

Shapiro S, Skinner EA, Kessler LG, et al: Utilization of health and mental health services. Arch Gen Psychiatry 1984; 41:971–982

Siegel JS, Taeuber CM: Demographic perspectives on the long-lived society. Daedalus 1986; 115(1):77–117

Spitzer RL, Endicott J: Schedule for Affective Disorders and Schizophrenia—Life-Time Version. New York, New York State Department of Mental Hygiene, Biometrics Research, 1978

Srole L, Fischer AK: The Midtown Manhattan Longitudinal Study vs. "The Mental Paradisde Lost" doctrine. Arch Gen Psychiatry 1981; 37:209–221

Strauss JS, Gabriel KR, Kokes R et al: Do psychiatric patients fit their diagnoses? Patterns of symptomatology as described with a biplot. J Nerv Ment Dis 1979; 167:105–113

Swartz M. Blazer D, Woodbury M, et al: Somatization disorder in a U.S. southern community: use of a new procedure for analysis of medical classification . Psychol Med 1986; 16:595–609

Teeter RB, Garetz FK, Miller WR, et al: Psychiatric disturbances of aged patients in skilled nursing homes. Am J Psychiatry 1976; 133:1430–1434

Warheit GJ, Hodzer CE, Schwart JJ: An analysis of social class and racial differences in depressive symptomatology: a community study. J Health Soc Behav 1973; 14:291–299

Weinstein MC, Feinberg HV: Clinical Decision Analysis. Philadelphia, W.B. Saunders, 1980

Weissman MM, Klerman GL: Epidemiology of mental disorders. Arch Gen Psychiatry 1978; 25:705–715

Wing JK: Patients with psychiatric disorders, in Community Mental Health: An International Perspective. Edited by Williams RN, Ozarin LD. San Francisco, Jossey-Bass, 1968

Wing JK, Cooper JE, Sartorius N: The Description and Classification of Psychiatric Symptoms: An Instruction Manual for the PSE nad CATEGO system. London, Cambridge University Press, 1974

The Diagnostic Workup in Late Life

Chapter 10

The Psychiatric Interview
of the Geriatric Patient

Dan G. Blazer, M.D., Ph.D.

The foundation of the diagnostic workup of the older adult suffering from a psychiatric disorder is the diagnostic interview. Unfortunately, in this age of increasing technology in the laboratory and standardization of interview techniques, the art of the clinical interview has suffered. The core of the psychiatric interview will be reviewed in this chapter, including history taking, assessment of the family, and the mental status examination. To supplement the clinical interview, structured interview schedules and rating scales of value in the assessment of older adults are described as well. Finally, techniques for communicating effectively with older adults are outlined.

History

The elements of a diagnostic workup of the elderly patient are presented in Table 1. To obtain historical information, the older adult should first be interviewed (if feasible). Then permission can be asked of the patient to interview family members. If available, family members from at least two generations can expand the perspective of the older adult's impairment. If the patient has difficulty providing an accurate or understandable history, the clinician should concentrate especially on eliciting those symptoms or problems perceived as being most disabling by the older adult and fill the historical gap with data from the family.

The *Diagnostic and Statistical Manual of Mental Disorders (Third Edition-Revised) (DSM-III-R)* (American Psychiatric Association 1987) has provided the clinician with a useful catalogue of symptoms and behaviors of

Table 1.   Psychiatric Interview of the Geriatric Patient

History

- Symptoms
- Present episode, including onset, duration, and change in symptoms over time
- Past history of medical and psychiatric disorders
- Family history of depression, alcohol abuse/dependence, psychoses, and suicide

Physical Examination

- Evaluation of neurologic deficits, possible endocrine disorders, occult malignancy, cardiac dysfunction, and occult infections

Mental Status Examination

- Disturbance of consciousness
- Disturbance of mood and affect
- Disturbance of motor behavior
- Disturbance of perception (hallucinations, illusions)
- Disturbance of cognition (delusions)
- Disturbance of self-esteem and guilt
- Suicidal ideation
- Disturbance of memory and intellience (memory, abstraction, calculation, aphasia, and knowledge)

---

psychiatric interest. Symptoms are bits of data, the most visible part of the clinical picture and generally the part that is most easily agreed on among different clinicians. Given that clinicians obtain equivalent information, symptoms should be defined such that minimal disagreement arises as to the presence or absence of a symptom. The decision as to whether those symptoms form a syndrome or derive from a particular etiology must be determined independently of obtaining symptomatic data.

Even so, clinicians may suffer bias when communicating with the older adult regarding psychiatric symptoms. As recognized by many insightful clinicians, such as Eisenberg (1977), physicians diagnose and treat diseases, that is, abnormalities in the structure and function of body organs and systems. Patients suffer illnesses—experiences of disvalued changes in states of being and in social function. Disease and illness do not maintain a one-to-one relationship. Factors that determine who becomes a patient and who does not can only be understood by expanding horizons beyond symptoms. In other words, patienthood is a social state (Eisenberg and Kleinman 1981). During the process of becoming a patient, the older adult, usually with the advice of others, forms a self-diagnosis of his or her problem and a judgment is made regarding the degree of ill-being. Since there are few uniform, satisfactory definitions of illness (or ill-being), definitions of well-being or wellness mean different things to different people. To some, illness is perceived when a specific discomfort is experienced. To others, illness re-flects a general perception of physical or social alienation and despair. The historical background and the values of the older adult within a social class and culture contribute to the formation of constructs regarding the nature of the problem, the cause, and the possibility for recovery.

For this reason, the clinician must take care to avoid accepting the patient's explanation for a given problem or set of problems. Statements such as "I guess I'm just getting old and there's nothing really to worry about" or "Most people slow down when they get to be my age" can lull the clinician into complacency in the face of a treatable psychiatric disorder (if they do not depress the clinician). On the other hand, the advent of new and disturbing symptoms in an older adult between each office visit can exhaust the clini-cian's patience to the point that adequate pursuit of the problem is derailed. For example, the hypochondriacal older adult who suffers from increased difficulty with awakenings during the night may insist that this symptom be treated with a sedative and plead with the clinician not to allow continual suffering. In the clinician's view, however, the symptom is a normal accompa-niment of old age and therefore should be accepted. Distress over a change in functioning, such as changes in sexual functioning, may overwhelm the elder and, especially if the clinician is perceived as unconcerned, precipitate self-medication or even a suicidal attempt.

To avoid biased attitudes when eliciting reports by the older adult (and therefore missing the symptoms and signs of a treatable psychiatric disorder), the initial interview with the older adult must include a review of the more important psychiatric symptoms in a relatively structured format. Common symptoms that should be reviewed include excessive weakness or lethargy, depressed mood or the blues, memory problems, difficulty concentrating, helplessness, hopelessness, uselessness, isolation, suspicion of others, anxiety and agitation, sleep problems, and appetite problems. Critical symptoms that should be reviewed include the presence or absence of suicidal thoughts, profound anhedonia, impulsive behavior, delusions and hallucinations, and confusion.

The review of symptoms is most valuable when it is considered within the context of symptom presentation. When did the symptom begin? How long has it lasted? Has its severity changed over time? Are there physical or environmental events that precipitate the symptom? What means, if any, have been taken to correct the symptom? Have any of these interventions proved successful? Do the symptoms vary during the day (diurnal varia-tion)? Do they vary during the week or with seasons of the year? Do the symptoms form clusters; that is, are they associated with one another? Which symptoms appear ego syntonic and which symptoms appear ego dystonic? As symptoms are reviewed, a window in time facilitates focus on the present illness. A 1-month or 6-month window enables the patient to review symptoms and events within time, an approach not usually taken by the distressed elder who concentrates on immediate sufferings.

Next, the clinician must review the past history of symptoms and episodes. The patient should be asked if he or she has suffered from a similar episode in the past. How long did the episode(s) last? When did it (they) occur? How many times in the patient's lifetime has such an episode occurred? Unfortunately, the older adult may not equate present distress with past episodes that symptomatically are similar. The perspective of the family is especially valuable when linking current and past episodes. Other psychiatric and medical problems should be reviewed as well, especially medical illnesses that have led to hospitalization and the use of medication. Not infrequently, the older adult experienced a major illness or trauma in childhood or as a younger adult, but this information is viewed as of no relevance to the present episode and is dismissed by the older adult. Probes to elicit these data are essential. Older adults do not spontaneously connect their present distress with past problems. They may ignore or even forget past psychiatric difficulties, especially if these difficulties were disguised. For example, mood swings in early or middle life may have been covered by periods of excessive and productive activity, episodes of excessive alcohol intake, or vague, undiagnosed physical problems. Periods of overt disability in usual activities may flag those previous episodes. Elders sometimes become angry or irritated when the clinician continues to probe. Reassurance regarding the importance of obtaining this information will generally suffice, except for that patient who cannot tolerate the discomfort and distress, even for brief periods. Elders suffering chronic and moderately severe anxiety who have a hysterical personality style, as well as the distressed Alzheimer's patient, tolerate their symptoms poorly.

Next, the distribution of psychiatric symptoms and illnesses within the family should be determined. The older person who suffers from symptoms consistent with senile dementia or primary degenerative dementia has a high probability of a family history of dementia. The genogram remains one of the best means for evaluating the distribution of mental illness and other relevant behaviors through the family tree. This genogram should include both parents, blood-related aunts and uncles, brothers and sisters, spouse(s), children, grandchildren, and great-grandchildren. A history should be obtained of institutionalization, significant memory problems in family members, hospitalization for a nervous breakdown or depressive disorder, suicide, alcohol abuse and dependence, use of electroconvulsive therapy, long-term residence in a mental health facility (and possibly a diagnosis of schizophrenia), and mental health services use by family members (Blazer 1984). Of relevance to the pharmacologic treatment of certain disorders in older adults (especially depression) is the tendency of individuals within a family to respond therapeutically to the same pharmacologic agent. If the older adult suffers from a depressive disorder and other family members (biological relatives) have been treated effectively for depression, the clinician should determine what pharmacologic agent was used to treat the depression. A positive response to nortriptyline in a family member of the depressed elder could render nortriptyline the drug of choice in treating that depressed elder, if side effects are not at issue (Ayd 1975).

Mendlewicz et al. (1975) remind us that accurate genetic information can be better obtained when family members from more than one generation are interviewed. Many psychiatric disorders present with a variety of symptoms, and therefore asking the patient or one family member for a history of depression would be insufficient. Research of the genetic expression of psychiatric disorders in families requires the investigator to interview directly as many family members as possible to obtain a true determination of case distribution through the family. Such detailed family assessment is not feasible for clinicians, yet a telephone call to more than one affected relative may become a standard of clinical assessment as the genetics of psychiatric disorders are clarified.

Psychiatric disorders occur within a biomedical and psychosocial context. The clinician naturally will determine what medical problems the patient has suffered, but could ignore a variation in the relative contribution of these medical disorders to psychopathology. The psychosocial contribution to the onset and continuance of the problem is just as likely to be overlooked. Has the spouse of the older adult undergone a change? Are the middle-aged children managing stress, such as the stress of caring for a disabled parent and financing their children through college simultaneously? Are the grandchildren placing emotional stress on the elderly patient and family because of adjustment problems in adolescence and young adulthood? Has the economic status of the older adult deteriorated? Has the availability of medical care changed? Though many psychiatric disorders are biologically driven, they do not occur in a psychosocial vacuum. Environmental precipitants remain important in the web of causation leading to the onset of an episode of emotional distress.

Next, it is essential to evaluate the medication history of the older adult. Most elders take a variety of medicines simultaneously, and the potential for drug–drug interaction is high. Some medications prescribed for older persons can exacerbate or produce depressive symptoms, such as propranolol (a ß blocker) or antihypertensive agents (such as alphamethyldopa). Antianxiety agents and sedative hypnotics can precipitate episodes of confusion and depression. Antidepressant agents, such as the tricyclics, may adversely interact with other drugs, such as clonidine. Simultaneous administration of clonidine and a tricyclic may lead to poorly controlled episodes of hypertension with confusional episodes and possibly an exacerbation of a multi-infarct dementia. The physician, a nurse, a social worker, or a paraprofessional should carefully determine present and past medication use via a historical inventory and a review of medicine containers brought to the office.

Family Assessment

Clinicians working with older adults must be equipped to evaluate the dysfunctional family. Just as an elevated white blood cell count is not pathognomonic of a particular infectious agent and yet is critical to the diagnosis, the complaint that "my family no longer loves me" does not reveal the specific problems within the family but does highlight the necessity to assess the potential of that family to provide care and support for the older adult (Blazer 1984). The nature of the family structure in interaction, the presence or absence of a crisis within the family, and the type and amount of support available to the older adult are the basic goals of a comprehensive diagnostic family workup.

The genogram detailing the distribution of illnesses across a family has already been described. A family-tree review for roles of individuals in the family and the availability of members to provide care to the older adult is equally important. For clinical purposes, the family consists not only of individuals genetically related but also of those who have developed relationships and are living together as if they were related (Miller and Miller 1979). Many older adults will have close relationships with friends, especially if a spouse dies, that are virtually familial. Garetz (1979) has described certain roles filled by family members when the older adult suffers from a mental or physical illness. These roles are helpful in evaluating and planning individual and family intervention. Modified somewhat (Blazer and Kaplan 1983), they include the following:

1. *Facilitator*—that individual in the family who resists medical or psychiatric treatment in order to maintain the stability achieved within a family secondary to the dysfunction in the older adult. This family member can present obstacles to therapeutic intervention though he or she may believe that he or she is helpful. Children wishing to obtain financial control of a family business for a parent may facilitate organic brain dysfunction.
2. *Victim*—the individual(s) in a family who perceive(s) the disorder of the older adult as a threat to self. The victim is usually in frequent contact with the disabled elder and therefore is in frequent contact with the clinician. The clinician may be criticized by the victim because of the burden of the illness. A sibling, forced for economic reasons to care for a disabled and demanding elder, will often in turn place demands on the clinician.
3. *Manager*—that family member who takes charge of a family during a crisis. He or she is usually calm, may be overly intellectual, and tends to organize and orchestrate family activities, often from a distance. The manager can be most helpful to the clinician in arranging tangible supports but is less able to provide the emotional support to the older adult or family members suffering as a result of a psychiatric disorder.

4. *Caretaker*—family member or members who nurture the disabled older adult. Such persons may provide inexhaustible help to a severely disordered elder, sometimes maintaining an older adult in the home far beyond the point at which institutionalization is indicated, such as in advanced primary degenerative dementia. Often avoiding opportunities for respite, caretakers may wear themselves to exhaustion and have few meaningful activities beyond caretaking. If the older adult dies, these individuals often suffer a tremendous void that may manifest itself in a severe and prolonged grief reaction.

5. *Escapee*—a family member who may withdraw from usual interactions within the family and who is therefore blamed for not demonstrating care and concern for the older person. A child frequently fills the role of escapee, especially if he or she has moved a good distance from the family. The escapee may become involved in altruistic endeavors, such as religious or civic activity locally, or may become devoted to his or her own nuclear family and therefore have little if any time and energy for the impaired elder. Families faced with the prospect of caring for a previously independent parent are often fraught with conflict and use the escapee to diffuse tensions within. In turn, the escapee may function well outside the family and therefore resist being drawn back into the stressed and conflicted family, despite a desire to be of help to the older adult.

6. *The identified patient*—the older person with the problem that is perceived to precipitate a family crisis. The identified patient may suffer only minimal problems and be content with his or her current state, yet provides an admission pass for the entire family to seek help from the clinician. The needs and problems of the older adult may quickly be set aside as family conflicts emerge during the diagnostic interview.

A primary goal of the clinician, as advocate for the psychiatrically disordered older adult, is to facilitate family support for the elder during a time of disability. At least four parameters of support are important for the clinician to evaluate as the treatment plan evolves. These include (1) availability of family members to the older person over time, (2) the tangible services provided by the family to the disordered elder, (3) the perception of family support by the older adult (and subsequently the willingness of the older adult to cooperate and accept support), and (4) tolerance by the family for specific behaviors that derive from the psychiatric disorder.

The clinician should ask the older person, "If you become ill, is there a family member to take care of you for a short period of time?" Next, the availability of family members to care for the older adult over an extended period of time can be determined. If a particular member is designated the primary caretaker, plans for respite should be discussed. Given the increased focus on short hospital stays and documented levels of greater impairment on discharge, the availability of family members becomes essential to the effective care of the older adult following hospitalization for a psychiatric, or combined medical and psychiatric, disorder.

What specific tangible services can be provided to the older adult by family members? Even the most devoted spouse is limited in the delivery of certain services because he or she may not drive (and therefore cannot provide transportation) or is not physically strong enough to provide certain types of nursing care. Generic services of special importance in the support of the psychiatrically impaired older adult at home include transportation; nursing services (such as administering medications at home); physical therapy; checking services or continual supervision; homemaker and household services; meal preparation; administrative, legal, and protective services; financial assistance; living quarters; and coordination of the delivery of services. These services have been termed "generic" because they can be defined in terms of their activities regardless of who provides the service. Assessing the range and extent of service delivery by the family to the functionally impaired elder provides a convenient barometer of the economic, social, and emotional burdens of the geropsychiatric patient on the family.

Regardless of the level of service provided by the family to the older person, for these services to be effective it is beneficial for the older person to perceive that he or she lives in a supportive environment. These intangible supports include the perception of a dependable network, participation or interaction in the network, a sense of belonging to the network, intimacy with network members, and a sense of usefulness to the family (Blazer and Kaplan 1983). Usefulness may be of less importance to some older adults in that they believe they have contributed to the family for many years and therefore deserve reciprocal service delivery in their waning years. Unfortunately, family members, frequently stressed across generations, may not recognize this reciprocal responsibility.

Family tolerance of specific behaviors may not correlate with overall support. Every person has a level of tolerance for specific behaviors that are especially difficult. Sanford (1975) found that the following behaviors were tolerated in decreasing frequency by families of impaired elders: incontinence of urine (81 percent), personality conflicts (54 percent), falls (52 percent), physically aggressive behavior (44 percent), inability to walk unaided (33 percent), daytime wandering (33 percent), and sleep disturbance (16 percent). This frequency may appear counterintuitive, for incontinence is generally considered particularly aversive to family members. Yet the outcome of incontinence can be corrected easily enough. A few nights of no sleep, however, can easily extend family members beyond their capabilities of serving a parent, sibling, or spouse.

The Mental Status Examination

Physicians and other clinicians are at times hesitant to perform a structured mental status examination, fearing the effort will insult or irritate the patient.

Perhaps the exam is also viewed as an unnecessary waste of time. Nevertheless, the mental status examination of the psychiatric patient in later life is central to the diagnostic workup (Blazer 1982). Mood and affect can usually be assessed by observing the patient during the interview. Affect is the feeling tone, pleasurable or unpleasurable, that accompanies the patient's cognitive output (Linn 1980). Affect may fluctuate during the interview; however, the older person is more likely to demonstrate a constriction of affect. Mood, the state that underlies overt affect and is sustained over time is usually apparent by the completion of the interview. For example, the affect of a depressed older adult may not reach the degree of dysphoria seen in younger persons (as evidenced by crying spells or protestations of uncontrollable despair), yet the depressed mood is usually sustained and discernible from beginning to end.

Psychomotor retardation or underactivity is characteristic of major depression and severe schizophreniform symptomatology and some variants of primary degenerative dementia. Psychiatrically impaired elders (except in some more advanced cases of dementia) are more likely to exhibit hyperactivity or agitation. The depressed will appear uneasy, move their hands frequently, and have difficulty remaining seated through the interview. The mild to moderately demented patients, especially those suffering from multi-infarct dementia, are easily distracted, arise from a seated position, and walk around the room or even out of the room. Pacing is often observed when the older adult is admitted to a hospital ward. Agitation can usually be distinguished from anxiety, for the individual does not complain of a sense of impending doom or dread. Movement generally relieves the immediate discomfort yet does not correct the underlying disturbance in psychomotor dysfunction. Occasionally, the motorically retarded older adult may in fact be suffering from a disturbance in consciousness, having reached an almost stuporous state. He or she may not be easily aroused, but when aroused, responds by grimacing or withdrawal.

Perception is the awareness of objects in relations that follow stimulation of peripheral sense organs (Linn 1980). Disturbances of perception include hallucinations—false sensory perceptions not associated with real or external stimuli. For example, the paranoid older adult may perceive invasion of her house at nighttime by individuals who disrupt her belongings and abuse her sexually. Hallucinations may often take the form of false auditory perceptions, false perceptions of movement or body sensation (such as palpitations), and false perceptions of smell, taste, and touch. The severely depressed elder may suffer from frank auditory hallucinations that condemn or encourage self-destructive behavior.

Disturbances in thought content are the most common disturbances of cognition noted in the psychiatrically impaired elder. The depressed patient often develops beliefs that are inconsistent with the objective information obtained from family members about the patient's abilities and social resources. In a series of recent studies, Meyers et al (1985) have found delusional depression to be more prevalent among older depressed patients. Forty-five percent of 161 patients with Research Diagnostic Criteria (RDC) (Spitzer et al. 1978a) for endogenous depression were found to be delusional. These delusions include beliefs such as "I've lost my mind," "My body is deteriorating," "I have an incurable illness," or "I have caused some great harm." Even after elders recover from the depression, they may still experience periodic recurrences of delusional thoughts, which can be most disturbing to an otherwise rational older adult. Elders appear less likely to suffer from delusions of self-remorse, guilt, or persecution.

Even if delusions are not obvious, preoccupation with a particular thought or idea is common among the depressed elderly. Such preoccupation is closely associated with obsessional thinking or irresistible intrusion of thoughts into the conscious mind. Though the older adult rarely acts on these thoughts compulsively, the guilt-provoking or self-accusing thoughts may occasionally become so difficult that the older adult will seek to take his or her own life.

Evaluation of the content and process of cognition may uncover disturbances such as problems with structure of associations, the speed of associations, and the content of thought. Thinking is a goal-directed flow of ideas, symbols, and associations initiated in response to environmental stimuli, a perceived problem, or a task that requires progression to a logical or reality-based conclusion (Linn 1980). The compulsive or schizophrenic older adult may pathologically repeat the same word or idea in response to a variety of probes, as may the patient suffering with primary degenerative dementia. Some demented older adults exhibit circumstantiality or the introduction of many apparently irrelevant details to cover a lack of clarity and memory problems. Such interviews can be most frustrating because they proceed at such a slow pace. On other occasions, elders appear incoherent, with no logical connection to their thought, or irrelevant answers are produced. The intrusion of thoughts from previous conversations into current conversation is a prime example of the disturbance in association found in primary degenerative dementia (e.g., Alzheimer's disease). This symptom is not typical of other dementias, such as the dementia of Huntington's disease. Even paranoid older adults, however, in the absence of dementia, generally do not demonstrate a significant disturbance in the structure of associations.

Although thoughts of death are common in late life, spontaneous revelations of suicidal thoughts are rare. A stepwise probe is the best means of assessing the presence of suicidal ideation (Blazer 1982). First, the clinician should ask the patient if he or she has ever thought life not worth living. If so, has the patient considered acting on that thought? If so, how would the patient attempt to inflict such harm? When definite plans are revealed, the clinician should probe to determine if the implements for a suicide attempt are available. For example, if the patient has considered shooting himself, the clinician should ask, "Do you have a gun available and loaded at home?" Suicidal ideation in an older adult is always of concern, but intervention is necessary when suicide has been considered seriously and the implements are available.

Although older adults may not complain of memory problems, they are more likely to suffer problems with memory, concentration, and intellect. Formal testing of cognitive status, as described below, is usually indicated. Yet there are brief, informal means of testing cognitive functioning that should be included in the diagnostic workup. As the clinician proceeds through an evaluation of memory and intellect, it must be remembered that poor performance may reflect psychic distress or a lack of education as opposed to mental retardation or dementia. In order to rule out the potential confounding of agitation and anxiety, testing can be performed on more than one occasion.

Testing of memory is based on three essential processes: (1) registration (the ability to record an experience in the central nervous system), (2) retention (the persistence and permanence of a registered experience), and (3) recall (the ability to summon consciously the registered experience and report it) (Linn 1980). Registration, apart from recall, is difficult to evaluate directly. Occasionally, events or information that the older adult denies remembering will appear spontaneously during other parts of the interview. Otherwise, techniques such as hypnosis, narcoanalysis, and psychoanalysis are the usual means of determining if registration has occurred. Registration usually is not impaired, except in the more severe dementing illnesses.

Retention, on the other hand, can be blocked by both psychic distress and brain dysfunction. Lack of retention is especially relevant to the unimportant data often asked for on a mental status examination. For example, requesting the older adult to remember three objects for 5 minutes will frequently reveal a deficit if the older adult has little motivation to attempt the task. Disturbances of recall can be tested directly in a number of ways. The most common are tests of orientation to time, place, person, and situation. Most persons continually orient themselves via radio, television, and reading material as well as conversing with others. Some elders may be isolated through sensory impairment or social isolation, and therefore poor orientation would represent more the physical and social environment as opposed to brain dysfunction.

Immediate recall can be tested by asking the elder to repeat a word, phrase, or series of numbers, but may also be tested in conjunction with cognitive skills by requesting a word to be spelled backwards or elements of a story to be recalled.

During the mental status examination, intelligence can be assessed only superficially. Tests of simple arithmetic calculation and fund of knowledge, supplemented by portions of well-known psychiatric tests, are helpful. A capacity for abstract thinking is often tested by asking the patient to interpret a well-known proverb, such as "A rolling stone gathers no moss." A more accurate test of abstraction, however, is the request to classify objects into a common category. For example, the elder is asked to inform as to the similarity between an apple and a pear. Whereas naming objects from a category (such as fruits) is retained despite moderate and sometimes marked declines in cognition, the opposite process of classifying two different objects into a common category is not as well retained. The classic test for calculation is to ask a patient to subtract 7 from 100 and to repeat this operation. Usually five calculations are sufficient to determine the ability of the older adult to complete this task. If this task is failed by the elder, a less exacting test is to request the patient to subtract 3 from 20 and to repeat this operation until 0 is reached. These examinations must not be rushed, for elders may not perform as well when they perceive a pressure in time.

Rating Scales and Standardized Interviews

Rating scales and standardized or structured interviews have progressively been incorporated into the diagnostic assessment of the psychiatric patient. Such rating procedures have increased in popularity in parallel with the need for systematic, reproducible diagnoses for third-party carriers (part of the impetus for the dramatic change in nomenclature evidenced in *DSM-III-R*) as well as a standard assessment of change in clinical status. A thorough review of all instruments that are used is not possible. Therefore, selected instruments are presented and evaluated in this section that either have special relevance to the geriatric patient or have been widely used.

Cognitive Dysfunction and Dementia Schedules

Two interviewer-administered cognitive screens have been popular in both clinical and community studies. The first is the Short Portable Mental Status Questionnaire (SPMSQ), a derivative of the Mental Status Questionnaire developed by Kahn and Goldfarb in 1960 (Pfeiffer 1975; Kahn et al. 1960). The SPMSQ consists of 10 questions assessing orientation, memory, fund of knowledge, and calculation. For most older adults in the community, two or fewer errors indicate intact functioning; three or four errors represent mild impairment; five to seven errors represent moderate impairment; and eight or more errors, severe impairment. The ease of administration and the epidemiologic data that have been accumulated using this instrument render it useful for both clinical and community screens. The Mini-Mental State Examination (Folstein et al. 1975) is a 30-item instrument that assesses orientation, registration, attention and calculation, recall, and language. It requires 5 to 10 minutes to administer and includes more items of clinical significance than does the SPMSQ. Seven to 12 errors suggest mild to moderate cognitive impairment; 13 or more errors, severe impairment.

A number of clinical assessment procedures for dementia have emerged in recent years. The most widely used and one of the first to appear is the scale suggested by Blessed et al. (1968), usually called the Blessed Dementia Scale. In contrast to the screening scales, clinical judgment is required to assess changes in performance of everyday activities (such as handling money, household tasks, and shopping); changes in eating and dressing habits; changes in personality, interests, and drive; tests of information (orientation and recognition of persons); memory (memory of past information such as occupation, place of birth, and town where the individual worked); and concentration (calculation task). A score is assigned to each of these tasks and a summary score is tabulated. The score has correlated well with the cerebral changes of primary degenerative dementia.

A dementia scale for assessing the probability that the dementia is secondary to multiple infarcts is that suggested by Hachinski et al. (1975). In a study of cerebral blood flow in primary degenerative dementia compared with multi-infarct dementia, certain clinical features were determined to be more associated with a multi-infarct dementia, and each assigned a score. These items, along with their scores, are as follows: abrupt onset = 2, stepwise deterioration = 1, fluctuating course = 2, nocturnal confusion = 1, relative preservation of personality = 1, depression = 1, somatic complaints = 1, emotional incontinence = 1, history of hypertension = 1, history of strokes = 2, evidence of associated atheroscleosis = 1, focal neurologic symptoms = 2, and focal neurologic signs = 2. A score of 7 or greater was highly suggestive of multi-infarct dementia. Given the frequent overlap of multiple small infarcts and primary degenerative dementia and the difficulty of assessing these items effectively, most investigators have ceased to rely on the Hachinski scale clinically.

Depression Schedules

A number of self-rating depression scales have been used to screen for depression throughout the life cycle, most of which have been studied in older populations. The Zung Self-Rating Depression Scale (Zung 1965) is probably the most widely use, at least until recent years. The initial popularity of the Zung scale was probably due to the availability of data for persons throughout the life cycle, especially the elderly (Zung 1967). Few randomly sampled community populations have been surveyed with the Zung Self-Rating Depression Scale, and therefore normative community standards are deficit. This 20-item scale, which ranks persons from 0 to 3 in terms of the severity of each of the 20 symptoms assessed, can be used by most older adults, though the four anchor points may create problems for some elders with mild cognitive impairment. Freedman et al. (1982) found peak symptom levels in 65- to 69-year-old females and 70- to 74-year-old males.

The most widely used of the current instruments in community studies is the Center for Epidemiologic Studies Depression Scale (CES-D) (Radloff 1977). This instrument, because of the normative population data, has replaced the Zung scale in recent years as a common instrument for screening depression. The scale is similar in format to the Zung scale. In a factor-analytic study of the CES-D in a community population, three factors were identified: an enervation factor, a positive affect factor, and an interpersonal relationship factor (Ross and Mirowsky 1984). The disaggregation of these factors and exploration of their interaction is a significant step forward in understanding the behavior of symptom scales like the CES-D in older populations. For example, are the enervation items truly associated with a course of depressive episodes similar to that described for major depression with melancholia, whereas the positive affect items are more associated with life satisfaction scores?

A scale widely used in clinical studies, but which has been less studied in community populations, is the Beck Depression Inventory (BDI) (Beck et al. 1961). The reliability of the BDI has been demonstrated to be good in both depressed and nondepressed older samples (Gallagher et al. 1982). The instrument consists of 21 symptoms and attitudes that are rated on a scale of 0 to 3 in terms of intensity. In another study by Gallagher et al. (1983), the BDI misclassified only 16.7 percent of subjects diagnosed as suffering from a major depression by RDC.

The Geriatric Depression Scale (GDS) was developed because of the problem the above scales present to older persons who had difficulty selecting one of four forced-response items (Yesavage et al. 1983). This 30-item scale permits patients to rate items as either present or absent and includes such symptoms as cognitive complaints, self-image, and losses. Items selected were thought to have relevance to late-life depression. The GDS has not been used in community populations and remains to be well standardized.

Another instrument, similar to the GDS, is the Carroll Rating Scale for Depression (Carroll et al. 1981). This instrument consists of 52 items scored either as "Yes" or "No" and which follow those areas assessed for the Hamilton Rating Scale for Depression (see below). Though not used extensively in older populations, the instrument has the same advantage as the GDS in being the forced-response type with yes/no answers.

Of the interviewer-rated scales, the Hamilton Rating Scale for Depression (Hamilton 1960) is by far the most commonly used. Though no formal normative data exist, the advantage of basing ratings on clinical judgment has rendered this scale popular to rate outcome in clinical trials. For example, a reduction in the Hamilton score to one-half the initial score or to below a certain value would indicate partial or complete recovery from an episode of depression. In one study of this scale in older adults, Hodern et al. (1963) found, for female depressed patients, that agitation, delayed insomnia, loss of weight, and depressed mood were more severe in the elderly compared with younger age groups.

A newer scale that is receiving considerable attention clinically, but which remains to be standardized in both clinical and community populations, is the Montgomery-Asberg Rating Scale for Depression (Montgomery and Asberg 1979). This scale follows the pattern of the Hamilton scale and concentrates on 10 symptoms of depression and calls for the clinician to rate each of these on a 0 to 6 scale (for a range of scores between 0 and 60). The symptoms include apparent sadness, reported sadness, inattention, reduced sleep, reduced appetite, concentration difficulties, lassitude, inability to feel, pessimistic thoughts, and suicidal thoughts. This scale theoretically is an improvement over the Hamilton scale in that it appears to differentiate better between responders and nonresponders to intervention for depression. The instrument does not include many somatic symptoms that tend to be more common in older adults, and therefore may be of greater value in tracking the core symptoms of depressive illness.

General Assessment Scales

A number of general assessment scales of psychiatric status (occasionally combined with functioning in other areas) have been found useful in both community and clinical populations.

One of the more frequently used scales is the Global Assessment Scale (Spitzer et al. 1978b). The rater makes, on the basis of clinical judgment, a single rating, ranging from 0 to 100, that best describes the lowest level of functioning in the week prior to the rating. The scale has not been standardized for older adults, but its common use in psychiatric studies suggests the need for standardization.

A similar scale is the Brief Psychiatric Rating Scale (BPRS) (Overall and Gorham 1962). In this scale, 16 relatively independent symptom areas, including somatic concern, anxiety, depressive mood, unusual thought content, and suspiciousness, are rated from "not present" to "extremely severe." A summary score is obtained. Symptom profiles on the BPRS have been shown to be different in older populations. Among older adults, depressive mood more often occurs in association with motor retardation, emotional withdrawal, and blunted affect, whereas depressive mood is usually accompanied by anxiety in younger patients (Beller and Overall 1984). In another study, Overall and Beller (1984) found five distinct phenomenologic types in a geriatric population: agitated dementia, retarded dementia, anxious depression, withdrawn depression, and paranoid psychosis.

Shader et al. (1974) developed an 18-symptom scale with each symptom rated along a 7-point scale, called the Sandoz Clinical Assessment–Geriatric. The scale has been shown to distinguish psychopathology in older persons, but the discrimination between subgroups of psychiatrically disordered older adults remains to be tested. This scale has not been used as frequently as other scales in recent years. The Geriatric Mental State Schedule (Copeland et al.

1976) is an adaptation of the Present State Examination (PSE) (Wing et al. 1974) and the Psychiatric Status Schedule (Spitzer et al. 1968), a semi-structured interviewing guide that inventories symptoms associated with psychiatric disorders. More than 500 ratings are made on the basis of information obtained by a highly trained interviewer who elicits symptoms from the month prior to the evaluation. Data are computerized in order to derive psychiatric diagnoses (Copeland et al. 1986). The instrument measures depression, impaired memory, selected neurologic symptoms (such as aphasia), and disorientation.

The Comprehensive Assessment and Referral Evaluation (CARE) is a hybridized assessment procedure developed for older adults that borrows items from a variety of sources (Gurland et al. 1977). Dimensional scores are obtained in memory–disorientation, depression–anxiety, immobility–incapacity, isolation, physical–perceptual difficulty, and poor housing–income. The goal of CARE is to provide a comprehensive assessment of the older adult that bridges the professional disciplines. The instrument has not been used extensively, though it has been used in cross-national studies. For example, Herbst and Humphrey (1980) used CARE in a study of hearing impairment in relation to mental status. The investigators found a relation between deafness and depression independent of age and socioeconomic status.

The Older Americans Resources and Services (1978; OARS) Multidimensional Functional Assessment Questionnaire is administered by a lay interviewer and obtains data in order to produce functional impairment ratings in five dimensions: mental health, physical health, social functioning, economic functioning, and activities of daily living. In one community survey (Blazer 1978a), 13 percent of persons in the community suffered from mental health impairment. The OARS instrument has been used widely in both community and clinical surveys and was developed in order to integrate functional measures across a series of parameters relevant to older adults. With the recent emphasis placed on discrete psychiatric disorders, however, the instrument has not been used as widely by mental health workers as might have occurred otherwise.

Any discussion of clinical rating scales should include the Abnormal Involuntary Movements Scale (AIMS) (National Institute of Mental Health 1975). Given the increased incidence of tardive dyskinesia among older adults, coupled with the need for better documentation for this dreaded outcome of prolonged prescription of antipsychotic agents, regular ratings on the AIMS by clinicians are becoming essential for the practice of inpatient and outpatient geriatric psychiatry. The scale consists of seven ratings of movement disorders, each of which is rated from "none" to "severe." Three items are devoted to a global judgment: severity of abnormal movements, incapacitation due to abnormal movements, and the patient's awareness of abnormal movements. Current problems with teeth or dentures are also assessed. Procedures are described to increase the reliability of this rating scale.

Structured Interviews

A number of structured interviews are now available for both clinical and community diagnosis. These interview schedules have increased the reliability of the identification of particular symptoms and psychiatric diagnoses. Unfortunately, the richness inherent in the unstructured interview tends to be lost if one adheres closely to the structured interview. Comments made by the patient during the evaluation that could trace relevant associations must be ignored in order to push through the interview schedule. Most of these interviews require more time than the traditional unstructured first session with the patient.

The oldest of the currently used interview schedules is the PSE (Wing et al. 1974). As noted above, the Geriatric Mental State Schedule is a variant of the PSE. The PSE is actually not an interview at all, but rather a list of definitions of behaviors or symptoms of psychiatric interest, ranging from specific delusions to general changes in affect. The clinician scores whether or not the symptom is present, and a computer algorithm provides a diagnosis. Suggested questions for eliciting the symptoms are available, but not obligatory. Only 54 questions are required during the interview, though many additional probes are provided to track positive responses. The interview schedule provides an excellent education for many psychiatrists in the meaning of various symptoms of relevance to working with older adults. Nevertheless, the focus on 1 month prior to the evaluation date and the association of the symptoms with the International Classification of Diseases classificatory system (as opposed to *DSM-III-R*) render the evaluation less popular with American investigators.

The most frequently used instrument in the United States is the Schedule for Affective Disorders and Schizophrenia (SADS) (Spitzer and Endicott 1975). This instrument is easily adaptable to the RDC and the *DSM-III-R*. Though specific questions are suggested for probing most areas of interest, the interviewer has the flexibility to ask additional questions and can use whatever data are available in order to assign a diagnosis. The interviewer must have clinical training but does not have to be a psychiatrist. Many of the symptoms may not be relevant to older adults (especially the extensive probes for psychotic symptoms), and the interview frequently takes 2½ to 3 hours to administer. Nevertheless, the experience gained by the clinician in using this instrument can be translated into a more effective clinical practice.

A recent addition to the schedules available is the Diagnostic Interview Schedule (DIS) (Robins et al. 1981). This highly structured interview, which can be administered by a lay interviewer and is computer scored, allows psychiatric diagnoses to be made according to *DSM-III-R* criteria, Feighner criteria (Feighner et al. 1972), and RDC. The DIS probes for the presence or absence of symptoms or behaviors relevant to a series of psychiatric disorders, the severity of these symptoms, and the putative cause of the symptoms. Diagnoses of cognitive impairment, schizophrenia or schizophreniform disorder, major depression, generalized anxiety, panic disorder, agoraphobia, obsessive–compulsive disorder, dysthymic disorder, somatization disorder, alcohol abuse and/or dependence, and drug abuse and/or dependence can be made from Axis I of *DSM-III-R*. Antisocial personality disorder from Axis II can also be made. The instrument has proved reasonably reliable in clinic populations for both current and lifetime diagnoses.

The range of disorders probed by the DIS, coupled with its relative ease of administration (it generally takes 45 to 90 minutes to administer to an older adult), has rendered it popular in clinical studies. In addition, community-based comparative data are available on a large sample from the Epidemiologic Catchment Area study (Regier et al. 1984; Myers et al. 1984). The instrument can be supplemented with additional questions to probe for specific symptoms (such as probing for melancholic symptoms and additional data regarding sleep disorders for depressed older adults). No problems have arisen when the instrument is used among older adults in the community. The memory decay that occurs in the elderly in general is no more a problem with this instrument than with other instruments. Nevertheless, the instrument is of less value in the study of institutional populations, because memory problems cannot be circumvented by clinical judgment. Supplementary data can be added to the instrument for developing a standardized diagnosis.

Communicating with the Older Patient

The clinician working with the older adult should be cognizant of those factors in both the patient and him- or herself that may produce barriers to effective communication (Blazer 1978b). Many older persons suffer from a relatively high level of anxiety yet do not complain of this symptom. Stress deriving from a new situation, such as visiting a clinician's office or being interviewed in a hospital, may intensify the anxiety and subsequently impair effective communication. Perceptual problems, such as hearing and visual impairment, may exacerbate disorientation and complicate the communication of problems to the clinician. The elderly are more likely to withhold information than to chance answers that may be incorrect. In other words, older persons tend to be more cautious. They frequently take longer to respond to inquiries and resist the clinician who attempts to rush through the historical interview.

The elderly patient may perceive the physician unrealistically, on the basis of previous experiences (i.e., transference). Though sometimes accepting the role of a child and viewing the physician as parent, the patient initially is more likely to view the clinician as the idealized child who can provide reciprocal care to the previously capable but now impaired parent. Splitting between the physician and children of the patient may subsequently occur. The clinician can perceive the older adult patient incorrectly because of preconceived fears of aging and death or previous negative experiences with his or her own parents. For a clinician to work effectively with older adults, these personal feelings should be discussed during training (and afterwards) in order to provide better patient care.

Once physician and patient attitudes are recognized, certain techniques have proved to be valuable, in general, in communicating with the elderly patient. These techniques should not be implemented indiscriminantly, however, for the variation among older adults is significant. First, the older person should be approached with respect. The clinician should knock before entering a patient's room and greet the patient by surname (Mr. Jones, Mrs. Smith) rather than by given names, unless he or she wishes to be addressed by a given name.

After taking a position near the older person, near enough to reach out and touch the patient, the clinician should speak clearly and slowly and use simple sentences. Because of hearing problems, older patients may understand conversation better over the telephone than in person. By placing the receiver against the mastoid bone, the patient can take advantage of preserved bone conduction in the presence of otosclerosis.

The interview should be paced so that the older person has time enough to respond to questions. Most elders are not uncomfortable with silence, because it gives them an opportunity to formulate their answers to questions and elaborate certain points they wish to emphasize. Nonverbal communication is frequently a key to effective communication with elders, for the older person may be reticent to reveal affect verbally. Changes in facial expression, gestures, postures, and long silences may clue the clinician to issues that are unspoken.

One key to successful communication with an older adult is a willingness to continue working with that person as a professional. Most elders do not require large segments of time from clinicians. Those who are more demanding can usually be controlled through structure in the interview. Yet older adults in the 1980s, possibly unlike their children and grandchildren, place much stress on loyalty and continuity.

References

American Psychiatric Association: Diagnostic and Statistical Manual of Mental Disorders (Third Edition-Revised). Washington, DC, American Psychiatric Association, 1987

Ayd FJ: Treatment-resistant patients: a moral, legal and therapeutic challenge, in Rational Psychopharmacotherapy and the Right to Treatment. Edited by Ayd FJ. Baltimore, Ayd Medical Communications, 1975

Beck AT, Ward CH, Mendelson M, et al: An inventory for measuring depression. Arch Gen Psychiatry 1961; 4:53–63

Beller SA, Overall JE: The Brief Psychiatric Rating Scale (BPRS) in geropsychiatric research: II. Representative profile patterns. J Gerontol 1984; 39:194–200

Blazer D: The OARS Durham surveys: description and application, in Multidimensional Functional Assessment: The OARS Methodology—A Manual (Second Edition). Durham, NC, Duke University Center for the Study of Aging and Human Development, 1978a

Blazer D: Techniques for communicating with your elderly patient. Geriatrics 1978b; 33(11):79–80, 83–84

Blazer DG: Depression in Late Life. St Louis, C.V. Mosby, 1982

Blazer DG: Evaluating the family of the elderly patient, in A Family Approach to Health Care in the Elderly. Edited by Blazer D, Siegler IC. Menlo Park, CA, Addison-Wesley, 1984

Blazer DG, Kaplan BH: The assessment of social support in an elderly community population. American Journal of Social Psychiatry 1983; 3:29–36

Blessed G, Tomlinson BE, Roth M: The association between quantitative measures of dementia and of senile change in the cerebral grey matter of elderly subjects. Br J Psychiatry 1968; 114:797–811

Carroll BJ, Feinberg M, Smouse PE, et al: The Carroll Rating Scale for Depression: I. Development, reliability and validation. Br J Psychiatry 1981; 138:194–200

Copeland JRM, Kelleher MJ, Kellet JM, et al: A semi-structured clinical interview for the assessment of diagnosis and mental state in the elderly: the Geriatric Mental State Schedule. Psychol Med 1976; 6:439–449

Copeland JRM, Dewey ME, Griffiths-Jones HM, et al: A computerized psychiatric diagnostic system and case nomenclature for elderly subjects: GMS and AGECAT. Psychol Med 1986; 16:89–99

Eisenberg L: Disease and illness: distinctions between professional and popular ideas of sickness. Cult Med Psychiatry 1977; 1:9–23

Eisenberg L, Kleinman A: Clinical social science, in The Relevance of Social Science for Medicine. Edited by Eisenberg L, Kleinman A. Boston, D. Reidel, 1981

Feighner JP, Robins E, Guze SB, et al: Diagnostic criteria for use in psychiatric research. Arch Gen Psychiatry 1972; 26:57–63

Folstein MF, Folstein SE, McHugh PR: "Mini-Mental State": a practical method for grading the cognitive state of patients for the clinician. J Psychiatr Res 1975; 12:189–198

Freedman N, Bucci W, Elkowitz E: Depression in a family practice elderly population. J Am Geriatr Soc 1982; 30:372–377

Gallagher D, Nies G, Thompson LW: Reliability of the Beck Depression Inventory with older adults. J Consult Clin Psychol 1982; 50:152–153

Gallagher D, Breckenridge J, Steinmetz J, et al: The Beck Depression Inventory and Research Diagnostic Criteria: congruence in an older population. J Consult Clin Psychol 1983; 51:945–946

Garetz FR: Responses of families to health problems in the elderly. Paper presented at the annual meeting of the American Geriatrics Society, New York, 1979

Gurland B, Kuriansky J, Sharpe L, et al: The Comprehensive Assessment and Referral Evaluation (CARE)—rationale, development and reliability. Int J Aging Hum Dev 1977; 8:9–42

Hachinski VC, Iliff LD, Zilhka E, et al: Cerebral blood flow in dementia. Arch Neurol 1975; 32:632–637

Hamilton M: A rating scale for depression. J Neurol Neurosurg Psychiaty 1960; 23:56–62

Herbst KG, Humphrey C: Hearing impairment and mental state in the elderly living at home. Br Med J 1980; 281:903–905

Hodern A, Holt NF, Burt CE, et al: Amitriptyline in depressive states: phenomenology and prognostic considerations. Br J Psychiatry 1963; 109:815–825

Kahn RL, Goldfarb AI, Pollack M, et al: Brief objective measures for the determination of mental status in the aged. Am J Psychiatry 1960; 117:326–328

Linn L: Clinical manifestations of psychiatric disorders, in Comprehensive Textbook of Psychiatry (Third Edition, Volume 1). Edited by Kaplan HI, Freedman AM, Sadock BJ. Baltimore, Williams & Wilkins, 1980

Mendlewicz J, Fleiss JL, Cataldo M, et al: Accuracy of the family history method in affective illness: comparison with direct interviews in family studies. Arch Gen Psychiatry 1975; 32:309–314

Meyers BS, Greenberg R: Late-life delusional depression. J Affective Disord 1986; 11:133–137

Meyers BS, Greenberg R, Varda M: Delusional depression in the elderly, in Treatment of Affective Disorders in the Elderly. Edited by Shamoian CA. Washington, DC, American Psychiatric Press, 1985

Miller KT, Miller JL: The family as a system. Paper presented at the annual meeting of the American College of Psychiatrists, New York, 1979

Montgomery SA, Asberg M: A new depression scale designed to be sensitive to change. Br J Psychiatry 1979; 134:382–389

Myers JK, Weissman MM, Tischler GL, et al: Six-month prevalence of psychiatric disorders in three communities: 1980 to 1982. Arch Gen Psychiatry 1984; 41:954–967

National Institute of Mental Health: Development of a Dyskinetic Movement Scale (Publication No. 4). Rockville, MD, National Institute of Mental Health, Psychopharmacology Research Branch, 1975

Older Amerians Resources and Services: Multidimensional Functional Assessment: The OARS Methodology—A Manual (Second Edition). Durham, NC, Duke University Center for the Study of Aging and Human Development, 1978

Overall JE, Beller SA: The Brief Psychiatric Rating Scale (BPRS) in geropsychiatric research: I. Factor structure on an inpatient unit. J Gerontol 1984; 39:187–193

Overall JE, Gorham DR: The Brief Psychiatric Rating Scale. Psychol Rep 1962; 10:799–812

Pfeiffer E: A Short Portable Mental Status Questionnaire for the assessment of organic brain deficit in elderly patients. J Am Geriatr Soc 1975; 23:433–441

Radloff LS: The CES-D Scale: a self-report depression scale for research in the general population. Applied Psychological Measurement 1977; 1:385–401

Regier DA, Myers JK, Kramer M, et al: The NIMH Epidemiologic Catchment Area program: historical context, major objectives, and study population characteristics. Arch Gen Psychiatry 1984; 41:934–941

Robins LN, Helzer JE, Croughan J, et al: National Institute of Mental Health Diagnostic Interview Schedule: its history, characteristics, and validity. Arch Gen Psychiatry 1981; 38:381–389

Ross CE, Mirowsky J: Components of depressed mood in married men and women: the CES-D. Am J Epidemiol 1984; 119:997–1004

Sanford JRA: Tolerance of debility in elderly dependents by supporters at home: its significance for hospital practice. Br Med J 1975; 3:471–473

Shader RI, Harmatz JS, Salzman C: A new scale for clinical assessment in geriatric populations: Sandoz Clinical Assessment—Geriatric (SCAG). J Am Geriatr Soc 1974; 22:107–113

Spitzer RL, Endicott J: Schedule for Affective Disorders and Schizophrenia (SADS) (Second Edition). New York, New York State Psychiatric Institute, 1975

Spitzer RL, Endicott J, Cohen GM: Psychiatric Status Schedule (Second Edition). New York, New York State Department of Mental Hygiene, Evaluation Unit, Biometrics Research, 1968

Spitzer RL, Endicott J. Robins E: Research Diagnostic Criteria: rationale and reliability. Arch Gen Psychiatry 1978a; 35:773–782

Spitzer RL, Gibbon M, Endicott J; The Global Assessment Scale (GAS). New York, New York State Department of Mental Hygiene, Evaluation Unit, Biometrics Research, 1978b

Wing JK, Cooper JE, Sartorius N: The Measurement and Classification of Psychiatric Symptoms. London, Cambridge University Press, 1974

Yesavage JA, Brink TL, Rose TL, et al: Development and validation of a geriatric depression screening scale: a preliminary report. J Psychiatr Res 1983; 17:37–49

Zung WWK: A self-rating depression scale. Arch Gen Psychiatry 1965; 12:371–379

Zung WWK: Depression in the normal aged. Psychosomatics 1967; 8:287–292

Chapter 11

Use of the Laboratory in the Diagnostic Workup of the Older Adult

Dan G. Blazer, M.D., Ph.D.
Ewald W. Busse, M.D.
Wade E. Craighead, Ph.D.
Don Evans, M.A.

The laboratory diagnosis of psychiatric disorders, except for the dementias, is a relatively new concept. This chapter considers the usefulness of a series of biomedical and psychologic laboratory tests. Other evaluation procedures are presented elsewhere in this text, especially self-rated and clinician rating symptom screens and diagnostic interviews. Virtually all of these laboratory diagnostic procedures are considered high technology and therefore are rapidly changing. Consequently, the reader must be alert to the relative value of these tests within the clinical setting and their limitations.

Some tests have clearly moved from research settings to an almost uniformly accepted role in general clinical practice. For example, the thera-peutic monitoring of tricyclic antidepressant (TCA) plasma levels is now a standard diagnostic test available to virtually all clinicians practicing in devel-oped countries. Other tests, such as magnetic resonance imaging (MRI), are in transition from research use to clinical use. Limitations in widespread use of these tests include cost and a lack of appropriate data regarding the utility of these tests.

As yet, there is no pathognomonic test for a primary psychiatric illness, though many laboratory tests provide the information needed to diagnose a physical illness that presents primarily with psychiatric symptoms (e.g., an abnormal thyroid panel and elevated thyroid-stimulating hormone (TSH) document hypothroidism as a cause of lethargy and depression). For this reason, a routine medical laboratory screen is indicated for all seriously ill psychiatric patients. Some diagnostic tests provide a direct indication of psychiatric disorder, such as the presence of cerebral atrophy on an MRI scan in the dementia patient. Most, however, are indirect "markers" of pathophysiology, including an abnormal dexamethasone suppression test (DST), an abnormal electroencephalogram (EEG), a shortened rapid eye movement (REM) latency from a polysomnogram, decreased cerebral blood flow, and a high score on the Minnesota Multiphasic Personality Inventory (MMPI). These markers can be of value in the clinical setting by providing complementary data to the history and physical examination.

Psychiatrists and other mental health care providers must become informed users of the laboratory in the future if they are to perform effectively as diagnosticians. Laboratory tests are subject to the same bias as clinical diagnostic procedures—a lack of reliability and validity. Therefore, for most diagnostic tests, such as the DST, certain methodologic criteria must be met if the test is to prove a useful marker of an illness. Shelps and Schechter (1984) suggest a series of methodologic criteria, which are modified slightly below:

1. Is there a well-defined gold standard?
2. Are "positive" and "negative" clearly defined for the diagnostic tests?
3. Is the test an "independent test"? For example, is the interpretation of performance of the diagnostic test blind to other clinical information?
4. In presentation of the usefulness of the test, are the data clearly displayed in tabular form?
5. Are sensitivity and specificity defined and used correctly in the presentation?
6. Are limitations for use of the test clearly stated?
7. Are guidelines provided for appropriate use?
8. Has the cost/benefit ratio or cost effectiveness of the test been discussed?
9. Have the procedures for performing the test been described in sufficient detail to permit replication?

The above questions relate primarily to the usefulness of a test in establishing a diagnosis in a setting where the clinical decision is to determine if an individual has or does not have a particular disorder. With the advent of the *Diagnostic and Statistical Manual of Mental Disorders (Third Edition)* (*DMS-III;* American Psychiatric Association 1980) and subsequently the revised third edition (*DSM-III-R;* American Psychiatric Association 1987) the "presence or absence" of a specific psychiatric disorder is the frequent decision made by the clinician.

To assess validity, a test is compared to a gold standard (such as a clinical diagnosis) that highlights four characteristics of the test. These characteristics are outlined in Figure 1.

Sensitivity is defined as the number of persons with a disorder who also exhibit a positive test result divided by the total number of individuals with the disorder (a/a + c). Specificity is defined as the number of individuals not suffering from a disorder with a negative test result divided by the total number of individuals not suffering from the disorder (d/b + d). The positive predictive value is the proportion of patients with positive test results who suffer from the disorder (a/a + b). The negative predictive value is the proportion of individuals with a negative test result who do not suffer from the disorder (d/c + d). Obviously, the percentage of individuals in the study population who actually suffer from the disorder will affect these values. For example, as prevalence falls in the study population, the positive predictive value must fall along with it, and negative predictive value must rise.

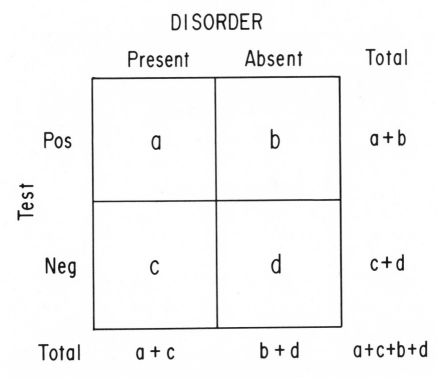

Figure 1. Data required to evaluate the usefulness of a diagnostic test.

When diagnostic tests are sensitive, relatively easy to administer, and not costly, they can be used as screening procedures. To date, there are no useful biomedical screens for primary psychiatric disorders. Nevertheless, screening scales, such as the Center for Epidemiology Studies Depression Scale (CES-D; described in Chapter 13), may be implemented in populations, such as a geriatric evaluation and treatment clinic. If there is strong clinical suspicion that a disorder is present, but further information is required to justify the suspicion, a specific test is indicated. Such tests may be more expensive, but when abnormal should essentially confirm the presence of the disease (e.g., multi-infarct dementia confirmed by an MRI scan).

Although these means of evaluating the performance of a test have traditionally been documented in tabular form with the introduction of tests, the evaluation of the usefulness of a test is a more complex process. For one, diagnostic tests are usually not performed in isolation. When multiple tests are used, the accumulation of abnormal results tends to confirm the presence of a disorder. These tests are least helpful when one is positive and the others are normal.

Biomedical tests are subject to another bias—a lack of reliability that directly affects validity. The modern geriatric psychiatrist has become familiar with the laboratory procedures for performing assays of hormones, metabolites of neurotransmitters, and concentrations of pharmacologic agents. Adequate laboratory assays that are reliable must be available to the clinician if these tests are to be useful. In addition, the range of normality and abnormality may vary from one laboratory to another. It is therefore essential for tests to be interpreted within the framework of the laboratory in which they are performed. Additional sources of variability must be explored in the future because many of these tests for pathophysiology are complex. For example, the variation in metabolism of dexamethasone across subjects may significantly alter the results of the DST.

Laboratory tests are used not only as procedures for screening and confirming diagnoses. Other uses include the potential of a test to predict response to therapy. For example, abnormalities in a thyroid function test, even in the absence of overt hyperthyroidism or hypothyroidism, may indicate an increased likelihood of supplemental thyroid preparations, such as Cytomel, as an adjunct to TCA therapy in the treatment-resistant depressed older adult. Tests may also predict clinical course. The DST, if abnormal during the initial phases of an episode that fails to normalize in the presence of improved clinical function, suggests an increased likelihood of rapid relapse (Schweitzer et al. 1987).

Given the variety of laboratory tests available, coupled with increasing restrictions on the overall cost of a diagnostic workup, geriatric psychiatrists and other clinicians working with psychiatrically impaired older adults must select appropriate batteries of tests that can provide optimal complementary information at reasonable cost for their patients. Which tests are justified in the routine workup of a depressed or demented older adult? What is the relative cost of tests, both monetary and in terms of burden upon patients already subjected to multiple diagnostic procedures? To what extent do diagnostic tests contribute to clinical decision making?

The following discussion of specific diagnostic tests is of necessity cursory. Nevertheless, it is hoped that these discussions will be of value in selecting an appropriate battery of tests in the diagnostic workup of the psychiatrically impaired older adult.

Polysomnography

The development of multiple monitoring of sleep and somatic function coupled with the increased flexibility of these methods has ushered in a new era in the diagnosis of sleep disorders. Diagnostic units for the investigation of sleep complaints have emerged in almost every major metropolitan area. The core diagnostic procedure used in sleep disorders units is the polysomnogram. This all-night, multiple monitoring of sleep and somatic function during sleep has proved both reliable and sensitive for recording the stages of sleep and concomitant physiologic functioning. Three basic recording variables are included in the polysomnogram—the sleep EEG, the electrooculogram (to measure eye movements during sleep), and submental electromyogram (to measure venilatory air exchange at the nairs in the mouth as well as respiratory effort). Additional monitors can be added for more specialized investigation, such as the electrocardiogram (ECG), electrodes placed over the anterior tibialis muscles (to measure leg movements), and venus catheterization to measure blood oxygen saturation. In specialized laboratories, video recording of sleep behaviors and postures are included as well as transducers to measure penile tumescence.

For years, the availability of the sleep laboratory to the clinician was limited because of the logistic difficulties that required a patient to sleep for 2 to 3 nights in a sleep laboratory (with constant monitoring by a laboratory technician) in order to obtain adequate data. Recently, portable units have been developed that permit the connection of electrodes attached to the scalp with a unit no larger than a portable tape recorder that may be carried to the home (or hospital room) of the patient being studied. These sleep tracings can later be evaluated in a shorter period of time via the use of computer-assisted monitoring.

Nevertheless, the polysomnogram remains of limited use in the general diagnostic workup of the depressed and/or demented older adult. An adequate polysomnogram requires a drug-free state for at least 7 days and preferably 10 to 14 days. The more severely depressed and demented older adult, especially those who are difficult to control behaviorially, require ongoing medication. Though medication could be withheld within a hospital setting, the advent of a diagnostic-related group approach to hospital care has limited the time available for hospitalization of older adults. Nevertheless, the polysomnogram will persist as a valuable diagnostic procedure for the study of the psychiatrically impaired older adult. Good studies of sensitivity and specificity for elders, however, remain to be published. The use of polysomnography in the diagnosis of sleep disorders and affective disorders is discussed in Chapters 6, 14, and 15.

The Electrocardiogram

The ECG is the most frequent screen of cardiovascular disease, when combined with a recording of blood pressure. The ECG is a graphic description of the electrical activity of the heart, which is recorded from the body surface by electrodes positioned to reflect activity from a variety of spatial perspectives. Cardiovascular disease can present with psychiatric manifestations in the older adult. For example, congestive heart failure and pulmonary edema may present with confusion and agitation. Transient ischemic attacks or arrhythmias may be present with episodes of acute confusion. Yet the most valuable use of electrocardiography in the diagnostic workup of the older adult is in screening for cardiovascular disease that would preclude the use of certain biologic therapies such as antidepressant medications or electroconvulsive therapy, and monitoring of the effect of these therapies on cardiovascular function.

The TCAs are well known to be cardiotoxic after an overdose, and their use has been considered unsafe, even in therapeutic doses, in patients with cardiovascular disease. Glassman and Bigger (1981) document that the most common cardiovascular complications of the TCAs is orthostatic hypotension, and patients with ventricular arrhythmias are likely to have their arrhythmias improve with therapy. Veith et al. (1982) found that TCAs had no effect on left ventricular ejection fractures at rest or during maximal exercise and that premature ventricular contractions were reduced by imipramine.

Nevertheless, TCAs near or above therapeutic plasma levels frequently prolong the P-R interval and the QRS complex. Though not dangerous, they should be monitored by an ECG before drug therapy is instituted and after therapy is discontinued. If patients have preexisting bundle branch block, those patients are at some danger for increased A-V or H-V block. Therefore, these elderly adults should be monitored frequently, probably in the hospital, when initially prescribed TCAs.

Cardiotoxicity is rarely a problem with antipsychotic agents as well. Orthostatic hypertension is the most common difficulty and can be induced by the less potent phenothiazines, such as thioridazine. Neuroleptic drugs also produce nonspecific T-wave changes on ECG, but once again these changes are not known to be of clinical significance. Nevertheless, it is generally recommended that low-potency neuroleptics not be used when conduction defects are identified initially on the ECG. Whenever a patient is sent for a routine ECG while on TCAs or neuroleptic agents, this fact should be indicated so the ECG can be interpreted correctly.

Clinical Chemistry Screen

A clinical chemistry screen is routine for virtually all hospital admissions and for most baseline outpatient visits. The yield on these screens is usually low for identifying the cause of psychiatric disorder, but the low cost and potential for correcting undetected medical illness render them of value to the psychiatrist.

The laboratory may be of most value in the diagnostic workup of the patient with cognitive impairment. The clinician must search for potentially reversible dementias, that is, dementias secondary to thyroid dysfunction, vitamin B_{12} deficiency, substance abuse, and infection. The Council on Scientific Affairs for the American Medical Association (1986) provided a consensus report on those laboratory tests that should be included in the diagnostic workup of the dementia patient. This evaluation includes blood count, electrolytes, blood sugar, blood urea nitrogen, creatinine, liver function tests, thyroid function tests, serologic tests for syphilis, toxicology screen, B_{12} and folate concentrations, sedimentation rate, and urinalysis. When a toxicology screen is not available, it is often helpful to obtain blood concentrations of all the medicines the patient is taking.

Abnormal sodium and chloride levels can lead to dehydration that can progress to delirium, lethargy, and convulsions. Overhydration may also evoke delirium and lethargy as well as weakness and muscular twitching. Respiratory or metabolic acidosis (an increased CO_2 level) may lead to drowsiness and weakness, which may be mistaken for a chronic depression or dementia. Respiratory alkalosis secondary to hyperventilation may lead to symptoms of lightheadedness, feelings of unreality, and paresthesias.

Among the electrolyte abnormalities, potassium disorders are the most critical to identify. Though they rarely present with psychiatric symptoms, the presence of a flaccid paralysis and paresthesias or muscular twitching may portend the onset of a severe cardiac arrhythmia and cardiac failure. Increased calcium resulting from hyperparathyroidism can lead to paranoid ideation and a variety of mental changes, as can hypocalcemia secondary to hypoparathyroidism. The mental changes of the latter may range from agitation to frank psychosis. Hyperinsulinism, causing a hypoglycemia, may initially be manifested by anxiety, perspiration, weakness, and shortness of breath. The symptoms of hyperglycemia (usually adult-onset diabetes) include lethargy, which may lead to diabetic coma and ketoacidosis.

The monitoring of thyroid function is especially important. Three test values are available in most laboratories and, for the psychiatric patient, a fourth test is generally suggested. The traditional components of the thyroid panel are a direct assay of thyroxine (T_4) by radioimmunoassay, a triiodothyronine (T_3) uptake, and the calculation of a free index. A combination of results of the thyroid panel and TSH assist in the diagnosis of both clinical and subclinical hypothyroidism. Subclinical hypothyroidism is not an uncommon cause of depressive symptoms in older adults.

The Thyrotropin-Releasing/Thyroid-Stimulating Hormone Test

The thyrotropin-releasing hormone (TRH) stimulation test is the most sensitive of the clinical tests for the thyroid disorder. The test assesses the functional state of the TSH-secretory mechanism. The interpretation of this test is described in Chapter 13 as it relates to the diagnosis of depression. After a drug-free period of 7 days, subjects are fasted overnight. The test begins at 9:00 A.M. and subjects lay recumbent. 0.5 mg of TRH are injected and TSH is recorded at intervals of 30 minutes for 3 hours. In addition to its value in identifying depression, a blunted TSH response to TRH is seen in functionally euthyroid patients with toxic goiters and occasionally in patients with pituitary hypothyroidism. Factors that may influence TSH response in normal subjects are thought to be relatively uncommon (Loosen and Prange 1982), but poor nutrition clearly contributes to an abnormal response. Elevated serum cortisol also appears to reduce TSH response both in patients with endocrine disorders and in normal subjects, though there is no evidence that serum cortisol elevation accounts for the TSH blunting seen in depressed patients.

Davies et al. (1985) found a blunted TSH response to TRH common in sick elderly patients but, contrary to initial hypothesis, did not find that patients with cardiac arrhythmias were more likely to exhibit a blunted response.

The Dexamethasone Suppression Test

The DST is discussed in detail in Chapters 12 and 13 as it assists in the diagnoses of dementia and depression respectively. This test, which existed for the diagnosis of Cushing's syndrome for years, has only recently been applied to the diagnosis of psychiatric disorders, specifically depression. The test became more valuable in psychiatry when the dose of dexamethasone was decreased from that usually recommended for the Cushing's syndrome test. The procedure used is to administer 1 mg of dexamethasone orally at 11:00 the night before the test. Venus blood samples are drawn for cortisol at 3:00 P.M. and 10:00 P.M. the next day, though an 8:00 A.M. cortisol has also been used. An abnormal DST result is defined as a plasma cortisol following dexamethasone administration at a level greater than 5 μg/dl.

The laboratory assay is critical to test performance. Good precision and accuracy of a given laboratory at the low end of plasma cortisol levels are essential. A number of exogenous factors may lead to a false positive result. These include medications (phenytoin, barbiturates, and carbamazepine), endocrine factors (Cushing's disease or pregnancy), major medical problems (serious infections or cancer), metabolic problems (recent withdrawal from alcohol, rapid weight loss, malnutrition, or nausea and vomiting), neurologic problems (multi-infarct dementia), increased intracranial pressure, and other factors (including the questionable effect of an unstable circadian rhythm). False negative results may occur when synthetic corticosteriods are used and possibly with the use of some benzodiazepines.

The DST has been the laboratory test most carefully scrutinized of all for its sensitivity and specificity, not to mention its clinical usefulness. Because it is so widely used as an adjunct to other diagnostic procedures, the necessity of an accurate diagnosis is essential. Better use of the test may result when the test is limited to the identification of major depression with melancholia (or endogenous depression) diagnosed by standardized procedures.

Cerebrospinal Fluid

Cerebrospinal fluid (CSF) investigations associated with geriatric mental disorders have focused on biochemical components in the CSF that may correlate with alterations within the brain including neurotransmitters and neuropeptides. These investigations have been enhanced by modern biochemical methods that can measure constituents using small amounts of CSF. Such studies are complicated by the fact that the content of lumbar spinal fluid may be quite different from that of intracranial CSF; furthermore, these changes may not reflect what is transpiring within the brain (Gottfries 1983).

In degenerative diseases of the central nervous system the proteins of the CSF are of particular interest (Harrington et al. 1986). Again, the variation in the site of origin that is within the blood or brain complicates the interpretation of these findings.

Aluminum is believed to accumulate within the brain of those persons with Alzheimer's disease, but increased aluminum is not consistently found in CSF.

Lumbar puncture is a procedure that should be done if the geriatric psychiatrist suspects a brain infection, trauma, or bleeding from an intracranial blood vessel. The Council on Scientific Affairs (1986) of the American Medical Association reports that in the workup of patients with dementia, some routinely do a lumbar puncture while others do it selectively. Similarly, another report indicates that this procedure should be done selectively and only if the clinician feels it is diagnostically justified.

Imaging

Plain radiographs continue to compose a significant portion of the bulk of diagnostic imaging. The clinician often requests plain skull films since they are useful in revealing the presence of intracranial masses, skull fractures, and bone changes.

During the last decade, a number of new imaging techniques are enhancing the research and diagnostic skills of the geriatric psychiatrist. These procedures are indeed windows into the brain. The following discussion will be limited to four diagnostic procedures. Since the clinical applications of these procedures appear in chapters throughout this book, this section includes the scientific basis of the procedure and reference to the historical background. It is presented in the hope of providing the clinician with an appreciation and understanding of the procedure that will not only benefit the clinician, but may be useful in providing the patient with sufficient information to ensure informed consent.

The architecture of the brain plays an important role in the functional imaging of the brain. The cerebral cortex has approximately four times the blood flow and the glucose metabolism of the white matter. Consequently, tracers that measure blood flow or glucose metabolism are all taken up predominantly by the cerebral cortex. Because the cortex is so thin, 4 to 8 mm, and because of the deep invaginations that carry two layers of cortex deep into the cerebrum, images obtained with these tracers reflect both the cerebral architecture and the limitations of the spatial resolution of the instrumentation (Holman 1985). As a result, the cerebral cortex appears much thicker on the images than it really is. The deep invaginations of gray matter create large islands of gray matter that must be taken into consideration when interpreting pictures.

Computed Tomography

Computed tomography (CT), originally called computerized axial tomography (CAT), was developed in England in 1972 by Hounsfield (1973) and was introduced into clinical use by Ambrose (1973). This radiologic scanning procedure has proved to be of considerable value for viewing the body, including the skull and its contents. Computed tomography is often said to be the "ultimate x-ray." Actually CT is a general term for several x-ray techniques that result in pictures of designated layers or slices of an organ such as the brain. The CT scanner uses a small beam of x-ray that rotates around the patient's skull or part of the body in a fixed plane. A computer converts the information generated by the beam into a cross-sectional x-ray picture. The resulting picture looks like a slice through the brain that permits many parts of the brain to be easily identified.

Computed tomographic imaging is essentially structural, while other types of imaging that will be discussed add a functional dimension. Pictures with CT permit evaluation of cerebral atrophy, ventricular size, and an estimation of the amount of CSF and distinguishes between gray and white matter. Such measures have been used to determine the effect of normal aging and to contrast these findings with diseases of the brain. The CT scans of so-called normal elderly subjects often indicate cortical cerebral atrophy. It appears that this loss of gray matter is an integral aspect of normal aging and is especially evident in the very old (Goldstein et al. 1985). This atrophy is not consistently related to intellectual decline; consequently, its significance is unclear. Similarly mild to moderate ventricular dilatation is common in the elderly. Only when these two findings exceed mild to moderate levels can they be related to dementia. The ventricular dilation, the increase in CSF, and the reduced brain tissue volume in the elderly are well documented by CT scan. Such gross anatomical changes would logically be reflected in a reduction of cerebral metabolic rates of glucose and oxygen. When these measures are carried out by positron emission tomography (PET), no reduction has been reported. One explanation has been offered and that is that some brain tissue is actually redundant and essentially nonfunctioning. Such an explanation may also be relevant to the poor correlation of PET results with intellectual changes.

Magnetic Resonance Imaging

Magnetic resonance imaging was originally called nuclear magnetic resonance (NMR). The name was changed because the term "nuclear" produced some apprehension in patients who falsely expected that the procedure would expose them to harmful radiation. Actually the principle underlying MRI has been used by chemists for three decades. The nuclei of certain identifiable atoms (isotopes) behave like tiny spinning magnets. This permits identification of these atoms by the use of an MRI scanner. In clinical use, it is a large doughnut-shaped magnet with a strength of 3,000 to 25,000 times the earth's natural magnetic field.

The stable isotopes of hydrogen and phosphorus are commonly used in MRI. Isotopes are forms of a single element that differ only in weight owing to a different number of neutrons in the nuclei. Such isotopes have identical chemical properties of the common atom. For example, the hydrogen isotope reacts with oxygen to form water, and the phosphorus isotope is incorporated into the metabolic processes that transpire in various tissues.

When these isotopes, acting as tiny spinning magnets, are placed in a static magnetic field generated by the previously described MRI apparatus, the nuclei will line up in the direction of that field. However, the nuclei are spinning and therefore also wobble. Different molecules can be identified because the nuclei wobble at different frequencies.

The second step is to use an alternating field applied at right angles to the first field. This moves some nuclei into a new alignment. Only the nuclei in resonance with this oscillating field, that is, only the nuclei wobbling at the same frequency as the field, will be realigned. When the second field is turned off, the realigned nuclei return to their original positions, releasing detectable signals that a computer can process and display as numerical data or as an image. This tells how much of a certain substance is present and also what kind of chemical and physical environment surrounds it. To further clarify, during the first exposure to a strong magnetic field the nuclei align themselves parallel to the field and their axes wobble randomly around it. When the second right angle magnetic field is applied, it is an oscillating one that makes the nuclei in the continuous field wobble or move in unison.

When the second oscillating field is turned off, the synchronized movement introduces a voltage that can be picked up and recorded. Gradually, on the order of milliseconds, the synchrony of the nuclei spin diminishes and the nuclei once again resume their random wobble, but they continue to be aligned with the first continuous magnetic field.

Measurements may be taken at various intervals during the MRI procedure (Bensen et al. 1985). For example, a measure can be taken at $T1$. $T1$ is the spin lattice relaxation time. This is the time needed for protons to relax back to their previous position. $T1$ is the time constant for the longitudinal component of magnetization to reach its equilibrium. $T1$ measures the difference between gray and white matter. This is possible because of the difference in fat and water ratio in the two tissues. There is a significant difference between the $T1$ of Alzheimer's disease and that of normal controls. Furthermore, $T1$ is altered by both multi-infarct dementia and Alzheimer's disease. It permits recognition of pathology in both white and gray matter. $T2$ represents spin-spin relaxation time. $T2$ is the time constant for the transverse component of magnetization to reach its equilibrium.

Magnetic resonance imaging has certain advantages. No radiation is involved and no contrast dye is needed. It produces high-resolution images and distinguishes normal from abnormal tissues. It can obtain pictures from parts of the body that are usually not accessible by the CT scan. The MRI procedure is limited by the patient's condition because the patient must remain perfectly motionless for extended periods of time and is surrounded by the previously described large doughnut-like structure. In addition, this large magnetic device must be housed in a large area devoid of iron and lined with copper. The copper shield is necessary to block any external inteference. The intense large magnetic field used in the procedure requires that personnel, as well as patients, do not carry, wear, or have imbedded within their bodies certain metals.

Positron Emission Tomography

Positron emission tomography is an exciting research technique and clinical evaluation procedure. In vivo studies of cerebral perfusion and metabolism and identification of their anatomical distribution are possible with PET.

The quantitative PET technique requires the integration of three components:

1. Compounds labeled with positron-emitting radioisotopes (unstable isotopes) to serve as tracers for physiologic processes. The isotopes are either injected into the patient or inhaled by the patient.
2. A position tomograph, which is a scanner for detecting tissue distribution of the tracer. Emissions produced by the positrons are measured by a circular array of radiation detectors and are recorded by a computer.
3. A tracer kinetic model is necessary. These are mathematical models that follow the labeled compounds through various so-called compartments noting when the tracer is in a certain compartment of a metabolic sequence. It is a way to quantify a physiologic process. An example of a compartment model is that of oxygen metabolism. The first compartment is oxygen in the plasma; the second is the oxygen metabolic processes that take place within the tissue.

Positrons are relatively short lived (unstable isotopes). Frequently used are the radioisotopes of carbon (^{11}C which has a high half-life of 20 minutes), nitrogen (^{13}N, with a half-life of 10 minutes), and oxygen (^{15}O, with a half-life of 2 minutes).

Fluoride (^{18}F) is a positron emitter tracer that does not naturally occur in the body. ^{18}F is often preferred because it has a long half-life of 110 minutes. ^{18}F is first produced by a cyclotron and then incorporated into a molecule. ^{18}F-2-deoxy-2 fluoro-D-glucose is the tracer compound often used to study the rate of glucose utilization. Other labeled compounds are used for measuring specific processes (Ferris et al. 1981).

The question arises as to what is a positron. It is often held to be one of the fundamental fragments that compose anatomic nuclei. An emitted positron is an antielectron and an antimatter. When it strikes an electron, annihilation takes place whereby two photons are formed. The photons (gamma rays) strike the detectors and the event is recorded (Phelps 1983). The data collected in this manner are used to form a tomographic image. These images are cross-sectional and are a picture of the distribution of tissue concentrations. The pictures are developed in accord with the principles of CT (Phelps and Mazziotta 1985). Positron emission tomography has been used to observe the physiologic processes associated with perception, learning, recall, and so forth. The technique has been used to study epilepsy, Parkinson's disease, senile dementia, schizophrenia, affective disorders, and Down's syndrome.

It is generally agreed that in Alzheimer's disease there is a decrease in metabolic activity in the temporal and parietal regions (D Sullivan, personal communication, 1987). In some cases, hypometabolism is widespread. Some decrease is seen in the thalamus and in the striatum, but the decrease is less than that in the cortex.

Phelps (1983) has reported a number of other PET observations. In patients with partial seizure disorders the epileptogenic focus in 70 percent of patients shows a decrease in glucose utilization while dormant, but very high glucose utilization during seizure switches. As to manic depressive illness, during the depressive phase the entire brain shows a reduction in glucose metabolism. Manic studies could not be satisfactorily completed because of the inability to control the patient (Phelps and Mazziotta 1985).

Symptomatic patients with Huntington's disease are reported to have reduced glucose metabolism in the caudate nuclei. It is possible that this reduction can be detected prior to the appearance of onset of symptoms (Mazziotta et al. 1987). This study needs further attention.

Rapaport (1986) reports that age differences are not found for the regional cerebral metabolic rates for glucose metabolism measured by PET. Right and left asymmetries appear early in Alzheimer's disease and are likely to be consistent with changes in specific brain function.

Single Photon Emission Computed Tomography

Single photon emission computed tomography (SPECT) is similar to PET in that it provides information concerning the function of the brain and other organs of the body. The usual procedure is to inject into a vein a small amount of a radioactive compound. Examples are ^{123}I or ^{133}Xe. They are used to label a number of compounds. The patient lies on a table between two SPECT cameras that are similar to Geiger counters. The cameras encircle the target for 10 to 20 minutes and record the amount of radioactivity given off. A computer converts this information into color or black-and-white cross-sectional images (Drayer 1986).

Although it is claimed that the information produced by SPECT is less detailed than that produced by PET or CT, the procedure is considerably less costly. Further, if its clinical value can be clearly demonstrated, it can be used in community hospitals and is not confined to major medical centers as are MRI and PET (Drayer and Friedman 1983).

In the SPECT procedure the emitting substance is a photon. A photon is a mass of energy; it is not a particle such as a neutron, proton, or electron. When a photon decays, it creates a positron and an electron as well as other fragments. The existence of a photon that is not a particle was originated by Max Planck who first discovered that heat radiation is absorbed or given out in the form of tiny packets of energy called quanta. This is known as Planck's quantum theory. Einstein in 1905 expressed conviction that light must behave in the same way, since each color of light is made of up packets containing different amounts of energy. Later, after further study, these light quanta were named photons.

Radioisotopes that are commercially available often omit only one photon per disintegration. Dual-photon-emitting isotopes are also available.

Dual-photo isotopes are positron emitters. They are short lived; they are technologically difficult and costly (Lassen 1985).

^{133}Xe is a single photon emitter and was used by Busse and Obrist to measure regional cerebral blood flow (see Chapter 6).

Electroencephalography

Aging changes of the EEG awake and asleep are reviewed in Chapter 6. With advancing age, brain wave changes are associated with alteration of brain function. Abnormalities occur that have diagnostic implications; some of these are described below.

Electroencephalographic Sleep in Psychotic Depression

Psychotic depression is considered a distinct subtype of major affective disorder in both the Research Diagnostic Criteria and in *DSM-III-R*. Persons with psychotic depression tend to be middle aged or older and their severe depression is accompanied by evidence of psychomotor disturbances as well as many other signs of depression. They often show a poorer clinical response to treatment with TCAs. A familial factor is not uncommon. Thase et al. (1986) compared 27 psychotic patients to 79 nonpsychotic subjects. Sleep in psychotic depression was characterized by increased wakefulness, decreased REM sleep percentage, and decreased REM activity. Psychotic subjects were more likely to have extremely short sleep-onset REM latency. These EEG abnormalities tended to increase with the duration of the illness. Patients with recent-onset depressions were characterized by marked initial insomnia, increased stage 1 sleep percentage, and long REM latencies. This contrasted with patients of longer duration who had extremely short REM latencies.

To summarize, patients with psychotic depression were found to have a significant decreased generation of REM sleep. It is generally accepted that endogenous depressions are accompanied by characteristic EEG sleep abnormalities including sleep continuity disturbances, diminished slow-wave sleep, shortened REM latency, and altered distribution of REM density and time. On the basis of these studies, we believe that there is a difference between psychotic depression and nonpsychotic depressive reactions.

Electroencephalogram Findings in Mixed Depression and Dementia

A frequent diagnostic and therapeutic problem involves the elderly person who manifests mixed symptoms of depression and dementia. It is estimated that 20 percent of elderly persons with depression also have deficits suggesting organic dementia. Depressive symptoms are not uncommon in patients with Alzheimer's disease. Routine EEG findings do not appear to differentiate between those who will show clinical improvement and those who will deteriorate. Electroencephalograms were found to be normal or only mildly abnormal in seven of eight patients who showed clinical improvement (Reynolds et al. 1986). Of the eight patients who deteriorated, five were found to have normal or mildly abnormal EEGs. A single markedly abnormal patient with depression showed an infarct on CT scan. Sleep EEGs were not studied.

Rae-Grant et al. (1987) point out that many studies have examined EEG changes in patients with dementing disorders. However, there have been serious methodologic problems such as the need for a well-defined diagnostic classification and with ultimate pathologic variation. In addition, it is important to study such patients and subjects over a period of years and the EEG studies must be correlated with clinical, psychologic, and laboratory observations. Correlations must be done at regular intervals throughout the study.

Although one would expect a progressive change in the EEG paralleling the progression of the dementia, this is not always true. Furthermore, there are some patients who remain at a plateau for long periods of time (Gordon 1968).

Rae-Grant et al. (1987) studied 318 patients with dementia and 159 control subjects. The subjects were matched for sex and age. The sample of those with dementia was reduced to 139 patients representing Alzheimer-type disease. Under this broad classification they included dementia of the Alzheimer's type, senile dementia of the Alzheimer's type, and a mixed type of dementia (the latter being those with an ischemic score of 4 to 7).

On a qualitative basis, the EEG findings in this study were not unlike those in previous reports; that is, there was a general slowing of the alpha rhythm with the appearance of slow waves and the presence of focal abnormalities. The EEG studies were significantly more abnormal than those of the controls. Focal abnormalities of the type often associated with aging were not significantly different between patients and control subjects. Focal abnormalities for age appeared in the first EEGs of 13 percent of patients and 14 percent of control subjects. Over a span of 4 years it appears that the survivors of the dementia group had an increasing tendency to have EEGs that remained relatively unchanged. In fact, a small percentage of EEGs from patients with dementia showed improvement. It was concluded that EEGs do not show a consistent progression to slower and more malignant rhythms, but vary in progression and pattern. There was a parallel between the worsening of the EEG and mental deterioration as measured by psychological testing. The EEGs did not discriminate between those with early-onset dementia, that is dementia of the Alzheimer's type, and senile dementia of the Alzheimer's type.

As to autopsy findings, severe EEG alterations correlated well with the presence of more severe neuronal loss in the hippocampi and with an increase in granulovacuolar ratio.

The Psychodiagnostics Laboratory

How to Use the Laboratory

The psychodiagnostics laboratory may be used for a number of valuable clinical activities. The primary services provided by a psychodiagnostics laboratory include neuropsychologic testing, intelligence testing, personality testing, and testing for specific disorders. These activities provide information pertinent to both Axis I and Axis II diagnoses as well as the patient's status on various personality constructs.

The most effective use of the psychodiagnostics laboratory is achieved when the question to be asked of the assessment is formulated properly and clearly. The referring clinician needs to know what he or she wants from the clinical assessment and the report of that assessment. The diagnostician must receive the proper question regarding the patient in order to know what assessment instrument to employ and how best to report back the obtained information to the referring clinician. The proper formulation of the question also assists the diagnostician in determining the testability of the patient. A clear statement of the purpose of the diagnostic evaluation allows the evaluator to determine if the patient is capable of completing the psychodiagnostic process necessary to obtain the requested assessment information. For example, the request for an evaluation of a hearing- or sight-impaired or extremely confused person should note those limitations.

The effective use of the psychodiagnostics laboratory can also be facilitated by developing an ongoing working relationship with a specific laboratory and/or the person doing the assessments and reports. This relationship will provide for efficient and effective communication. It will allow for clear communication of the question being asked of the assessment and will over time provide for the expedient transfer of information, formatting of reports, and scheduling of patients.

The following material provides a sampling and brief overview of some of the instruments that are generally available for use in a psychodiagnostics laboratory. The listing is in no way exhaustive, but merely provides some examples of what is available. It is beyond the scope of this chapter to provide a detailed description of the assessment instruments or a thorough evaluation of their usefulness and psychometric properties.

Neuropsychologic and Intelligence Testing

The major contributions of a neuropsychologic evaluation fall into three broad categories (Golden 1983). The first of these is diagnosis. Included in this category are (1) identifying the presence of brain injury or related disorder, including differentiating between emotional problems and brain dysfunction; (2) specifying the nature of the deficits caused by brain damage, including localizing the injury to specific areas of the brain; and (3) helping to determine the cause of the brain dysfunction.

The second important contribution is tracking changes in functioning over time. This is especially useful when examining the efficacy of a particular course of treatment or monitoring the course of a progressive illness.

The third area is assisting in the planning of a rehabilitation program. This relatively new area holds considerable promise. Both the knowledge of brain function and the ability to assess it are rapidly increasing. As the understanding of brain-behavior relationships improves so will efforts to provide specific rehabilitative procedures that maximally benefit the individual.

As outlined previously, neuropsychologic assessment may address a variety of questions. A selected sample of common types of evaluation and typical instruments employed are described herein. In addition, two of the most widely used comprehensive neuropsychologic batteries will be briefly reviewed.

Screening.   The Mini-Mental State Examination (Folstein et al. 1975) is an abbreviated mental status examination in which each area to be evaluated is represented by only a few questions (Lezak 1983). Areas evaluated include orientation, verbal reception, attention and calculation, language, and figure construction. It is quite brief and can be administered in 5 to 10 minutes. Because of its brevity, it can be especially useful in diagnostic screening or in following the course of a condition. Both the administration and scoring are standardized and its use it easily learned.

Intellectual assessment.   One of the most widely used intelligence tests is the Wechsler Adult Intelligence Scale–Revised (WAIS–R), an updated version of the original published in 1955 (Lezak 1983). Another frequently used test in the Stanford-Binet Intelligence Scale (Terman and Merrill 1973). Although both tests have proven value for intellectual assessment, the WAIS–R is described here because of its inclusion in the Halstead-Reitan Neuropsychological Battery.

The WAIS was initially designed as a measure of "general" intelligence; it is actually a composite test consisting of a number of subtasks. A review of intellectual functioning in which the WAIS or WAIS–R serves as the major instrument is often sufficient to demonstrate adequate intellectual functioning or provide an indication of the nature of altered function. For all but the most severely impaired adults, the WAIS–R can comprise a substantial portion of the neuropsychologic examination.

The WAIS–R is composed of 11 different subtests divided into two categories, Verbal and Performance. The six Verbal tests are Information, Comprehension, Arithmetic, Similarities, Digit Span, and Vocabulary. The five Performance tests include Digit Symbol, Picture Completion, Block Design, Picture Arrangement, and Object Assembly.

After administration and scoring of each of the subtests, they are adjusted for age effects on the basis of established norms. The results of the test consist of 11 age-corrected subscale scores and age-corrected composite scores for Verbal IQ, Performance IQ, and Overall IQ. Additionally, the results can be used to provide both an estimate of premorbid functioning and useful information regarding the possible nature and location of observed deficits. Proper use of the WAIS–R as a neuropsychologic assessment tool requires a combination of skills. In addition to a knowledge of how specific aspects of brain functioning affect test performance, the clinician must take other potential influences into account by using available behavioral, historic, and psychologic information.

Memory assessment.   Memory is essential for an individual's adequate functioning. One test that evaluates several important aspects of memory is the Revised Wechsler Memory Scale (Russell 1975). It consists of the Logical Memory and Visual Reproduction subtests of the original instrument and an additional recall trial after a half-hour delay. Together they provide indices of both immediate and delayed recall for verbal and figural material. Severity-of-impairment scores are easily derived from available norms, and these scores have been found useful in discriminating between normal controls and patients with organic cognitive impairment (Lezak 1983).

Neuropsychologic batteries.   A vast number of tests are available to evaluate specific cognitive functions. In many instances the selected use of a small number of these is adequate to answer a given referral question. However, another approach is the use of neuropsychologic test batteries, which provide a comprehensive evaluation of cognitive functioning. The Halstead-Reitan Neuropsychological Battery continues to be the most widely used and most extensively validated battery (Meier 1985). It consists of a number of independent tests. Several versions exist (Golden 1979); however, most consist of the following:

1. The WAIS,
2. The MMPI,
3. The Halstead Category Test,
4. The Speech Sounds Perception Test,
5. The Seashore Rhythm Test,
6. The Tactual Performance Test,
7. The Trail Making Test,
8. The Reitan-Klove Sensory–Perceptual Examination,
9. The Reitan–Indiana Aphasia Examination,
10. The Lateral Dominance Examination,
11. The Halstead Finger Tapping Test.

The MMPI (to be discussed later) is included to evaluate emotional factors that could contribute to deficits in test performance.

The Luria-Nebraska Neuropsychological Battery differs from the Halstead-Reitan in several ways (Anastasi 1982). It requires less time to administer—$2\frac{1}{2}$ hours as opposed to 6 or more hours for the Halstead-Reitan. Its content, materials, administration, and scoring are more highly standardized. Although less established and not as thoroughly researched thus far, it compares favorably to the Halstead-Reitan (Osmon 1983). Further modifications will undoubtedly be forthcoming to address problems such as a weakness in the memory function evaluation. Primary summary scores are provided in the following areas: motor functions, rhythm, tactile functions, visual function, receptive speech, expressive speech, writing, reading, arithmetic, memory, and intellectual processes.

Personality Assessment

Information for personality assessments is usually obtained from the patient via one of the following three formats: paper-and-pencil instruments, interviews, and projective procedures. Following discussion of the most widely used personality assessment instruments in each of these formats, recent assessment procedures evaluating a patient's status on a specific personality trait or disorder will be noted.

Paper-and-pencil instruments. The most widely used personality assessment instrument is the MMPI, developed by Hathaway and McKinley of the University of Minnesota in the 1940s. It is composed of 566 items to which the patient responds in a true–false format. If a statement does not apply, the patient simply makes no answer. The MMPI has recently undergone extensive revisions with the development of appropriate norms from adolescence and on up the life span.

The MMPI is a criterion-keyed, empirically developed instrument originally designed to discriminate between various clinical groups (Axis I diagnoses) and a control group of about 700 "normals." It provides scores on a number of clinical scales that correspond to the equivalent of Axis I diagnoses current at the time the instrument was developed. It also includes various correction scales for lying, faking, and so on. Over the many years of its employment in the clinical setting, it has gradually come to be seen as of less value for specific clinical judgment and of more value in providing information regarding a patient's status on scales or patterns of scales of personality traits. It is probably most valuable to the clinician when the diagnostician reports on the various patterns of personality scales or traits for which the individual achieves a deviant score or set of scores.

There are a number of limitations of the MMPI that should be noted (see

Anastasi 1982; Cronbach 1984). In general, these are that some of the scales have low reliabilities, the size and representativeness of the normal sample have been questioned, and there appears to be a lack of appropriate validity for most of the specific clinical scales. It is not surprising that the personality clinical scales do not predict the current classification system given the substantial revisions in the classification system since the MMPI was developed. Nevertheless, the MMPI may serve useful functions for the clinician. It is most useful as a diagnostic aid for the trained clinician. The pattern of abnormal clinical scales may suggest both the general form and the level of severity of pathology, which can be evaluated further in clinical work. In some cases, the MMPI report may call attention to pathology that the clinician otherwise might not note or at least might not note early on in the work with a specific patient. Thus, so long as the clinician does not take either a clinical report or a computerized report of clinical diagnostic scales as representing valid clinical classification data, the MMPI may continue to be of usefulness to the clinician.

The other paper-and-pencil personality inventory that may be useful to clinical practice is the Millon Clinical Multiaxial Inventory–II (MCMI–II, National Computer Systems 1987). It is a 1987 revision of Theodore Millon's mid-1970s personality assessment scale (Millon 1982). It is designed to be used with individuals ages 17 and older, is written at an eighth-grade level, and takes about one half-hour to complete. The MCMI–II is composed of 175 items in a true-false format. The instrument provides scores for 9 clinical syndromes (Axis I diagnoses) and 13 personality disorders (Axis II diagnoses). The reliabilities of the individual scales are generally adequate, although marginal in some cases (National Computer Systems 1987). In additional to the 22 clinical and personality scales, the MCMI–II also has corrective scales for deceptive type responses and a validity index that is designed to detect random or confused response patterns. The instrument is distributed by National Computer Systems, and they make available computerized reports that either simply summarize the individual scale scores or provide a more exhaustive clinical interpretive report.

The MCMI–II is not as exhaustive with regard to Axis I diagnoses as the MMPI. It probably does not go far beyond the information gathered in standard clinical interviews and intervention sessions. Since it is quite similar to MCMI–I it is likely to continue to be of questionable validity in regard to Axis I diagnoses because of the overlap ot items, intercorrelations, and the multidimensional nature of the clinical syndrome scales (Choca et al. 1986). On the other hand, it may be considerably useful for Axis II diagnosis. It probably can best be used as an efficient "first pass" at personality psychopathology diagnoses. Its ultimate validity relative to clinical diagnosis of Axis II disorders remains to be adequately demonstrated. Furthermore, there are not yet clinical outcome studies that demonstrate the prognostic capabilities of either the MCMI–I or the MCMI–II.

Interviews.   Several interviews have been developed to assess personality disorders. Perhaps the most sophisticated and useful of these instruments is the Structured Interview for the *DSM–III* Personality Disorders developed by Pfohl and his colleagues at the University of Iowa Medical Center (Pfohl et al. 1982; Stangl et al. 1985).

The SIDP consists of 160 questions grouped around themes such as self-esteem and social interaction skills, as opposed to being grouped around the *DSM–III* personality disorders themselves. The interviewer simply asks each question on the structured interview and scores the response. When the interview is completed, the inteviewer then employs an algorhithm designed by the SIDP developers to determine the presence or absence of each of the *DSM–III* personality disorders.

The interview takes between 60 and 90 minutes to complete. Zimmerman et al. (1986) have demonstrated that the reliability and validity of the SIDP can be enhanced by briefly interviewing an informant regarding the patient and his or her behavior. Stangl et al. (1985) report Kappas for many of the personality disorders included in the SIDP. Most of the Kappas were indicative of adequate reliabilities for the scales. However, a few of them were below .70, indicating that they were barely acceptable or even unacceptable, for example, .45 for avoidant personality disorder. This interview is currently being revised, partially to address the low reliabilities of several of the scales and partially in order to update it to make it match better with *DSM–III–R*.

There are a number of other interviews available to assess personality disorders. Perhaps the most promising of these (but less developed than the SIDP) is the Tridimensional Interview of Personality Style (TIPS) developed by Cloninger (1987). This interview is built around his recent model of personality and personality disorders, and it very likely will prove to be of clinical and theoretical significance. Cloniger (1987) also has developed the Tridimensional Personality Questionnaire, which is a self-report instrument developed from the TIPS and is designed to assess personality disorders via the paper-and-pencil format. Cloninger's instruments need further psychometric refinement before they will be of general clinical and research usefulness.

Projectives.   Projective assessment techniques can be distinguished from other forms of psychodiagnostic testing by the use of a relatively unstructured task. Test stimuli are usually vague and only general instructions are given. The hypothesis on which projective tests are based is that the lack of structure present in the task requires the individual to provide the structure. The projections from the person are observed by the examiner and assumed to reflect the characteristic thought processes and other aspects of personality organization. Although the person being tested is aware of being evaluated, the projective tests are generally less transparent than other forms of inquiry (see Anastasi 1982).

Projective techniques for assessing individuals are available in a wide variety of forms. Only two of the major instruments will be described here. In general, when the psychometric properties of this class of instruments are evaluated they are quite weak (Cronbach 1984). However, they may be clinically useful when administered and interpreted by an experienced and skilled examiner. They continue to enjoy popular and widespread use, even though they possess poor psychometric properties.

Hermann Rorschach, a Swiss psychiatrist, was the first to demonstrate that patients of differing types respond to inkblots differently (Cronbach 1984). The task of the respondent is to describe what he or she sees in the inkblot. The materials consist of a set of 10 cards, each with a symmetric blot so irregular as to allow a wide range of interpretations. Some of the cards are black and white while others include colors.

Several available scoring systems attempt to address the criticisms regarding the poor psychometric properties of projectives. Most share counting the number of responses, location, determinants, and content. Beyond these there is considerable variability in the scoring procedures.

The Thematic Apperception Test (TAT) elicits open or disguised statements about beliefs, attitudes, and motives (Anastasi 1982). This task requires the test taker to tell a story based on a picture presented by the examiner. The person is instructed to describe what is happening, what led up to the scene, and the outcome. It is presumed that persons taking the test project themselves into the scene, identifying with a character. The TAT consists of 19 pictures in black and white and one blank white card. Some of the cards are suggested for one sex or the other. Usually a subset (approximately 10) of the cards is administered. Although formal scoring systems are available, the most common method of interpretation is the impressionistic approach (Cronbach 1984). The interpreter considers recurrent themes, reflected attitudes, stylistic issues, and concern for detail and accuracy. This information is used to form hypotheses to describe the person's personality, motives, drives, defenses, and emotional conflicts.

Assessment of specific disorders.   During recent years there has been an increasing emphasis in psychologic assessment on the evaluation of specific disorders. Thus, a number of assessment batteries have been developed that focus on the clinical evaluation of disorders such as major depression, anxiety, and antisocial behavior. Although it is beyond the scope of this chapter to review the various assessment instruments available, a quick overview of a possible depression assessment battery will illustrate the potential utility of the psychodiagnostics laboratory as a resource for obtaining pertinent clinical information for specific disorders. The major interview available to evaluate the presence of a major depressive disorder is the Schedule of Affective Disorders and Schizophrenia (Endicott and Spitzer 1978). Clinical rating scales that can be based on this interview include the

Hamilton Depression Rating Scale (Hamilton 1960) and the Montgomery-Asberg (1979). Both of these scales have demonstrated adequate reliability and give a good indication of the clinician's judgment of the level of the severity of the depression. In addition to these instruments, there are several self-report measures of depression that give a good measure of the patient's experienced level of depression. Perhaps the two most useful instruments in this regard are the Beck Depression Inventory (Beck et al. 1961) and the Carroll Rating Scale (Carroll et al. 1981). Information from these three types of clinical assessments provides the clinician with a very thorough indication of the presence or absence of a major depressive episode and the level of severity of that disorder. Similar instruments are also available for the specific assessment of most other types of psychiatric disorders.

References

Ambrose J: Computerized transverse axial scanning—clinical application. Br J Radiol 1973; 46:1023–1047

Anastasi A: Psychological Testing. New York, Collier Macmillan, 1982

Beck AT, Ward CH, Mendelson M, et al: An inventory for measuring depression. Arch Gen Psychiatry 1961; 4:561–571

Bensen J, Mutch W, Smith F, et al: The relationship between Parkinson's disease and dementia: a study using proton NMR imaging parameters. Br J Psychiatry 1985; 147:380–382

Carroll BJ, Feinberg M, Smouse PE, et al: The Carroll Rating Scale for Depression: I. Development, reliability and validation. Br J Psychiatry 1981; 138:194–200

Choca JP, Peterson CA, Shanley LA: Factor analysis of the Millon Clinical Multiaxial Inventory. Consult Clin Psychol 1986; 54:253–255

Cloninger CR: A systematic method for clinical description and classification of personality variants: a proposal. Arch Gen Psychiatry 1987; 44:573–588

Council on Scientific Affairs of the American Medical Association: Dementia. JAMA 1986; 256:2234–2238

Cronbach LJ: Essentials of Psychological Testing. New York, Harper & Row, 1984

Davies AB, Williams J, John R, et al: Diagnostic value of thyrotrophian–releasing hormone test in elderly patients with atrial fibrillation. Br Med J 1985; 291:773–777

Drayer B: Radiology—"windows" into the living body. Duke Health Line, Spring 1986; pp. 4–6

Drayer B, Friedman JR: In vivo quantification of regional cerebral blood flow: validation of the HIPDm SPECT. American Journal of Neural Radiology 1983; 4:572–576

Endicott J, Spitzer R: A diagnostic interview: the Schedule for Affective Disorders and Schizophrenia. Arch Gen Psychiatry 1978; 35:837–844

Ferris S, Mony J, Wolf A et al: Positron emission tomography in the study of aging and senile dementia Neurobiol Aging 1981; 1:127–131

Folstein MF, Folstein SE, McHugh PR: Mini–mental state. J Psychiatr Res 1975; 12:189–198

Glassman AH, Bigger JT: Cardiovascular effects of therapeutic doses of tricyclic antidepressants; a review. Arch Gen Psychiatry 1981; 38:815–820

Golden CJ: Clinical Interpretations of Objective Psychological Tests. New York, Grune & Stratton, 1979

Golden CJ: The neuropsychologist in neurological and psychological populations, in Foundations of Clinical Neuropsychology. Edited by Golden CJ, Vincente PJ. New York, Plenum Press, 1983

Goldstein SJ, Wekstein D, Kirkpatrick C, et al: Imaging the centenarian brain: a computed tomographic study. J Am Geriatr Soc 1985; 33:579–584

Gordon EB: Serial EEG studies in presenile dementia. Br J Psychiatry 1968; 114:779–780

Gottfries C–G: Biochemical changes in blood and cerebrospinal fluid, in Alzheimer's disease. Edited by Reisberg B. New York, Free Press, 1983

Hamilton M: A rating scale for depression. J Neurol, Neurosurg Psychiatry 1960; 23:56–62

Harrington MG, Merril CR, Asher DM et al: Abnormal proteins in the cerebrospinal fluid of patients with Creutzfeldt–Jakob disease. N Engl J Med 1986; 315:279–283

Holman BL: Anatomy and function of the brain, in Radionuclide Imaging of the Brain, Contemporary Issues in Nuclear Imaging (Volume 1). Edited by Holman BL. New York, Churchill Livingstone, 1985

Hounsfield CN: Computerized transverse axial scanning (tomography)—description of a system. Br J Radiol 1973; 46:1016–1022

Lassen NA: Measurement of regional cerebral blood flow in humans with single–photon emitting radioisotope, in Brain Imaging and Brain Function. Edited by Sokoloff L. New York, Raven Press, 1985

Lezak MD: Neuropsychological Assessment (second edition). New York, Oxford University Press, 1983

Loosen PT, Prange AJ: Serum thyrotrophian response to thyrotropin–releasing hormone in psychiatric patients: a review. Am J Psychiatry 1982; 139:405–416

Mazziotta JC, Phelps, ME, Pahl JJ, et al: Glucose metabolism and Huntington's disease. N Engl J Med 1987; 316:357–362

Meier MJ: Review of the Halstead–Reitan neuropsychological test battery, in The Ninth Mental Measurements Yearbook (Volume 1). Edited by Mitchel JV Jr. Lincoln, NE, University of Nebraska Press, 1985

Millon T: Millon Clinical Multiaxial Inventory Manual. Minneapolis, MN, National Computer Systems, 1982

Montgomery S, Asberg M: A new depression scale designed to be sensitive to change. Br J Psychiatry 1979; 134:382–389

National Computer Systems: Millon Clinical Multiaxial Inventory–II. Minneapolis, MN, National Computer Systems, 1987

Osmon DC: The use of test batteries in clinical neuropsychology, in Foundations of Clinical Neuropsychology. Edited by Golden CJ, Vincente PJ. New York, Plenum Press, 1983

Pfohl B, Stangl D, Zimmerman M: The Structured Interview for DSM–III Personality Disorders (SIDP), 1982. Available from B. Pfohl, M.D., Department of Psychiatry, University of Iowa, 500 Newton Rd, Iowa City, IA 52242

Phelps, M: Positron computed tomography for studies of myocardial and cerebral function. Ann Intern Med 1983; 98:339–359

Phelps ME, Mazziotta JC: Positron emission tomography: human brain function and biochemistry. Science 1985; 228:799–809

Rae–Grant A, Blume W, Lau C et al: The electroencephalogram in Alzheimer–type dementia. Arch Neurol 1987; 50–54

Rapaport SI: Positron emission tomography in normal aging and Alzheimer's disease. Gerontology 1986; 32(Suppl 1):6–13

Reynolds CR III, Kupfer DJ, Hoch CC, et al: Two-year follow-up of elderly patients with mixed depression and dementia. J Am Geriatr Soc 1986; 34:793–799

Russell EW: A multiple scoring method for the assessment of complex memory functions. J Consult Clin Psychol 1975; 43:800–809

Schweitzer I, McGuire KP, Gee AH, et al: Prediction of outcome in depressed patients by weekly monitoring with the dexamethasone suppression test. Br J Psychiatry 1987; 151:780–784

Shelps SB, Schecter MT: The assessment of diagnostic tests: a survey of current medical research. JAMA 1984; 252:2418–2422

Stangl D, Pfohl B, Zimmerman M, et al: A structured interview for DSM–III personality disorders: a preliminary report. Arch Gen Psychiatry 1985; 42:591–596

Terman LM, Merrill MA: The Stanford–Binet Intelligence Scale. Manual for Third Revision, Form L–M. Boston, Houghton Mifflin, 1973

Thase ME, Kupfer DJ, Ulrich RF: Electroencephalographic sleep in psychotic depression. Arch Gen Psychiatry 1986; 43:886–893

Veith RC, Raskind MA, Caldwell JH, et al: Cardiovascular effects of trycyclic antidepressants in depressed patients with chronic heart disease. N Engl J Med 1982; 306:954–959

Zimmerman M, Pfohl B, Stangl D, et al: Assessment of DSM–III personality disorders: the importance of interviewing an informant. J Clin Psychiatry 1986; 47:261–263

Psychiatric Disorders in Late Life

Chapter 12

Organic Mental Disorders

Murray A. Raskind, M.D.

The organic mental disorders as a group are the most prevalent psychiatric disorders of later life. They are also the most costly both in terms of financial resources dedicated to patient care and in terms of morbidity, mortality, and the stress patients place on the community. Approximately one-half of beds in community nursing homes are devoted to dementia patients, and the cost of this care has been estimated to be 25 billion dollars per year (Katzman 1986). The prevalence and burden of the organic mental disorders will only increase (unless effective treatments or preventive measures are found) as the proportion of elderly persons in the United States population increases over the next 50 years.

Although the clinical management of the organic mental disorders has often been associated with pessimism or even therapeutic nihilism, such a stance is becoming much less common. Many organic mental disorders are symptomatically treatable, and even the irreversibly demented patient can benefit from an appropriate therapeutic regimen. Furthermore, advances in our understanding of the pathophysiology of at least some organic mental disorders (e.g., primary degenerative dementia of the Alzheimer's type) raise hopes for rational effective therapies in the not too distant future.

This chapter will present the phenomology, differential diagnosis, pathophysiology and pathogenesis (where known) of the major organic mental disorders of later life. The chapter will also review diagnostic and therapeutic

This work was supported in part by the Veterans Administration.

313

approaches to these disorders and discuss some areas of controversy as well as areas in which future research is expected to produce helpful new knowledge.

Classification: The Diagnostic and Statistical Manual of Mental Disorders (Third Edition-Revised)

The classification of the organic mental disorders in this chapter will conform with the *Diagnostic and Statistical Manual of Mental Disorders (Third Edition-Revised) (DSM-III-R)* published in 1987 by the Task Force on Nomenclature and Statistics of the American Psychiatric Association. The *DSM-III*, published in 1980, provided both clinicians and researchers with an important tool for diagnosis of and communication about psychiatric disorders in general and the organic mental disorders specifically. The *DSM-III* classification of the organic mental disorders has been widely influential in psychiatry as well as other medical specialties and associated health disciplines. The revisions in *DSM-III-R* further clarify and strengthen this diagnostic instrument. In the *DSM-III-R* "organic mental syndromes" are distinguished from "organic mental disorders." Organic mental syndrome refers to a group of signs and symptoms without reference to etiology; in contrast, organic mental disorder describes a particular mental syndome in which the etiology is either known or can be presumed with a reasonable degree of certainty. These organic etiologic factors are at least potentially demonstrable by currently available laboratory procedures (such as computerized tomography of the brain or measurement of a chemical toxin in body tissues), physical examination, or medical history. The organic factor responsible for an organic mental disorder of later life is most commonly a primary disease of brain tissue (such as Alzheimer's disease or multiple cerebral infarctions), but systemic illnesses secondarily affecting the brain (such as myxedema or uremia) also commonly occur, particularly as etiologic agents in delirium. The term "disorder" should be used when a physical disorder underlying the behavioral constellation of signs and symptoms is known.

It should be noted that the term "organic *brain* syndrome" used in *DSM-III* has been dropped from *DSM-III-R* and replaced with the term "organic *mental* syndrome." Despite the historic use of the dichotomy between "organic mental disorders," which implies disordered brain anatomy or physiology, and "functional mental disorders" which implies psychologic or social etiologic factors, it should be recognized that this distinction is becoming increasingly artificial as our knowledge of the biology of the major "functional" psychiatric illnesses increases.

The organic mental syndromes are numerous, and a complete discussion of all organic mental syndromes is beyond the scope of this chapter. Rather, discussion will focus on the organic mental syndromes of primary importance in the geriatric population. These are (1) dementia, (2) amnestic syndrome, (3) delirium, and (4) organic mood syndrome. Each syndrome will be described with the diagnostic criteria from *DSM-III-R* included, and the specific organic mental disorders associated with the syndromes will be discussed.

Dementia

The essential feature of the dementia syndrome is impairment in short- and long-term memory associated with impairment in at least one other aspect of intellectual function such as abstract thinking, impaired judgment, aphasia, or personality. The *DSM-III-R* criteria for the diagnosis of dementia (see Table 1) place a greater emphasis than did *DSM-III* on impairment of memory as the primary deficit in dementia. This change from *DSM-III*, which more broadly emphasized "loss of intellectual abilities," appears to be an improvement in specificity and is more consistent with the typical clinical presentation. Memory impairment is usually the initial and most prominent symptom in dementing disorders. In the early stages of the progressive dementias of later life, memory loss tends to be more marked for recent events. The patient may be obviously repetitious in conversation, become lost in new environments, and fail to keep track of appointments and obligations. As the dementia progresses, remote and highly learned memory traces are also lost and the patient may be unable to recognize immediate family members. Impairment in abstract thinking is manifested by reduced capacity for generalization, synthesis, differentiation, logical reasoning, and concept formation. Impaired judgment is often an early sign of dementia and may cause great consternation to family members and other associates, especially if the presence and nature of an underlying dementing disorder is not yet fully appreciated.

The most common personality change in late-life progressive dementing disorders is apathy. A previously nurturant, caring, and responsive spouse, parent, or friend becomes self-centered and loses interest in and empathy for the needs of others, while requiring ever greater care from others. Other personality changes commonly seen in late-life progressive dementing disorders include increased dependency on the spouse or other care provider, manifested by anxious clinging behavior, and exaggeration of premorbid personality traits such as obsessional and compulsive features. Premorbid personality traits may also be altered so that a previously compliant and well-modulated patient may become impulsive, irritable, and occasionally physically abusive. Inappropriate sexual and antisocial behaviors occasionally occur, but far more commonly the patient loses interest in sexuality, and antisocial behavior is limited to occasional angry outbursts when the patient does not comprehend why his or her activity is being limited by a care provider.

Table 1. DSM-III-R Diagnostic Criteria for Dementia

A. Demonstrable evidence of impairment in short- and long-term memory. Impairment in short-term memory (inability to learn new information) may be indicated by inability to remember three objects after five minutes. Long-term memory impairment (inability to remember information that was known in the past) may be indicated by inability to remember past personal information (e.g., what happened yesterday, birthplace, occupation) or facts of common knowledge (e.g., past presidents, well-known dates).

B. At least one of the following:

    (1) impairment in abstract thinking, as indicated by inability to find similarities and differences between related words, difficulty in defining words and concepts, and other similar tasks

    (2) impaired judgment, as indicated by inability to make reasonable plans to deal with interpersonal, family, and job-related problems and issues

    (3) other disturbances of higher cortical function, such as aphasia (disorder of language), apraxia (inability to carry out motor activities despite intact comprehension and motor function), agnosia (failure to recognize or identify objects despite intact sensory function), and "constructional difficulty" (e.g., inability to copy three-dimensional figures, assemble blocks, or arrange sticks in specific designs)

    (4) personality change, i.e., alteration or accentuation of premorbid traits

C. The disturbance in A and B significantly interferes with work or usual social activities or relationships with others.

D. Not occuring exclusively during the course of Delirium.

E. Either (1) or (2):

    (1) there is evidence from the history, physical examination, or laboratory tests of a specific organic factor (or factors) judged to be etiologically related to the disturbance

    (2) in the absence of such evidence, an etiologic organic factor can be presumed if the disturbance cannot be accounted for by any nonorganic mental disorder, e.g., Major Depression accounting for cognitive impairment

Criteria for severity of Dementia:

    Mild: Although work or social activities are significantly impaired, the capacity for independent living remains, with adequate personal hygiene and relatively intact judgment.

    Moderate: Independent living is hazardous, and some degree of supervision is necessary.

Table 1. DSM-III-R Diagnostic Criteria for Dementia, continued

---

Severe: Activities of daily living are so impaired that continual supervision is required, e.g., unable to maintain minimal personal hygiene; largely incoherent or mute.

Note. Reprinted with permission from the *Diagnostic and Statistical Manual of Mental Disorders (Third Edition-Revised).* Copyright © 1987 American Psychiatric Association.

Aphasia (disordered language due to structural brain damage) is a prominent feature of Alzheimer's disease (AD) and also occurs in other cortical dementing disorders. In AD the aphasia is of the fluent variety, usually beginning with anomia and paraphasias, but often progressing to global loss of speech and comprehension of spoken language. Aphasia is more prominent in early-onset AD but also occurs in late-onset AD. Aphasia in multi-infarct dementia (MID) depends on the location of infarcted brain tissue. A nonfluent or expressive aphasia is commonly present in MID if the dominant middle cerebral artery area has been involved. In the presence of such an aphasia, accurate evaluation of cognitive function is extremely difficult. Apraxia (inability to carry out motor activities despite intact comprehension and motor function) is common in AD. This symptom can be extremely distressing to care providers, who may attribute the inability to dress or use eating utensils to stubbornness and "passive-aggressive" behavior if the apraxia is not fully understood as a reflection of structural brain damage.

Associated Features of the Dementia Syndrome

Associated features of dementia resemble behaviors common to the "functional" psychiatric disorders and include depression, psychotic (delusional and hallucinatory) features, and sleep disorder. Several authors have reported increased rates of depressive symptomology in patients suffering from dementia. Reifler et al. (1982) reported that 23 percent of outpatients with dementia suffered from a coexistent depression. The rate of depression was highest in the mildly demented patients and decreased as the dementia became more severe. In a large outpatient dementia population, Reding et al. (1985) reported a similar prevalence of depression. Fifteen percent of 156 demented outpatients met *DSM-III* criteria for either major depressive disorder or dysthymic disorder. In this study, depression was more common in demented patients with AD (19 percent) than in patients with MID (6 percent).

Psychotic signs and symptoms such as hallucinations and persecutory delusions as well as other false beliefs not explainable by memory impairment alone are also common in patients suffering from dementia. Reisberg et al. (1987) have recently reported severe behaviorial disturbances in 33 AD outpatients. Common symptoms included delusions of theft (48 percent), agitation (48 percent), day–night disturbance (42 percent), motor restlessness (36 percent), violence (30 percent), verbal outbursts (24 percent), tearful episodes (24 percent), delusions of "one's house is not one's home" (21 percent), delusions of abandonment (21 percent), suspiciousness (21 percent), and paranoia (21 percent).

Some apparently delusional phenomena appear directly related to memory loss. A patient will forget the location of an object or forget having eaten a meal. When the misplaced object is perceived as missing, or the food eaten at a forgotten meal is discovered to be absent from the refrigerator, accusations of theft may result. Such "delusions of theft" based on defective memory are common causes of interpersonal turmoil in both the home and long-term care settings. Other psychotic phenomena, such as bizarre delusions or auditory and visual hallucinations, more closely resemble those manifested in schizophrenia. Although occurring in uncomplicated dementia, these latter symptoms should prompt evaluation for a superimposed delirium.

Finally, the importance of sleep disorder in dementia disorders should not be underestimated. Of the problems which cause eventual failure of the family to continue to provide care in the community, sleep disorder is among the most important. Prinz et al. (1982) have described the frequency and severity of disrupted diurnal sleep rhythms of patients with AD even in the early stages of the disorder. Clinically, these disrupted sleep rhythms present as nocturnal restlessness and wandering, behaviors that deprive the care provider of needed rest and may lead to eventual extrusion of the dementia patient from the home setting.

Differential Diagnosis of Dementia

Delirium may be mistaken for dementia, since both manifest impairment of memory and other intellectual abilities. However, in dementia the patient is alert (except in very late stages of dementia), whereas in delirium the patient's attention and level of consciousness are impaired. The symptoms and signs of the delirious patient are more likely to fluctuate than are those of the dementia patient. Furthermore, delirium usually clears within days (provided the etiologic agent has been removed) and rarely lasts longer than one month. However, some illnesses causing delirium, such as uremia or chronic hypnotic intoxication, can be of long duration, thus complicating differential diagnosis. Furthermore, delirium frequently complicates a dementing disorder, thus making it essential to keep in mind the possibility of concurrent diagnoses with special attention to possible reversible etiologies of a delirium superimposed on an irreversible dementing disorder. Further aspects of delirium will be discussed below.

Perhaps the differential diagnostic problem that has received the most attention is the differentiation of depression from dementia in the cognitively impaired elderly person. It should be emphasized at the outset of this discussion that depression superimposed on a dementing disorder is more common than a pure depressive disorder presenting with severe enough cognitive disturbance to mimic the dementia syndrome. This latter so-called depressive pseudodementia (Kiloh 1961) does occur, however, and can present diagnostic difficulties. Although the term "depressive pseudodementia" has been justly criticized by Reifler (1982), it will be used in this discussion both for historical purposes and for its widespread acceptance among practicing clinicians (Wells 1979). Depressive pseudodementia is usually distinguishable from a true dementia by a careful history and clinical examination (Post 1975). Depression usually begins with dysphoric mood, loss of interest and pleasure in the environment, decreased energy and activity level, changes in appetite and sleep pattern, increased somatic complaints, and decreased self-esteem. It is unusual for cognitive changes to occur in depression before the other symptoms and signs of depression have become obvious. In contrast, the patient with dementia will have exhibited memory loss and other cognitive deficits before signs and symptoms of depression appear. Clinical examination is also helpful in this differential diagnostic problem. The depressed patient is more likely to give "don't know" answers than to demonstrate clear memory deficits. Often, if the depressed patient can be motivated to attempt cognitive tasks, performance improves dramatically. Furthermore, aphasia is not present in the depressed patient. Persistently confusing diagnostic problems are usually resolved by several weeks of inpatient hospitalization and careful observation by hospital staff. A therapeutic trial of somatic antidepressant therapy can also resolve the problem.

Neuroendrocrine approaches the differential diagnosis of depression and dementia have not proved as valuable in clinical practice as one would have anticipated from initial reports. The finding that early escape of plasma cortisol from suppression by dexamethasone appeared to differentiate endogenous depression from other "functional" psychiatric disorders (Carroll et al. 1981) raised hopes that the overnight dexamethasone suppression test (DST) could be useful in differentiating depression from dementia (Rudorfer and Clayton 1981; McAllister et al. 1982). That is, a positive DST (early escape of plasma cortisol from dexamethasone suppression) would suggest the diagnosis of depression in the cognitively impaired patient, and therefore help identify depressive pseudodementia as well as depression complicating a dementing disorder. Because depression and dementia have several signs and symptoms in common (e.g., sleep disturbance, impaired concentration, agitation or retardation, and loss of interest in the environment), the data obtained from the clinical interview of the forgetful and often aphasic dementia patient can be difficult to interpret, an objective biologic measure that could help diagnose depression in the demented patient would be of obvious value. However, before the DST could be accepted as a valid diagnostic tool for differentiating depression from dementia, it had to be demonstrated that dementing illnesses per se were not associated with a positive DST. Although a few studies suggested possible applicability of the DST to this diagnostic problem (Carnes et al. 1983; Grunhaus et al. 1983), the majority of studies found that the common dementing disorders (AD and MID) have a high incidence of "positive" DST results even in patients who are free of diagnosable depression. Spar and Gerner (1982) and Raskind et al. (1982a) demonstrated a positive DST in approximately 50 percent of nondepressed dementia patients. These results have been confirmed by other investigators (McKeith 1984; Balldin et al. 1983; Abou-Saleh et al. 1987).

Another neuroendocrine test that has been applied to the diagnosis of depression, at least in cognitively intact younger adults, has been the response of thyrotropin-stimulating hormone (TSH) to its hypothalmatic releasing factor thyrotropin-releasing hormone (TRH). A blunted TSH response to TRH has been associated with depression in several studies (Loosen and Prange 1982). As with the DST, a blunted TSH response to TRH is only useful in discriminating between depression and a dementing illness if such a blunted TSH response occurs at a substantially lower frequency in dementing illnesses than in depression. Several recent studies have addressed this issue in patients with AD. The majority of studies report no difference in the TSH response to TRH in nondepressed AD subjects compared with normal elderly control subjects (Lampe et al. in press; Peabody et al. 1986; El-Sobky et al. 1986). However, Sunderland et al. (1985) reported a significantly lower mean increase in TSH concentrations in plasma following a TRH infusion in AD subjects as well as a higher incidence of a blunted TSH response (7 of 15 AD subjects vs. 0 of 10 control subjects) in AD. Further studies of the TRH stimulation test comparing depressed dementia patients with nondepressed dementia patients would be helpful in clarifying this area.

Another issue relevant to the differential diagnosis of depression and dementia is the question of whether a depressive disorder appearing for the first time in later life may be an early manifestation of an underlying dementing disorder. Although such a belief was once widespread, the classic psychogeriatric epidemiologic studies of Kay (1962) and Post (1972), in which patients with late-onset depression were carefully followed over time, suggested that such late-onset depression was not an early manifestation of a dementing disorder. Specifically, these two studies found that patients with late-life depressive disorder developed a dementing disorder at no higher frequency than occurred in the general population. On the other hand, a recent 3-year prospective study (Reding et al. 1985) of 44 elderly outpatients demonstrated that 16 (57 percent) of 28 of the depressed, nondemented patients went on to develop frank dementia. Thirteen of these 16 patients had subtle signs of organic neurologic disease. The discrepancies between the earlier British studies, suggesting that late-life depression was not related to dementing disorders, and the recent American study reporting a high incidence of development of dementia following the diagnosis of late-life depression are perhaps due to different diagnostic methods as well as the fact that the British subjects were psychiatrically hospitalized and the American subjects were outpatients.

Chronic schizophrenia in an elderly patient, particularly one who has spent many years institutionalized, may superficially resemble dementia. Difficulties in examining a withdrawn, socially impaired, and often uncooperative schizophrenic patient may further cloud the diagnostic issue. A history of chronic psychiatric illness beginning in early adulthood together with the presence of schizophreniform thought disorder, bizarre delusions and hallucinations, and grossly intact memory greatly favor the diagnosis of schizophrenia. Of course, schizophrenia and dementia may coexist in the same patient.

The Course of Dementia

It was previously implied by the *DSM-II* (American Psychiatric Association 1968) nomenclatural term "chronic organic brain syndrome" that the dementia syndrome had a persistent course. The *DSM-II* further implied that the onset of dementia was gradual. Although such assumptions are generally valid regarding the major dementing disorders of later life, the dementia syndrome can have an acute onset. For example, dementia secondary to acute hypoxia has an acute onset and runs a stable if not gradually improving course, as opposed to the insidious onset and progressively deteriorating course of AD. Furthermore, the course of dementia may be reversible, and in some fortunate cases patients actually may be restored to their previous level of cognitive function (e.g., successful surgical treatment of normal pressure hydrocephalus). Thus, the course of the dementia syndrome depends on the nature of the underlying dementing disorder.

Epidemiology of Dementia

Prevalence studies of dementia in late life are in relative agreement that about 4 percent of the population over age 65 suffers from a dementing illness severe enough to impair the ability to live independently (Mortimer 1983). Although the prevalence of dementia among younger persons is unknown, it is certainly much less common. Among this 4 percent of persons over age 65 suffering from dementia, at least two-thirds of them are demented secondarily to AD. Incidence studies of late-life dementia indicate that approximately 1 percent of those over age 65 become demented each year. A marked increase in prevalence occurs between ages 70 and 85. Although the incidence rates may become constant at approximately age 75, the greater reduction in expected survival duration among early-onset patients probably contributes to the sharply rising prevalence rate with age. The cumulative morbidity risk to the general population of developing severe dementia is probably close to 20 percent by the age of 80.

Diseases Causing the Dementia Syndrome

Primary Degenerative Dementia of the Alzheimer Type

The majority of patients with late-life dementia of insidious onset and a progressive deteriorating course are suffering from AD (Katzman 1976). The *DSM-III* term "primary degenerative dementia" has been modified to "primary degenerative dementia of the Alzheimer type" in *DSM-III-R*. This entity is referred to as AD in this chapter for simplicity and for concordance with the usage of this specific disease term in the general medical and neurologic literature. The *DSM-III-R* criteria for this disorder are listed in Table 2.

Alzheimer's disease is a combined clinical and neuropathologic diagnosis, which can definitely be made only when a patient meeting clinical criteria for AD is found at brain biopsy or postmortem neuropathologic examination to have the histopathologic changes of AD (numerous neuritic plaques and neurofibrillary tangles in the hippocampus and neocortex). If a psychiatrist practicing in the 1950s were to examine the scientific literature today, he or she would be mystified at the emphasis given to what was considered 30 years ago to be a relatively uncommon "presenile" dementing disorder. That AD would be considered the most important neuropsychiatric disorder of later life would be difficult to comprehend. This "epidemic" of AD can be attributed largely to increased knowledge of the correct etiology of dementia in later life. Prior to the studies of Blessed et al. (1968) the large number of persons who developed dementia in their 70s, 80s, and 90s were

Table 2.   DSM-III-R Diagnostic Criteria for Primary Degenerative
            Dementia of the Alzheimer Type

A.   Dementia (see Table 1)
B.   Insidious onset with a generally progressive deteriorating course
C.   Exclusion of all other specific causes of Dementia by history, physical
     examination, and laboratory tests

---

believed to have become demented from cerebrovascular insufficiency. Blessed et al. (1968) performed a careful neuropathologic and neurohistologic study of elderly demented patients compared with elderly persons who were cognitively intact at death. In more than half of these elderly "senile dementia" patients, the only neuropathologic lesions were the neuritic plaques and neurofibrillary tangles described by Alzheimer in two presenile onset dementia patients in 1907. Furthermore, the number of neuritic plaques in a given volume of brain tissue correlated significantly with cognitive function measured antemortem. A significantly positive although less robust correlation was found between neurofibrillary tangle count and antemortem cognitive function. That is, the greater the number of the classic neurohistologic lesions of AD, the more cognitively impaired was the patient before death. Only in approximately 15 percent of demented patients could their cognitive impairment be attributed to sequelae of cerebrovascular disease as measured by volume of infarcted brain tissue, and in another approximately 15 percent of patients, the lesions of AD and cerebrovascular disease coexisted. That cerebrovascular disease accounts for even this large a minority of cases of late-life dementia has recently been challenged by Brust (1983). It is now widely accepted that the majority of patients developing dementia in later life are suffering from AD (Katzman 1986).

Course of Alzheimer's disease. Alzheimer's disease begins insidiously. Subtle difficulties in memory are almost always the first symptom. Personality changes manifested by loss of interest and apathy often occur soon thereafter. Memory impairment gradually worsens and deficits in other cognitive abilities such as judgment, abstract reasoning, calculation, and visual/spatial skills appear. Sometimes early, but more often in the middle stages of AD, a fluent type of aphasia begins with difficulty naming objects or choosing the right word to express an idea (anomia). The aphasia is progressive in many patients, especially those with early-onset disease, who totally lose useful speech. Apraxia (the inability to perform a well-learned activity despite understanding the nature of the task and having intact motor function) also occurs and can be a tremendous problem for care providers. In the later stages of the illness, patients develop severe disruption of their sleep/wake cycle, and tend to wander, become episodically agitated and irritable, and lose the ability to attend to their personal needs, such as dressing, feeding, and personal hygiene. Motor deficits usually do not occur until the late stages of the illness and are predominantly manifested by rigidity. Myoclonic jerks develop in a substantial minority of patients (Hauser et al. 1986; Mayeux et al. 1985), particularly those with early-onset disease, and can erroneously suggest Creutzfeldt-Jakob disease. Seizures of several types may occur in the late stages of the illness. The terminal stages of AD are marked by inability to ambulate, speak, or attend to any personal needs. The course of AD can vary from 2 to 20 years. Many patients with very advanced disease live for extended periods of time if good nursing care is provided for them. Alzheimer's disease has a poor prognosis and significantly shortens life expectancy. In a 20-year follow-up study of hospitalized patients, Kay (1962) reported a mean life expectancy of 2.6 years for men and 2.3 years for women with no patients surviving to the end of the follow-up period. This mortality compared with a mean survival of 8.7 years for men and 10.9 years for women in a control group of nondemented elderly persons. Barclay et al. (1985) reported a 50 percent survival of 3.4 years for 199 AD patients diagnosed in an outpatient clinic. A 5-year follow-up study (Heyman et al. 1987) of 92 patients with early-onset AD revealed a cumulative mortality rate after entry into the study of 24 percent compared with an expected rate of 9.5 percent. The 5-year cumulative rate of admission to nursing homes for these originally community-based patients was 63 percent. Not surprisingly, greater impairments in language ability, cognitive function, and overall ratings of dementia at intake predicted subsequent institutional care and death. Risk of institutionalization and death was greater in younger onset patients with severe cognitive impairment compared with older individuals with the same degree of impairment.

Possible subtypes of Alzheimer's disease.   Although the neurohistologic features of AD do not differentiate between patients with early-onset (presenile) and late-onset (senile) disease, controversy still exists as to whether AD is a unitary entity or contains heterogeneous subgroups. Several clinicians have considered early-onset disease to be marked by more aphasic symptoms and a more malignant course. Seltzer and Sherwin (1983) recently documented a greater prevalence of aphasic disturbances in early-onset AD compared with late-onset AD. Mayeux et al. (1985) reviewed 121 consecutive patients and described four subgroups: a subgroup with relatively early onset, myoclonus, severe intellectual decline, and frequent late-stage mutism; a subgroup with extrapyramidal symptoms, severe intellectual and functional decline, and frequent psychotic symptoms; a benign group with little or no progression over a 4-year period; and a more typical group with gradual progression of intellectual and functional decline but without other distinguishing features. Bird et al. (1983) provided further evidence for myoclonic subgroup with early onset. In their neuropathologically examined series, patients with myoclonus had an earlier onset and very low levels of brain choline acetyltransferase (CAT) activity. Neurochemical differences between early and late onset subgroups in AD have been more extensively investigated by Roseor et al. (1984). These investigators compared brain neurochemical parameters of 49 patients who had died with AD to 54 patients who had died from non-dementing illnesses. As expected, the AD group exhibited noticeably reduced cholinergic activity manifested by reductions of the cholinergic marker enzyme choline acetyltransferase in the cerebral cortex. In addition, the AD patients showed reduced concentrations of norepinephrine, γ-aminobutyric acid (GABA), and somatostatin. Interesting differences existed between AD patients who died in their ninth and tenth decades as compared with younger patients who had died in their seventh and eighth decades. The group with younger age of death had widespread and severe cholinergic deficits together with deficiencies in brain content of norepinephrine, GABA, and somatostatin. In contrast, the older patients had a relatively restricted cholinergic deficit with reduced concentrations of choline acetyltransferase confined to the temporal lobe and hippocampus. In addition, the older group did not manifest deficiencies in norepinephrine, GABA, or somatostatin. Taken together, these data support the possibility of distinct subgroups in AD, particularly the concept of early-onset versus late-onset AD being different entities. However, these differences may be quantitative rather than qualitative. A large dose of the same etiologic factor could produce a more widespread and malignant disease at an earlier age. The failure to find differences in the gross or microscopic neuropathology in early-onset versus late-onset AD supports this latter possibility.

Accuracy of antemortem diagnosis of Alzheimer's disease. Recent neuropathologic studies have demonstrated that the antemortem diagnosis of AD, if based on standard diagnostic criteria such as those of *DSM-III* or those of the National Institute of Neurologic, Communicative Diseases and Stroke–Alzheimer's Disease and Related Disorders Association (NINCDS-ADRDA) work group (McKahnn et al. 1984) will be accurate more than 80 percent of the time. Sulkava et al. (1983) reported that of 27 autopsy patients fulfilling *DSM-III* criteria for primary degenerative dementia, 22 met neuropathologic criteria for AD. No patients had MID. Of the five patients with non-AD neuropathology, one had Parkinson's disease, two had hippocampal and subcortical neuronal loss and gliosis, and two had nonspecific neuropathologic abnormalities. Molsa et al. (1985) reported that 20 of 28 patients diagnosed as AD antemortem had only the neuropathologic stigmata of AD at autopsy. An additional three subjects had both AD and MID neuropathologically. It should be noted that these investigators' criteria for MID were the presence of any ischemic lesions, either macroscopically or microscopically, and the absence of neocortical tangles. These criteria may have overdiagnosed MID (Brust 1983). Risse et al. (1986) reported neuropathologic findings in 21 AD patients evaluated consecutively antemortem and diagnosed by *DSM-III* criteria for primary degenerative dementia. Seventeen of 21 patients had AD neuropathologically. Of the remaining four patients, one had Parkinson's disease and three had extensive subcortical or combined subcortical and cortical gliosis, neuronal loss, and atrophy. Among 11 patients with predominantly early-onset AD and mild to moderate dementia undergoing cortical biopsy, Fox et al. (1985) documented neuritic plaque counts diagnostic of AD by histologic criteria (Khachaturian 1985) in all cases. This report needs replication before its implications can be accepted. The exclusion by these investigators of patients with aphasia, apraxia, or visual agnosia (clinical features that are commonly present in AD, especially in early-onset patients) makes the generalizability of these findings uncertain.

A specific chemical antemortem diagnostic marker for AD measurable in blood or cerebrospinal fluid would be very useful in both clinical care and research. Attempts to identify such a marker have been frustrating to date (Hollander et al. 1986), but recent studies (Davies and Wolozin 1987) have described an antigen that may prove to be specific to AD. These investigators raised monoclonal antibodies against human nucleus basalis tissue. One of these antibodies recognized a 68,000-dalton protein that appears to accumulate only in brain tissue from patients with AD and Down's syndrome. Furthermore this "A68" antigen is measurable in cerebrospinal fluid and in preliminary studies (Wolozin and Davies in press) appears only in cerebrospinal fluid from AD patients. The diagnostic as well as possible pathophysiologic significance of the A68 antigen awaits further studies.

Pathophysiology of Alzheimer's disease. Attempts to understand the pathophysiology of AD have focused on two areas: understanding the biochemical nature of neuritic plaques and neurofibrillary tangles (the histopathologic hallmarks of AD); and understanding changes in brain neurotransmitter systems that may mediate clinical expression of the disorder. Recent advances in protein biochemistry and successful solubilization of plaques and tangles have led to major progress in the first area. Careful neurochemical and cytochemical studies in postmortem and in some cases brain biopsy tissue have led to advances in the second area as well.

Neurofibrillary tangles are bundles of submicroscopic filaments wound into a paired helical structure that accumulate in neuronal cell bodies and are readily demonstrated by silver staining and other staining techniques. Neuritic plaques are composed of clusters of degenerating nerve terminals that surround a core of proteinaceous material that has the chemical and ultrastructural characteristics of amyloid protein. These extracellular neuritic plaques and intraneuronal neurofibrillary tangles are characteristically found in the temporal and parietal lobe association areas, the hippocampus, the entorhinal cortex and the amygdala as well as in many subcortical brain structures. It should be emphasized that qualitatively indistinguishable lesions are found in small numbers in normal older adults. The neurohistologic diagnosis of AD is based on large numbers of these lesions widely distributed throughout the brain.

Chemical analysis of the neurofibrillary tangle was inhibited for many years by the insolubility of these structures. Recent success in solubilization of neurofibrillary tangles in formic acid has led to studies demonstrating cytoskeletal proteins such as the microtubule-associated phosphoprotein tau in neurofibrillary tangles (Selkoe 1986). Studies of the amyloid found in neuritic plaques and the congophilic angiopathy of AD have also been productive. The vascular amyloid protein of congophilic angiopathy was sequenced by Glenner and Wong (1984) to position 28, and knowledge of this protein sequence has led to advances in the molecular genetics of AD. Subsequent solubilization of neuritic plaque core amyloid protein has revealed an amino acid composition similar to the vascular amyloid protein (Masters et al. 1985). Further studies have suggested that amyloid fibrils in neuritic plaques, amyloid fibrils in blood vessels, and the intraneuronal paired helical filaments of neurofibrillary tangles are composed of the same protein (Masters et al. 1985; Kidd et al. 1985). Other investigators, however, have presented immunologic data suggesting that the vascular and plaque amyloid in AD are chemically different from neurofibrillary tangles (Selkoe et al. 1986). Much further work is necessary to understand the chemical nature and ultimately the origin of these complex histologic structures.

Attempts to discover abnormalities in brain neurotransmitter systems in AD that might be correctable by pharmacologic treatment with subsequent symptomatic improvement received impetus from the successful application of such a strategy to Parkinson's disease. In Parkinson's disease, the discovery of a dopaminergic deficit has led to effective symptomatic treatment with dopaminergic-enhancing drugs. That such a strategy might succeed in AD became plausible in the late 1970s with the discovery of a specific deficit in the central cholinergic system in postmortem tissue from AD patients (Davies and Maloney 1976; Perry et al. 1978) manifested by substantial decreases in the synthetic enzyme for acetyl choline, choline acetyltransferase, in hippocampus and cortex in AD patients compared with age-matched normal controls. The cholinergic deficiency hypothesis was strengthened by Whitehouse et al. (1982), who demonstrated extensive neuronal damage in the nucleus basalis of Meynert in AD brain tissue. This basal forebrain nucleus is the source of cholinergic neurons projecting to the neocortex. This finding led to speculation that damage to the nucleus basalis of Meynert was a primary lesion in AD. Others believe that deterioration of the nucleus basalis of Meynert is secondary to cortical pathology. Pearson et al. (1983) compared cholinergic neurons in the nucleus basalis of Meynert in AD and age- and sex-matched normal brains. Cholinergic neuronal bodies in AD were substantially smaller but not decreased in number. The persistence of shrunken cholinergic neurons is similar to that seen in an experimental animal study of retrograde cellular degeneration in the nucleus basalis following primary damage to the cerebral cortex (Sofroniew et al. 1983). Furthermore, cortical choline acetyltransferase activity in AD is far greater than the loss of cells from the nucleus basalis of Meynert (Perry et al. 1982). In brain biopsy tissue from AD patients, reduction in cortical choline acetyltransferase activity is significantly correlated with senile plaque frequency (Neary et al. 1986b). In this study of 17 patients, however, the highest correlation between severity of dementia as determined by mental test performance was with pathologic changes in large cortical neurons (cell loss, reduction in nuclear and nucleolar volume, and cytoplasmic ribonucleic acid content). It has been speculated that at least some of these large cortical neurons that may play a hitherto unrecognized role in the pathophysiology of AD are glutamate neurons (Hardy et al. 1987). Further support for the relationship between cholinergic neurons and neuritic plaques comes from a study in which plaques from monkeys aged 4 to 31 years were stained for acetylcholinesterase, a marker for presynaptic cholinergic neurons (Struble 1982). Both immature and mature plaques were rich in acetylcholinesterase activity, but as the plaque matured the amount of amyloid increased and the number of neurites and the activity of acetylcholinesterase decreased. End-stage plaques were rich in amyloid and lacked acetylcholinesterase. These observations suggest an association between cholinergic innervation and the evolution of the neuritic plaque in this animal model. In contrast to the clear presynaptic cholinergic abnormalities in AD, most studies have found postsynaptic muscarinic receptors (the predominant species of cholinergic receptors in the brain) to be relatively unchanged from those of normal age-matched controls (Davis and Wolozin 1987). The persistence of such postsynaptic muscarinic cholinergic receptors has provided further rationale for attempts to enhance the activity of remaining presynaptic cholinergic neurons or to directly stimulate these postsynaptic receptors. A recent study has documented substantial decreases in postsynaptic nicotinic cholinergic receptors in AD (Whitehouse et al. 1986).

Although it is not clear whether the cholinergic deficit in AD is a primary or secondary phenomenon, the cholinergic deficiency hypothesis has generated pharmacologic strategies to enhance cholinergic activity as a potential means of improving memory in AD. Results of these trials have been disappointing compared with the success of dopaminergic enhancement in Parkinson's disease, but attempts to find an effective treatment via manipulation of the cholinergic system may yet prove at least partially successful (see below). The difficulty encountered by investigators attempting to improve symptoms in AD with purely cholinergic interventions may be based on the recently described deficits in multiple other brain neurotransmitter systems. Studies in postmortem tissue have suggested decreased brain noradrenergic activity in AD. Cell counts in the locus ceruleus, the major noradrenergic (norepinephrine) projection nucleus to the central nervous system, are reduced in AD, particularly in early-onset patients (Bondareff et al. 1987; Tomlinson et al. 1981). Studies have demonstrated decreased norepinephrine content in hypothalamus, caudate, and cerebral cortex (Mann et al. 1982; Adolfson et al. 1979). However, the noradrenergic deficiency hypothesis is not as clearly supported as is the cholinergic deficiency hypothesis. The content of the primary brain metabolite of norepinephrine, 3-methoxy-4-hydroxyphenylglycol (MHPG), is elevated in several brain areas in which norepinephrine content is decreased (Winblad et al. 1982). In cortical biopsy tissue from temporal lobe of AD patients, MHPG concentration was increased in early-onset patients (Francis et al. 1985). Cerebrospinal fluid concentrations of norepinephrine and MHPG are elevated in early-onset AD patients with advanced disease (Raskind et al. 1984). These studies are compatible with increased norepinephrine turnover in patients with early-onset AD. The apparent contradiction between dramatic cell loss in the locus ceruleus and increased norepinephrine turnover in the central nervous system in early-onset AD may represent increased activity of remaining noradrenergic neurons (Hollander et al. 1986).

Several central nervous system neuropeptides are also deficient in AD. Somatostatin, a neuropeptide primarily found in intrinsic cortical neurons, has been consistently demonstrated to be reduced in neocortex and hippocampus (Davies et al. 1980; Ferrier et al. 1983; Rossor et al. 1984). Somatostatin may be specifically reduced in parietal association cortex (Tamminga et al. 1985). Cerebrospinal fluid concentrations of somatostatin are also decreased in AD (Wood et al. 1982; Francis et al. 1984; Soininen et al. 1984; Serby et al. 1984; Raskind et al. 1986). Although the functional significance of extrahypothalamic somatostatin is unclear, when injected intracerebroventricularly, somatostatin increases the excitability of the cerebral cortex and produces arousal in animals (Ioffe et al. 1978; Reichlin 1983). Of further interest is the coexistence of acetylcholinesterase activity (a marker of presynaptic cholinergic neurons) and somatostatin in neurons cultured from rat cerebrum (Delfs et al. 1984). Furthermore, somatostatin-containing neurons contain neurofibrillary tangles (Roberts et al. 1985), and somatostatin has been detected in neuritic plaques (Morrison et al. 1985).

Vasopressin is a neuropeptide that enhances learning in animal models (DeWied and Versteeg 1979; Kovacs et al. 1979). Although the central versus peripheral site of action of vasopressin has been controversial, it appears clear that at least a component of the positive effect of vasopressin on learning is mediated centrally (DeWied et al. 1984). Measurements of vasopressin concentrations in cerebrospinal fluid in AD have consistently demonstrated reduced concentrations (Sorensen et al. 1983; Sundquist et al. 1983; Mazurek et al. 1986a; Raskind et al. 1986). Measurements of the concentration of vasopressin in AD brain tissue have revealed significantly lower concentrations in globus pallidus (Rossor et al. 1984) and in hippocampus, nucleus accumbens, and globus pallidus interna (Mazurek et al. 1986b). That decreases in vasopressin concentrations in AD are not merely indications of nonspecific diffuse neuronal degeneration is suggested by the finding of normal concentrations in AD of oxytocin, a neuropeptide produced in cell bodies in the same hypothalamic areas as vasopressin (Raskind et al. 1986). In fact, oxytocin concentrations may be elevated in hippocampal and temporal cortical brain tissue in AD (Mazurek et al. 1987). This finding is of interest given reports that centrally administered oxytocin impairs learning in animal models (Bohus et al. 1978; Kovacs et al. 1979). Several studies have reported decreased concentrations of corticotropin-releasing factor (CRF) in AD (Bissette et al. 1985; DeSouza et al. 1986). The latter study also found reciprocal increases in CRF receptor binding in cortical areas in which CRF concentrations were reduced, suggesting a neurotransmitter role for CRF in brain and a modulation of brain CRF receptors associated with altered CRF content. Taken together, the abnormalities in brain neuropeptides in AD highlight the complexity of the multiple neurochemical lesions that involve not only classic neurotransmitters such as acetylcholine and norepinephrine, but also more recently described neurotransmitters and neuromodulators whose function is only beginning to be understood.

Genetics of Alzheimer's disease. Much controversy surrounds the exact nature of the genetic transmission of AD. It is well established that in certain unusual families, AD is transmitted in an autosomal-dominant manner with early onset of illness in affected family members being the rule (Cook et al. 1979). Detecting a genetic pattern of transmission in AD is complicated by the late age of expression of AD, raising the possibility that most relatives at risk will die of some other disorder before AD will ever be expressed. This phenomenon makes most AD patients appear to be "sporadic." Heston (1981) reported that if one evaluates the empirical risks to relatives, a large proportion of cases of AD are isolated. However, he found that the risk to siblings of AD probands with onset before age 70 and who had an affected parent was in the range of an autosomal-dominant trait (approaching 50 percent).

Using a different approach, a recent study (Breitner and Folstein 1984) investigated AD patients with aphasia and found the 90-year lifetime risk of AD among the pooled first-degree relatives of such probands exceeded 50 percent, thus suggesting autosomal-dominant transmission. Relatives of the AD probands without aphasia were at low risk for AD, which was no greater than that of the general population. It should be noted that this study was performed in a nursing home population composed predominantly of late-onset AD patients in their eighth and ninth decades of life.

In a recent study of predominantly early-onset AD patients who met NINCDS criteria for AD, Mohs et al. (1987) demonstrated that first-degree relatives of patients showed a 46 percent cumulative incidence of probable AD by 86 years of age. This risk was four times that for a control population. As in the previous study, these investigators applied the Kaplan-Meier Life Table method to estimate a specific cumulative incidence of AD in relatives of AD probands and controls. The actual prevalence of cognitive impairment among relatives of AD probands was 14 percent and among control relatives 4.3 percent.

The issue of the presence of aphasia indicating possible autosomal-dominant transmission still remains a possibility given that aphasia is present in the great majority of AD patients with early onset (such as those in the study of Mohs et al.) whereas late-onset AD patients (such as those studied by Breitner and Folstein) probably have a higher proportion of patients with minimal or no aphasia (Seltzer and Sherwin 1983). These nonaphasic AD patients may represent a form of AD with nondominant transmission.

Data from a recent twin study (Nee et al. 1987) suggest that AD cannot be entirely accounted for by a single autosomal gene. These investigators studied 22 twin pairs in which one or both twins had AD. Seven monozygotic pairs were concordant for AD, but 10 monozygotic pairs were discordant. Two dizygotic pairs were concordant for AD, while three dizygotic pairs were discordant. It should be remembered, however, that previous twin studies have shown that the expression of AD in monozygotic twins can occur more than 10 years apart (Cook et al. 1979) and that some of these monozygotic twin pairs currently discordant may become concordant over time. Even if this qualification is kept in mind, however, some nongenetic factor is necessary to explain the differential age of expression of the AD phenotype.

An important aspect of the genetics of AD is the observation that persons with Down's syndrome (Trisomy 21) who live into middle age develop the classic neurohistologic features of AD with widespread neuritic plaques and neurofibrillary tangles in the hippocampus and neocortex. This subject has recently been reviewed by Karlinsky (1986). In addition, Down's syndrome patients over 35 years of age manifest the cholinergic deficiency seen in AD (Godridge et al. 1987). Although controversy exists as to whether these neurohistologic and neurochemical changes are accompanied by frank dementia in middle-aged Down's syndrome patients, the evidence suggests that having three copies of chromosome 21 predisposes to very early onset AD.

Pathogenesis of Alzheimer's disease: molecular genetic studies. Using genetic linkage analysis with restriction fragment length polymorphism deoxyribonucleic acid (DNA) markers, St. George Hyslop et al. (1987) studied four large kindreds with histologically proved familial AD. Results indicated that the familial AD gene mapped to chromosome 21, the chromosome which is trisomic in Down's syndrome. However, the familial AD gene was not located in the region of chromosome 21 associated with the Down's syndrome phenotype. Tanzi et al. (1987) used a complementary DNA probe for the amyloid beta protein originally isolated from AD cerebrovascular amyloid by Glenner and Wong (1984). The amyloid beta protein gene locus also mapped to chromosome 21. Regional localization of the amyloid beta protein gene suggested it is located in the vicinity of the gene defect responsible for familial AD; it further suggested that the amyloid beta protein gene may be involved in the pathogenesis of familial AD. Goldgaber et al. (1987) used an oligonucleotide probe corresponding to the first 20 amino acids of the amyloid beta protein to map the gene encoding the protein that forms amyloid in AD to chromosome 21 and to demonstrate that this gene is highly conserved in evolution. Although these reports taken together suggest that both a gene for the amyloid protein and a gene for familial AD are located on chromosome 21, much work remains to be done to demonstrate that these genes are in fact identical and to isolate the gene and demonstrate the abnormal gene product responsible for the phenotypic expression of AD.

Other than the genetic risk for AD and the increased risk for AD in Down's syndrome, epidemiologic studies have revealed few factors that appear to predispose toward the development of AD. One potential risk factor that has been noted at a significantly higher rate in AD patients than normal controls in case control studies is a remote history of head trauma severe enough to cause loss of consciousness (Mortimer et al. 1985; Heyman et al. 1984). Although found significantly more frequently in AD patients than controls, such a history of head trauma occurs in fewer than 25 percent of AD subjects and its link to a possible pathogenetic mechanism is not clear.

Aluminum. Several lines of evidence suggest that aluminum, the third most common element in the earth's crust, may play a role in the pathophysiology or even pathogenesis of AD. The severe encephalopathy seen in chronic dialysis patients with high plasma levels of aluminum secondary to high concentrations of aluminum in dialysate solution suggests that aluminum can impair cognitive and other neurologic functions in humans (Sideman and Manor 1982). Furthermore, neurofibrillary changes can be induced in rabbits by injecting aluminum into the central nervous system (Wisniewski et al. 1980). Several studies (Crapper et al. 1973; Trapp et al. 1978) have reported increased concentrations of aluminum in postmortem brain tissue from patients with AD. Using x-ray spectrometry at the histologic level, Perl and Brody (1980) demonstrated focal intraneuronal accumulations of aluminum within neurofibrillary-tangle-bearing neurons in hippocampal tissue from patients with AD. Tangle-free neurons from the same AD material as well as neurons from nondemented age-matched controls failed to show similar degrees of aluminum accumulation. Furthermore, aluminosilicate accumulations have been reported in the cores of neuritic plaques (Candy et al. 1986). Although these data provide circumstantial evidence for a neurotoxic role of aluminum in AD, other studies cast doubt on this hypothesis. Several investigators have failed to find differences in brain aluminum concentrations between AD patients and age-matched controls (McDermott et al. 1977; Markesbery et al. 1981). Delaney (1979) found no difference in cerebrospinal fluid aluminum concentrations between patients with AD and patients with other neurologic disorders. On balance, however, the possibility that aluminum is somehow involved in the pathophysiology or even pathogenesis of AD deserves further investigation.

Dementia in Parkinson's Disease

The high prevalence of dementia in Parkinson's disease was not fully appreciated until the functional life of Parkinson's disease was extended by the introduction of L-dopa and other specific dopaminergic-enhancing therapies. These patients generally present with memory impairment and slowness of thinking with preserved language function although aphasia and apraxia may also occur (Perry et al. 1985). Sweet et al. (1975) reported that dementia was found in approximately one-third of 100 Parkinson's disease patients followed for a 6-year period while being treated with L-dopa. Lieberman et al. (1979) reported that 32 percent of 520 Parkinson's disease patients evaluated over an 8-year period had moderate to marked dementia. The demented patients were somewhat older than the nondemented patients (70.4 years vs. 65.5 years), and the incidence of dementia in Parkinson's disease was 10 times higher than in normal age-matched controls.

It has been proposed that the dementia seen in Parkinson's disease actually could be attributed to the concurrent presence of AD in these patients. This hypothesis received some support from a study by Hakim and Mathieson (1979) in which 34 cases of Parkinson's disease diagnosed at autopsy were found to have more neuritic plaques, neurofibrillary tangles, granulovacuolar degeneration, and cortical cell loss than were present in control subjects who had died from trauma or cerebral infarction. This study can be criticized because patients were not diagnosed as having Parkinson's disease antemortem and because the neuropathologic stigmata of Parkinson's disease (cell loss and Lewy bodies in the substantia nigra) have been documented in a substantial percentage of patients with clear-cut AD (Leverenz and Sumi 1984).

That the dementia of Parkinson's disease is in fact not usually secondary to concomitant AD has received support from several recent studies. Chui et al. (1984) reported careful histopathologic studies of cerebral cortex, hippocampus, substantia nigra, locus ceruleus, and nucleus basalis of Meynert in four parkinsonian patients whose dementia had been carefully documented neuropsychologically antemortem. In these patients, dementia was associated with severe neuronal loss in subcortical nuclei, but significant numbers of neuritic plaques or neurofibrillary tangles were not documented in hippocampus or cerebral cortex.

Recent studies (Perry et al. 1985; Ball 1984) have confirmed that the dementia of Parkinson's disease usually occurs in the absence of substantial AD type changes in the cortex. Perry et al. (1985) suggest that the cognitive deficits in Parkinson's disease may be related to abnormalities in central nervous system cholinergic systems. In their parkinsonian subjects, choline acetyltransferase reductions in temporal neocortex correlated with the degree of mental impairment. Furthermore, choline acetyltransferase activity correlated with the number of neurons in the nucleus basalis of Meynert, suggesting that primary degeneration of basal forebrain cholinergic neurons may be related to the dementia of Parkinson's disease. Cash et al. (1987) have suggested that damage to the locus ceruleus, the nucleus whose neurons provide the majority of noradrenergic innervation to the central nervous system, is related to dementia of Parkinson's disease. They found that norepinephrine and its metabolite MHPG were decreased in the locus ceruleus of 7 demented Parkinson's disease patients compared with 13 age-matched control patients who were free of psychiatric or neurologic disease. In contrast, in eight nondemented Parkinson's disease patients there was no difference in norepinephrine or MHPG in the locus ceruleus compared with the control population. Reductions in brain CRF have also been reported in Parkinson's disease (Whitehouse et al. 1987). If one accepts that neuritic plaques and neurofibrillary tangles are the biologic substrates of the dementia of AD, then the dementia of Parkinson's disease appears to be qualitatively different. It is intriguing, however, that similar neurochemical systems (cholinergic, noradrenergic, CRF) are damaged in both disorders.

Multi-Infarct Dementia

As recently as the early 1960s, it was widely believed that most elderly patients with dementia were cognitively impaired secondary to cerebrovascular disease. This erroneous notion was dispelled by the landmark study of Blessed et al. (1968), which definitively demonstrated that AD was the principle cause of dementia in later life. However, Tomlinson et al. (1970), using the same neuropathologic material, demonstrated that cerebrovascular dementia, defined as dementia resulting from enough loss of brain tissue secondary to repeated episodes of cerebral infarction to impair cognitive functions globally, was still an important cause of late-life dementia. Using a "cut-off" of more than 50-ml volume of infarction, these investigators found that 17 percent of 50 demented elderly people had definite or probable arteriosclerotic dementia and an additional 18 percent had a combination of arteriosclerotic dementia and AD. On the basis of this carefully studied but small sample of demented patients, subsequent investigators have accepted multiple cerebral infarctions as the basis of dementia in late life if cerebral infarctions can be demonstrated radiologically antemortem or at autopsy. However, the contribution of location of infarcts and quantity of infarcted tissue to the ultimate production of dementia awaits further careful clinical pathologic studies (Kase 1986). It remains possible that multi-infarct dementia, a term introduced by Hachinski et al. (1974), continues to be overdiagnosed in elderly demented patients (Brust 1983).

The *DSM-III-R* includes diagnostic criteria for MID (see Table 3). The typical course of MID includes a relatively abrupt onset with stepwise deterioration in cognitive function. "Patchy" deterioration in the early stages of the illness leaves some intellectual functions relatively intact. Patients with MID are usually more aware of their deficits than patients with AD, and may have a higher incidence of depression complicating their illness (Cummings and Benson 1983). The "typical" neuropathologic features of MID are variable. Some patients have multiple infarcts of the cerbral cortex. These patients often present with hemiparesis, aphasia, and hemisensory findings. In the presence of a dense aphasia, the presence of dementia may be difficult to document accurately. Other patients have lesions involving the perforating

Table 3. Diagnostic Criteria for Multi-infarct Dementia

A. Dementia (see Table 1).

B. Stepwise deteriorating course with "patchy" distribution of deficits (i.e., affecting some functions, but not others) early in the course

C. Focal neurologic signs and symptoms (e.g., exaggeration of deep tendon reflexes, extensor plantar response, pseudobulbar palsy, gait abnormalities, weakness of an extremity, etc.).

D. Evidence from history, physical examination, or laboratory tests of significant cerebrovascular disease that is judged to be etiologically related to the disturbance.

Note. Reprinted with permission from the *Diagnostic and Statistical Manual of Mental Disorders (Third Edition-Revised).* Copyright © 1987 American Psychiatric Association.

arteries with production of small "lacunes" in subcortical structures commonly including the basal ganglia, internal capsule, thalamus, and brainstem. These patients present with gait disturbance, rigidity, pseudobalbar palsy, emotional incontinence, and paucity of speech and motor activity. A third entity, presumably secondary to ischemia of cortical white matter, has been termed "Binswanger's disease." That Binswanger's disease is in fact a different entity from multiple lacunar infarctions is debatable (Roman 1985). To increase the confusion, magnetic resonance imaging scans are finding radiolucent areas in cortical white matter, the nature of which remains unclear pending neuropathologic correlation. However, these findings are being reported as compatible with Binswanger's disease in some centers.

Despite these controversies, it is reasonably clear that multiple cerebral infarctions and other ischemic sequelae of cerebrovascular insufficiency produce or contribute to dementia in elderly persons. Hachinski et al. (1975) proposed a diagnostic rating scale for diagnosing MID that has gained wide acceptance. The Hachinski scale derives an ischemic score from 13 items based on clinical observation. A score of 7 or above on the scale suggests MID and a score of 4 or below suggests AD. The Hachinski ischemic score was partially validated by Rosen et al. (1980) in a retrospective study of 14 neuropathologically examined patients who met neuropathologic criteria for either AD, MID, or mixed AD and MID and who had been documented on neuropsychologic testing antemortem to have been moderately or severely demented. The Hachinski score was derived retrospectively by chart review and information from family and medical staff. The ischemic score clearly differentiated patients with AD from those with MID but patients with mixed

MID and AD were not differentiable from persons with MID alone. Eight features were found to be characteristic of MID in this study. Of primary importance were abrupt onset, stepwise deterioration, history of stroke, focal neurologic signs, and focal neurologic symptoms. A history or presence of hypertension was of secondary importance but still differentiated MID from AD. Hypertension is an accepted risk factor for the development of MID and is clearly more common in MID patients than in AD patients (St. Clair and Whalley 1983). Of questionable importance were somatic complaints and emotional incontinence.

Two recent studies support the concept of MID as a valid entity. Rogers et al. (1986) prospectively studied 181 neurologically normal elderly volunteers (mean age 71 years) who included a large percentage (49 percent) preselected for risk factors for stroke such as hypertension. Over the course of the study, 5.5 percent of the patients developed MID and 3.3 percent developed AD. The higher incidence of MID probably reflected the preselection of half of the volunteers for the presence of stroke risk factors. Of the 88 volunteers at risk for stroke, 11.4 percent developed MID within 7 years. Of interest was the finding that in MID patients, cerebral blood flow values as measured by the xenon inhalation technique began to decline approximately 2 years before the onset of MID symptoms. In contrast, in the AD patients cerebral blood flow levels remained normal until symptoms of dementia appeared and declined rapidly thereafter. Survival rates in AD and MID also appear to differ. Barclay et al. (1985) over a 5-year period followed 199 patients with AD and 69 patients with MID as defined by a Hachinski ischemic score greater than 6. Both diagnostic categories had comparable progression of behavioral and cognitive impairment and institutionalization rate at follow-up. However, 50 percent survival rate from diagnosis was only 2.6 years for MID patients compared with 3.4 years for AD patients. Fifty percent survival from estimated onset of disease was 6.7 years for MID patients and 8.1 years for AD patients. Thus, MID patients have a higher mortality than AD patients, which raises the question of whether controlling known risk factors for MID would slow the progression of the disorder. This question is particularly relevant for hypertension, a known risk factor for stroke and a treatable condition. To study this question Meyer et al. (1986) followed 52 MID patients prospectively for a mean interval of 22 months. Among hypertensive patients with MID, improved cognitive function and clinical course correlated with control of systolic blood pressure within the upper limits of normal (135 mm Hg mercury to 150 mm Hg). However, if systolic blood pressure was reduced below this level, MID patients deteriorated. Furthermore, normotensive patients with MID manifested improved cognition with cessation of cigarette smoking. This study suggests the value of carefully reducing systolic blood pressure, keeping in mind that too vigorous control of hypertension in MID patients can result in accelerated deterioration rather than improvement.

Pick's Disease

Pick's disease is a progressive dementing disorder of middle and later life that is difficult to differentiate from AD antemortem, but the neuropathology and neurochemistry of which bear little relation to those of AD. The gross pathology demonstrates frontotemporal atrophy. Microscopic changes include neuronal loss, gliosis, and the presence of Pick's bodies (masses of cytoskeletal elements) inside neuronal cell bodies. The cholinergic and somatostatinergic deficits of AD are not present in Pick's disease (Wood et al. 1983). Although Pick's disease is a rare neuropathologic diagnosis in most centers, it was found to be relatively common in one Scandinavian series (Sjogren et al. 1952) and accounted for 5 percent of progressive dementing disorders in a Minnesota series (Heston et al. 1987). Although the neuropathologic differences between AD and Pick's disease are clear, these two illnesses appear to share specific antigens in degenerating neurons (Rasool and Selkoe 1985). Clinically, it has been suggested that Pick's disease shows affective disturbances and excessive eating resembling aspects of the Klüver-Bucy syndrome (Cummings and Duchen 1981; Constantinidis et al. 1974). Heston et al. (1987) confirmed that excessive eating may be a feature of Pick's disease but that affective changes were not striking in their patients, and most cases were clinically indistinguishable from AD antemortem. These investigators also found evidence for a genetic component in Pick's disease.

A recent study using positron emission tomography (PET) (Kamo et al. 1987) found a sharply decreased cortical metabolic rate for glucose in the frontal lobes of a Pick's disease patient who had extensive gliosis and neuronal loss in the frontal lobes postmortem. This PET pattern was sufficiently distinctive to suggest that PET scan may be a useful antemortem diagnostic test to distinguish Pick's from AD.

Normal-Pressure Hydrocephalus

Normal-pressure hydrocephalus is probably the most important disorder producing a truly correctable dementia syndrome. This syndrome was described by Adams et al. (1965). The classical clinical presentation included the triad of dementia, gait disorder, and urinary incontinence associated with ventricular dilatation in the absence of evidence of persistently elevated intracranial pressure. Although the etiology of normal-pressure hydrocephalus in most patients is unclear, a substantial minority result from previous subarachnoid hemorrhage, meningitis, or other neurologic insults. The demonstration that some or all aspects of the syndrome were occasionally reversible by a cerebroventricular shunt created widespread enthusiasm for surgical treatment, which was performed in large numbers of patients with dementia (many of whom did not have normal-pressure hydrocephalus but rather were suffering from AD and had ventricular dilatation secondary to shrinkage of cortical tissue). Recent more careful patient selection appears to have led to improved outcome in recently reported series. Thomasen et al. (1986) recently evaluated 40 patients with normal-pressure hydrocephalus neuropsychologically before and 12 months after a ventriculoatrial shunt procedure. Cognitive function improved in 16 patients, was unchanged in 19, and deteriorated in 5. Known cause of normal-pressure hydrocephalus, short history, and absence of gyral atrophy were among factors associated with a good postoperative outcome. The severity of ventricular dilatation relative to the degree of sulcal enlargement on head computed tomographic scan helps differentiate normal-pressure hydrocephalus from cerebral atrophy secondary to AD or other primary degenerative dementing disorders. Isotope cisternography is also helpful if the classic cerebrospinal fluid dynamic aberrations are demonstrated, but its diagnostic capacity is certainly not absolute. It has been suggested (Wikkelso et al. 1982) that drainage of 20 to 40 ml of cerebrospinal fluid by lumbar puncture with subsequent transient clinical improvement indicates patients most likely to respond to a shunt procedure. This finding is of interest but awaits a controlled evaluation before it can be accepted. Because gait disturbance is a primary diagnostic feature of normal-pressure hydrocephalus, especially in the setting of mild dementia, patients with other diseases that complicate gait evaluation, such as those with severe arthritis (Rasker 1985) may be at risk of a missed diagnosis of a potentially correctable dementing disorder. Meyer et al. (1985) prospectively evaluated 10 patients with dementia due to normal-pressure hydrocephal and then performed serial follow-up evaluations at intervals up to 8 months following a ventricular shunting procedure. Cerebral blood flow in both white and grey matter progressively increased for 3 months after shunting and remained increased except for one case complicated by chronic alcoholism. Clinical recovery correlated with improved cerebral perfusion. The majority of patients showed improvement in urinary continence and gait as well as activities of daily living. Cognitive function as measured by the Mini-Mental State Exam was the last factor to improve. It must be kept in mind when evaluating the literature on surgical intervention of normal-pressure hydrocephalus that none of the reports are of controlled trials. Although understandable, given the difficulty of adequately controlling for an invasive surgical procedure, lack of appropriate controls hinders interpretation of therapeutic efficacy.

Metabolic Dementing Disorders

Although metabolic disorders most commonly produce delirium, they can, especially if persistent, produce dementia. Hypothyroidism can produce a dementia that is often accompanied by irritability, paranoid ideation, and depression. Although anecdotal reports suggest that dementia secondary to thyroid deficiency can be correctable (Whybrow et al. 1969), in a recent careful follow-up study of thyroid-deficient patients diagnosed in an outpatient dementia clinic (Larson et al. 1984) none of their hypothyroid patients had a completely reversible dementia. Three of these four hypothyroid patients followed for 2 years developed progressive cognitive deterioration consistent with AD. In the fourth hypothyroid patient the dementia did not show progression.

Vitamin B_{12} deficiency can present with dementia even in the absence of megaloblastic anemia (Strachan and Henderson 1965). Cognitive improvement with vitamin B_{12} replacement therapy is variable and no controlled trials of such replacement therapy are available. Wieland (1986) anecdotally reported a mildly demented patient with a low serum B_{12} blood level who demonstrated "dramatic clinical improvement" with administration of vitamin B_{12}. Gross et al. (1986) presented two case reports suggesting modest improvements in cognitive function, mood, and activities of daily living following parenteral vitamin B_{12}. Both patients had pernicious anemia documented by abnormal Schilling tests. Again, such anecdotal reports are only suggestive of some modest efficacy of B_{12} replacement in dementia presumably secondary to B_{12} deficiency.

A metabolic cause of dementia that deserves greater emphasis is multiple hypoglycemic episodes of iatrogenic origin in diabetic patients treated with hypoglycemic medications. The theoretic advantages of rigid blood glucose control in the elderly diabetic patient must be balanced against the risks of hypoglycemic damage to brain tissue. This problem is particularly difficult in the unsupervised patient who is either unwilling or unable to maintain an adequate and regular diet.

Infectious Dementing Disorders

Although rare in the elderly population, infectious dementing disorders should be considered in the differential diagnosis of dementia. Creutzfeldt-Jakob disease is a rapidly fatal degenerative disease of the central nervous system usually afflicting persons in middle and late middle life. Patients present with a rapidly progressive dementia accompanied by myoclonic jerks, seizures, ataxia, rigidity, and other signs of widespread brain involvement. Neuropathologic exam reveals spongiform changes, neuronal loss, and gliosis. The disease is caused by a "slow virus" with a prolonged latency between exposure to and expression of the disease. It has been transmitted from human to human by corneal transplants, by implantation of contaminated stereotactic electroencephalogram electrodes and through parenteral administration of growth hormone prepared from pooled human pituitary glands. Death within 2 years from onset of symptoms is the rule in this disorder. The rapid course helps differentiate Creutzfeldt-Jakob disease patients from AD patients, who may also have prominent myoclonic jerks (Mayeux et al. 1985; Risse et al. 1986). A recent report suggests that abnormal proteins in the cerebrospinal fluid of patients with Creutzfeldt-Jakob disease may be helpful in differential diagnosis of this disorder (Harrington et al. 1986). Although dementia secondary to neurosyphilis is rare in this age of widespread antibiotic administration, the prolonged latency for the development of general paresis (up to 20 years) raises the possibility of this previously common dementing disorder occasionally being diagnosed in the current era. Because the Venereal Disease Research Laboratory Test is negative in nearly one-third of patients with late syphilis, the more sensitive fluorescent treponemal antibody absorption test should be obtained if late syphilis is suspected. Treatment with high doses of penicillin may be effective, but it is possible for the disease to progress despite adequate antibiotic therapy (Wilner and Brody 1968).

The virus (HTLV-III) that causes acquired immune deficiency syndrome (AIDS) attacks neuronal cells of the brain as well as lymphoid cells of the immune system (Gajdusek et al. 1985). The subacute encephalitis, which occurs in approximately one-third of patients with AIDS (Snider et al. 1983; Price et al. 1986), is characterized in its early stages by subtle cognitive changes that may progress to severe dementia in several weeks or months. In its early stages, the AIDS dementia complex can mimic depression, but patients eventually develop clear dementia often accompanied by other neurologic signs and symptoms (Carne and Adler 1986). In 20 percent of AIDS dementia complex patients reported by Navia et al. (1986a), the disease ran a more protracted indolent course with patients eventually exhibiting a picture of severe dementia, mutism, incontinence, paraplegia, and in some cases myoclonus. The bulk of evidence suggests that this syndrome is caused by direct HTLV-III brain infection as opposed to brain infection by opportunistic agents (Navia et al. 1986b).

Clinical Evaluation of the Cognitively Impaired Older Patient

The clinical evaluation of the cognitively impaired patient is based on a careful history obtained from the patient as well as from friends or relatives who can accurately describe the onset, progression, and nature of signs and symptoms. The second most important part of the evaluation is a careful mental status examination with evaluation of the patient's orientation, memory, ability to calculate, aphasia, apraxia, and visual spatial skills. In addition, the mental status examination must assess mood, presence of hallucinations and delusions, impulse control, and level of consciousness and cooperation. A physical examination, including a screening neurologic evaluation with special attention to localizing signs, is also essential. An inventory of current medications either prescribed or obtained without prescription should always be obtained and a urine specimen analyzed for the presence of drugs if there is any question as to the reliability of the drug history. Behavioral toxicity from a variety of medications both psychiatric and general medical may be the most common etiology of reversible cognitive and behavioral impairments in the elderly cognitively impaired patient (Larson et al. 1984). Laboratory tests for electrolyte imbalance and metabolic disorders as well as systemic medical illnesses that can impair cognitive function should be included in the diagnostic evaluation. Although the routine inclusion of a head computed tomographic scan is debatable (Larson et al. 1984), this noninvasive procedure can detect intracranial mass lesions such as resectable tumors and subdural hematomas, which, albeit unusual, can make the difference between a functional life and chronic institutionalization in the individual patient. The computed tomographic scan can also help identify normal-pressure hydrocephalus and MID.

Cognitive rating scales are supplemental to the history, mental status examination, physical examination, and laboratory evaluation of the cognitively impaired elderly patient for purposes of diagnosis, but they are important for the establishment of a quantified baseline of cognitive function to which one can refer over time. The Mini-Mental State Exam developed by Folstein et al. (1975) is a brief instrument that is surprisingly comprehensive. This instrument assesses orientation, registration and recall of information, attention and calculation, aphasia, apraxia, and visual spatial skills. It is not particularly useful in the differential diagnosis of the various dementing disorders; nor does it help localize brain lesions. However, as a routine clinical tool it has gained wide acceptance and has become a standard means of expressing the level of cognitive impairment in the dementia patient both in the clinical setting and in research studies. The Information-Memory-Concentration Test of Blessed et al. (1968) is another widely used brief test that has the advantage of significant correlation with neuritic plaque counts in AD patients. The Mini-Mental State Exam is highly correlated with the Blessed Test (Thal et al. 1986), and probably would correlate positively with the neurohistologic lesions of AD if such a study were undertaken. If a more comprehensive yet reasonably concise cognitive rating instrument is necessary, the Dementia Rating Scale developed by Mattis (1976) is a battery specifically designed for patients with some degree of cognitive impairment. It is a reliable instrument that correlates well with the functional capacity of AD patients (Vitaliano et al. 1984). A rating scale for global impairment developed by Reisberg (1982) has also found wide use, particularly for gross characterization of stage of illness in research studies.

It has previously been thought that a careful evaluation such as that outlined in Table 4 would reveal potentially correctable underlying disorders in 10 to 30 percent of dementia patients (Marsden and Harrison 1972; Fox et al. 1975; Freeman 1976; Victoratos et al. 1977). These studies were mainly performed in early-onset dementia patients who were evaluated in the inpatient setting. A perhaps more realistic yield of truly correctable disorders impairing cognitive function following comprehensive diagnostic evaluation in later onset dementia patients in an outpatient clinic has been reported by

Table 4. Evaluation of Cognitive Impairment

History from patient and relative or friend
Mental status exam
Physical and neurologic exam
Medication inventory/urine toxicology
Electrocardiogram
Head computed tomography scan
Complete blood count
Serum Venereal Disease Research Laboratories Test
Serum sodium, potassium, chloride bicarbonate, calcium
Serum blood urea nitrogen, creatinine, bilirubin, albumin/globulin
Serum B_{12}
Serum triiodothyronine/thyroxine, thyroid stimulating hormone
Serum glucose (fasting)
Brief cognitive test (e.g., Mini-Mental State Examination)

Larson et al. (1984). Of 107 unselected elderly outpatients referred for evaluation of global cognitive impairment of at least 3 months' duration, only 15 had potentially reversible causes for their dementias, of which hypothyroidism and drug toxicity were the most common causes. The six patients with potentially reversible dementia secondary to medication side effects formed the largest single group. Only three patients with potentially reversible dementia, in fact, proved to return to normal mental status examination at follow-up. One patient had a subdural hematoma, another had mixed drug toxicity, and a third had rheumatoid cerebrovasculitis. The first two patients presented with subtle and mild mental status abnormalities only. Of the 13 patients with potentially reversible dementia available for follow-up over a 2-year period, 3 of 4 patients with hypothyroidism, 1 patient with subdural hematoma, and even 4 of 6 patients with medication toxicity developed progressive deterioration consistent with AD. Alzheimer's disease was confirmed at autopsy in two of these patients. Of greater therapeutic benefit was the recognition of other treatable disorders complicating dementia in 48 patients. Treatment of these complicating conditions (e.g., depression, Parkinson's disease, and congestive heart failure) appeared to result in symptomatic improvement although dementia persisted.

Pharmacologic Treatment of Agitated Behaviors in Dementia

The secondary behavioral features of dementia, such as depression, hallucinations, and delusions, appear to be responsive to treatment. Somatic treatment interventions will be discussed first and psychosocial therapies will be discussed subsequently.

The successful treatment of psychotic signs and symptoms by neuroleptic drugs in nonelderly schizophrenic patients raised great hopes in the 1950s and 1960s that these potent drugs might dramatically improve function and relieve symptoms in elderly demented patients whose illness was complicated by agitated behaviors such as pacing, violent outbursts, delusions, hallucinations, and irritability. Although neuroleptics are widely prescribed to elderly patients in long-term care facilities (Prien and Caffe 1977), their efficacy in this population has not lived up to early expectations. A review of the limited number of reasonably designed placebo-controlled trials of neuroleptics in elderly patients suffering from dementia suggests a definite but limited role for these drugs in the treatment of the behaviorally disturbed dementia patient. These studies have recently been reviewed by Raskind et al. (1987).

Two recent well-designed placebo-controlled studies of neuroleptic medications in behaviorally disturbed dementia patients are worth reviewing in detail. In both of these studies, diagnoses conformed to *DSM-III* criteria for dementia. In addition to cognitive and activities of daily living impairments, inclusion criteria in these studies required that patients exhibit at least three of the following signs and symptoms: agitation, anxiety, delusions, depressed mood, hallucinations, hostility, irritability and sleep distuburbance. The first study (Petrie et al. 1982a) evaluated haloperidol (mean dose = 4.6 mg/day), loxapine (mean dose = 22 mg/day), and placebo in 64 demented inpatients (mean age = 73 years) who were residents in a large state psychiatric hospital. Although active neuroleptic treatment was significantly more effective than placebo for suspiciousness, hallucinatory behavior, excitement, hostility, and uncooperativeness, only 32 percent of loxapine-treated patients, 35 percent of haloperidol-treated patients, and 9 percent of placebo-treated patients were globally rated as moderately or markedly improved. These percentages contrast with figures of 60 to 70 percent moderately or markedly improved reported in non-placebo-controlled studies of neuroleptics in similar patient populations (Salzman 1987).

Barnes et al. (1982) came to fairly similar conclusions in a study of thioridazine (mean dose = 63 mg/day), loxapine (mean dose = 11 mg/day), and placebo in 53 demented nursing home patients whose mean age was 83 years. Improvement with active medication was significantly greater than with placebo for anxiety, excitement, and uncooperativeness. However, suspiciousness and hostility in these very elderly nursing home patients improved significantly over time with placebo to such a degree that the differences between improvement in these symptoms with active drug and placebo were not significant. Only one-third of the patients in this study manifested either marked or moderate global improvement and the greatest global improvement was noted in patients with the most severe baseline symptoms.

Although neuroleptic medications are commonly administered to elderly demented patients on a chronic maintenance basis, this practice has not been prospectively evaluated. A few studies, however, have systematically observed patients following discontinuation of long-term neuroleptic treatment. In one study (Barton and Hurst 1966), following substitution of neuroleptic drugs by placebo treatment, statistically significant but modest deterioration in mean group ratings was noted for agitation, overactivity, resistiveness, and noisiness. However, only 8 of the 50 subjects demonstrated a greater than 10 percent deterioration in their total behavioral ratings. The investigators interpreted this finding as suggesting the possibility that maintenance neuroleptic medication was being overprescribed in their population. It should be noted, however, that their 3-week placebo period may not have been an adequate drug-free interval to demonstrate maximal behavioral deterioration. In a recent study, Risse et al. (1987) substituted placebo for maintenance neuroleptic medication in nine male dementia patients (mean age = 65 years) who had received neuroleptic treatment for at least 90 consecutive days at a mean dose of 430 mg/day (chlorpromazine equivalent) for the control of agitated behaviors. One patient developed severe agitation by the third drug-free week and neuroleptic treatment was reinstituted. Of the remaining eight patients, however, only one was more agitated, two were unchanged, and five tended to be less agitated by the end of the 6-week placebo period. Tardive dyskinetic movements were more pronounced during the placebo period, but no change in cognitive function could be detected on the Mini-Mental State Exam between placebo period and maintenance neuroleptic treatment.

The limited data available from reasonably designed studies of neuroleptic drugs in elderly dementia patients suggest a definite but limited role in dementia patients with such complicating disturbed behaviors as agitation, irritability, and classically psychotic symptoms (delusions and hallucinations). Furthermore it appears that maintenance neuroleptic medications may be required in only a minority of the patients in whom they have been prescribed for agitated behaviors. The robust placebo responses in the acute treatment trial of Barnes et al. (1982) suggest that nonpharmacologic treatment strategies may also be effective in agitated dementia patients. The potential adverse effects of these drugs (sedation, orthostatic hypotension, pseudoparkinsonian rigidity and tremor, and tardive dyskinesia) in elderly patients should not be underestimated. Because the neuroleptics have antimuscarinic activity at brain muscarinic cholinergic receptors, they have potential for further exacerbating the cholinergic deficiency in AD and thus further compromising cognitive function. Such central anticholinergic effects may sometimes have clinical relevance (Steele et al. 1986), and cognitive function should be assessed before and during neuroleptic treatment to monitor this possible adverse effect.

Other classes of drugs besides the neuroleptics have been used to treat agitated behaviors in demented patients. Non-placebo-controlled trials (Kirven and Montero 1973; Cervara 1974) have suggested limited efficacy for benzodiazepines in the behaviorally disturbed dementia patient. β-Blocker drugs such as propranolol have been anecdotally suggested to control aggressive and agitated behavior in elderly dementia patients (Yudofsky 1981; Jenike 1983), and the antidepressant drug trazodone has also been anecdotally cited as effective in the treatment of the disturbed dementia patient (Simpson and Foster 1986).

Pharmacologic Treatment of Depression in Dementia

That substantial depressive symptomatology (Lazarus et al. 1987) as well as diagnosable depressive disorder (Reifler et al. 1982) is present in patients with late-life dementing disorders is well established. Uncontrolled studies suggest that standard tricyclic antidepressant therapy is effective in the treatment of depression complicating AD (Reifler et al. 1986). In a double-blind placebo-controlled study, Reifler et al. (1987) evaluated the antidepressant efficacy of imipramine in patients with AD who were suffering from a concomitant major depressive disorder diagnosed by *DSM-III* criteria. In this 8-week study (mean imipramine dose = 83 mg/day, mean plasma imipramine/desipramine concentration = 119 ng/ml) Hamilton Depression Rating Scale scores dropped from 19.3 pretreatment to 11.5 at the end of the treatment period in the imipramine group and from 18.6 to 10.8 in the placebo group. The degree of improvement did not differ between groups. Cognitive function as measured by the Mini-Mental State Examination did not change in the imipramine group (16.9 pretreatment vs. 18.7 posttreatment) or in the placebo-treated depressed AD patients (18.0 pretreatment vs. 19.3 posttreatment). There was decreased cognitive function in the depressed AD patients treated with imipramine on the more comprehensive Mattis Dementia Rating Scale (111 pretreatment vs. 104 posttreatment) suggesting a mild adverse effect of imipramine on cognitive function. This study suggests that mild to moderate depression in moderately demented AD patients can be successfully ameliorated, but that the tricyclic antidepressant drug was not the specific therapeutic agent. Although tricyclic antidepressant plasma concentrations were somewhat lower than those suggested as therapeutic in younger nondemented depressed patients (Glassman et al. 1977), these plasma concentrations are similar to those associated with efficacy as compared to placebo in a study of depressed patients with ischemic heart disease (Veith et al. 1982; Raskind et al. 1982b). That tricyclic antidepressants may be specifically effective in dementia patients with more severe depressions or depressions with more endogenous features has not been ruled out by this limited study. On the other hand, these results underscore the need for adequate controls in any treatment evaluations in these subject populations. For example, the encouraging report that monoamine oxidase inhibitor antidepressant drugs may be effective in depressed AD patients (Jenike 1985) must be validated in placebo-controlled trials before being accepted as a guide for clinical practice.

Cognitive-Acting Drugs in Alzheimer's Disease

Rational attempts pharmacologically to enhance cognitive function in AD have focused on the documented deficiency in presynaptic cholinergic neurons innervating hippocampus and neocortex. The first strategy, administration of the acetylcholine precursors choline or lecithin (phosphatidyl choline), unfortunately failed to produce improvement in cognitive function in clinical trials (Boyd et al. 1977; Thal et al. 1981; Brinkman et al. 1982). A somewhat more successful strategy has attempted to prolong the synaptic activity of acetylcholine released from presynaptic cholinergic neurons by administering centrally active cholinesterase inhibitor drugs. Intravenous administration of the cholinesterase inhibitor physostigmine briefly improved cognitive function in AD patients with mild or moderate disease (Davis et al. 1979). On the basis of these results, treatment with oral physostigmine, a more convenient dosage form with longer duration of activity, was evaluated in several studies. Although significant cognitive improvement was demonstrated in several studies (Mohs et al. 1985; Thal et al. 1983), such improvement was modest and not all studies of oral physostigmine have demonstrated clinical efficacy (Jotkowitz 1983; Schmechel et al. 1984), perhaps because of the low bioavailability of oral physostigmine (Whelpton and Hurst 1985). The most encouraging results for cholinesterase inhibitor therapy have been reported recently by Summers et al. (1986), who administered the centrally active oral anticholinesterase, tetrahydroaminoacridine for extended periods to patients with AD. These investigators demonstrated substantial improvement both in activities of daily living and in psychometrically documented cognitive function in a double-blind placebo-controlled crossover study lasting an average of 12.6 months. This study has generated great interest, and a large multicenter clinical trial attempting to replicate these findings is currently being conducted.

Cholinergic agonist therapy has also been attempted. Christie (1981) showed limited cognitive improvement following an acute intravenous infusion of the direct muscarinic agonist arecoline. Harbaugh et al. (1984) administered a continuous intracranial infusion of the muscarinic agonist bethanechol delivered by a totally implantable infusion system to patents with biopsy-documented AD. Unfortunately, this fairly invasive treatment did not result in reproducible cognitive improvement. Given the complexity of the role of the central cholinergic system in memory, the multiple neurotransmitter abnormalities in AD, and the crudity of our current pharmacologic attempts to mimic normal central cholinergic function, the results of clinical trials to date should not be overly discouraging. Future approaches with combined therapies or more precise methods of mimicking normal cholinergic enhancement of memory function may prove more successful.

Other rational attempts to improve cognitive function in AD have focused on the neuropeptide vasopressin, which improves learning in animal models and the concentration of which is decreased in cerebrospinal fluid and in some brain areas in AD (see above). Modest cognitive improvement with intranasally administered vasopressin peptides has been reported in several studies (Weingartner 1981; Kaye et al. 1982), but other investigators have failed to confirm these positive findings (Tinklenberg et al. 1981; Chase et al. 1982). Because vasopressin peptides do not cross the blood-brain barrier, it is not surprising that peripheral administration lacks substantial efficacy. It should also be noted that DDAVP and lysine vasopressin, the vasopressin peptides used in several studies, bind only weakly to the subclass of vasopressin receptors found in brain (Dorsa and Raskind 1985), and therefore even if they were able to enter the central compartment they would be only weakly active at the brain vasopressin receptors presumably involved in the modulation of memory.

Other drugs have been used to treat cognitive and functional impairments in dementia patients on a more empiric basis. Ergoloid mesylates, papaverine, cyclandelate, and other agents have been suggested as cognitive-enhancing drugs, with several studies, especially of the ergoloid mesylates, suggesting improvement in functional status as compared to placebo. This area has recently been reviewed by Hollister and Yesavage (1984). Unfortunately, it has been difficult to document cognitive improvement of these agents psychometrically, and reported positive results are usually of modest degree and limited to patients with mild dementia.

Psychosocial Therapies

For the greater part of their illness, elderly patients with AD or another progressive dementing illness of later life will be cared for at home by family. The demands on these caregivers are very great. The unending burden of providing supervision and care for these patients has been documented in the *The 36-Hour Day* (Mace and Rabins 1981). Supporting the morale and treatment skills of the family is a critical factor in providing optimal care to the patient and keeping the patient in the community as long as possible. Excessive stress on the care-providing family is a major factor in the decision ultimately to institutionalize the demented patient. Successful intervention to reduce stress and increase coping skills by providing information about the biology, behavioral manifestations, and course of the dementing illness can be extremely helpful. It is particularly important for families to understand the effects of the illness on the patient's behavior and personality. Knowing that such problems as passivity, loss of empathy, wandering, and emotional liability are not deliberate and willful acts, but rather the results of a structurally damaged brain helps to dispel the caregiver's anger and fosters appropriate expectations. In the case of AD, families appreciate accurate information about the effectiveness (or lack thereof) of the many dietary and pharmacologic treatments promoted in the lay literature and about the heritability of the disease. That ongoing research offers hope for the future is an important message to communicate. In addition, families should understand that the course of AD is highly variable and that many patients do well for periods of years at home. Patients and families appear to benefit from an emotionally supportive psychotherapeutic relationship with their physician or other health care provider. The patient and his or her family should be followed at regular intervals assessing cognitive function, activities of daily living, and specific problems at each visit. The importance of regularly scheduled visits, even if they are no more frequent than once every 3 or 4 months (as opposed to "return as needed"), cannot be over emphasized. Brief supportive psychotherapy provided at these visits allows exploration and resolution of some of the frustration and grief attendant to caring for the patient with a dementing illness (Rabins et al. 1982). Families find it helpful to learn that their feelings and reactions are normal responses to an extremely difficult situation. Caregivers should also be encouraged to maintain frequent contact with family and friends in an effort to increase social support (Zarit et al. 1980). Respite care, time away from the patient for the family to renew their strength and enthusiasm for care, is increasingly available both on an outpatient basis in the form of adult day care and more extended inpatient care for several days or weeks in nursing homes or hospitals. Unfortunely, current respite resources are not adequate to meet the needs. It must be emphasized to caregivers that attention to their own needs improves their ability to care for their loved one.

In addition to individual counseling, family members can derive great benefit from membership in peer support groups such as those sponsored by the Alzheimer's Disease and Related Disorders Association. Such organizations have been established in most communities around the nation. In addition to acting as political advocacy groups, they offer group meetings that can be of great therapeutic benefit to the family (Barnes et al. 1981). Participants gain emotional support and learn new strategies of responding to the dementia patient by hearing what other members have done successfully in similar situations. These groups can be the best sources of information about community resources such as adult day care centers, nursing homes that offer respite, and home care chore services. The support groups are also sources of knowledge concerning attorneys or other professionals particularly helpful in the areas of guardianship, wills, and laws pertaining to public benefits for demented patients.

Nonpharmacologic interventions are also important once the patient's disease has progressed to institutionalization. Wandering is one of the greatest problems facing institutions caring for demented patients, particularly in

AD patients whose cognitive function is severely impaired but whose motor function remains intact. Such aimless wandering at all hours of the day and night can be disruptive and pose the threat of the patient's inadvertently leaving the facility and coming to harm. Pharmacologic approaches to the wandering patient are generally unsuccessful. In fact, akathisia, an adverse effect of neuroleptic drugs manifested by restless pacing and the inability to sit still, can exacerbate wandering if neuroleptic drugs are prescribed. It is increasingly clear that patients and facilities caring for them benefit from a secure area in which patients can wander at any hour without harming themselves or causing disruption to others. Such an environmental strategy can dramatically decrease the need for questionably effective pharmacologic interventions and their attendant adverse effects.

Reality orientation is a behavioral and educational approach originally developed for "psychogeriatric" institutionalized patients among whom were many elderly persons which chronic schizophrenia who had spent much of their adult lives in psychiatric institutions (Taulbee and Folsom 1966). The relevance of reality orientation to persons who have been psychiatrically well until developing a late-life dementing disorder has not been clarified. Reality orientation therapy includes both informal repeated presentation of basic information to patients during routine patient/staff interactions as well as more formal "classroom" orientation, in which patients and a therapist meet daily using a large board with oversized letters to attempt to "learn" such facts as the date, the time, the place, the patient's name, the weather report, the next meal, and other discrete daily events. As with pharmacologic interventions, uncontrolled studies of reality orientation have claimed wide-ranging improvement in patient behavior and cognitive function. However, in controlled studies gains have been much more modest. A recent review of the literature on reality orientation (Powell-Proctor and Miller 1982) suggests a number of problems and shortcomings in our knowledge of the efficacy of this treatment modality. Most studies have not carefully defined the extent, cause, or duration of dementia in their subject populations, making it impossible to determine which patients are most likely to benefit from treatment. While most studies have demonstrated modest but statistically significant improvement in the accuracy of responses to the orientation questions that form the basis of the reality orientation sessions, the practical value of such improvement is unclear. Most studies have not demonstrated that improvement in orientation generalizes to improvement in other cognitive functions, ward behavior, or activities of daily living. Furthermore, gains quickly disappear when treatment is withdrawn. Best results with reality orientation seem to depend on tailoring the specific contents of therapy to individual attributes of the patient. Little benefit can be expected in patients with advanced dementia. Enthusiastic and regular interaction of staff members with patients probably contributes a great deal to the success of treatment and can help create and maintain a positive therapeutic approach to the care of institutionalized patients. On the other hand, an overly zealous and rigid advocacy of reality orientation may be more harmful than helpful.

The application of classic behavioral techniques to the treatment of the demented patients has received little attention, perhaps because of the tacit assumption that an intact memory is a prerequisite for successful behavior modification. A recent pilot study of stimulus control in the modification of problem behaviors in elderly demented patients offers some hope that classic behavioral techniques can be applied to these patients (Hussian 1982). In this study, supernormal environmental stimuli were effective in controlling high-frequency problem behaviors exhibited by severely demented, institutionalized elderly patients. The use of color cues significantly decreased wandering behavior, and stereotyped behavior such as repetitive picking, vocalizations, and rubbing were modified by the use of discriminate stimuli. The application of classic behavioral modification techniques to the demented patient is an area that deserves further investigation.

Amnestic Syndrome

The essential feature of the amnestic syndrome is impairment in both short- and long-term memory secondary to a specific organic factor that is usually bilateral structural damage to diencephalic and medial temporal areas of the brain such as the mammillary bodies, fornix, and hippocampus. The diagnostic criteria for amnestic syndrome in *DSM-III-R* are listed in Table 5. In amnestic syndrome remote events are better recalled than more recent events and the patient is usually disoriented to time and often to place. Confabulation, the verbal production of imagined information to cover up memory gaps, is classically described in amnestic syndrome, but the actual prevalence of confabulation in amnestic syndrome as compared with either dementia or delirium is not known.

The *DSM-III-R* stipulates that the diagnosis cannot be made if the memory impairment is accompanied by a delirium in which the patient's ability to maintain and shift attention is impaired. More controversial exclusions in *DSM-III-R* are impairment in abstract thinking, impaired judgment, other disturbances of higher cortical function, or personality change. The implication being that if these latter signs or symptoms are present, the correct diagnosis should be dementia. Because chronic alcoholism with the subsequent development of Korsakoff's syndrome is the most common disorder producing the amnestic syndrome, and because most chronic alcoholic patients demonstrate impairment in at least some higher cortical functions when tested neuropsychologically, the logical distinction between amnestic syndrome and dementia becomes blurred (Lishman 1981).

The most common etiology of amnestic syndrome is multiple episodes of acute Wernicke's encephalopathy caused by thiamine deficiency in chronic alcoholics, ultimately producing Korsakoff's psychosis. The acute encephalop-

Table 5.   DSM-III-R Diagnostic Criteria for Amnestic Syndrome

A. Demonstrable evidence of impairment in both short- and long-term memory; with regard to long-term memory, very remote events are remembered better than more recent events. Impairment in short-term memory (inability to learn new information) may be indicated by inability to remember three objects after five minutes. Long-term memory impairment (inability to remember information that was known in the past) may be indicated by inability to remember past personal information (e.g., what happened yesterday, birthplace, occupation) or facts of common knowledge (e.g., past presidents, well-known dates)

B. Not occurring exclusively during the course of Delirium, and does not meet the criteria for Dementia (i.e., no impairment in abstract thinking or judgment, no other disturbances of higher cortical function, and no personality change).

C. There is evidence from the history, physical examination, or laboratory tests of a specific organic factor (or factors) judged to be etiologically related to the disturbance.

Note. Reprinted with permission from the *Diagnostic and Statistical Manual of Mental Disorders (Third Edition-Revised).* Copyright © 1987 American Psychiatric Association.

athy classically presents with confusion, nystagmus, lateral gaze palsy, and ataxia reflecting structural damage to the brain tissue adjacent to the third and fourth ventricles. Thiamine is specifically therapeutic, and a transketolase deficiency may predispose toward development of the syndrome in thiamine-deficient patients (Blass and Gibson 1977). This treatable acute syndrome may be more difficult to detect than in an earlier era. Harper (1979) reported that of 51 cases of Wernicke's encephalopathy diagnosed at autopsy, only 7 had been suspected antemortem, despite the fact that the great majority of patients had been known alcoholics.

The cognitve disorders of alcoholism have recently been reviewed in a comprehensive manner by Lishman (1981), who presents a cogent case for the existence of a true dementing disorder secondary to chronic alcoholism in a substantial number of alcoholic patients who suffer cognitive impairment. Not only are deficits in higher cortical function common in chronic alcoholics, but neuropsychologic testing even in sober alcoholics without obvious dementia consistently reveals difficulties in new learning, abstract thinking, and visuospatial functions (Tarter 1980). Furthermore, Brewer and Perett (1971) have reported cortical atrophy or ventricular enlargement in a high percentage of alcoholic patients with significant correlations between the severity of cortical changes and cognitive impairment. Lishman (1981) evaluated computed tomographic scans in 100 male alcoholics clinically free of Korsakoff's psychosis and 50 healthy age-matched control subjects. The alcoholic subjects had significantly greater evidence of cortical atrophy as measured by sulcal widening, sylvian-fisher widening, and ventricular enlargement. This study suggests that chronic alcoholism has a widespread deleterious effect on brain tissue that extends beyond the classic periventricular areas described in the Wernicke/Korsakoff syndrome. That chronic alcohol administration can severely damage neuronal tissue in the absence of malnutrition has been demonstrated in experimental animals (Riley and Walker 1978).

An interesting possible neurochemical lesion has been described in Korsakoff's psychosis involving the brain noradrenergic system (McEntee et al. 1984). These investigators reported decreased concentrations of MHPG in patients with Korsakoff's psychosis, which increased toward normal in four patients who recovered from amnesic symptoms (Mair et al. 1986). This group also reported decreased concentrations of the neuropeptide arginine vasopressin in Korsakoff's psychosis, with concentrations of the peptide increasing in recovered Korsakoff's patients. These investigators suggest that the periventricular lesions in Korsakoff's psychosis damage ascending noradrenergic fibers from the locus ceruleus to more rostral brain areas involved in cognitive function. The locus ceruleus is frequently damaged histologically in the Wernicke/Korsakoff syndrome (Victor and Adams 1971).

Delirium

Delirium includes the spectrum of clinical pictures of diverse organic etiologies whose most prominent feature is a disorder of attention (Table 6). Essential features are rapid onset of fluctuating disturbances of attention, memory, and orientation. Also present are reduced wakefulness or insomnia, perceptual disturbances, and changes in psychomotor activity. This organic brain syndrome is synonymous with "metabolic encephalopathy" and roughly equivalent to the terms "acute brain syndrome" and "acute organic brain syndrome."

The disorder of attention is manifested by impaired ability to sustain attention to environmental stimuli, to engage in goal-directed thinking or to perform goal-directed behavior. The patient is unable to carry on a conversation without becoming distracted and can barely sustain attention long enough to watch television or read. Thinking may be either slowed or accelerated and can become completely disorganized. The patient frequently loses his or her train of thought, switches from subject to subject, and may become completely incoherent. In contrast to dementia, disorders of memory and orientation are secondary rather than primary. Because the patient cannot

Table 6. DSM-III-R Diagnostic Criteria for Delirium

A. Reduced ability to maintain attention to external stimuli (e.g., questions must be repeated because attention wanders) and to appropriately shift attention to new external stimuli (e.g., perseverates answer to a previous question).

B. Disorganized thinking, as indicated by rambling, irrelevant, or incoherent speech.

C. At least two of the following:

(1) reduced level of consciousness, e.g., difficulty keeping awake during examination

(2) perceptual disturbances: misinterpretations, illusions, or hallucinations

(3) disturbance of sleep-wake cycle with insomnia or daytime sleepiness

(4) increased or decreased psychomotor activity

(5) disorientation to time, place, or person

(6) memory impairment, e.g., inability to learn new material, such as the names of several unrelated objects after five minutes, or to remember past events, such as history of current episode of illness

D. Clinical features develop over a short period of time (usually hours to days) and tend to fluctuate over the course of a day.

E. Either (1) or (2):

(1) evidence from the history, physical examination, or laboratory tests of a specific organic factor (or factors) judged to be etiologically related to the disturbance

(2) in the absence of such evidence, an etiologic organic factor can be presumed if the disturbance cannot be accounted for by any nonorganic mental disorder, e.g., Manic Episode accounting for agitation and sleep disturbance

Note. Reprinted with permission from the *Diagnostic and Statistical Manual of Mental Disorders (Third Edition-Revised).* Copyright © 1987 American Psychiatric Association.

attend to stimuli, he or she is unable to register and retain new information. There is often little if any recall of the delirious episodes once the delirium has resolved, although patients may report the episode as a "bad dream." Level of consciousness can vary from drowsiness or stupor in conditions such as hepatic or renal failure to excessive alertness and severe insomnia in sedative drug or alcohol withdrawal. Vivid dreams and nightmares are common and may merge with hallucinations occurring in periods of wakefulness. Perceptual disturbances include misinterpretation, illusions, or hallucinations. Delusions and hallucinations are commonly visual, but can frequently be auditory or occur in other modalities of sensation. Acute paranoid episodes can present serious management problems and endanger the safety of the patient.

Associated features include the range of affective responses. Fear, anxiety, and anger commonly accompany delusional ideation and may precipitate attempts at escape from the immediate environment or destructive rage episodes. Less frequently euphoria is present. Depression may also occur, raising the risk of suicidal behavior. It is common for sensory misperceptions and fearfulness to reach greatest intensity at night.

The onset of delirium is usually rapid and duration brief. An episode of delirium can last for hours or days but rarely persists for greater than 1 month. In the absence of complications, clearing of the delirium leaves the patient's previous level of functioning intact. In some cases, depending on the etiology of the delirium, a dementia may persist after the delirium has cleared. Cognitive impairment often fluctuates, and lucid intervals may occur, especially during the daytime hours.

Etiologic factors are numerous. They include acute neurologic disorders, general medical illness, drug ingestion, drug withdrawal in a dependent person, postoperative states, and less well-understood phenomena such as sensory deprivation and the coronary care unit syndrome (see Table 7).

Differential diagnosis includes acute functional psychoses such as manic disorder, depressive disorder psychotic type, schizophrenia, and schizoaffective disorder. Absence of an organic cause, history of past psychiatric illness, and the pattern of onset of the present illness episode are helpful in differential diagnosis. Furthermore, signs and symptoms of delirium are typically shifting, poorly systematized, and accompanied by fluctuations in level of awareness and impaired memory and orientation. The electroencephalogram often demonstrates generalized slowing of background activity in delirium, a finding not present in psychotic disorders. Differentiating dementia from delirium is usually straightforward, but delirium can be superimposed on a preexisting dementia even if only for a period of hours, and the clinical picture may be confusing. Furthermore, the elderly patient with dementia is at increased risk for the development of delirium from any of a number of causes.

Treatment of Delirium

Treatment should be directed toward the disorder underlying the delirium. Frequently, however, the underlying disorder is either not clearly discernible or not completely correctable, and symptomatic treatment be-

Table 7. Etiologies of Delirium

Systemic Illness	**Neurologic Disorders**
Congestive heart failure	Cerebrovascular accident
Pulmonary insufficiency	Head trauma
Renal insufficiency	Subarachnoid hemorrhage
Hepatic insufficiency	Meningitis (acute and chronic)
Lupus erythematosus	Intracranial mass lesion
Infection	Neurosyphilis
Burns and multiple trauma	Seizure
Acquired immune deficiency	
syndrome	**Pharmacologic Adverse Effects**
	Bromide
Metabolic Disorders	Levodopa
Hypothyroidism	Digitalis
Hyperadrenalcorticism	Anticholinergic drugs
Hypoadrenalcorticism	Antipsychotics
Hypercalcemia	(phenothiazines, etc.)
Hypoglycemia	Tricyclic antidepressants
	Antispasmodics
Miscellaneous	(Belladonna, etc.)
Withdrawal from addiction to	Antiparkinsonian
alcohol, sedatives, hypnotics	anticholinergics
Postoperative state (particularly	Corticosteroids
cardiac surgery)	Cimetidine
Intensive care unit syndrome	Sedatives, hypnotics

comes necessary if agitation, anxiety, delusions, hallucinations, or other behavioral symptoms interfere with patient management or threaten patient safety. Mild anxiety and agitation may respond to reassurance from an attendant family member, a nurse regularly caring for the patient, or a physician whose role is clear to the patient. The environment should be structured to provide consistency of stimulation at a moderately low level. A nightlight can be helpful in those patients whose delirium is exacerbated by darkness. The delirious patient is at risk for self-injury and therefore a physically secure and carefully monitored environment is essential.

Although it is ideal to avoid adding medications to the delirious patient's regimen, pharmacologic intervention is sometimes necessary. If the delirium is secondary to withdrawal from a central nervous system depressant drug such as alcohol, barbiturate, or benzodiazepine, treatment with a cross-tolerant sedative hypnotic drug such as a medium-duration barbiturate or benzodiazepine is indicated. Dosage must be titrated for the individual patient and the proper route of administration chosen for the individual drug. In delirium not secondary to withdrawal from cortical depressant drugs, low doses of neuroleptic medication can be helpful. With the neuroleptics, hypotension and lowered seizure threshold are possible and must be kept in mind. The goal in using psychotropic medication in delirium is control of symptoms without adding to disturbed brain function with sedative or anticholinergic psychotropic drug effects.

Organic Mood Syndrome, Depressed Type

Organic mood syndrome, depressed type, is a disturbance of mood resembling major depressive disorder that can be clearly attributed to an underlying organic factor and that does not meet criteria for delirium or dementia (see Table 8). Etiologic factors of organic mood disorder depressed type overlap those for delirium, and both syndromes may coexist in a specific patient. Causes of the syndrome are listed in Table 9. Toxic and metabolic factors frequently underlie this syndrome. Antihypertensive drugs, particularly those that reduce central noradrenergic activity, have been associated with this syndrome. Reserpine, especially in the high doses prescribed before other effective antihypertensive agents were available, frequently induced depression in older men with a past history of depressive disorder. Depression associated with alphamethyldopa, clonidine, and ß blockers (Petrie et al. 1982b) has also been reported.

Although potent diuretics such as the thiazides and furosemide do not affect mood, secondary hypokalemia can present as depression. Alcohol may precipitate depression in heavy drinkers, particularly toward the end of a binge drinking episode. The barbiturates, benzodiazepines, and neuroleptic drugs have also been associated with depressive disorder.

Metabolic disorders can present as depression. Overt hypothyroidism can cause depression (Whybrow et al. 1969). A recent report (Haggerty et al. 1986) suggests that even subclinical hypothyroidism manifested only by an elevated level of TSH may be associated with depression and dementia. In this report, patients treated with thyroid replacement showed substantial improvement in mood but only limited improvement in cognitive function. Cushing's syndrome, although a rare disorder, is associated with depression in a majority of cases (Cohen 1980; Kelly et al. 1980). Hyperparathyroidism with resultant hypercalcemia can present with features of retarded depression, as can other medical illnesses that cause hypercalcemia (e.g., multiple myeloma, metastatic carcinoma, sarcoidosis). Organic mood disorder, depressed type, associated with a specific drug or metabolic disorder should first be treated by correcting the metabolic disturbance or removing the pharmacologic agent.

Recent studies suggest a strong relationship between two dementing

Table 8. DSM-III-R Diagnostic Criteria for Organic Mood Syndrome (Depressed Type)

A. Prominent and persistent depressed mood.

B. There is evidence from the history, physical examination, or laboratory tests of a specific organic factor (or factors) judged to be etiologically related to the disturbance.

C. Not occurring exclusively during the course of Delirium.

Note. Reprinted with permission from the *Diagnostic and Statistical Manual of Mental Disorders (Third Edition-Revised).* Copyright © 1987 American Psychiatric Association.

Table 9. Etiologies of Organic Mood Syndrome, Depressed Type

Systemic Illness
Congestive heart failure
Pulmonary insufficiency
Renal insufficiency
Hepatic insufficiency
Lupus erythematosus
Acute intermittent porphyria
Pancreatic carcinoma
Acquired immune deficiency
  syndrome

Metabolic Disorders
Hypothyroidism
Hyperadrenalcorticism
Hypokalemia
Hypercalcemia

Neurologic Disorders
Parkinson's disease
Intracranial mass lesion
Huntington's chorea
Stroke

Pharmacologic Adverse Effects
Reserpine
Alpha methyldopa
Clonidine
Propranolol
Bromide
Ethanol
Barbiturates
Diazepam
Glucocorticoids
Digitalis

disorders of later life and depression. In both Parkinson's disease and stroke, depression appears to be more than a reaction to disability and may well be a function of abnormal brain physiology. Robins (1976) compared depressive symptomatology in 45 parkinsonian patients and 45 chronically disabled control patients with a significantly more severe grade of physical handicap. Depressive symptomatology was significantly greater in the parkinsonian patients and was unaffected by the severity of disability. Rabins (1982) diagnosed a depressive syndrome in 46 percent of parkinsonian patients. Mayeux et al. (1986) evaluated 49 consecutive patients with Parkinson's disease and found major depression or dysthymic disorder in 40 percent. Biochemical evaluation revealed evidence for serotoninergic deficiency in depressed Parkinson's disease patients compared with nondepressed Parkinson's disease patients. The 1 mg overnight dexamethasone suppression could not distinguish between depressed and nondepressed parkinsonian patients in this study.

Depression is common and persistent following stroke (Robinson et al. 1984). Furthermore, the frequency of depression following stroke may be related to specific location of the infarct (Robinson and Szetela 1981; Ross and Rush 1981). Of particular interest is a recent pharmacologic trial (Lipsey et al. 1984) in which the efficacy of the tricyclic antidepressant nortriptyline was assessed in poststroke depression in 34 patients, half of whom had major depression and half of whom had dysthymic disorder. There was a significantly greater improvement in depression in patients treated with nortriptyline than in a similar group of placebo-treated patients. This study is the only placebo-controlled clinical trial evaluating antidepressant efficacy in organic mood disorder, depressed type. Other such studies would be extremely valuable.

References

Abou-Saleh MT, Spalding EM, Kellet JM, et al: Dexamethasone suppression test in dementia. J Am Geriatr Soc 1987; 35:271

Adams RD, Fisher CM, Hakim S, et al: Symptomatic occult hydrocephalus with "normal" cerebrospinal-fluid pressure: a treatable syndrome. N Engl J Med 1965; 273:117–126

Adolfsson R, Gottfries CG, Roos BE, et al: Changes in brain catecholamines in patients with dementia of Alzheimer type. Br J Psychiatry 1979; 135:216–223

American Psychiatric Association: Diagnostic and Statistical Manual of Mental Disorders (Second Edition). Washington, DC, American Psychiatric Association, 1968

American Psychiatric Association: Diagnostic and Statistical Manual of Mental Disorders (Third Edition). Washington, DC, American Psychiatric Association, 1980

American Psychiatric Association: Diagnostic and Statistical Manual of Mental Disorders (Third Edition-Revised). Washington, DC, American Psychiatric Association, 1987

Ball MJ: The morphological basis of dementia in Parkinson's disease. Can J Neurol Sci 1984; 11:180–184

Balldin J, Gottfries CG, Karlsson I, et al: DST and serum prolactin in dementia. Br J Psychiatry 1983; 143:277–281

Barclay LL, Zemcor A, Blass JP, et al: Survival in Alzheimer's disease and vascular dementias. Neurology 1985; 35:834–840

Barnes RF, Raskind MA, Scott M, et al: Problems of families caring for Alzheimer patients: use of a support group. J Am Geriatr Soc 1981; 29:80–85

Barnes R, Veith R, Okimoto J, et al: Efficacy of antipsychotic medications in behaviorally disturbed dementia patients. Am J Psychiatry 1982; 139:1170–1174

Barton R, Hurst L: Unnecessary use of tranquilizers in elderly patients. Br J Psychiatry 1966; 112:989–990

Bird TD, Stranahan S, Sumi SM, et al: Alzheimer's disease: choline acetyltransferase activity in brain tissue from clinical and pathological subtypes. Ann Neurol 1983; 14:284–293

Bissette G, Reynolds G, Kilts CD, et al: Corticotropin-releasing factor-like immunoreactivity in senile dementia of the Alzheimer type. JAMA 1985; 254:3067–3069

Blass JP, Gibson GE: Abnormality of a thiamine-requiring enzyme in patients with Wernicke-Korsakoff syndrome. N Engl J Med 1977; 297:1367–1370

Blessed G, Tomlinson BE, Roth M: The association between quantitative measures of dementia and of senile change in the cerebral grey matter of elderly subjects. Br J Psychiatry 1968; 114:796–811

Bohus B, Koracs GL, DeWied D: Oxytocin, vasopressin and memory: opposite effects on consolidation and retrieval processes. Brain Res 1978; 157:414–417

Bondareff W, Mountjoy CQ, Roth M, et al: Age and histopathologic heterogeneity in Alzheimer's disease. Arch Gen Psychiatry 1987; 44:412–417

Boyd WD, Graham-White J, Blackwood G, et al: Clinical effects of choline in Alzheimer senile dementia. Lancet 1977; 2:711

Brewer C, Perrett L: Brain damage due to alcohol consumption: an air-encephalographic, psychometric, and electroencephalographic study. Br J Addict 1971; 66:170–182

Breitner JCS, Folstein MF: Familial Alzheimer dementia: prevalent disorder with specific clinical features. Psychol Med 1984; 14:63–80

Brinkman SD, Smith RC, Meyer JS, et al: Lecithin and memory training in suspected Alzheimer's disease. J Gerontol 1982; 37:4–9

Brust JCM: Vascular dementia—still overdiagnosed. Stroke 1983; 14:298–300

Candy JM, Klinowski J, Perry RH, et al: Aluminosilicates and senile plaque formation in Alzheimer's disease. Lancet 1986; 1:354–356

Carne CA, Adler MW: Neurological manifestations of human immunodeficiency virus infection. Br Med J 1986; 293:462–463

Carnes M, Smith JC, Kalin NH, et al: The dexamethasone suppression test in demented outpatients with and without depression. Psychiatr Res 1983; 9:337–344

Carroll BJ, Feinberg M, Greden JF, et al: A specific laboratory test for the diagnosis of melancholia. Arch Gen Psychiatry 1981; 38:15–22

Cash R, Dennis T, L'Heureux R, et al: Parkinson's disease and dementia: norepinephrine and dopamine in locus ceruleus. Neurology 1987; 37:42–46

Cervara AA: Psychoactive drug therapy in the senile patient: controlled comparison of thioridazine and diazepam. Psychiatric Digest 1974; 35:15–21

Chase TN, Durso R, Fedio P, et al: Vasopressin treatment of cognitive deficits in Alzheimer's disease, in Alzheimer's Disease: A Report of Progress in Research. Edited by Corkin S, Davis KL, Growden JH, et al. New York, Raven Press, 1982

Christie JE, Shering A, Ferguson J, et al: Physostigmine and arecoline: effects of intravenous infusions in Alzheimer's presenile dementia. Br J Psychiatry 1981; 138:46–50

Chui HC, Mortimer JA, Slager U, et al: Pathological correlates of dementia in Parkinson's disease. Presented at the annual scientific meeting of the Gerontological Society, San Francisco, 1984

Cohen, SI: Cushing's syndrome: a psychiatric study of 29 patients. Br J Psychiatry 1980; 136:120–124

Constantinidis J, Richard J, Tissot R: Pick's disease, histological and clinical correlations. Eur Neurol 1974; 11:207–218

Cook RH, Ward B, Austin J: Studies in aging of the brain: IV. Familial Alzheimer's disease. Neurology 1979; 29:1402–1412

Crapper DR, Krishnan SS, Dalton AJ: Brain aluminum distribution in Alzheimer's disease and in experimental neurofibrillary degeneration. Science 1973; 180:511–513

Cummings JL, Benson DF: Dementia: A Clinical Approach. Boston, Butterworth, 1983

Cummings JL, Duchen LW: Kluver-Bucy syndrome in Pick's disease: clinical and pathologic correlations. Neurology 1981; 31:1415–1422

Davies P, Maloney AJF: Selective loss of central cholinergic neurons in Alzheimer's disease. Lancet 1976; 2:1403

Davies P, Wolozin BL: Recent advances in the neurochemistry of Alzheimer's disease. J Clin Psychiatry 1987; 48(5):23–30

Davies P, Katzman R, Terry RD: Reduced somatostatin-like immunoreactivity in cerebral cortex from cases of Alzheimer disease and Alzheimer senile dementia. Nature 1980; 288:279–280

Davis KL, Mohs RC, Tinklenberg JR: Enhancement of memory by physostigmine. N Engl J Med 1979; 301:946

Delaney JF: Spinal fluid aluminum levels in patients with Alzheimer's disease. Ann Neurol 1979; 5:580–581

Delfs JR, Zhu C-H, Dichter MA: Coexistence of acetylcholinesterase and somatostatin-immunoreactivity in nerves cultured from rat cerebrum. Science 1984; 223:61–63

DeSouza ED, Whitehouse PJ, Kuhar MJ, et al: Reciprocal changes in corticotropin-releasing factor (CRF)-like immunoreactivity and CRF receptors in cerebral cortex of Alzheimer's disease. Nature 1986; 319:593–595

DeWied D, Versteeg HG: Neurohypophyseal principles and memory. Fed Proc 1979; 38:2348–2354

DeWied D, Gaffori O, van Ree JM, et al: Central target for the behavioral effects of vasopressin neuropeptides. Nature 1984; 308:276–278

Dorsa DM, Raskind MA: Vasopressin in neuropsychiatric disorders, in Vasopressin. Edited by Schrier RW. New York, Raven Press, 1985

El Sobky A, Shazly M, Darwish AK, et al: Anterior pituitary response to thyrotrophin releasing hormone in senile dementia (Alzheimer type) and elderly normals. Acta Psychiatr Scand 1986; 74:13–17

Ferrier IN, Cross AJ, Johnson JA, et al: Neuropeptides in Alzheimer-type dementia. J Neurol Sci 1983; 62:159–170

Folstein MF, Folstein SE, McHugh PR: Mini-Mental State: a practical method for grading the cognitive state of patients for the clinician. J Psychiatr Res 1975; 12:189–198

Fox JH, Topel JL, Huckman MS: Dementia in the elderly—a search for treatable illnesses. J Gerontol 1975; 30:557–564

Fox JH, Penn R, Clasen R, et al: Pathological diagnosis in clinically typical Alzheimer's disease. N Engl J Med 1985; 313:1419–1420

Francis PT, Bowen DM, Neary D, et al: Somatostatinlike immunoreactivity in lumbar cerebrospinal fluid from neurohistologically examined demented patients. Neurobiol Aging 1984; 5:183–186

Francis PT, Palmer AM, Sims NR, et al: Neurochemical studies of early-onset Alzheimer's disease. N Engl J Med 1985; 313:7–11

Freeman FR: Evaluation of patients with progressive intellectual deterioration. Arch Neurol 1976; 33:658–659

Gajdusek DC, Amyx HL, Gibbs CJ, et al: Infection of chimpanzees by human T-lymphotropic retroviruses in brain and other tissues from AIDS patients. Lancet 1985; 1:55–56

Glassman AH, Perel JM, Shostak M, et al: Clinical implications of imipramine plasma levels for depressive illness. Arch Gen Psychiatry 1977; 34:197–204

Glenner GG, Wong CW: Alzheimer disease: initial report of the purification and characterization of a novel cerebrovascular amyloid protein. Biochem Biophys Res Commun 1984; 120:885–890

Godridge H, Reynolds GP, Czudek C, et al: Alzheimer-like neurotransmitter deficits in adult Down's syndrome brain tissue. J Neurol Neurosurg Psychiatry 1987; 50:775–778

Goldgaber D, Lerman MI, McBride OW, et al: Characterization and chromosomal localization of a cDNA encoding brain amyloid of Alzheimer's disease. Science 1987; 235:877–879

Gross JS, Weintraub NT, Neufeld RR, et al: Pernicious anemia in the demented patient without anemia or macrocytosis: a case for early recognition. J Am Geriatr Soc 1986; 34:612–614

Grunhaus L, Dilsaver S, Greden JF: Depressive pseudo dementia: a suggested diagnostic profile. Biol Psychiatry 1983; 18:215–221

Hachinski VC, Larson NA, Marshall J: Multi-infarct dementia. Lancet 1974; 2:207–210

Hachinski VC, Iliff LD, Zilhka E, et al: Cerebral blood flow in dementia. Arch Neurol 1975; 32:632–637

Haggerty JJ, Evans DL, Prange AJ: Organic brain syndrome associated with marginal hypothyroidism. Am J Psychiatry 1986; 143:785–786

Hakim AM, Mathieson G: Dementia in Parkinson's disease: a neuropathologic study. Neurology 1979; 29:1209–1214

Harbaugh RE, Roberts DW, Coombs DW, et al: Preliminary report: intracranial cholinergic drug infusion in patients with Alzheimer's disease. Neurosurgery 1984; 15:514–518

Hardy J, Cowburn R, Barton A, et al: Glutamate deficits in Alzheimer's disease. J Neurol Neurosurg Psychiatry 1987; 50:356–357

Harper C: Wernicke's encephalopathy: a more common disease than realized. J Neurol Neurosurg Psychiatry 1979; 42:226–231

Harrington MG, Merril CR, Asher DM et al: Abnormal protein in the cerebrospinal fluid of patients with Creutzfeldt-Jakob disease. N Engl J Med 1986; 315:279–283

Hauser WA, Morris MA, Heston LL, et al: Seizures and myoclonus in patients with Alzheimer's disease. Neurology 1986; 36:1226–1230

Heston LL, Mastri AR, Anderson VE, et al: Dementia of the Alzheimer type: clinical genetics, natural history and associated conditions. Arch Gen Psychiatry 1981; 38:300–301

Heston LL, White JA, Mastri AR: Pick's disease: clinical genetics and natural history. Arch Gen Psychiatry 1987; 44:409–411

Heyman A, Wilkinson NE, Stafford JA, et al: Alzheimer's disease: a study of epidemiologic aspects. Ann Neurol 1984; 15:335–341

Heyman A, Wilkinson WE, Hurwitz MD, et al: Early-onset Alzheimer's disease: clinical predictors of institutionalization and death. Neurology 1987; 37:980–984

Hollander ER, Mohs RL, Davis KL: Antemortem markers of Alzheimer's disease. Neurobiol Aging 1986; 7:367–386

Hollister LE, Yesavage J: Ergoloid mesylates for senile dementias: unanswered questions. Ann Intern Med 1984; 100:894–898

Hussian RA: Stimulus control in the modification of problematic behavior in elderly institutionalized patients. International Journal of Behavioral Geriatrics 1982; 1:33–42

Ioffe S, Havlicek V, Friesen H, et al: Effect of somatostatin and L-glutamate on neurons of the sensorimotor cortex in awake habituated rabbits. Brain Res 1978; 153:414–418

Jenike MA: Treating the violent elderly patient with propranolol. Geriatrics 1983; 38:29–31

Jenike MA: Monoamine oxidase inhibitors as treatment for depressed patients with primary degenerative dementia (Alzheimer's disease). Am J Psychiatry 1985; 142:763–764

Jotkowitz S: Lack of clinical efficiency of chronic oral physostigmine in Alzheimer's disease. Ann Neurol 1983; 14:690–691

Kamo H, McGeer PL, Harrop R, et al: Positron emission tomography and histopathology in Pick's disease. Neurology 1987; 37:439–445

Karlinsky H: Alzheimer's disease in Down's syndrome. J Am Geriatr Soc 1986; 34:728–734

Kase CS: "Multi-infarct" dementia: a real entity? J Am Geriatr Soc 1986; 34:482–484

Katzman R: The prevalence and malignancy of Alzheimer disease: a major killer. Arch Neurol 1976; 33:217–218

Katzman R: Alzheimer's disease. N Engl J Med 1986; 314:964–973

Kay DWK: Outcome and cause of death in mental disorders of old age. Acta Psychiatr Scand 1962; 38:249–276

Kaye WH, Weingartner H, Gold P, et al: Cognitive effects of cholinergic and vasopressin-like agents in patients with primary degenerative dementia, in Alzheimer's Disease: A Report of Progress in Research. Edited by Corkin S, Davis KL, Growden JH, et al. New York, Raven Press, 1982

Kelly WF, Checkley SA, Bender DA, Cushing's syndrome, tryptophan and depression. Br J Psychiatry 1980; 136:125–132

Khachaturian ZS: Diagnosis of Alzheimer's disease. Arch Neurol 1985; 42:1097–1105

Kidd M, Allsop D, Landon M: Senile plaque amyloid in Alzheimer's disease are all deposits of the same protein. Lancet 1985; 1:278

Kiloh LG: Pseudo-dementia. Acta Psychiatr Scand 1961; 37:336–351

Kirven LE, Montero EF: Comparison of thioridazine and diazepam in the control of non-psychotic symptoms associated with senility: double-blind study. J Am Geriatr Soc 1973; 21:546–551

Kovacs GL, Bohus B, Versteeg DHG, et al: Effect of vasopressin and oxytocin on memory consolidation: sites of action and catecholaminergic correlates after local microinjection into limbic midbrain structures. Brain Res 1979; 175:303–314

Lampe TH, Plymate SR, Risse SC, et al: TSH responses to two TRH doses in men with Alzheimer's disease. Psychoneuroendocrinology, in press

Larson, EB, Reifler BV, Featherstone HJ, et al: Dementia in elderly outpatients: a prospective study. Ann Intern Med 1984; 100:417–423

Lazarus LW, Newton N, Cohler B, et al: Frequency and presentation of depressive symptoms in patients with primary degenerative dementia. Am J Psychiatry 1987; 144:41–45

Leverenz, J, Sumi SM: Prevalence of Parkinson's disease in patients with Alzheimer's disease. Neurology 1984; 34 (Suppl)

Lieberman, A, Dziatolowski M, Kupersmith M, et al: Dementia in Parkinson disease. Ann Neurol 1979; 6:355–359

Lipsey JR, Robinson RG, Pearlson GD, et al: Nortriptyline treatment of post-stroke depression: a double-blind study. Lancet 1984; 1:297–300

Lishman WA: Cerebral disorder in alcoholism: syndromes of impairment. Brain 1981; 104:1–20

Loosen PT, Prange AJ: Serum thyrotropin response to thyrotropin-releasing hormone in psychiatric patients: a review. Am J Psychiatry 1982; 139:405–416

Mace NL, Rabins PV: The 36-hour day. Baltimore, John Hopkins University Press, 1981

Mair RG, Langlais PJ, Mazurek MF: Reduced concentrations of arginine vasopressin and MHPG in lumbar CSF of patients with Korsakoff's psychosis. Life Sci 1986; 38:2301–2306

Mann DA, Yates PO, Hawkes J: The noradrenergic system in Alzheimer and multi-infarct dementias. J Neurol Neurosurg Psychiatry 1982; 45:113–119

Markesbery WR, Ehmann WD, Hussain TIM, et al: Instrumental neutron activation of brain aluminum in Alzheimer disease and aging. Ann Neurol 1981; 10:511–516

Marsden CD, Harrison MJG: Outcome of investigation of patients with presenile dementia. Br Med J 1972; 2:249–252

Masters CL, Multhaup G, Sims G, et al: Neuronal origin of a cerebral amyloid. EMBO J 1985; 4:2757–2763

Mattis S. Mental status examination for organic mental syndrome in the elderly patient, in Geriatric Psychiatry. Edited by Bellack R, Karasu TB. New York, Grune & Stratton, 1976

Mayeux R, Stern Y, Spanton S: Heterogeneity in dementia of the Alzheimer type: evidence of subgroups. Neurology 1985; 35:453–461

Mayeux R, Stern Y, Williams JBW, et al: Clinical and biochemical features of depression in Parkinson's Disease. Am J Psychiatry 1986; 143:756–759

Mazurek KMF, Beal MF, Bird ED, et al: Vasopressin in Alzheimer's disease: a study of postmortem brain concentrations. Ann Neurol 1986a; 20:665–670

Mazurek MF, Growden JH, Beal MF, et al: CSF vasopressin concentration is reduced in Alzheimer's disease. Neurology 1986b; 36:1133–1137

Mazurek MF, Beal MF, Bird Ed, et al: Oxytocin in Alzheimer's disease: postmortem brain levels. Neurology 1987; 37:1001–1003

McAllister TW, Ferrell RB, Price TRP, et al: The dexamethasone suppression test in two patients with severe depressive pseudodementia. Am J Psychiatry 1982; 139:479–481

McDermott JR, Smith AI, Iqbal K, et al: Aluminum and Alzheimer's disease. Lancet 1977; 2:710–711

McEntee WJ, Mair RG, Langlais PJ: Neurochemical pathology in Korsakoff's psychosis. Neurology 1984; 34:648–652

McKeith IG: Clinical use of the DST in a psychogeriatric population. Br J Psychiatry 1984; 145:389–393

McKhann G, Drachman D, Folstein M, et al: Clinical diagnosis of Alzheimer's disease. Neurology 1984; 34:939–944

Meyer JS, Kitigawa Y, Tanahashi N, et al: Evaluation of treatment of normal-pressure hydrocephalus. J Neurosurg 1985; 62:513–521

Meyer JS, Judd BW, Tawaklna T, et al: Improved cognition after control of risk factors for multi-infarct dementia. JAMA 1986; 256:2203–2209

Mohs RC, Davis KL, Tinklenberg JR, et al: Choline chloride effects on memory in the elderly. Neurobiol Aging 1980; 1:21–25

Mohs RC, Davis BM, Johns CA, et al: Oral physostigmine treatment of patients with Alzheimer's disease. Am J Psychiatry 1985; 142:28–33

Mohs RC, Breitner JCS, Silverman JM, et al: Alzheimer's disease: morbid risk among first degree relatives. Arch Gen Psychiatry 1987; 44:405–408

Molsa PK, Paljarvi L, Rinne J, et al: Validity of clinical diagnosis in dementia: a prospective clinicopathological study. J Neurol Neurosurg Psychiatry 1985; 48:1085–1090

Morrison JH, Rogers J, Scherr S, et al: Somatostatin immunoreactivity in neuritic plaques of Alzheimer's patients. Nature 1985; 314:90–91

Mortimer JA: Alzheimer's disease and senile dementia: prevalence and incidence, in Alzheimer's Disease: The Standard Reference. Edited by Reisberg B. New York, Free Press, 1983

Mortimer JA, French LR, Hutton JT, et al: Head injury as a risk factor for Alzheimer's disease. Neurology (NY) 1985; 35:264–267

Navia BA, Cho ES, Petito CK, et al: The AIDS dementia complex: II. Neuropathology. Ann Neurol 1986a; 19:525–535

Navia BA, Jordan BD, Price RW: The AIDS dementia complex: I. Clinical features. Ann Neurol 1986b; 19:517–524

Neary D, Snowden JS, Bowen DM: Neuropsychological syndromes in presenile dementia due to cerebral atrophy. J Neurol Neurosurg Psychiatry 1986a; 49:163–174

Neary D, Snowden JS, Mann DMA, et al: Alzheimer's disease: a correlative study. J Neurol Neurosurg Psychiatry 1986b; 49:229–237

Nee LE, Eldridge R, Sunderland T, et al: Dementia of the Alzheimer type: clinical and family study of 22 twin pairs. Neurology 1987; 37:359–363

Peabody CA, Minkoff JR, Davies HD, et al: Thyrotropin releasing hormone stimulation test and Alzheimer's disease. Biol Psychiatry 1986; 21:553–556

Pearson RCA, Sofroniew MV, Cuello AC, et al: Persistence of cholinergic neurons in the basal nucleus in a brain with senile dementia of the Alzheimer's type demonstrated by immunohistochemical staining for choline acetyltransferase. Brain Res 1983; 289:375–379

Perl D, Brody A: Alzheimer's disease: spectrometric evidence of aluminum accumulation in neurofibrillary tangle-bearing neurons. Science 1980; 208:297–299

Perry EK, Curtis M, Dick DJ, et al: Cholinergic correlates of cognitive impairment in Parkinson's disease: comparisons with Alzheimer's disease. J Neurol Neurosurg Psychiatry 1985; 48:413–421

Perry EK, Tomlinson BE, Blessed G, et al: Correlation of cholinergic abnormalities with senile plaques and mental test scores in senile dementia. Br Med J 1978; 2:1457–1459

Perry RH, Candy JM, Perry EK, et al: Extensive loss of choline acetyl transferase activity is not reflected by neuronal loss in the nucleus of Meynert in Alzheimer's disease. Neurosci Lett 1982; 33:311–315

Petrie, WM, Ban TA, Berney S, et al: Loxapine in psychogeriatrics: a placebo- and standard-controlled clinical-investigation. J Clin Psychopharmacol 1982a; 2:122–126

Petrie WM, Mafucci RJ, Woosley RL: Propranolol and depression. Am J Psychiatry 1982b; 139:92–94

Post F: The management and nature of depressive illness in late life: a follow-through study. Br J Psychiatry 1972; 121:393–404

Post F: Dementia, depression, and pseudodementia, in Psychiatric Aspects of Neurologic Disease. Edited by Benson DF, Blumer D. New York, Grune & Stratton, 1975

Powell-Proctor L, Miller E: Reality orientation: a critical appraisal. Br J Psychiatry 1982; 140:457–463

Price RW, Navia BA, Cho E-S: AIDS encephalopathy. Neurol Clin 1986; 4:285–301

Prien F, Caffe EM: Pharmacologic treatment of elderly patients with organic brain syndrome: a survey of twelve Veterans Administration hospitals. Compr Psychiatry 1977; 18:551–560

Prinz P, Peskind E, Vitaliano P, et al: Changes in sleep and waking EEG in nondemented and demented elderly. J Am Geriatr Soc 1982; 30:86–93

Rabins P: The psychopathology of Parkinson's disease. Compr Psychiatry 1982; 12:421–428

Rabins PV, Mace NL, Lucas MJ: The impact of dementia on the family. JAMA 1982; 248:333–335

Rasker JJ, Jansen ENH, Jaan J, et al: Normal-pressure hydrocephalus in rheumatic patients. N Engl J Med 1985; 312:1239–1241

Raskind MA, Peskind E, Rivard MF, et al: Dexamethasone suppression test and cortical circadian rhythm in primary degenerative dementia. Am J Psychiatry 1982a; 139:1468–1471

Raskind MA, Veith R, Barnes R, et al: Cardiovascular and anti-depressant effects of imipramine in the treatment of secondary depression in patients with ischemic heart disease. Am J Psychiatry 1982b; 139:1114–1117

Raskind MA, Peskind ER, Halter JB, et al: Norepinephrine and MHPG levels in CSF and plasma in Alzheimer's disease. Arch Gen Psychiatry 1984; 41:343–346

Raskind MA, Peskind ER, Lampe TH, et al: Cerebrospinal fluid vasopressin, oxytocin, somatostatin, and beta-endorphin in Alzheimer's disease. Arch Gen Psychiatry 1986; 43:382–388

Raskind MA, Risse SC, Lampe TH: Dementia and antipsychotic drugs. J Clin Psychiatry 1987; 48:16–18

Rasool CG, Selkoe DJ: Sharing of specific antigens by degenerating neurons in Pick's disease and Alzheimer's disease. N Engl J Med 1985; 312:700–705

Reding M, Haycox J, Blass J: Depression in patients referred to a dementia clinic: a three year prospective study. Arch Neurol 1985; 42:894–896

Reichlin S: Somatostatin. N Engl J Med 1983; 309:1556–1563

Reifler BV: Arguments for abandoning the term pseudodementia. J Am Geriatr Soc 1982; 30:665–668

Reifler BV, Larson E, Hanley R: Coexistence of cognitive impairment and depression in geriatric outpatients. Am J Psychiatry 1982; 139:623–629

Reifler BV, Larsen E, Teri L, et al: Dementia of the Alzheimer's type and depression. J Am Geriatr Soc 1986; 34:855–859

Reifler BV, Teri L, Raskind M, et al: A double-blind trial of a tricyclic antidepressant in Alzheimer's patients with and without depression. Presented at the annual meeting of the American Psychiatric Association, Chicago, 1987

Reisberg B, Ferris SH, DeLeon MJ, et al: The Global Deterioration Scale for assessment of primary degenerative dementia. Am J Psychiatry 1982; 139:1136–1139

Reisberg B, Borenstein J, Salob SP, et al: Behavioral symptoms in Alzheimer's disease: phenomenology and treatment. J Clin Psychiatry 1987; 48(5):9–15

Riley JN, Walker DW: Morphological alterations in hippocampus after long-term alcohol consumption in mice. Science 1978; 201:646–648

Risse SC, Raskind MA, Lampe TH, et al: Research clinical diagnostic criteria for Alzheimer's disease with neuropathologic correlation: a prospective study. Presented at annual meeting of the Academy of Neurology, New Orleans, 1986

Risse SC, Cubberly L, Lampe TH, et al: Acute effects of neuroleptic withdrawal in elderly dementia patients. J Geriatr Drug Ther 1987; 2:65–77

Roberts GW, Crow TJ, Polak JM: Location of neuronal tangles in somatostatin neurons in Alzheimer's disease. Nature 1985; 314:91–94

Robins AH: Depression in patients with Parkinsonism. Br J Psychiatry 1976; 128:141–145

Robinson RG, Szetela B: Mood change following left hemisphere brain injury. Ann Neurol 1981; 9:445–453

Robinson RG, Starr LB, Price TR: A two year longitudinal study of past stroke mood disorders: prevalence and duration at six months followup. Br J Psychiatry 1984; 144:256–262

Rogers RL, Meyer JS, Mortel KF, et al: Decreased cerebral blood flow procedes multi-infarct dementia but follows senile dementia of Alzheimer type. Neurology 1986; 36:1–6

Roman GC: The identity of lacunar dementia and Binswanger disease. Medical Hypotheses 1985; 16:389–391

Rosen WG, Terry RD, Fuld PA, et al: Pathological verification of ischemic score in differentiation of dementias. Ann Neurol 1980; 7:486–488

Ross ED, Rush AJ: Diagnosis and neuroanatomical correlates of depression in brain damaged patients. Arch Gen Psychiatry 1981; 38:1344–1354

Rossor MN, Iversen LL, Reynolds GP: Neurochemical characteristics of early and late onset types of Alzheimer's disease. Br Med J 1984; 288:961–964

Rudorfer MV, Clayton PV: Depression, dementia and dexamethasone suppression (letter to editor). Am J Psychiatry 1981; 138:701

Salzman C: Treatment of the elderly agitated patient. J Clin Psychiatry 1987; 48(Suppl):19–22

Schmechel DE, Schmitt F, Horner J, et al: Lack of effect of nal physostigmine and lecithin in patients with Alzheimer's disease. Neurology 1984; 34:280

Selkoe DJ: Altered structural proteins in plaques and tangles: what do they tell us about Alzheimer's disease? Neurobiol Aging 1986; 7:425–432

Selkoe DJ, Abraham CR, Podlishy MB, et al: Isolation of low-molecular-weight proteins from amyloid plaque fibers in Alzheimer's disease. J Neurochem 1986; 146:1820–1834

Seltzer B, Sherwin I: A comparison of clinical features in early- and late-onset primary degenerative dementia. Arch Neurol 1983; 40:143–146

Serby M, Richardson SB, Tevente S, et al: CSF somatostatin in Alzheimer's disease. Neurobiol Aging 1984; 223:61–63

Sideman S, Manor D: The dialysis dementia syndrome and aluminum intoxication. Nephron 1982; 31:1–10

Simpson PM, Foster D: Improvement in organically disturbed behavior with trazodone treatment. J Clin Psychiatry 1986; 47:191–193

Sjogren T, Sjogren H, Lindgren AGH: Morbus Alzheimer and Morbus Pick. Acta Psychiatr Scand 1952; 82 (Suppl 82):1–66

Snider WD, Simpson DM, Nielsen S: Neurological complications of acquired immune deficiency syndrome. Ann Neurol 1983; 14:403–418

Sofroniew MV, Pearson RCA, Eckenstein F, et al: Retrograde changes in cholinergic neurons in the basal forebrain of the rat following cortical damage. Brain Res 1983; 289:370–374

Soininen HS, Jolkkonen JT, Reinikainen KJ, et al: Reduced cholinesterase activity and somatostatinlike immunoreactivity in the cerebrospinal fluid of patients with dementia of the Alzheimer types. J Neurol Sci 1984; 63:167–172

Sorenson PS, Hammer M, Vorstrup S, et al: CSF and plasma vasopressin concentrations in dementia. J Neurol Neurosurg Psychiatry 1983; 46:911–916

Spar JE, Gerner R: Does the dexamethasone suppression test distinguish dementia from depression? Am J Psychiatry 1982; 139:238–240

St. Clair D, Whalley LJ: Hypertension, multi-infarct dementia and Alzheimer's disease. Br J Psychiatry 1983; 143:274–276

St. George Hyslop PH, Tanzi RE, Polinsky JL, et al: The genetic defect causing familial Alzheimer's disease maps on chromosome 21. Science 1987; 235:885–889

Steele C, Lucas MJ, Tune L: Haloperidol versus thioridazine in the treatment of behavioral symptoms in senile dementia of the Alzheimer's type: preliminary findings. J Clin Psychiatry 1986; 47:310–312

Strachan RW, Henderson JG: Psychiatric syndromes due to avitaminosis B_{12} with normal blood and bone marrow. QJ Med 1965; 34:303–309

Struble RG, Cork LC, Whitehouse PJ, et al: Cholinergic innervation in neuritic plaques. Science 1982; 216:413–415

Sulkava R, Haltia M, Paetau A, et al: Accuracy of clinical diagnosis in primary degenerative dementia: correlation with neuropathological findings. J Neurol Neurosurg Psychiatry 1983; 46:9–13

Summers WK, Lawrence VL, Marsh GM, et al: Oral tetrahydroaminoacridine in long-term treatment of senile dementia, Alzheimer type. N Engl J Med 1986; 315:1241–1245

Sunderland T, Tariot PN, Mueller EA, et al: TRH stimulation test in dementia of the Alzheimer type and elderly controls. Psychiatry Res 1985; 16:269–275

Sundquist J, Forsling ML, Olsson JE, et al: Cerebrospinal fluid arginine vasopressin in degenerative disorders and other neurological diseases. J Neurol Neurosurg Psychiatry 1983; 46:14–17

Sweet RD, McDowell FH, Feigenson JS, et al: Mental symptoms in Parkinson's disease during chronic treatment with levodopa. Neurology 1975; 26:305–310

Tamminga CA, Foster NL, Chase TN: Reduced brain somatostatin levels in Alzheimer's disease. N Engl J Med 1985; 313:1294–1295

Tanzi RE, Gusella JF, Watkins PC, et al: Amyloid B protein gene: cDNA, mRNA distribution and genetic linkage near the Alzheimer locus. Science 1987; 235:880–884

Tarter RE: Brain damage in chronic alcoholics: a review of the psychological evidence, in Addiction and Brain Damage. Edited by Richter D. London, Creon Holm, 1980

Taulbee LR, Folsom JC: Reality orientation for geriatric patients, Hosp Community Psychiatry 1966; 17:133–135

Thal LJ, Rosen W, Sharpless NS, et al: Choline chloride fails to improve cognition in Alzheimer's disease. Neurol Aging 1981; 2:205–208

Thal LJ, Fuld PA, Masur DM, et al: Oral physostigmine and lecithin improve memory in Alzheimer's disease. Ann Neurol 1983; 13:491–496

Thal LJ, Grundman M, Golden R: Alzheimer's disease: a correlation analysis of the Blessed Information-Memory-Concentration Test and the Mini-Mental State Exam. Neurology 1986; 36:262–264

Thomasen AM, Borgesen SE, Bruhn P, et al: Prognosis of dementia in normal-pressure hydrocephalus after a shunt operation. Ann Neurol 1986; 20:304–310

Tinklenberg JR, Pfefferbaum A, Berger PA: 1-Desamino-D-arginine-vasopressin in cognitively impaired patients. Psychopharmacol Bull 1981; 17:206–207

Tomlinson BE, Blessed G, Roth M: Observations on the brains of demented old people. J Neurol Sci 1970; 11:205–242

Tomlinson BE, Irving D, Blessed G: Cell loss in locus coeruleus in senile dementia of Alzheimer type. J Neurol Sci 1981; 49:419–428

Trapp GA, Miner GD, Zimmerman RL, et al: Aluminum levels in brain in Alzheimer's disease. Biol Psychiatry 1978; 13:709–718

Veith RC, Raskind MA, Caldwell JH, et al: Cardiovascular effects of the tricyclic antidepressants in depressed patients with chronic heart disease. N Engl J Med 1982; 306:954–959

Victor M, Adams RD: The Wernicke-Korsakoff Syndrome. Philadelphia, F.A. Davis, 1971

Victoratos GC, Lonman JAR, Herzberg L: Neurological investigation of dementia. Br J Psychiatry 1977; 130:131–133

Vitaliano PP, Breen AR, Russo J, et al: The clinical utility of the dementia rating scale for assessing Alzheimer patients. J Chron Dis 1984; 37:743–753

Weingartner H, Gold P, Ballenger JC, et al: Effects of vasopressin on human memory functions. Science 1981; 211:601–603

Wells CE: Pseudodementia. Am J Psychiatry 1979; 136:895–890

Whelpton R, Hurst P: Bioavailability of oral physostigmine. N Engl J Med 1985; 313:1293–1294

Whitehouse PJ, Price DL, Struble RG, et al: Alzheimer's disease and senile dementia: loss of neurons in the basal forebrain. Science 1982; 215:1237–1239

Whitehouse PJ, Martino AM, Antuono PG, et al: Nicotinic acetylcholine binding sites in Alzheimer's disease. Brain Res 1986; 371:146–151

Whitehouse PJ, Vale WW, Zweig RM, et al: Reductions in corticotropin releasing factor-like immunoreactivity in cerebral cortex in Alzheimer's disease, Parkinson's disease and progressive supranuclear palsy. Neurology 1987; 37:905–909

Whybrow PC, Prange AJ Jr, Treadway CR: Mental changes accompanying thyroid gland dysfunction. A reappraisal using objective psychological measurement. Arch Gen Psychiatry 1969; 20:48–53

Wieland RG: Vitamin B_{12} deficiency in the nonanemic elderly. J Am Geriatr Soc 1986; 34:618–619

Wikkelso G, Andersson H, Blomstrand C, et al: The clinical effect of lumbar puncture in normal pressure hydrocephalus. J Neurol Neurosurg Psychiatry 1982; 45:64–69

Wilner E, Brody JA: Prognosis of general paresis after treatment. Lancet 1968; 2:1370–1371

Winblad B, Adolfsson R, Carlsson A, et al: Biogenic amines in hairs of patients with Alzheimer's disease, in Alzheimer's Disease: A Report of Progress in Research. Edited by Corkin S, Davis KL, Growden JH, et al. New York, Raven Press, 1982

Wisniewski HM, Sturman JA, Shek JW: Aluminum chloride induced neurofibrillary changes in the developing rabbit: A chronic animal model. Ann Neurol 1980; 8:479–490

Wolozin BL, Davies P: Alzheimer related neuronal protein A68: Alzheimer specific accumulation and detection in cerebrospinal fluid. Ann Neurol 1987; 22:521–526

Wood PL, Etienne P, Lal S, et al: Reduced lumbar CSF somatostatin levels in Alzheimer's disease. Life Sci 1982; 31:2073–2079

Wood PL, Nair NP, Etienne P, et al: Lack of cholinergic deficit in the neocortex in Pick's disease. Prog Neuropsychopharmacol Biol Psychiatry 1983; 7:727

Yudofsky S: Propanolol in the treatment of rage and violent behavior in patients with chronic brain syndromes. Am J Psychiatry 1981; 138:218–230

Zarit SH, Reever KE, Bach-Peterson J: Relatives of the impaired elderly: correlates of feelings of burden. Gerontologist 1980; 20:649–655

Chapter 13

Affective Disorders in Late Life

Dan G. Blazer, M.D., Ph.D.

The themes of aging and depression often coalesce. Frequent questions surrounding these themes include the following: Do persons become more depressed as they grow older? Does depression become more difficult to treat with increased age? Is depression more difficult to identify in the older adult? The answers to these questions rest in part with the definition of late-life depression. Depression in late life is not a unitary construct. Depending on how depression is defined, the answers to questions regarding late-life depression will change.

Depression can be construed in at least three ways, each of which has clinical relevance for older adults. First, depression can be viewed as a unitary phenomenon with the various manifestations of depression forming a continuum. Sir Aubrey Lewis (1934) noted that the various classifications of depression are "nothing more than attempts to distinguish between acute and chronic, mild and severe " (p. 1). Kendell (1976) has argued for the unitary view in more recent years. Though the extremes of the continuum are different, precise boundaries can be found between these extremes. Depression symptom checklists, such as the Self-Rating Depression Scale (Zung 1965), the Center for Epidemiologic Studies Depression Scale (CES-D) (Radloff 1977), and the Beck Depression Inventory (Beck et al. 1961), would therefore be useful in distinguishing the degree to which an individual suffers from depression in late life.

Most modern investigators, however, find it difficult to conceive of depression as phenomenologically homogeneous. Therefore, a categorical approach, exemplified in the *Diagnostic and Statistical Manual of Mental Disorders (Third Edition-Revised)* (American Psychiatric Association 1987), has been of more interest to modern clinicians. By viewing the affective disorders as a group of distinct entities or independent syndromes, with each of the categories mutually exclusive, the diagnosis and management of depression is allied with the traditional medical model. Given the availability of excellent, but potentially dangerous, biologic therapies, the use of the categorical approach has been adopted by most geriatric psychiatrists. Specific therapies can be prescribed for distinct diagnostic entities.

The third approach to the conceptualization of the depressed elder is a functional approach. Depressive symptoms become severe enough to be identified as a case worth clinical attention when function is impaired. Social function, especially the performance of role responsibilities, has been targeted as a critical in monitoring treatment. An example of the functional approach can be found in many surveys of community subjects (Langner and Michael 1963; *Multidimensional Functional Assessment* 1978). For the family, function is critical element, because they do not view symptom remission alone, but rather, a return to social involvement and improved life satisfaction as an essential marker of improvement. An older adult who sleeps better, has a better appetite, and ceases to be suicidal may be determined improved by the clinician but little improved by the family if social isolation and disinterest in the social environment persist after appropriate therapy. Axis V of the *DSM-III-R* partially assesses the impact of a disorder on social functioning.

The categorical approach to diagnosis—that is, a focus on Axis I of *DSM-III-R*—is adopted, for the most part, through the remainder of this chapter. Nevertheless, the reader must recognize that other constructs of depression must complement the categorical approach if it is to be effective in the diagnosis and treatment of older adults. Depressive symptoms that do not cluster in such a way as to fit the procrustean bed of a given diagnostic system may nevertheless be of clinical significance. Social and physical functioning, both during and following therapy, are at least as important in assessing the success of therapeutic intervention as the remission of a series of symptoms.

The Epidemiology of Late-Life Depression

General comments on the epidemiology of psychiatric disorders in late life have been reported in Chapter 9. In a recent study, investigators at Duke University Medical Center attempted to untangle the different subtypes of depression in late life in a community survey (Blazer et al. 1987). More than 1,300 older adults living in both urban and rural communities who were 60 years of age or older were screened for depressive symptomatology. Of the 27 percent reporting depressive symptoms, 19 percent were suffering from a mild dysphoria only. Symptomatic depression, that is, subjects with more severe depressive symptoms, made up 4 percent of the population. These individuals were primarily suffering from stressors, such as physical illness and stressful life events. Only 2 percent were suffering from a dysthymic disorder, and less than 1 percent (0.8 percent) were suffering from a current major depressive episode. No cases of current manic episodes were identified. Finally, 1.2 percent suffered from a mixed depression and anxiety syndrome. These data suggest that the traditional *DSM-III-R* depressive categories do not capture most depressed older adults in the community population.

In a study of psychiatric inpatients (Blazer et al. in press), subjects in both middle life and late life were identified as suffering from a major depressive episode with melancholia. Criteria symptoms for depression and symptoms specifically associated with melancholic or endogenous depression did not differ across age groups. The syndrome of major depression with melancholia is relatively common in inpatient service among older adults and is easily enough recognized.

How does one reconcile these seemingly disparate results? "Depression in late life" remains a generic term that captures many constructs, some of which are well defined and others of which are ill defined. The burden of depression in the elderly, as noted above in the frequency of significant depressive symptoms in community populations, is unquestioned. Many older persons with atypical presentations of depression do not meet criteria for major depression. Nevertheless, the usual reasons given for not identifying a severely depressed older adult in the clinical setting—pseudodementia, somatization, denial of depressive symptomatology, poor response to antidepressant medication, or masked depression—do not apply to most severely depressed elders, such as the melancholic older adult. The *DSM-III-R* and similar nomenclatures may therefore work for some, but not all, depressive syndromes in late life.

Manic episodes in late life are uncommon but not unseen. In a study of 6-month prevalence of psychiatric disorders in three communities (Myers et al. 1984), no person over the age of 65 was found to suffer from a current manic episode (out of more than 3,000 elders interviewed). One reason for the very low prevalence in community populations may be the inability of structured instruments to identify the atypical presentation of manic episodes among the elderly. When mania does occur, the syndrome may be so severe that the elder is hospitalized and therefore would not be located during a community inquiry.

Snapshot prevalence studies do not adequately represent late-life depression within the context of historical trends. The 20-year follow-up of the Midtown Manhattan study in New York illustrates the importance of cohort analysis (Srole and Fischer 1980). Nearly 700 of the original 1,660 adults interviewed initially between the ages of 20 and 59 were reinterviewed 20 years later using an identical instrument. This mental health impairment scale actually assessed primarily depressive symptomatology. Though in both 1954 and 1974 the highest rates of mental health impairment were found among the elderly (22 percent for the 50- to 59-year-olds, compared with 7 percent for the 20- to 29-year-olds in 1954), the prevalence of mental health impairment did not increase with age longitudinally. For example, from age 50–59 to age 70–79, depression remained almost constant (22 percent in 1954 vs. 18 percent in 1974). How can these findings be explained? Cohort effects may influence the distribution of depressive symptoms across the life cycle more than the effects of aging. The burden of depressive symptoms within a birth cohort may remain relatively constant through the life cycle.

An additional parameter of late-life affective disorders is the outcome from these disorders. The epidemiology of suicide has already been discussed in Chapter 9. The association between depressive symptoms and all-cause mortality among older participants in the Epidemiology Catchment Area study in North Carolina did not reveal a relationship between depressive symptoms and mortality when other known causes of mortality were included in a logistic analysis (Fredman et al. unpublished data). When age, activities of daily living, sex, and cognitive impairment were controlled, neither the diagnosis of major depression nor the accumulation of significant depressive symptoms at baseline predicted mortality 2 years following the initial interview of more than 1,600 community respondents 60 + years of age.

The association between late-life depression and mortality, however, is intuitively attractive, for older persons are thought to experience loss of meaningful roles and emotional support through retirement, widowhood, death of friends, low economic and material well-being, and increased isolation and loneliness (Atchley 1972; Fassler and Gavira 1978). In other community-based prospective longitudinal studies, depressed persons did have a significantly higher mortality rate than the nondepressed, but in most of these studies only age was controlled as a potential confounder (Enzell 1984; Kay and Bergmann 1966; Markush et al. 1977; Persson 1981).

Long-term follow-up of survivors of severe episodes of late-life depression are relatively scarce, given the frequency and clinical importance of the disorder. The typical course of major depression throughout the life cycle is remission and relapse. In patients who have a history of recurrent episodes, new episodes tend to exhibit similar symptoms and last for about as long as prior episodes. As individuals age, however, they may experience more frequent episodes and these episodes can merge into a chronic condition. Classic studies of depression suggest the duration of major depression throughout the life cycle to be approximately 9 months, if untreated (Dunner 1985). Post (1972) argued that the episodes of depression in late life may last longer than at earlier stages of the life cycle.

Most clinicians and clinical investigators report that more than 70 percent of patients suffering from major depression and treated with antidepressant medications will recover from the index episode of depression. Prediction of recovery from a depressive episode is enhanced through use of the dexamethasone suppression test (DST) (Carroll et al. 1981; Greden et al. 1983). Return to normal suppression of cortisol from a nonsuppression state often precedes clinical improvement and therefore bodes a good prognosis.

In contrast, if nonsuppression persists, patients, even if they improve clinically, are more likely to experience an early relapse (Greden et al. 1980). For predicting long-term follow-up, however, the DST has proved to be of less value (Zimmerman et al. 1987). The literature on the long-term outcome of depressive disorders and traditionally used to evaluate treatment response is equally sparse (Cadoret et al. 1980; Keller and Shapiro 1981). Even less has been reported in outcome by age group (Blazer et al. unpublished data; Cole 1983; Murphy 1983; Post 1972).

A general impression has emerged, however, that older persons have a poor prognosis if they suffer from depression. For example, Post (1972), in evaluating a follow-up study of 92 depressed older adults for 3 years, found that only 26 percent had sustained a recovery from depression, 37 percent experienced a recurrence after recovery, 25 percent experienced recurrent attacks within the context of chronic depressive symptoms (i.e., partial recovery), and 12 percent remained ill throughout the course of follow-up. Murphy (1983) reviewed the outcome of 124 patients with a Feighner diagnosis (Feighner et al. 1972) of primary depression over a 1-year period. Thirty-five percent recovered and remained well, 19 percent recovered but experienced a relapse, 29 percent remained ill throughout the follow-up, and 14 died. Cole (1983), however, found that older adults with primary depression without cognitive impairment and serious physical illness were more likely to remain well if they recovered when their first onset of depression was after the age of 60.

In a direct comparison of middle-aged and elderly patients hospitalized suffering from major depression, little difference was found between middle-aged and older adults in recovery (Blazer et al., unpublished data). Of the 44 older adults (60+ years of age), 48 percent had not recovered from the depressive episode leading to hospitalization, 27 percent had recovered completely from the index episode but suffered a recurrence of another episode of major depression, and 25 percent had recovered completely without a recurrence. Of the 35 middle-aged patients, 46 percent had not recovered from the index episode, 45 percent had recovered completely but suffered a recurrence of another episode, and 9 percent had recovered completely and remained recovered. Significant depressive symptoms at the time of follow-up (a score of 16 or higher on the CES-D) were reported by 59 percent of the elderly, but only 43 percent of the middle-aged subjects. This 1- to 2-year follow-up suggests that in terms of recovery and remission, older adults do not differ from their middle-aged counterparts. If they do recover, however, elders appear to suffer a residual of depressive symptoms. Whether these symptoms result from the major depressive episode or whether they were present before the onset of the depressive episode is unknown.

Persons suffering from a dysthymic disorder (depressive neurosis) experience a more chronic course than persons suffering with major depression. By *DSM-III-R* definition, these individuals must experience their symptoms at least 2 years. An undetermined percentage of community-dwelling (and possibly institutionalized) elders (possibly as high as 4 to 8 percent) suffer moderately severe depressive symptoms for longer than 2 years, though they report intermittent periods lasting longer than a few days when they are relatively free of depressive symptoms. The severity of their symptoms is not so great as to meet criteria for a diagnosis of major depression, and the intermittent symptom-free periods disqualify them from the diagnosis of dysthymic disorder. Nevertheless, these individuals suffer a chronic depression. Other older adults suffer from chronic depressions secondary to medical or even psychiatric disease, such as anxiety, alcoholism, and obsessive–compulsive disorder. Each of these disorders contributes to the residual of depression in the ambulatory elderly.

Although few factors have been demonstrated to predict long-term outcome from episodes of major depression, a few studies have suggested a relationship between social support assessment during an index episode and outcome from psychologic distress and depression. Intuitively, the availability of adequate support should enhance the recovery from a severe or moderately severe psychiatric disorder such as major depression. Holahan and Moos (1981), in a study of 493 community respondents, found that decreases in social support from family and work environments were related to increases in psychologic maladjustment over a 1-year follow-up period. In a longitudinal study, however, Henderson and Moran (1983) found no relationship between objective measures of support and the onset or the remission of substantial neurotic symptoms in a longitudinal community survey.

In a similar study (George et al., in press) 104 inpatients diagnosed as suffering from major depression were followed for 1 to 2 years following their hospitalization. Fifty-three of these patients were 60 years of age or older. Thirty-three reported that they had recovered from the index episode and scored lower than 10 on the CES-D at follow-up. Subjects who reported an adequate social support network at the time of the index depressive episode were 2.3 times more likely to have recovered than those who reported an impaired social network (44 percent vs. 19 percent). In a multiple regression analysis, social support remained a predictor of recovery from major depression when age, sex, and the initial CES-D score were controlled.

Personality pathology is another measurable phenomenon that is known to be associated with outcome. Weissman et al. (1978), among others, have noted that outcome from major depression is compromised. Unfortunately, there are no published reports of personality as a predictor of major depression outcome in the elderly. In addition, extant studies are confounded by the interaction of depressive symptomatology and personality variables at baseline assessment; that is, a depressed affect may influence the underlying personality. Given the stability of personality in late life, longitudinal studies of personality relationships to both the onset and outcome of major depression would be most helpful.

The outcome of bipolar disorder in the elderly remains virtually unknown. Winokur (1975), in a long-term follow-up study of 500 patients in Iowa, found there was a tendency for bipolar disorder to occur in clusters over time and speculated that early-onset bipolar illness may "burn itself out" with time. Shulman and Post (1980), in a study of elderly bipolar patients, found few of the existing cases to have their onset early in life. Cutler and Post (1982), in a review of a small number of untreated patients with severe and prolonged bipolar disorder, found a tendency for more rapid recurrences late in the history of the illness with decreasing periods of normality. In other words, if bipolar disorder reemerges in the later years, then the episodes of mania, or mania mixed with depression, may once again tend to cluster as the disorder typically clusters at earlier periods of life. Most clinicians who have worked with bipolar patients in late life recognize the tendency for these disorders to recur frequently for periods of time, only to remit for an extended period.

Risk Factors

The etiology of late-life affective disorders is undoubtedly multifactorial. Twin and family studies, along with recent studies of molecular genetics, provide strong evidence for a heritable contribution to the etiology of major depression and bipolar disorder (Egeland et al. 1987; Slater and Cowie 1971). Evidence that these genetic factors weigh heavily in the etiology of bipolar disorders in late life is virtually nonexistent, though the biologic nature of this disorder would suggest some genetic contribution. Evidence from studies of unipolar depression in late life suggests that the genetic contribution is weaker than at earlier stages of the life cycle (Hopkinson 1964; Mendlewicz 1976; Schulz 1951). For example, Hopkinson found the risk for immediate relatives of patients with onset of depression that occurred later than age 50 to be 8.3 percent, compared with 20.1 percent for relatives of patients who had onset before the age of 50. Stenstedt (1959) found the risk for affective disorder among relatives of probands falling ill for the first time at the age of 60 or over to be 4 to 5 percent, higher than expected but lower than the risk among relatives of manic–depressive probands earlier in life.

Associated with the genetic predisposition for depression is the observation that major depression is more common in females (Myers et al. 1984). Most studies that consider the distribution of major depression across the life span confirms the persistence of the 2:1 ratio of females to males into late life. However, there is no evidence for a genetic predisposition, that is, a sex-linked mode of inheritance, that would favor females in the onset of major depression. Nevertheless, even in the best-controlled studies, the sex difference in the prevalence of the more severe depressions persists. Whatever factor or factors that are operable persist into the later years.

Another contributing factor to late-life depression may be selective changes that occur in the activity and metabolism of neurotransmitters with aging. For example, Robinson et al. (1971) analyzed the concentrations of norepinephrine and serotonin in the hindbrains of 55 psychiatrically normal subjects who died at various ages. The concentrations of both neurotransmitters decreased with age, but the metabolite 5-hydroxyindoleacetic acid and the enzyme monoamine oxidase were found to increase with age.

Dysregulation of the hypothalamic–pituitary–adrenal (HPA) axis is also thought to contribute to a predisposition for depression. An association between increased cortisol concentrations and depression has been documented for many years: There is an increase throughout the 24-hour circadian excretion of cortisol in depressed patients (Sachar 1975). This led Carroll et al. (1981) to propose the DST as a laboratory test for melancholic depression. In a large study of males and females between the ages of 20 and 78, Rosenbaum et al. (1984) found that 18 percent of persons over the age of 65 were nonsuppressors of cortisol after administration of DST, compared with 9.1 percent of younger subjects. Whether this higher prevalence of nonsuppression reflects an increased propensity of older persons to suffer disregulation of the HPA axis, or whether it may result from difficulty in absorbing or metabolizing dexamethasone, remains to be discovered.

Dysregulation of the thyroid axis as well as in growth hormone release has also been implicated in the etiology of depression in later life. Blunted responses of thyroid-stimulating hormone (TSH) to the administration of thyrotropin-releasing hormone (TRH) are found in many normal elderly subjects, however (Snyder and Utiger 1972), and in depressed patients (Targum et al. 1982). Secretion of growth hormone occurs only during sleep in the elderly and may cease altogether (Finkelstein et al. 1972). Drugs known to stimulate α-adrenergic receptors, such as clonidine, also affect the release of growth hormone, a response that has been shown to be blunted in endogenous depression (Checkley et al. 1981).

Despite these numerous neurotransmitter and neuroendocrine changes that are common to old age and depressive illness, the relatively low prevalence of major depression and bipolar disorder in late life militates against the assumption that older persons are uniquely predisposed to the onset of melancholic or endogenous depressions. If so, protective factors that are yet to be discovered may also be operative in late life.

A relatively new putative contributor to the etiology of depressive disorders is desynchronization of circadian rhythms. The cyclicity of depressive disorders suggests an underlying disruption of the normal biochemical and physiologic circadian rhythms. Vogel et al. (1980) note that the clinical features of depression, especially insomnia and diurnal variation of mood, suggest abnormalities in biologic rhythms. The disruption of the sleep cycle with age (though this is the only circadian rhythm known to be dramatically affected by age) suggests the possibility of circadian problems contributing to the etiology of depression in late life. As age increases, there is a gradual diminution in total sleep time and a decrease in sleep continuity (Kupfer 1984; Ulrich et al. 1980). Endocrine secretion patterns, also associated with depression, are known to be less affected by the aging process (Lakatua et al. 1984).

Finally, social factors must be considered in the development of a risk model for depression in late life. Pfifer and Murrell (1986) examined the additive and interactive roles of six sociodemographic factors, three being from the domain of social resources and three being categories of life events, in the development of depressive symptoms. In a probability sample of more than 1,200 persons age 55 and older, 66 developed significant depressive symptoms (as measured by the CES-D scale) 6 months after an initial evaluation. Health and social support played both an additive and an interactive role in the onset of depressive symptoms, life events had weak effects, and sociodemographic factors did not contribute to depression onset. A weak support network in the presence of poor physical health placed older persons at an especial risk for the onset of depressive symptoms. It must be recognized, however, that depressive symptoms are not analogous to the onset of a major depressive episode. Though the relationship between stressful life events and the onset of major depression across the life cycle has been established in a number of cross-sectional studies (Lloyd 1980), the relationship weakens when persons are studied longitudinally, as observed by the Pfifer and Murrell study.

The interaction of social support and depression is more complex. Social support may contribute to the onset of major depression, it may contribute to the outcome of major depression, or it may in turn be affected by the depressive symptoms. Blazer (1983) tested the hypothesis that a major depressive disorder contributes to a decline in social support by studying 331 community subjects selected at random. Impaired support was associated with the presence of major depressive disorder at baseline. Thirty months later, however, the surviving subjects whose social supports had improved were nearly three times more likely to have been depressed earlier than those whose social supports did not improve. In other words, major depressive disorder was a significant predictor of improvement in supports at follow-up.

The Diagnosis and Differential Diagnosis of Late-Life Affective Disorders

Four clinical entities are listed under the affective disorders in *DSM-III-R* relevant to the clinical manifestations of depression in the elderly. They are (1) bipolar disorder (manic, depressed, and mixed), (2) major depression (single episode, recurrent, with or without melancholia, with or without psychotic features), (3) dysthymic disorder (depressive neurosis), and (4) atypical depression. Other *DSM-III-R* disorders, such as bereavement, adjustment disorder with depressed mood, and the organic affective syndrome, are manifested by a depressive symptom picture. Still other psychiatric disorders exhibit depressive symptomatology as a central component of the clinical picture on occasions, such as organic mental disorders, paranoid disorders, sleep disorders, and hypochondriasis. Physical illnesses (Axis III disorders) that frequently result in depressive symptoms include hypothyroidism, cancer, cardiovascular disease, hypertension, stroke, chronic pain syndromes, and Parkinson's disease.

For a patient to qualify for a diagnosis of manic episode (bipolar disorder), *DSM-III-R* requires the inclusion of at least three classic manic symptoms, such as overactivity, pressure of speech, distractibility, decreased sleep (without feeling a need for sleep), overspending, and grandiosity. Mood, however, can be either elevated or irritable and may be labile or mixed in the affective presentation. Post (1978) found that most elderly patients suffering from a bipolar disorder exhibited a depressive admixture with manic symptomatology. Spar et al. (1979) reported that manic elders are atypical in presentation, with dysphoric mood and denial of classic manic symptoms. Shulman (1986) described the special problem of manic delirium. During a full-blown manic episode, cognitive functioning is difficult to test, yet perseverative behavior, catatonic-like symptoms, and even negativistic symptoms may emerge. The patient in manic delirium can demonstrate the delirium-like symptom of picking at imaginary objects. In general, manic patients in late life are less likely to experience euphoria, though such cases are not absent. The differential diagnosis between a manic episode and an agitated depressive episode often cannot be disentangled except by virtue of a thorough examination of the longitudinal course and therapeutic response to medications.

First-onset episodes of major depression in late life are common and often go untreated for months or even years. For this reason, many investigators have suggested that late-life depression is "masked" (Davies 1965; Lesse 1974; Salzman and Shader 1972). Recent studies, however, suggest that older persons admit many feelings of sadness on self-rating scales for depression (Epstein 1976; Zung and Green 1972). In a recent study (Blazer et al. 1987) of hospitalized patients diagnosed as suffering from major depressive episodes with melancholia, the criteria symptoms for depression and symptoms specifically associated with melancholia (or endogenous depression) did not differ between individuals in middle life and late life. Melancholic depression was a relatively frequent syndrome identified in the elderly and was symptomatically similar to that found among persons in middle age. Community surveys confirm that *DSM-III-R* major depression is identified among the elderly when usual case-finding methods are applied across the life cycle (Myers et al. 1984).

There are variants of classic major depression among the elderly, however. One is the recently described seasonal affective disorder (Jacobsen et al. 1987). Diagnostic criteria for seasonal affective disorder include (1) a history of depression fulfilling Research Diagnostic Criteria (or *DSM-III-R* criteria) for major depression, (2) a history of at least 2 consecutive years of fall/winter depressive episodes remitting in the spring or summer, and (3) the absence of other major psychiatric disorder or psychosocial explanations for the seasonal mood changes. These disorders are most difficult to treat with usual therapies and may be perpetuated by the use of tricyclic antidepressants. Specifically, tricyclic antidepressants are thought to increase the likelihood of rapid cycling. In contrast, lithium carbonate or carbamazepine may be of some benefit in preventing the cyclic episodes. Light therapy, using high-intensity light to approximate the visual experience of a sunny day (usually in the morning), has been proved to be of some value in the treatment of these disorders.

Late-onset psychotic depression deserves special attention. Meyers et al. (1984) compared the prevalence of delusions between individuals who suffered the onset of depression before and after the age of 60 in 50 patients hospitalized for endogenous major depression. Depressives with onset after age 60 had delusions more frequently than did those with earlier onset. Individuals suffering from delusional depression tended to be older and to respond to electroconvulsive therapy (ECT) as opposed to tricyclic antidepressants. Delusions of persecution or having an incurable illness are more common than delusions associated with guilt. If guilt predominates the delusional picture, it usually involves some relatively trivial episode that occurred many years prior to the onset of the depressive episode, forgotten over time, but presently viewed as a major problem (Bridges 1986). For example, a one-time sexual liaison, forgotten or forgiven by the spouse, is resurrected by the patient with a fear of an ongoing venereal disease or cancer, or is associated with chronic and severe pain. Nihilistic delusions (delusions of nothingness) may occur more commonly in late life. Focus on the abdomen is common in the elderly patient suffering from a delusional or psychotic depression. Hallucinations are uncommon, however.

Every clinician who has worked with elderly patients has observed significant and unremitting depressive symptoms associated with apparent psychosocial causes. Verwoerdt (1976) suggests that "reactive depressions" become more frequent with aging (such as the depression associated with bereavement), whereas dysthymic disorder (depressive neurosis) seems to be less frequent in the later part of the life cycle. Recent community data, however, suggest that the prevalence of dysthymic disorder in the elderly is lower, but not dramatically lower as seen with major depression (Myers et al. 1984).

The psychologic mechanisms of late-life dysthymia usually do not include the classic mechanism of dysthymia, that is, self-reproach, guilt, and the turning inward of hostile feelings toward loss. Cath (1965) notes that manifest guilt in older persons is less prevalent, though reaction to loss is a common factor. Busse et al. (1954) suggested that among the elderly, introjection is seldom a mechanism for developing depression. Instead, late-life depression is associated with a loss of self-esteem that results from the older adult's inability to supply needs and drives or to defend him- or herself against threats to security. Levin (1965) noted the role of restraint as a mechanism in the neurotic depressions of later life. Though sexual satisfaction and interest in sexuality continue to be important for the older adult, sexual drive, though persistent, may not at times be as easily mobilized into behavior. Restraint may derive from either physical problems or lack of an available partner.

Other investigators have emphasized the cultural factors that may contribute to a dysthymic disorder in late life. Wigdor (1980) informs that the major resources in our culture lead to the development of habit patterns that emphasize activity and productivity; that is, ours is an achievement-oriented society. With retirement from the work force and cessation of parenting responsibilities, recognition, self-esteem, and confidence for many are withdrawn. These needs are not easily substituted. Erikson (1950) suggests that the primary developmental task for late life is the acquisition of integrity, and the means for achieving integrity is to resolve previous developmental crises that have persisted through the life cycle. In other words, striving for industry and generativity may continue to be important for the older adult. If the opportunities for realizing these productive urges are unavailable or the elder cannot reconcile previous generative disappointments, then despair will ensue.

Lazarus and Weinberg (1980), emphasizing the role of narcissistic pathology in the etiology of late-life depression, note that narcissism may manifest itself in "recurring depressions or defensive grandiosity in response to minor slights or disappointments, self-consciousness, overdependence on approval from others for maintenance of self-esteem, and the transitory periods of fragmentation and discohesiveness of the self" (p. 435). Associated with the depressive symptoms are an overconcern with physical appearance, possessions, and past accomplishments and the seeking of approval and reassurance from others.

In summary, dysthymic disorders in the elderly, though no more common than at other stages of the life cycle, are to be expected given the psychologic tasks that face older adults, coupled with a social environment that may restrain and devalue elders. That the elder maintains a sense of satisfaction and fulfillment given these inevitable losses and responses from others is a testimony to the resilience of older adults and a psychologic integration that permits a mature completion of life's developmental tasks.

Another subtype of depression in the elderly is most appropriately codified under *DSM-III-R* nomenclature as "atypical depression." This atypical depression, however, is not that usually described, that is, manifested by increased sleep, increased appetite, and known responsiveness to monoamine oxidase inhibitors. Rather, the atypical depressions in late life are more often intermittent and unexplained by psychosocial or clear biologic factors.

Two subcategories for *DSM-III-R* atypical depression empirically capture the symptom pattern frequently seen by clinicians working with depressed elders. First, the syndrome may fulfill the criteria for dysthymic disorder; however, there are intermittent periods of normal mood lasting more than a few months. The dysphoric older adult reports prolonged periods of depression usually lasting a period of months, but not extending for the entire 2 years required for *DSM-III-R* dysthymic disorder. Other elders fill the second criterion for atypical depression, that is, a brief episode of depression that does not meet the criteria for major affective disorder and is apparently not reactive to psychosocial stress (so that it cannot be classified as an adjustment disorder). These episodes do not meet criteria, for they do not last the full 2 weeks required for *DSM-III-R* diagnosis of major depression. Nevertheless, the symptoms can be moderately severe and most troubling to the older adult. The possibility that pharmacologic intervention will be effective in treating these atypical presentations of depression in late life cannot be eliminated. Nevertheless, the difficulty in describing the phenomenology of these syndromes must be overcome if effective drug trials can be implemented.

Bereavement is a universal human experience and therefore cannot be properly classified as a psychiatric disorder. Primary care physicians are likely to encounter the normal symptoms of grief, but these may be poorly recognized by the bereaved elder. Lindemann (1944), for example, suggests that the normal symptoms of bereavement include sensations of somatic distress such as tightness in the throat, shortness of breath, sighing respirations, lassitude, and loss of appetite. The bereaved are preoccupied with the image of the deceased and frequently can identify events from which they report guilt (often guilt at not having met the needs of the deceased). The grieving are often irritable and hostile, and change their usual patterns of conduct. These behavior changes are disturbing to the family and include a pressure of speech, restlessness, an inability to sit still, and a lack of capacity to initiate and maintain usual activities. Pathologic grief, in contrast, is delayed (an apparent denial of the loss) and/or distorted. Overactivity without a sense of loss, acquisition of symptoms belonging to the last illness of the deceased, frank psychosomatic illness, an alteration of relationships with family and friends, hostility toward specific persons (not uncommonly, family members), and persistent loss of patterns of social interaction can be seen. The *DSM-III-R* description of uncomplicated bereavement has not improved on Lindemann's classic description. A symptom picture of major depression usually presents with normal, uncomplicated bereavement, yet the syndrome is recognized by the older adult as normal to the occasion and does not seriously interfere with necessary function.

Among the common presentations of depression in late life is the onset of a depressed mood and expressions of hopelessness as a reaction to an identifiable stressor. The *DSM-III-R* category of adjustment disorder with depressed mood is reserved for those individuals who exhibit a maladaptive reaction to an identifiable stressor, yet the relationship of the syndrome to the stressful event is clear. Stressors for older adults include life events such as retirement, marital problems, difficulty with children, loss of a social role, or an ill-advised change of residence. Retirement is usually not a source of excessive stress for the older adult. Therefore, the onset of significant depressive symptomatology and withdrawal from activities following retirement may indicate a true adjustment disorder. Of much greater frequency, however, is the development of depressive symptomatology secondary to a physical illness. When an episode of depression accompanies a physical illness and exceeds dramatically the level of symptoms expected, then the diagnosis of adjustment disorder is indicated.

The final depressive category of relevance is the organic affective syndrome. The essential feature of this syndrome is a disturbance in mood resembling a major depressive episode due to a specific organic factor. The most common toxic factors to cause depressive symptoms in older adults are medications. Agents frequently prescribed to older adults that can precipitate depressive symptoms include β-blockers, benzodiazepines, alcohol, clonidine, reserpine, methyldopa, and even tricyclic antidepressants. Withdrawal of these agents permits a dramatic improvement in symptoms, though both patient and clinician may not associate these agents with the onset of the symptoms. Mild cognitive impairment is often observed in conjunction with the change in mood. Fearfulness, anxiety, irritability, and excessive somatic concerns may accompany the depressive symptoms as well. Metabolic disorders induce appreciable depressive symptoms, and these are properly classified in *DSM-III-R* under the category of the organic affective syndrome. For example, hyperthyroidism and hypothyroidism are known to present with depressive features. These disorders are included below in the discussion of physical illnesses that may contribute to a depressive episode.

The differential diagnosis of late-life depression must include not only other psychiatric and physical disorders but also the changes of normal aging. Some associate a depressed mood with aging. However, most longitudinal studies of depression and life satisfaction do not validate this assumption. Though Busse et al. (1954) found that elderly subjects were aware of more frequent and more annoying depressive periods than they had experienced earlier in life, only a small number admitted to severe and protracted periods of depression. Approximately 85 percent of the subjects in this study were able to trace the onset of these depressive episodes to specific stimuli. Epidemiologic data presented in Chapter 9 confirm that the frequency of severe late-life depression (major depression) is lower than at earlier stages of the life cycle.

Life satisfaction, morale, and adjustment were not found to decline in a 4-year longitudinal study of an elderly cohort (Palmore and Kivett 1977). Rather, life satisfaction is associated with health status, socioeconomic status, social participation, income, and living arrangements (Thomae 1980). Poor life satisfaction may be correlated with depressive symptoms, yet these two constructs must be considered independently. Severe clinical depression can occur within the context of satisfaction with one's life and adjustment to one's situation. On the other hand, dissatisfaction with life and demoralization may be manifested as poor self-esteem, helplessness and hopelessness, sadness, confused thinking, and so forth, yet never progress to the point at which the syndrome could adequately be described as meeting criteria for a psychiatric disorder. Rather, discouragement and dissatisfaction are typical of the elder who, as described by Frank (1973), "finds that he cannot meet the demands placed on him by the environment, and cannot extricate himself from his predicament" (p. 312).

The normal biologic changes of aging may interact with depressive symptomatology as well. Older persons, for example, spend more time lying in bed at night without attempting to sleep or unsuccessfully trying to sleep, and therefore complain of decreased sleep efficiency. The rapid eye movement (REM) sleep latency, a marker that has been associated with depression (see below), is also known to decrease slightly throughout life in both sexes (Dement et al. 1982). Elderly persons are notorious for complaining of poor appetite and reduced food intake. Munro (1981) found that caloric intake falls with aging. In addition, poor dentition may contribute to decreased food intake as well. Taste acuity also decreases with increasing years (Schiffman 1979). Lethargy is another common complaint of older adults.

Among the psychiatric disorders, the most common problem in the differential diagnosis of depression is with the organic mental disorders. Pseudodementia is a syndrome in which dementia is mimicked or caricatured by a functional psychiatric illness, most commonly depression (Wells 1979). Patients with pseudodementia respond on the mental status examination similarly to those who suffer from true degenerative brain disease. Though not rare in the elderly, Kiloh (1961) reminds the clinician that pseudodementia is "purely descriptive and carries no diagnostic weight" and yet these patients are in danger of inaccurate diagnosis and therapeutic neglect. Wells (1979) distinguishes depression presenting as pseudodementia from true dementia by the rapid onset of the cognitive problems in depression, the relatively short duration of symptoms, the consistent depressed mood associated with cognitive difficulties, and a tendency among the depressed to highlight disabilities as opposed to concealing (or attempting to conceal) them. The depressed older adult is more likely to respond with "I don't know" on the mental status exam, whereas the demented is more likely to attempt answers or to attempt to deflect the questions. Cognitive impairment in depression fluctuates from one exam to another, whereas cognitive impairment in dementia is relatively stable.

Of more clinical import, however, is the frequent overlap of depressive symptoms and symptoms of the organic mental disorders. Grinker et al.

(1961) noted impaired recent memory in 21 percent and poor remote memory in 14 percent of persons studied with depressive disorders of all ages. Reifler et al. (1982) studied 88 cognitively impaired elderly outpatients and found that depression was superimposed upon dementia in 17 (19 percent). Patients with greater cognitive impairment exhibited fewer symptoms of depression. When individuals were treated with an antidepressant medication, they responded with a remission of the depressive symptoms, yet the cognitive dysfunction persisted.

The diagnostic problems may be more complex, however. Specifically, there may be actual cerebral changes in depression that contribute to the dementia-like syndromes seen in some depressed older adults (Thielman and Blazer 1986). Though older adults may not spontaneously complain of difficulty with memory and concentration more frequently than persons at earlier stages of the life cycle in the presence of significant depressive symptoms, they do have more difficulty performing on mental status examinations (Blazer et al. 1986).

Given the propensity for older adults to exhibit more psychotic features during an episode of major depression, the appearance of an overt psychosis with delusional thinking suggests to many clinicians the onset of a major depressive episode. The discovery of paranoid ideation and delusions, however, may be evidence of a late-life schizophrenic disorder. Older adults suffering from late-life schizophrenic-like symptoms generally do not become profoundly depressed. Rather, they are distressed and focus all of their difficulties on a perceived hostile environment. Though family members or physicians are often surprised at the discovery of these symptoms, paranoid ideation and delusional thinking in a schizophrenic-like illness rarely begin suddenly but rather evolves gradually. An inquiry into the history of the disorder uncovers gradual withdrawal, bizarre comments, and often elaborate preparations to ensure safety (such as multiple locks on the door, bars on the windows, or stockpiling of food). The source of threat gradually moves from outside to within, such as a perception of being sexually molested, yet the paranoid elder rarely has a sense of poor self-worth.

Idiopathic sleep problems are often accompanied by depressive symptoms. The normal changes in sleep that mimic depressive sleep problems have been reviewed above. A number of sleep disorders also contribute to symptoms that mimic major depression. Delayed or advanced sleep phase syndrome, that is, the shift of the normal sleep cycle to later or earlier in the evening, is most disturbing to older persons who have previously viewed their sleep as a habitual given. The elder who, from boredom or other conditions, begins a night's sleep at 8:00 or 9:00 P.M. will awaken at 2:00 or 3:00 in the morning and thereby complain of "early morning awakening." In addition, the anxiety inherent when awakening to a darkened home with no activity exacerbates the discomfort associated with a sleep phase syndrome.

Sleep apnea syndrome, which is more common with aging, may not be recognized by the older adult (especially if he or she lives alone). A spouse or sleeping partner, however, cannot spend many nights with an apneic elder without recognizing that something is abnormal about the sleep pattern. However, the elder suffering from sleep apnea will only complain of lethargy and vague concerns regarding sleep, including excessive sleep.

Depressive disorders have been documented to be associated with a variety of physical illnesses, including cardiovascular disease (Dovenmuehle and Verwoerdt 1962), endocrine disturbances (Relkin 1969), Parkinson's disease (Asnis 1977), stroke (Post 1962), cancer (Whitlock and Siskind 1979), and chronic pain (Krishnan et al. 1985). In addition, depressive symptoms have been found to be frequent in surveys of medical inpatients (Harwin 1973; Schwab et al. 1965).

The association between depression and hypothyroidism has been well established. Though the profoundly life-threatening symptoms of myxedema —stupor or coma—are rarely missed in diagnosis, less severe symptoms and signs are common with normal aging and major depression. These include constipation, cold intolerance, psychomotor retardation, decreased exercise tolerance, and cognitive changes, as well as a depressed affect. Laboratory evaluation will generally reveal a depressed thyroxine and elevated serum TSH concentration. When this laboratory finding is identified, intervention for the thyroid difficulty must precede intervention for the depressive affect.

Depressive symptoms have also been associated with the development of cancer. Early in modern medicine, Guy (1759) thought women with melancholia to be more prone to develop breast cancer. Whitlock and Siskind (1979) studied 39 men and 90 women older than 40 years who had a primary diagnosis of depression. They were followed from 2 years and 4 months, to 4 years. During the follow-up period, nine men and nine women died, and six had cancer deaths, significantly higher than would have been expected.

Dovenmuehle and Verwoerdt (1962) found that 64 percent of 62 cardiac patients, 41 of whom were more than 60 years of age, developed moderate to severe depressive symptoms.

The impact of physical illness on emotion can be more direct. Evidence is emerging that a neurology of depression exists (Coffey 1987). The right hemisphere may be uniquely specialized for the perception, experience, and expression of emotion. Consistent differences have been observed in the emotional behavior of individuals who have suffered either left or right hemispheric damage. A left-sided stroke may be associated with depressive and even catastrophic responses manifested by combinations of dysphoria, episodes of crying, feelings of despair, hopelessness, anger, and self-depreciation (Gainotti 1972; Sackeim et al. 1982). A lesion of the right cerebral hemisphere is more often followed by a neutral or indifferent, or even euphoric, response with denial of deficits and social disinhibition. Though exceptions exist to these studies, the recognition that selective lesions of the brain may contribute to specific syndromes closely associated with the depressive disorders implies, in some cases, an anatomy of depression rather than generalized neurochemical abnormalities.

The association between chronic pain and depression has been established for many years (Blumer and Heilbronn 1982; Kraemlinger et al. 1983). The evidence for this association is based on the increased frequency of depression in chronic pain patients and the frequent report of pain by depressed patients, coupled with the high concurrence of biologic markers of depression and markers for chronic pain. Krishnan et al. (1985) found that most items on a typical depression rating scale, such as the Hamilton Depression Rating Scale, did not discriminate patients suffering from major depression from those suffering from chronic low back pain. Nevertheless, the items discriminated well between patients with and without depression. France et al. (1984), in an attempt to unravel the relationship between chronic pain and depression, found that 41 percent of patients with major depression were nonsuppressors of cortisol in response to a challenge with dexamethasone, yet all patients without major depression had normal DST results when studying a group of 42 patients with chronic pain. In general, chronic pain does not become more prevalent with aging, but a number of older persons do suffer from specific and rather severe chronic pain syndromes, such as cancer pain or severe osteoarthritis. The clinician must distinguish the chronic pain patient from the individual suffering from hypochondriasis, where the interrelationship with depressive symptoms may be different.

Depression is a frequent accompaniment of Parkinson's disease. Most older persons differ little in the physical symptoms and signs of paralysis agitans from persons observed at earlier ages. The major problems encountered in treating the parkinsonian older adult are secondary to either undue sensitivity to medications or the emotional state of the patient. The parkinsonian older adult may become disoriented and aggressive and experience ideas of persecution. More commonly, the elder withdraws socially and expresses helplessness and hopelessness regarding the future and considerable anger regarding the difficulties in adjusting doses of medication (Carter 1986). Slow movement, weakness, rigidity, and masked and unexpressive facial expressions suggest to the clinician a depressed affect associated with the progression of Parkinson's disease. Nevertheless, the appearance of depression may be more severe than the actual affect. Clinicians must be judicious in determining the necessity of pharmacologic intervention in the parkinsonian patient.

Hypochondriasis is a frequent confounder of the differential diagnosis of the depressed older adult. Though a depressed mood may be experienced by the hypochondriacal elder, the essential feature of hypochondriasis is an unrealistic interpretation of physical signs or sensations as abnormal, which in turn leads to a preoccupation with the fear or belief of suffering from a serious illness (APA 1980). A number of investigators have reported the prevalence of "hypochondriacal symptoms" to be elevated among the depressed elderly. De Alarcon (1964) found that of 152 patients suffering from depression, 65 percent of the men and 62 percent of the women reported concomitant hypochondriacal symptoms, the most common being constipation.

The concurrence of depressive symptoms and hypochondriacal symptoms may increase the risk of suicide. In de Alarcon's study, 24.8 percent of individuals with hypochondriacal symptoms attempted suicide, whereas only 7.3 percent of those free of such symptoms did so. Hypochondriasis as a disorder differs from hypochondriacal symptoms. True hypochondriasis can be distinguished from depression usually by the length of the episode (hypochondriasis usually persists from middle life), the degree to which the patient appears to suffer from symptoms (the depressed appear to suffer more), and the cyclicity of symptoms (atypical of hypochondriasis but typical of depression). The endogenously depressed older adult with many somatic complaints will generally tolerate antidepressant medications as well as other elders, whereas the hypochondriacal patient generally does not tolerate an antidepressant medication because of the anticholinergic side effects (Blazer 1984).

The Diagnostic Workup of the Depressed Older Adult

Of special importance in evaluating the depressed elder is the assessment of the length of the current depressive episode; the history of previous episodes; the history of drug and alcohol abuse; response to previous therapeutic interventions for the depressive illness; family history of depression, suicide, and/or alcohol abuse; and the degree to which the older adult appears to be suffering from the depressive symptomatology. The establishment of some indication of the risk for suicide is essential, for suicidal risk may determine the location of treatment. The physical examination must include a thorough neurologic examination to determine the presence of soft neurologic signs (such as a frontal release sign) or laterality. Weight loss and psychomotor retardation in the depressed older adult may lead, in some individuals, to a peroneal palsy, documented by electromyography and nerve conduction abnormalities (Massey and Bullock 1978). Because the older adult is less occupied with physical activities and therefore tends to sit, the peroneal nerve is subject to chronic trauma.

The laboratory workup of the depressed older adult should include a thyroid panel (triiodothyronine, thyroxine, and radioactive iodine uptake) along with TSH. A blood screen enables the clinician to identify the presence of an anemia. Usually the evaluation of red cell size and abnormalities on the smear enables the recognition of a potential deficit in B_{12} or folate. Although dementing illness is the most prominent outcome of a B_{12} deficiency, depressive symptoms may also result. The use of psychologic testing can assist the clinician in distinguishing permanent versus temporary cognitive deficits as well as identifying potential laterality of cognitive abnormalities. Nevertheless, in the midst of severe depressive illness, psychologic testing may be of less value. Therefore, timing the use of psychologic testing is essential to maximize the value of test results in clinical decision making.

The laboratory evaluation of depression has entered a new era in the 1980s. Depressive disorders that were identified exclusively by clinical signs and symptoms can now be delineated by a combination of these signs and symptoms with so-called biologic markers. Though no true laboratory test is available for the diagnosis of major depression (or even the subtypes of major depression), the use of the laboratory by clinicians as well as clinical investigators has increased dramatically.

The most used and the most debated of these laboratory tests is the DST. Based upon the recognition of hyperactivity of the HPA axis in depressive disorders, Carroll et al. (1981) suggested a modified DST as a diagnostic aid for endogenous depression or melancholia. One milligram of dexamethasone is administered at 11:00 P.M. The next day, blood samples for the determination of plasma cortisol are drawn at 4:00 P.M. and 11:00 P.M. For outpatients, only the 4:00 sample would be drawn. An increased plasma concentration of cortisol in either of the blood samples will signify an abnormal or positive result. The cutoff in most laboratories for normal plasma cortisol concentration following dexamethasone is 5 μg/dl with competitive protein-binding assays. In the original study by Carroll, the test was nearly 50 percent sensitive and more than 90 percent specific for endogenous depression. Since the initial introduction of the DST, many investigators have replicated these results. Two factors have emerged from these investigations, however. First, the DST may not be as specific as originally believed, since persons suffering from other psychiatric disorders also exhibited a positive DST. In addition, a number of conditions may contribute to false positive results, such as physical illness (Cushing's disease, pregnancy, diabetes mellitus), medications (barbiturates, meprobamate, phenytoin), low body weight, ongoing weight loss (which frequently accompanies depressive illness), and acute infectious illnesses with fever and dehydration.

The DST has been studied extensively in elderly populations. Magni et al. (1986) found a sensitivity of 73 percent for major depressive disorder among hospitalized depressed elders, with only 11 percent of the controls and 11 percent of the persons suffering from dysthymic disorder having an abnormal DST. Jenike and Albert (1984) found that among persons with mild cognitive impairment secondary to Alzheimer's disease, the DST was useful in distinguishing the depressed from nondepressed. When they included the more severely demented subjects, however, the DST was less specific. Tourigny-Rivard et al. (1981) did not find advanced age to affect the overnight DST in healthy normal adults and therefore suggested the test would be equally useful for the young and the elderly. In general, however, investigators believe that nonsuppression following dexamethasone increases gradually with age and therefore the usefulness of the DST probably diminishes with increasing age, especially after the age of 75.

A second biologic marker that has received increased attention is the use of sleep electroencephalogram (EEG) results to identify depression. Generally, two nights of sleep recording are obtained after patients have been drug free for 14 days, and mean data from the two nights are used for the study. Rapid eye movement density and REM latency have both been proposed as potential markers for depression (Kupfer et al. 1978). Compared with control subjects, endogenously depressed patients appear to show increased sleep discontinuity (i.e., a disruption of the sleep architecture), reduced slow-wave sleep (stages 3 and 4), shortened REM latency (the time between the onset of sleep and the first REM period), and increased REM density (the ratio of the sum of eye movements to the length of time of REM sleep). Those trends in the sleep EEG that appear to mark endogenous depression are, as described above, trends that often accompany the normal aging process. However, the combined use of sleep EEG tracings and other markers may help increase the probability of identifying the more biologically derived depressive disorders.

Attention has been recently directed to platelet tritiated-imipramine-binding density as a marker of depressive illness. A number of reports suggest that the maximal density of platelet imipramine-binding sites (β_{max}) is lower in unmedicated subjects suffering from a unipolar affective disorder (Asarch et al. 1981; Briley et al. 1980). In contrast to the decreased sensitivity of the DST with aging, tritiated imipramine binding may actually be a more specific test for endogenous depression in the elderly than in younger control subjects (Knight et al. 1986; Schneider et al. 1985). In the study by Knight and colleagues, comparing subjects between the ages of 35 and 50 with subjects 60+ years of age, the number of platelet tritiated-imipramine-binding sites was reduced in patients with major depression. The finding was especially robust in the elderly depressed but remained normal in other neuropsychiatric disorders such as Alzheimer's disease and schizophrenia.

Another marker that has been associated with depression throughout the life cycle is platelet monoamine oxidase activity. In a study by Schneider et al. (1986), platelet monoamine oxidase activity was found to be significantly higher in elderly depressed women than in sex- and age-comparable controls. There were no significant relationships between monoamine oxidase activity and duration of the current depressive episode, the lifetime duration of the illness, or family history.

Another potential marker for biologic depression is platelet α_2 adrenoceptors. This marker may also be of value in studying depression in late life, as neither binding capacity nor affinity of α_2 adrenoceptors on platelets is known to be correlated specifically with age (Buckley et al. 1986).

A more thoroughly studied marker that may have not only diagnostic but therapeutic implications is the blunted TSH response to TRH. Thyrotropin-releasing hormone stimulates the release of TSH from the anterior pituitary gland. The TRH test—the measurement of serum TSH concentration follow-ing administration of TRH—has become a standard test in endocrinology. Administration of synthetic TRH challenges the anterior pituitary to respond. The differential response in the serum TSH may characterize disorders of the HPA axis. Though TSH blunting is not specific to depression, a number of studies have found TSH to be blunted in depression (Gregoire et al. 1977; Loosen and Prange 1982). Once again, however, increasing age is known to be associated with a blunted TSH response to TRH (Snyder and Utiger 1972). Because of this abnormality, supplemental thyroid has been prescribed to depressed persons, with occasional beneficial response. For example, Cyto-mel (at 25 μg daily) could augment the therapeutic effect of the traditional tricyclic antidepressants. This augmentation may be valuable to some elders, since subclinical hypothyroidism occasionally contributes to depression in older adults. The first step, however, is a more thorough workup and the use of thyroid agents alone to determine if the depressive symptoms are solely determined by hypothyroidism.

Given the emergence of an ever-increasing list of potential markers—some to be investigated further, some yet to be discovered, and some that will be dropped from the list as not useful for clinical purposes—how is the clinician best to integrate these markers into clinical practice? First, their primary utility is in probing the biologic contribution to the depressive disorders of late life. None of these biochemical, neuroendocrine, or circa-dian abnormalities qualify as a biologic test for a psychiatric disorder at present. They may never reach this status, because the etiology of late-life depression is multidetermined, with no clear evidence that one factor is necessary for the symptoms to emerge. Nevertheless, these markers may be considered analogous to symptoms, in that they can be included in the data base collected in order to increase the probability of delineating a real psychopathologic entity that can be effectively diagnosed and treated, and whose outcome can be predicted.

Treatment

The treatment of depression in late life is four pronged: psychotherapy, pharmacotherapy, ECT, and family therapy. Since pharmacotherapy is cov-ered in some detail elsewhere, the remaining three therapeutic approaches are emphasized below.

Psychotherapy

Cognitive–behavioral therapy is the only psychotherapy that has been designed specifically to treat depression (Beck et al. 1979). Even the more recent interpersonal therapy (Klerman et al. 1984) is primarily a cognitive–be-havioral orientation to improving interpersonal relationships. The advantage of cognitive–behavioral therapy in treating the older adult is that it is directive and time limited, usually requiring between 10 and 25 sessions for completion. Cognitive–behavioral therapy has been studied specifically in the elderly (Gallagher and Thompson 1982; Steuer et al. 1984).

The goal of the behavioral and cognitive therapies is to change behavior and modes of thinking. This change is accomplished through behavioral interventions such as weekly activity schedules, mastery and pleasure logs, and graded task assignments. Cognitive approaches to restructuring negative cognitions or automatic thoughts include empirical reality testing of these cognitions, examining distortions (such as overgeneralizations, catastrophizing, and dichotomous thinking), and generating new ways of viewing one's life (Steuer et al. 1984). Depressed patients typically regard themselves and their present and future in somewhat idiosyncratic or negative ways. Such patients believe themselves to be inadequate or defective and believe that unpleasant experiences are caused by a problem with themselves and therefore they are worthless, helpless, and hopeless. This cognitive triad leads the older adult to believe that he or she is suffering from a never-ending depression and that nothing pleasant will ever happen again. The cognitive model presupposes that these symptoms of depression are consequences of negative thinking patterns.

Results from empirical studies (such as the studies of Gallagher and Thompson [1982] and Steuer et al. [1984]) suggest that compared with controls, those engaging in psychotherapy exhibit incremental improvement. Not only does the percentage of elders who respond to these treatments compare favorably to younger samples, the improvement appears equivalent to that secondary to medications, especially with nonendogenous depressions. Because drug therapy is not appropriate for some elders, cognitive–behavioral psychotherapy provides a viable alternative. In addition, evidence has emerged that suggests that the long-term benefit of cognitive–behavioral therapy may be greater than that of medications, especially if the medications are discontinued during the first year of treatment.

Pharmacotherapy

Details regarding the treatment of the older adult with psychopharmacologic agents are presented elsewhere. The tricyclic antidepressants remain the agents of choice, despite the advent of third-generation antidepressant medications. Medications that are effective yet relatively free of side effects (especially cardiovascular effects) are preferred. Nortriptyline and desipramine have become the more popular agents in recent years for treating endogenous or melancholic major depression in older adults, yet doxepin remains a favorite among many practitioners.

The dosage of antidepressant medication in late life should be case specific but generally is less than for persons in middle life. For example, 25 to

50 mg of nortriptyline orally at bedtime or 25 mg of desipramine orally twice a day are frequently adequate in relieving depressive symptoms. Plasma levels of the medications can be helpful in dosing. Unfortunately, good studies of thresholds and windows for drug use remain to be established.

If the tricyclic medications are ineffective, or side effects are too severe, trazodone is an alternative. Trazodone has advantages over the tricyclic antidepressants in that it is virtually free of anticholinergic effects. Nevertheless, the drug is not without side effects, such as excessive daytime sedation and occasionally priapism. Monoamine oxidase inhibitors provide another alternative to tricyclics. If monoamine oxidase inhibitors are considered when intolerance to side effects from the tricyclic antidepressants ensues, older adults usually do not tolerate the monoamine oxidase inhibitors better. If the depression is severe and ECT is contemplated, the use of a monoamine oxidase inhibitor precludes initiation of ECT until 10 days to 2 weeks following discontinuance of the drug. Such a delay may seriously impede effective clinical management of the suicidal elder.

Some clinicians prescribe low-dose stimulant medications, such as 5 mg of methylphenidate, in the morning to improve the mood of the apathetic older adult. The effectiveness of stimulants has not been conclusively demonstrated. Nevertheless, the agents are generally safe in low dosage, and rarely does the clinician encounter an elder with a propensity to abuse stimulants or to become addicted when given on a once-a-day basis.

Electroconvulsive Therapy

Electroconvulsive therapy continues as the most effective form of treatment available for the more severe major depressive episodes (Scovern and Kilmann 1980). The induction of a seizure appears to be that factor which is effective in reversing a major depression. Though the treatment has been established for many years, ECT is no longer used as much as it was immediately following its development in 1938 (Weiner 1982). Despite its effectiveness, ECT is not the treatment of choice initially for a major depression and should be prescribed only because other therapeutic modalities have been ineffective. However, ECT has been demonstrated to be effective in selected individuals, primarily those suffering from major depression with melancholia and especially those suffering from major depression with psychotic symptoms associated with agitation or withdrawal. Many older adults suffering from such syndromes do not respond to antidepressant medications or become toxic (they usually experience postural hypotension) when taking antidepressants. The presence of self-destructive behavior, such as a suicide attempt or refusal to eat, increases the necessity for intervening effectively and often renders ECT the treatment of choice.

If ECT is elected as an intervention, the clinician must first discuss in detail with the patient and the family the nature of the treatment and the reasons for a recommendation. Why is ECT necessary? What are the procedures that the patient will undergo during a course of ECT? How many treatments can be expected and how long will the hospitalization continue? Can ECT be performed on an outpatient basis? What are the risks and side effects of ECT? What kind of results, both immediate and long term, can be expected from the treatment? Even in the most severely depressed elder, careful and thoughtful discussion with the patient and family will usually result in a willingness by the patient (often with encouragement from the family) to undergo the course of treatments. Once treatment is begun, the fears of ECT usually remit.

The medical workup prior to ECT includes a complete medical history, physical examination, and consultation with a cardiologist if any cardiac abnormalities are recognized. A family history that includes a history of psychiatric disorder and/or suicide and treatment of family members with ECT is helpful. Laboratory examination includes a clinical blood count, a urinalysis, routine chemistries, chest and spinal x-rays (to document previous compression fractures), an electrocardiogram, and a computed tomographic scan (which is rapidly being replaced by magnetic resonance imaging [MRI]). An EEG and skull x-ray are not routinely required with computed tomography and MRI available. The presence of some abnormalities on MRI does not militate against the use of ECT, however. For example, a series of older adults suffering from major depression were found to have subcortical arteriosclerotic encephalopathy on MRI but promptly improved when undergoing ECT (C. E. Coffey et al., unpublished data, 1986).

To prepare for ECT, the older adult should be withdrawn from all medications, if possible. As noted above, any monoamine oxidase inhibitor must be withdrawn for 10 days to 2 weeks in order to avoid toxic effects of the monoamine oxidase inhibitor with the anesthetic used during ECT. Reserpine and anticholinesterases should also be withdrawn for at least 1 week. The use of lithium carbonate, tricyclic antidepressants, antipsychotics, or antianxiety agents (including the sedative–hypnotic agents) is not an absolute contraindication to ECT. Benzodiazepines, however, increase the seizure threshold. Generally, the use of a short-acting barbiturate, such as 500 mg of chloral hydrate orally at bedtime, is the most appropriate sedative–hypnotic and should not be given on the night preceding ECT, if possible. The use of low-dose haloperidol or thiothixene is probably the most appropriate means to control severe agitation or psychotic symptoms.

The basic techniques for ECT are well described. Thirty minutes prior to treatment, an anticholinergic agent is administered intramuscularly to prevent complications of cardiac arrhythmias and aspiration. Prior to treatment, a short-acting anesthetic, such as thiopental or methohexital, is administered until an eyelash response is no longer present. Then a muscle relaxant, such as succinylcholine, is administered to prevent severe muscle contractions. Investigators now are increasingly using a unilateral electrode placement to the nondominant cerebral hemisphere, since evidence has accumulated that there is less confusion following treatment with unilateral versus bilateral treatment. Nevertheless, unilateral electrode placement does not preclude the development of memory difficulties. Some question the efficacy of unilateral versus bilateral electrode placement, but no evidence has accumulated that clearly establishes bilateral electrode placement as superior to unilateral placement. The electrical stimulus is applied, and the seizure is monitored either by applying a tourniquet to one arm and observing the tonic and clonic movements in the extremity peripheral to the tourniquet or by direct EEG monitoring. Direct EEG monitoring is preferred, and a seizure lasting 25 seconds or more is required for optimal results.

Seizure duration varies with age. In a study of 228 ECT patients, Hinkle et al (1986) found that of patients over the age of 60, a greater percentage were likely to have a seizure of 30 seconds or less. The use of caffeine may increase the likelihood of inducing a seizure without the necessity of restimulation with higher electrical parameters (which could lead to increased central nervous system toxicity).

Treatments are generally administered three times per week, and usually 6 to 12 treatments are necessary for an adequate therapeutic response. A clear improvement is often noted after one of the treatments (with the patient reporting a remarkable improvement in mood and functioning following that treatment). Two or three treatments are generally given following the treatment leading to improvement. The risks and side effects of ECT in the elderly are similar to those in the general population. Cardiovascular effects are of the most concern and include premature ventricular contractions, ventricular arrhythmias, and transient systolic hypertension. Multiple monitoring during the treatment decreases the risk of one of these side effects leading (albeit infrequently) to permanent problems. Confusion and amnesia often result after a treatment, but the length of this confusional episode is brief. Some patients, however, even with the use of unilateral nondominant treatment, suffer from prolonged memory difficulties. Headaches are a common symptom with ECT but are usually responsive to nonnarcotic analgesics. Status epilepticus and compression fractures are some of the rare but more serious adverse effects.

What can the clinician expect in terms of outcome from the use of ECT in older adults? The overall success rate of ECT in drug nonresponders is usually 80 percent or greater, and there is no evidence that effectiveness is lower for older adults (Avery and Lubrano 1979). Unfortunately, the relapse rate with no prophylactic intervention following treatment may exceed 50 percent in the year following a course of ECT. This relapse rate can be lowered if tricyclic antidepressants or lithium carbonate are prescribed following the treatment. In a very few patients who exhibit a high likelihood of recurrence and/or a high toxicity to prophylactic medications, the use of maintenance ECT may be necessary. Weekly or monthly treatments (usually on an outpatient basis) are therefore prescribed, with careful monitoring of response and side effects.

Despite the effectiveness of ECT, few deny the treatment may lead to memory difficulties. In a study by Frith et al. (1983), 70 severely depressed patients were randomly assigned to receive eight real or sham ECT treatments and were divided on the basis of the degree of recovery from depression afterwards. Compared with a nondepressed control group, the depressed patients were impaired on a wide range of tests of memory and concentration prior to treatment, but afterwards performance on most tests had improved. Real ECT induced impairments of concentration, short-term memory, and learning, but significantly facilitated access to remote memories. At 6-month follow-up, all differences between real and sham ECT groups had disappeared.

Family Therapy

The final component of therapy for the elderly depressed patient is work with the family. Not only may family dysfunction contribute to the depressive symptoms experienced by the older adult, but family support is critical to a successful outcome in treating the depressed elder. A clinician must attend to (1) those members of the family who will be available to the elder, (2) the interaction of the older adult with family members and the interaction between other family members (both frequency and quality of interaction), (3) the overall family atmosphere, (4) family values regarding psychiatric disorder, (5) family support and tolerance of symptoms (such as expressions of wishing not to live), and (6) stressors encountered by the family other than the depression experienced by the elder (Blazer 1982).

Most depressed elders do not resist interaction between the clinician and family members. With the permission of the patient, the family should be instructed as to the nature of the depressive disorder and the potential risks resulting from depression in late life, especially suicide. Family members can assist the clinician in observing changes in behavior, such as an increase in discomfort (either physical or emotional), increased withdrawal and decreased verbalization, preoccupation with medications or weapons, and so forth. The family can assist in removing the implements of suicide from easy access. The family can also take responsibility for administering medications to an older adult who is unreliable or whose potential for suicide is high.

Family members can also benefit from simple instructions regarding means by which they may communicate with the elderly depressed patient. Methods of responding to expressions of low self-esteem and pessimism, such as paraphrase and expression of understanding without a sense of responsibility to intervene, can be especially effective. Families can be taught, for example, to acknowledge to the patient that "I hear what you are saying, and I understand." Behavioral techniques for dealing with demanding or overly dependent elders can be taught to families as well. A demand for constant attention by a family member from a depressed elder may require "weaning" the patient from continued contact.

When the symptoms of depression become so severe that hospitalization is required, family members are valuable in facilitating hospitalization. Without a proper alliance between the clinician and family, families may be resistant to hospitalizaton and undermine the attempts of the clinician to treat the older adult appropriately. It is usually necessary for the clinician to take responsibility for saying that hospitalization is essential, that the situation has reached the point at which the family has no choice. In such a situation, the clinician informs the patient of the necessity of hospitalization in the presence of the family, and the family in turn can support the clinician's position. In such a situation, the patient rarely resists hospitalization for long.

References

American Psychiatric Association: Diagnostic and Statistical Manual of Mental Disorders (Third Edition-Revised). Washington, DC, American Psychiatric Association, 1987

Asarch KB, Shih JC, Kulscàr A: Decreased 3H-imipramine binding in depressed males and females. Communications in Psychopharmacology 1981; 4:425–432

Asnis G: Parkinson's disease, depression, and ECT: a review and case study. Am J Psychiatry 1977; 134:191–195

Atchley RC: Social Forces in Later Life. Belmont, CA, Wadsworth Publications, 1972

Avery D, Lubrano A: Depression treated with imipramine and ECT: the DeCarolis study reconsidered. Am J Psychiatry 1979; 136:559–562

Beck AT, Ward CH, Mendelson M, et al: An inventory for measuring depression. Arch Gen Psychiatry 1961; 4:561–571

Beck AT, Rush AJ, Shaw BF, et al: Cognitive Therapy of Depression. New York, Guilford Press, 1979

Blazer DG: Depression in Late Life. St. Louis, C.V. Mosby, 1982

Blazer DG: Impact of late-life depression on the social network. Am J Psychiatry 1983; 140:162–166

Blazer DG: Hypochondriasis, in A Family Approach to Health Care in the Elderly. Edited by Blazer D, Siegler IC. Menlo Park, CA, Addison-Wesley, 1984

Blazer D, Bachar JR, Hughes D: Major depression with melancholia: a comparison of middle-aged and elderly adults. J Am Geriatr Soc 1987; 35:927–932

Blazer D, George L, Landerman R: The phenomenology of late life depression, in Psychiatric Disorders in the Elderly. Edited by Bebbington PE, Jacoby R. London, Mental Health Foundation, 1986

Blazer D, Hughes DC, George LK: The epidemiology of depression in an elderly community population. Gerontologist 1987; 27:281–287

Blazer D, Fowler N, Hughes D: Follow-up of hospitalized depressed patients: an age comparison. Unpublished data

Blumer D, Heilbronn M: Chronic pain as a variant of depressive disease: the pain-prone disorder. J Nerv Ment Dis 1982; 170:381–394

Bridges P: The drug treatment of depression in old age, in Affective Disorders in the Elderly. Edited by Murphy E. Edinburgh, Churchill Livingstone, 1986

Briley MS, Raisman R, Sechter D, et al: [³H]-imipramine binding in human platelets: a new biochemical parameter in depression. Neuropharmacology 1980; 19:1209–1210

Buckley C, Curtin D, Walsh T, et al: Ageing and platelet α₂-adrenoceptors (letter). Br J Clin Pharmacol 1986; 21:721–722

Busse EW, Barnes RH, Silverman AJ: Studies of the processes of aging: factors that influence the psyche of elderly persons. Am J Psychiatry 1954; 110:897–903

Cadoret R, Widener RB, Noth C: Depression in family practice: long-term prognosis in somatic complaints. J Fam Pract 1980; 10:625–629

Carroll BJ, Feinberg M, Greden JF, et al: A specific laboratory test for the diagnosis of melancholia: standardization, validity, and clinical utility. Arch Gen Psychiatry 1981; 38:15–22

Carter AB: The neurologic aspects of aging, in Clinical Geriatrics (Third Edition). Edited by Rossman I. Philadelphia, J.B. Lippincott, 1986

Cath SH: Some dynamics of middle and later years: a study in depletion and restitution, in Geriatric Psychiatry: Grief, Loss, and Emotional Disorders in the Aging Process. Edited by Berezin MA, Cath SH. New York, International Universities Press, 1965

Checkley SA, Slade AP, Schur E: Growth hormone and other responses to clonidine in patients with endogenous depression. Br J Psychiatry 1981; 138:51–55

Coffey CE: Cerebral laterality and emotion: the neurology of depression. Compr Psychiatry 1987; 28:197–219

Coffey CE, Hinkle PE, Weiner RD, et al: Electroconvulsive therapy of depression in patients with subcortical arteriosclerotic encephalopathy. Unpublished manuscript, Duke University, 1986

Cole MG: Age, age of onset and course of primary depressive illness in the elderly. Can J Psychiatry 1983; 28:102–104

Cutler NR, Post RM: Life course of illness in untreated manic–depressive patients. Compr Psychiatry 1982; 23:101–115

Davies BM: Depressive illness in the elderly patient. Postgrad Med 1965; 38:314–320

de Alarcon R: Hypochondriasis and depression in the aged. Gerontologia Clinica 1964; 6:266–277

Dement WC, Miles LE, Carskadon MA: "White paper" on sleep and aging. J Am Geriatr Soc 1982; 30:25–50

Dovenmuehle RH, Verwoerdt A: Physical illness and depressive symptomatology: I. Incidence of depressive symptoms in hospitalized cardiac patients. J Am Geriatr Soc 1962; 10:932–947

Dunner DL: Affective disorder: clinical features, in Psychiatry (Volume 1). Edited by Michels R, Cavenar JO. Philadelphia, J.B. Lippincott, 1985

Egeland JA, Gerhard DS, Pauls DL, et al: Bipolar affective disorders linked to DNA markers on chromosome 11. Nature 1987; 325:783–787

Enzell K: Mortality among persons with depressive symptoms and among responders in a health checkup. Acta Psychiatr Scand 1984; 69:89–102

Epstein LJ: Depression in the elderly. J Gerontol 1976; 3:278–282

Erikson E: Childhood and Society. New York, Norton, 1950

Fassler LB, Gavira M: Depression in old age. J Am Geriatr Soc 1978; 26:471–475

Feighner JP, Robins E, Guze SB, et al: Diagnostic criteria for use in psychiatric research. Arch Gen Psychiatry 1972; 26:57–63

Finkelstein JW, Roffwarg HP, Boyar RM, et al: Age-related change in the twenty-four-hour spontaneous secretion of growth hormone. J Clin Endocrinol Metab 1972; 35:665–670

France RD, Krishnan KRR, Houpt JL, et al: Differentiation of depression from chronic pain with the dexamethasone suppression test and *DSM-III*. Am J Psychiatry 1984; 141:1577–1578

Frank JD: Persuasion and Healing. Baltimore, Johns Hopkins University Press, 1973

Fredman L, Schoenbach VJ, Kaplan BH, et al: The association between depressive symptoms and mortality among older participants in the Epidemiologic Catchment Area–Piedmont Health Survey. Unpublished data

Frith CD, Stevens M, Johnstone EC, et al: Effects of ECT and depression on various aspects of memory. Br J Psychiatry 1983; 142:610–617

Gainotti G: Emotional behavior and hemispheric side of lesion. Cortex 1972; 8:41–55

Gallagher D, Thompson LW: Differential effectiveness of psychotherapies for the treatment of major depressive disorder in older adult patients. Psychotherapy: Theory, Research and Practice 1982; 19:42–49

George LK, Blazer DG, Hughes DC: Social support and the outcome of major depression. Br J Psychiatry, in press

Greden JF, Albala AA, Haskett RF, et al: Normalization of dexamethasone suppression test: a laboratory index of recovery from endogenous depression. Biol Psychiatry 1980; 15:449–458

Greden JF, Gardner R, King D, et al: Dexamethasone suppression test and antidepressant treatment of melancholia. Arch Gen Psychiatry 1983; 40:493–500

Gregoire F, Brauman H, de Buck R, et al: Hormone release in depressed patients before and after recovery. Psychoneuroendocrinology 1977; 2:303–312

Grinker RR, Miller J, Sabshin M, et al: The Phenomena of Depressions. New York, Harper & Row, 1961

Guy R: An Essay on Scirrhous Tumors and Cancer. London, J & A Churchill, 1759

Harwin B: Psychiatric morbidity among the physically impaired elderly in the community: a preliminary report, in Roots of Evaluation: The Epidemiological Basis for Planning Psychiatric Services. Edited by Wing JK, Häfner H. London, Oxford University Press, 1973

Henderson AS, Moran PAP: Social relationships during the onset and remission of neurotic symptoms: a prospective community study. Br J Psychiatry 1983; 143:467–472

Hinkle P, Coffey CE, Weiner R, et al: ECT seizure duration varies with age. Presented at the annual meeting of the American Geriatrics Society, Chicago, 1986

Holahan CJ, Moos RH: Social support and psychological distress: a longitudinal analysis. J Abnorm Psychol 1981; 90:365–370

Hopkinson G: A genetic study of affective illness in patients over 50. Br J Psychiatry 1964; 110:244–254

Jacobsen FM, Wehr TA, Sack DA, et al: Seasonal affective disorder: a review of the syndrome and its public health implications. Am J Public Health 1987; 77:57–60

Jenike MA, Albert MS: The dexamethasone suppression test in patients with presenile and senile dementia of the Alzheimer's type. J Am Geriatr Soc 1984; 32:441–444

Kay DWK, Bergmann K: Physical disability and mental health in old age: a follow-up of a random sample of elderly people seen at home. J Psychosom Res 1966; 10:3–12

Keller MB, Shapiro RW: Major depressive disorder: initial results from a one-year prospective naturalistic follow-up study. J Nerv Ment Dis 1981; 169:761–767

Kendell RE: The classification of depressions: a review of contemporary confusion. Br J Psychiatry 1976; 129:15–28

Kiloh LG: Pseudo-dementia. Acta Psychiatr Scand 1961; 37:336–351

Klerman GL, Weissman MM, Rounsaville BJ, et al: Interpersonal Psychotherapy of Depression. New York, Basic Books, 1984

Knight DL, Krishnan KRR, Blazer DG, et al: Titrated imipramine binding to platelets is markedly reduced in elderly depressed patients. Society for Neuroscience Abstracts 1986; 12:1251

Kraemlinger KG, Swanson DW, Maruta T: Are patients with chronic pain depressed? Am J Psychiatry 1983; 140:747–749

Krishnan KRR, France RD, Pelton S, et al: Chronic pain and depression: I. Classification of depression in chronic low back pain patients. Pain 1985; 22:279–287

Kupfer DJ: Neurophysiological markers: EEG sleep measures. J Psychiatr Res 1984; 18:467–495

Kupfer DJ, Foster FG, Coble P, et al: The application of EEG sleep for the differential diagnosis of affective disorders. Am J Psychiatry 1978; 135:69–74

Lakatua DJ, Nicolau GY, Bogdan C, et al: Circadian endocrine time structure in humans above 80 years of age. J Gerontol 1984; 39:648–654

Langner TS, Michael ST: Life Stress and Mental Health. Toronto, Free Press of Glencoe, 1963

Lazarus LW, Weinberg J: Treatment in the ambulatory care setting, in Handbook of Geriatric Psychiatry. Edited by Busse EW, Blazer DG. New York, Van Nostrand Reinhold, 1980

Lesse S: Masked Depression. New York, Jason Aronson, 1974

Levin S: Depression in the aged, in Geriatric Psychiatry: Grief, Loss, and Emotional Disorders in the Aging Process. Edited by Berezin MA, Cath SH. New York, International Universities Press, 1965

Lewis AJ: Melancholia: a historical review. J Ment Sci 1934; 80:1–42

Lindemann E: Symptomatology and management of acute grief. Am J Psychiatry 1944; 101:141–148

Lloyd C: Life events and depressive disorder reviewed: I. Events as predisposing factors. Arch Gen Psychiatry 1980; 37:529–535

Loosen PT, Prange AJ: Serum thyrotropin response to thyrotropin-releasing hormone in psychiatric patients: a review. Am J Psychiatry 1982; 139:405–416

Magni G, Schifano F, De Leo D, et al: The dexamethasone suppression test in depressed and non-depressed geriatric medical inpatients. Acta Psychiatr Scand 1986; 73:511–514

Markush RE, Schwab JJ, Farris P, et al: Mortality and community mental health: the Alachua County, Florida, mortality study. Arch Gen Psychiatry 1977; 34:1393–1401

Massey EW, Bullock R: Peroneal palsy in depression. J Clin Psychiatry 1978; 287:291–292

Mendlewicz J: The age factor in depressive illness: some genetic considerations. J Gerontol 1976; 31:300–303

Meyers BS, Kalayam B, Mei-Tal V: Late-onset delusional depression: a distinct clinical entity? J Clin Psychiatry 1984; 45:347–349

Multidimensional Functional Assessment: The OARS Methodology—A Manual (Second Edition). Durham, NC, Duke University Center for the Study of Aging and Human Development, 1978

Munro HN: Nutrition and aging. Br Med Bull 1981; 37:83–88

Murphy E: The prognosis of depression in old age. Br J Psychiatry 1983; 142:111–119

Myers JK, Weissman MM, Tischler GL, et al: Six-month prevalence of psychiatric disorders in three communities. Arch Gen Psychiatry 1984; 41:959–967

Palmore E, Kivett V: Change in life satisfaction: a longitudinal study of persons aged 46–70. J Gerontol 1977; 32:311–316

Persson G: Five-year mortality in a 70-year-old urban population in relation to psychiatric diagnosis, personality, sexuality, and early parental death. Acta Psychiatr Scand 1981; 64:244–253

Pfifer JF, Murrell SA: Etiologic factors in the onset of depressive symptoms in older adults. J Abnorm Psychol 1986; 95:282–291

Post F: The significance of affective syndromes in old age (Maudsley Monograph 10). London, Oxford University Press, 1962

Post F: The management and nature of depressive illness in late life: a follow-through study. Br J Psychiatry 1972; 121:393–404

Post F: The functional psychoses, in Studies in Geriatric Psychiatry. Edited by Isaacs AD, Post F. New York, Wiley, 1978

Radloff LS: The CES-D scale: a self-report depression scale for research in the general population. Applied Psychological Measurement 1977; 1:385–401

Reifler BV, Larson E, Henley R: Coexistence of cognitive impairment and depression in geriatric outpatients. Am J Psychiatry 1982; 39:623–626

Relkin R: Effect of endocrines on central nervous system: part I. NY State J Med 1969; 69:2133–2145

Robinson DS, Davies JM, Nies A, et al: Relation of sex and aging to monoamine oxidase activity of human plasma and platelets. Arch Gen Psychiatry 1971; 24:536–541

Rosenbaum AH, Schatzberg AF, MacLaughlin MS, et al: The DST in normal control subjects: a comparison of two assays and the effects of age. Am J Psychiatry 1984; 141:1550–1555

Sachar EJ: Neuroendocrine abnormalities in depressive illness, in Topics in Psychoendocrinology. Edited by Sachar EJ. New York, Grune & Stratton, 1975

Sackeim HA, Greenberg MS, Wiman AL, et al: Hemispheric asymmetry in the expression of positive and negative emotions. Arch Neurol 1982; 39:210–218

Salzman C, Shader RI: Responses to psychotropic drugs in the normal elderly, in Psychopharmacology in Aging. Edited by Eisdorfer C, Fann WE. New York, Plenum Press, 1972

Schiffman S: Changes in taste and smell with age: psychophysiological aspects, in Aging: Sensory Systems and Communication in the Elderly (Volume 10). Edited by Ordy JM, Brizzee K. New York, Raven Press, 1979

Schneider LS, Severson JA, Sloane RB: Platelet ^{3}H-imipramine binding in depressed elderly patients. Biol Psychiatry 1985; 20:1234–1237

Schneider LS, Severson JA, Pollock V, et al: Platelet monoamine oxidase activity in elderly depressed outpatients. Biol Psychiatry 1986; 21:1360–1364

Schulz B: Auszahlungen in der Verwandtschaft von nach Erkrankungsalter und Geschlecht gruppierten Manisch-Depressiven. Archiv fur Psychiatrie und Nervenkrankheiten 1951; 186:560–576

Schwab JJ, Clemmons RS, Bialow M, et al: A study of the somatic symptomatology of depression in medical inpatients. Psychosomatics 1965; 6:273–276

Scovern AW, Kilmann PR: Status of electroconvulsive therapy: review of the outcome literature. Psychol Bull 1980; 87:260–303

Shulman KI: Mania in old age, in Affective Disorders in the Elderly. Edited by Murphy E. Edinburgh, Churchill Livingstone, 1986

Shulman K, Post F: Bipolar affective disorder in old age. Br J Psychiatry 1980; 136:26–32

Slater E, Cowie V: The Genetics of Mental Disorder. London, Oxford University Press, 1971

Snyder PJ, Utiger RD: Response to thyrotropin releasing hormone (TRH) in normal man. J Clin Endocrinol Metab 1972; 34:380–385

Spar JE, Ford CV, Liston EH: Bipolar affective disorder in aged patients. J Clin Psychiatry 1979; 40:504–507

Srole L, Fischer AK: The Midtown Manhattan Longitudinal Study vs "The Mental Paradise Lost" doctrine: a controversy joined. Arch Gen Psychiatry 1980; 37:209–221

Stenstedt A: Involutional melancholia: an etiologic, clinical and social study of endogenous depression in later life, with special reference to genetic factors. Acta Psychiatr Neur Scand 1959; suppl 127:5–71

Steuer JL, Mintz J, Hammen CL, et al: Cognitive–behavioral and psychodynamic group psychotherapy in treatment of geriatric depression. J Consult Clin Psychol 1984; 52:180–189

Targum SD, Sullivan AC, Byrnes SM: Neuroendocrine relationships in major depressive disorder. Am J Psychiatry 1982; 139:282–286

Thielman SB, Blazer DG: Depression and dementia, in Dementia in Old Age. Edited by Pitt B. Edinburgh, Churchill Livingstone, 1986

Thomae H: Personality and adjustment to aging, in The Handbook of Aging and Mental Health. Edited by Birren J, Sloane RB. Englewood Cliffs, NJ, Prentice-Hall, 1980

Tourigny-Rivard M, Raskin DM, Rivard D: The dexamethasone suppression test in an elderly population. Biol Psychiatry 1981; 16:1177–1184

Ulrich RF, Shaw DH, Kupfer DJ: Effects of aging on EEG sleep in depression. Sleep 1980; 3:31–40

Verwoerdt A: Geropsychiatry. Baltimore, Williams & Wilkins, 1976

Vogel GW, Vogel F, McAbee RS, et al: Improvement of depression by REM sleep deprivation: new findings and a theory. Arch Gen Psychiatry 1980; 37:247–253

Weiner RD: The role of electroconvulsive therapy in the treatment of depression in the elderly. J Am Geriatr Soc 1982; 30:710–712

Weissman MM, Prusoff BA, Klerman GC: Personality and the prediction of long-term outcome in depression. Am J Psychiatry 1978; 135:797–800

Wells CE: Pseudodementia. Am J Psychiatry 1979; 136:895–900

Whitlock FA, Siskind M: Depression and cancer: a follow-up study. Psychol Med 1979; 9:747–752

Wigdor BT: Drives and motivations with aging, in The Handbook of Aging and Mental Health. Edited by Birren JE, Sloane RB. Englewood Cliffs, NJ, Prentice-Hall, 1980

Winokur G: The Iowa 500: heterogeneity and course in manic–depressive illness (bipolar). Compr Psychiatry 1975; 16:125–131

Zimmerman M, Coryell W, Pfohl B: Prognostic validity of the dexamethasone suppression test: results of a six-month prospective follow-up. Am J Psychiatry 1987; 144:212–214

Zung WWK: A self-rating depression scale. Arch Gen Psychiatry 1965; 12:63–70

Zung WWK, Green RL: Detection of affective disorders in the aged, in Psychopharmacology in Aging. Edited by Eisdorfer C, Fann WE. New York, Plenum Press, 1972

Chapter 14

Late-Life Schizophrenia and Paranoid Disorders

Caron Christison, M.D.
George Christison, M.D.
Dan G. Blazer, M.D., Ph.D.

Among the more frequent psychiatric symptoms presenting to the clinician working with the cognitively impaired or emotionally distressed older adult are suspiciousness, persecutory ideation, and paranoid delusions. Lowenthal (1964), in a study of older persons in the San Francisco community, found that 17 percent of those rated as psychiatrically impaired had symptoms of suspiciousness and 13 percent had delusions. Of the entire sample, 2.5 percent exhibited suspiciousness and 2 percent paranoid delusions. Christenson and Blazer (1984) found that 4 percent of an elderly community sample suffered from generalized persecutory ideation.

Yet, a recent series of epidemiologic studies in the United States (the Epidemiologic Catchment Area [ECA] studies) identified few cases of schizophrenia and/or schizophreniform disorder in the elderly, with rates generally below 0.1 percent (Myers et al. 1984). An examination of the ECA community studies, however, reveals that a primary reason for so few cases of schizophrenia is the early age of onset (age 45) required for the diagnosis of schizophrenia in the *Diagnostic and Statistical Manual of Mental Disorders (Third Edition-Revised) (DSM-III-R)* (American Psychiatric Association 1987). For more than 1,600 individuals 60 years of age and older in the ECA study at Duke University (a survey of urban and rural North Carolina), the unweighted prevalence of schizophrenia or schizophreniform disorder was 0.2 percent in the community (Blazer et al. in press). Nevertheless, nearly 8 percent of the

403

elderly sample reported at least one current symptom of schizophrenia; 4.3 percent reported severe delusional symptoms; and 5.4 percent, severe hallucinatory experiences.

The confusion and controversy surrounding the diagnosis of schizophrenia and schizophrenic symptoms in the elderly center on at least two factors: the definition of a case of schizophrenia in *DSM-III-R* (can a case of schizophrenia develop after the age of 45?) and the range of clinical conditions that may present with schizophrenic-like symptomatology. A number of authors suggest that a symptom picture virtually identical to *DSM-III-R* schizophrenia can have an onset after the age of 45 (Gold 1984; Rabins et al. 1984; Volavka 1985). The argument for these cases is straightforward. Symptom profiles do not vary except for the criterion requiring onset before age 45. Many patients who suffer from paranoid delusions of late onset respond well to traditional therapies for schizophrenia. The European literature (in which an age criterion has not been used) is often cited to support this contention. The argument for limiting the onset of schizophrenia to prior to the age of 45 and labeling late-onset psychosis as a separate disorder, such as atypical paranoid disorder, is that the vast majority of cases of schizophrenia develop before the age of 45.

Historical Perspectives

The controversy regarding schizophrenic-like illnesses in late life derives in part from the historical evolution of the term "late paraphrenia." Kraepelin (1919) used the term "paraphrenia" to describe a comparatively small group of patients characterized by marked paranoid delusions and many characteristics in common with dementia praecox. Kraepelin distinguished paraphrenia from dementia praecox, however, by stating that paraphrenic patients exhibited "far slighter development of the disorder of emotion and volition" and that the "dullness and indifference which so frequently form the first symptoms of dementia praecox" were not seen in paraphrenia until, perhaps, "the latest periods of the malady." The diagnostic entity paraphrenia subsequently fell into disuse because follow-up of Kraepelin's paraphrenic group revealed that the diagnosis was changed to schizophrenia in more than half the cases (Kolle 1931; Mayer-Gross 1932).

Roth (1955) reintroduced the term "paraphrenia," defining it as a syndrome characterized by a "well-organized system of paranoid delusions with or without auditory hallucinations existing in the setting of a well-preserved personality and affective response. . . . In the great majority of these patients, the illness commences after the age of 60" (p. 281). He used the term descriptively and in an empirical follow-up study demonstrated that the outcome of elderly patients suffering from paraphrenia differed from those with a diagnosis of affective disorder or dementia. Since the syndrome of paraphrenia did not appear to be the same as schizophrenia (though it resembled schizophrenia) and the syndrome was frequently found among the elderly, the term "late paraphrenia" emerged.

The existence of a group of patients with schizophrenic-like symptoms beginning in late life that are not due to affective or dementing illnesses has been evaluated in several studies. Baron et al. (1983) found that of 93 chronic schizophrenic patients, none became ill after the age of 40 (though the oldest subject in the study was only 48 years old). Studies such as this can be used to support the *DSM-III-R* age criterion for schizophrenia. Fish (1960), Essa (1982), and Marneros and Deister (1984), in contrast, each found a substantial number of subjects who experienced the onset of schizophrenic-like symptoms after the age of 50 (with many having the first onset of these symptoms after the age of 65).

Post (1966) identified three patterns of symptom presentation among paraphrenic patients in later life. The first was characterized by auditory hallucinations and false beliefs of persecution; the second, by understandable delusions (such as feelings of being observed or having one's conversation taped); and the third, by evidence of the so-called first-rank symptoms of schizophrenia as elucidated by Schneider (1959). Post believed the etiology of the paranoid state, whether due to organic causes, social isolation, or sensory loss, was not related to the symptom pattern. Like others, Post recognized that a poor premorbid history among some patients suggested they were borderline schizophrenic prior to the onset of the overt disorder in late life. Nevertheless, he emphasized that the overt symptoms of the disorder did manifest themselves first in late life.

The Differential Diagnosis of Schizophrenic-Like Illness in the Elderly

Eisdorfer (1980) has suggested some useful constructs for the differential diagnosis of late-life schizophrenic-like symptoms. These are (1) suspiciousness, (2) transitional paranoid reactions, and (3) paraphrenia (late-onset paranoia as suggested by Roth) or paranoia associated with schizophrenia of late onset. To these a fourth should be added—acute paranoid reactions secondary to affective illness. Because paranoid symptoms can be so dramatic in late-onset major depression, Meyers and Greenberg (1986) have suggested that delusional depressive older adults should be distinguished from their depressed but nondelusional counterparts.

Most older adults who demonstrate heightened suspiciousness, such as those that have been identified in community surveys (Christenson and Blazer 1984; Lowenthal 1964), never come into contact with a mental health professional. Such individuals offer vague complaints of external forces controlling their lives. On occasion, such beliefs can become focal, often addressed toward children. Feelings of being deserted by their children or that their children have plotted against them may become so severe that they force the children to seek counsel, yet these older adults continue daily activities with little difficulty. A sense of loss of control, coupled with an inability to evaluate the social milieu properly, provides adequate grounds for the development of mild suspiciousness.

The clinician is more likely to encounter suspiciousness associated with loss of memory and attention. Frequently a problem among patients in long-term care facilities who are suffering from a dementing illness, accusations can plague both family and staff. Such suspiciousness is usually disjointed, not focused, and not accompanied by emotional distress, except for brief episodes. Complaints of objects being stolen, medicines being swapped, misbehavior of attendants in other parts of the facility, and so forth are common symptoms of such suspiciousness. Inability to organize environmental stimuli and comprehend the frequently confusing activities of a hospital or long-term care facility may contribute to the onset of this disorder. Whether an underlying hostile and paranoid personality style contributes to such a disorder is not known.

Eisdorfer's second variety of paranoid disorder is transitional paranoid reaction. This derives from the work of Post (1973), who describes focal, narrow, and situational paranoid hallucinations. Such individuals are often females who live alone and who believe a plot exists against them. The focus of their hallucinations and delusional thinking usually begins outside the person's house and moves gradually inward, to complaints of noises in the basement and attic and progressing even to physical abuse or molestation (hence the transition from without to within). Factors that may contribute to this transitional paranoia include social isolation and perceptual difficulties (Eisdorfer 1980; Post 1965).

These transitional paranoid reactions may also accompany moderate to severe dementia, either primary degenerative dementia or multi-infarct dementia. Not infrequently, patients in long-term care facilities will complain of fragmented yet elaborately constructed plots against them. They imagine personnel have contrived to incinerate the facility if their room is overheated. Others protest plots by family members to dispossess them of their possessions, often the family home from which they have been moved to the institution. As the plot evolves in the elder's imagination, the threat moves closer to the individual. Similar to the suspiciousness associated with dementia, the emotions associated with these fragmented paranoid reactions may be strong at times but are not sustained.

Eisdorfer's final category is paraphrenia and paranoia associated with schizophrenic-like illness. Though Roth (1955) distinguishes late paraphrenia from paranoid schizophrenia, others would not make the distinction. Investigators who distinguish a syndrome of late-onset paraphrenia emphasize that the disorder is a primary disorder; that is, it is not due to affective illness or an organic mental disorder. Paranoid delusions and hallucinations are almost always apparent, yet the gross disturbances of affect, volition, or function seen in schizophrenia are not prominent. The course may be chronic, but deterioration to the extent observed in the course of schizophrenia or Alzheimer's disease is not characteristic. As can be seen, the distinction between transitional paranoid states and late paraphrenia is unclear, as is the distinction between late paraphrenia and classic paranoid schizophrenia.

Part of the difficulty in distinguishing the spectrum of paranoid symptomatology in late life derives from a poor understanding of the natural course of schizophrenia. Chronic institutionalization of schizophrenic patients in the past, coupled with increased mortality, has rendered community follow-up studies inadequate. Tsuang and Dempsey (1979) found that 200 persons developing schizophrenia before the age of 40 were four times more likely to die during the first 9 years after onset. Talbott (1981) documents that almost one-half of the patients who have been deinstitutionalized over the last 30 years are in nursing homes (about 750,000). Tsuang and Dempsey also found that among those survivors to late life who were diagnosed as schizophrenic early in life, 18 percent were hospitalized in a mental institution at follow-up and 48 percent were in nursing homes.

Factors Associated with Paranoid Symptoms in the Elderly

Cognitive Disorders

Transient cognitive disorders are probably the most important and frequent cause of paranoid symptoms in late life (Lipowski 1983). Confusion is one of the more common causes for referral of a patient to the geropsychiatrist. In a multicenter study in Great Britain, 35 percent of the patients aged 65 and older exhibited delirium on admission or developed it during the hospital stay under study (Hodkinson 1976). Transient cognitive disorders can result in a number of symptoms, including disordered perception, disordered thinking, impaired memory, decreased alertness, and psychomotor agitation or retardation. Problems with perception are manifested often by a reduced capability to distinguish actual environmental stimuli from imagery, dreams, and even hallucinations (Lipowski 1980). Patients report visits from relatives or friends who are deceased, travels to areas they remember in the past (even if they have not left the hospital bed), and conversations in which reality is intermixed with fantasy. Though acute delirium often precipitates a dramatic affective response to these perceptual abnormalities, the patient with chronic dementia can report illusions and hallucinations with little affect.

Cognitive dysfunction also contributes to disorganized and fragmented thinking. In the midst of an acute brain syndrome, paranoid ideation and delusions of persecution (often unconnected and transient) have been reported to occur in 40 to 55 percent of older adults (Simon and Cahan 1963). As described by Lipowski (1983), the elderly delirious patient, in contrast to the younger patient, is less likely to combine florid reports of hallucinations associated with delusional thinking. In contrast, an impoverished and incoherent thought process is accompanied by impaired reason and judgment associated with the general suspiciousness and isolated reports that are clearly delusional.

Gender

Female gender is another factor reported by most investigators to be associated with late paraphrenia. The increased propensity for females to suffer from paranoid symptoms in late life, even when age is adjusted, is in contrast to the 1:1 sex ratio in classic schizophrenia. In a study from Graylingwell Hospital of 42 patients with late paraphrenia, Kay and Roth (1961) found 39 females to suffer from the disorder, but only 3 males. Marneros and Deister (1984) found that among 1,208 first psychiatric admissions with schizophrenia, 85 percent were female among the group over the age of 50. Rabins et al. (1984) found an 11:1 ratio of females to males in a study of 35 patients over the age of 44.

A number of factors have been posited to explain the increased risk for females to develop late-onset schizophrenic symptoms. Some have suggested that females tend to develop schizophrenic symptoms later than males and therefore have a later "peak" of symptom manifestation. For example, Zigler and Levine (1981) found that men with schizophrenia are hospitalized about 5 years earlier than women. Seeman (1981) speculated that dropping estrogen levels in women may contribute to increased vulnerability. As evidence, she points out that hormonal instability during the postpartum period has been associated with high vulnerability to behavioral decompensation. Others have noted the greater likelihood of older women to survive to late life. Another suggestion is that older women with schizophrenic symptoms are more likely to come to the attention of health care providers. A review of the evidence, however, does not provide a satisfactory explanation of this empirical finding.

Social and Occupational Functioning

Another factor associated with schizophrenic-like symptoms in late life has been poor social and occupational adjustment. The majority of patients suffering from paraphrenia, according to most investigators, were capable of supporting themselves until retirement or the onset of their illness (Kay 1963). According to clinical experience, however, these individuals were more likely in earlier life to be isolated, to work in occupations that required little social interaction, and to be marginal in their social relations outside of work. Odegaard (1953) hypothesized that the prepsychotic personalities of patients suffering from late-onset schizophrenia tended to be schizoid or paranoid. Prepsychotic behavior was characterized by explosive tempers, adherence to minority religious sects, and, in the case of men, antisocial behavior. Marriages tended to be fragile, with frequent divorce, and the patients were described by their children as cold and unloving.

Another contributory factor may be the concurrent social isolation. The suspicious or paranoid older adult is often a loner. This can be due to loss of family and friends, coupled with a relatively isolated life-style. Prolonged social isolation is a fertile breeding ground for the gradual development of distorted thoughts that eventually progress to delusions regarding neighbors, the neighborhood, or the state of the world. To be isolated is to be uninformed, which encourages suspicion and can lead to fabrication of explanations of the unknown.

Sensory Impairment

A number of investigators have reported the association of schizophrenic-like symptoms in late life with sensory impairment. In a community study of older adults (Christenson and Blazer 1984), nearly 78 percent of subjects with persecutory ideations had impaired vision, compared with 51 percent without persecutory ideations. Hearing was impaired in 58 percent of the symptomatic subjects but only 36 percent of the nonsymptomatic subjects. Post (1966) found "deafness" in 30 percent of older adults with persistent paranoid symptoms, compared with 11 percent who were depressed and 7 percent of the normal community subjects. In a more detailed study, Cooper et al. (1974, 1976) found that when tested with audiometric devices, patients with paranoid psychosis had hearing losses of significantly greater magnitude than did patients with depressive disorders. Leuchter and Spar (1985) compared elderly psychotic inpatients with elderly nonpsychotic inpatients. Auditory impairment was more prevalent among the psychotic patients than controls (21 percent vs. 12 percent), and visual impairment was more common as well (34 percent vs. 18 percent). Psychotic symptoms, such as hallucinations, may fill in for stimuli that are absent for the patient with sensory impairment. With respect to the development of paranoid ideation, if an isolated elder does not hear speech clearly (especially when in a group situation), he may conclude that others are talking about him, or he may refer to himself fragments of speech that are partially heard (Zarit 1980).

Marital Status

Most studies suggest that the late-onset paranoid patient is more likely to have been married than the schizophrenic patient (Bridge and Wyatt 1980; Marneros and Deister 1984). However, this finding is confounded by functional impairment in the earlier onset schizophrenic group during the years when they are most likely to be married.

Family Psychiatric History

If late-onset schizophrenic-like symptoms are a subset of the schizophrenias, one would expect the prevalence of schizophrenia among family members to be comparable for early- and late-onset cases. Funding (1961), in a study of 148 patients with onset of paranoia after the age of 50, found the expectancy rate for schizophrenia among siblings to be 2.5 percent. This is greater than the approximately 1 percent reported for the general population, but less than the prevalences of nearly 10 percent reported among siblings for younger schizophrenic patients. Kay (1963), in a study of 57 patients with late-onset paranoid symptoms, discovered that 19 percent of the probands had at least one relative with schizophrenia. The risk among siblings was 4.9 percent and the risk for children, 7.3 percent. Age of onset of schizophrenia among these relatives was before the age of 40 in the large majority of cases. Rabins et al. (1984) found a higher likelihood of schizophrenia among family members of patients with paraphrenia than among age- and sex-matched controls with affective disorder. In the bulk of these investigations, the rate of schizophrenia in relatives of paraphrenic probands falls between that of the general population and that of relatives of schizophrenic probands. Certainly, late-onset paranoid disorders are more closely related to schizophrenia in terms of family history than to the affective disorders, but the genetic loading is not as prominent as for classic schizophrenia.

Intrapsychic Factors

A potential psychologic risk factor for late-onset paranoid symptoms is having primitive defense mechanisms for dealing with loss (Eisdorfer 1960, 1980). The older person with a long-standing propensity to use projection as a defense may expel grief and adjustment to loss from the process of working through internally. A tendency to see losses as due to external factors can contribute to suspiciousness and paranoia. Potential areas of loss include one's work, one's role in society, and one's functional capacity. Of particular importance, as described above, is the loss of perceptual ability and poorer cognitive capacity with associated attentional and mnemonic deficits. The characteristic of many of these losses is that they are not under the control of the older adult and may be almost imperceptible to the patient. Nevertheless, they challenge the elder's mastery of the world, leading to a search for an explanation to account for the losses.

Treatment of the Patient with
Schizophrenic Symptoms in Late Life

The core of effective management of the patient with late-onset schizophrenic-like symptoms is treatment with antipsychotic medications. Post

(1966) reported that those patients who improved the most clinically were those who received adequate treatment and maintenance with neuroleptic medications. Leuchter and Spar (1985) followed 15 patients who suffered from late-onset primary psychotic symptoms and found that the 10 patients treated with phenothiazines had significantly better outcome than those not treated. Other investigators report similar findings. The patients who have been followed in these treatment studies (when organic problems were not present) have an outcome as good as, if not better than, patients with schizophrenic symptoms earlier in life. For example, Post (1966) found that of 75 patients treated with either trifluoperazine (10 to 60 mg/day) or thioridazine (75 to 600 mg/day), 43 experienced a complete remission, whereas only 8 showed no response. With follow-up over several months to 3 years, the majority of these patients were maintained symptom free when they received adequate initial phenothiazine treatment and maintenance.

Unfortunately, the clinician treating the paranoid older adult with neuroleptic medication faces the fact that tardive dyskinesia due to long-term (and even short-term) treatment with antipsychotic medications is more prevalent in late life. Mukherjee et al. (1982) found age to be significantly correlated with tardive dyskinesia in 153 psychiatric outpatients. Age must be included— along with length of neuroleptic treatment, cumulative dose of neuroleptics, and the presence of an organic brain syndrome—as a factor that increases the likelihood of the development of tardive dyskinesia (DeVeaugh-Geiss 1982).

Although a higher dose of medication is required for more severe symptoms, initial starting doses (especially for outpatients with paranoid symptoms) range from 10 to 25 mg daily of thioridazine, 2 to 4 mg daily for thiothixene, and 1 to 3 mg daily for haloperidol. Choice of medication usually depends on what side effects the clinician wishes to avoid. Thioridazine is especially troublesome for the older person subject to postural hypotension, whereas haloperidol presents significant problems to the older person inclined to develop parkinsonian side effects. Also, the onset of akathisia in the already delusional patient may undermine initial efforts to encourage compliance with a medication in the older adult.

Most older persons, however, are willing to use a medication if it is explained that the medication will be of value in improving sleep and decreasing anxiety. Medication compliance is usually less a problem for the paranoid older adult than it is for paranoid patients at earlier stages of the life cycle. Most elders are trusting of their clinicians and are willing to adhere to the suggestions made for optimal therapy. When objections to medications occur, alliance with a family member is beneficial. Strong objection to medication or any intervention, however, may suggest the need for hospitalization.

Medications are not the sole intervention available for the paranoid older adult. Clinicians must work to establish a trusting, supportive relationship with the patient. Respect for the patient, a willingness to listen to whatever complaints and fears the patient experiences, and availability by telephone when crises occur contribute to an improved therapeutic alliance. A professional, matter-of-fact posture is valued by the distressed paranoid elder. He or she wants the attention of the clinician as the concerns are expressed. Most elders do not abuse the telephone, and therefore if a patient calls, a return phone call is important.

Of equal importance in treating the paranoid older adult is the development of relationships with persons in the patient's social environment. Family relations are self-evident, for family members are often the first to notice a deterioration in the patient's condition and therefore the first to contact the physician regarding the problem. In addition, police officers, neighbors, pharmacists, and so forth, can serve as valuable allies. Older persons with paranoia living in relatively contained communities are well known by these communities. Neighbors and contacts who have known the individual for years not only recognize a change in behavior, but also serve as valuable allies for limiting the destructiveness of this behavior. Paranoid symptoms can be tolerated by communities, more than many clinicians expect, when they are understood. The clinician and social worker must help to facilitate a network among these various contacts in the community. Needless phone calls to the police, investigations, neighborhood rifts, and so forth can be avoided when a network for supporting and caring for the paranoid older adult is allowed to become established around that elder. Fragmented neighborhoods and a fast-paced life-style, common in the latter part of the 20th century, render such a network less likely. Nevertheless, the capability exists for even transient participants in the patient's life to form a network.

Many young clinicians wish to confront the older paranoid patient with the lack of reason and false assumptions inherent in paranoid ideation. Unfortunately, such frontal attacks are of no value in managing the paranoid older adult and frequently result in severance of the therapeutic relationship. Clinicians must not be deceitful by pretending to agree with paranoid ideation when in fact they do not agree. Rather, statements such as "I don't see the situation as you do, but I can understand how you might view it as such and wish to help you nevertheless" can facilitate the therapeutic alliance. Even with the remission of paranoid symptoms, the older adult may not relinquish the belief that these symptoms were reasonable and real.

If behavior resulting from paranoid ideation becomes dysfunctional or dangerous, behavioral approaches may be required to constrain that behavior. These, for the outpatient, are usually best implemented by family and friends. Limiting the distance that the elder drives, limiting the use of the telephone, and obtaining guardianship (and therefore the ability to manage the elder's finances) are some of the constraints that can be applied for managing the paranoid older adult.

Finally, if physical health can be improved or if sensory deficits and social isolations can be alleviated, many paranoid symptoms will correct themselves. The "hard-core" paranoid will have more difficulty in social interactions, but the individual with transitional paranoid ideation or suspiciousness will do better with frequent social contacts. When hearing problems can be corrected or vision improved, increased function will often follow.

References

American Psychiatric Association: Diagnostic and Statistical Manual of Mental Disorders (Third Edition-Revised). Washington, DC, American Psychiatric Association, 1987

Baron M, Gruen R, Asnis L, et al: Age-of-onset in schizophrenia and schizotypal disorders: clinical and genetic implications. Neuropsychobiology 1983; 10:199–204

Blazer D, George LK, Hughes D: Schizophrenic symptoms in an elderly community population, in Epidemiology of Aging. Edited by Brody J, Maddox GL. New York, Springer, in press

Bridge TP, Wyatt RJ: Paraphrenia: paranoid states of late life: I. European research. J Am Geriatr Soc 1980; 28:193–200

Christenson R, Blazer D: Epidemiology of persecutory ideation in an elderly population in the community. Am J Psychiatry 1984; 141:1088–1091

Cooper AF, Kay DWK, Curry AR, et al: Hearing loss in paranoid and affective psychoses of the elderly. Lancet 1974; 2:851–854

Cooper AF, Garside RF, Kay DWK: A comparison of deaf and nondeaf patients with paranoid and affective psychoses. Br J Psychiatry 1976; 129:532–538

DeVeaugh-Geiss J (ed): Tardive Dyskinesia and Related Involuntary Movement Disorders: The Long-term Effects of Antipsychotic Drugs. Boston, John Wright, 1982

Eisdorfer C: Rorschach rigidity and sensory decrement in a senescent population. J Gerontol 1960; 15:188–190

Eisdorfer C: Paranoia and schizophrenic disorders in later life, in Handbook of Geriatric Psychiatry. Edited by Busse EW, Blazer DG. New York, Van Nostrand Reinhold, 1980

Essa M: Late-onset schizophrenia (letter). Am J Psychiatry 1982; 139:1528

Fish F: Senile schizophrenia. J Ment Sci 1960; 106:938–946

Funding T: Genetics of paranoid psychoses in later life. Acta Psychiatr Scand 1961; 37:267–282

Gold DD: Late age of onset schizophrenia: present but unaccounted for. Compr Psychiatry 1984; 25:225–237

Hodkinson HM: Common Symptoms of Disease in the Elderly. Oxford, Blackwell, 1976

Kay DWK: Late paraphrenia and its bearing on the aetiology of schizophrenia. Acta Psychiatr Scand 1963; 39:159–169

Kay DWK, Roth M: Environmental and hereditary factors in the schizophrenias of old age ("late paraphrenia") and their bearing on the general problem of causation in schizophrenia. J Ment Sci 1961; 107:649–686

Kolle K: Die primare Verrucktheit. Leipzig, Thieme, 1931

Kraepelin E: Dementia Praecox and Paraphrenia. Translated by Barclay RM. Edited by Robertson GM. Huntington, NY, Robert E. Krieger, 1971 (original 1919)

Leuchter AF, Spar JE: The late-onset psychoses: clinical and diagnostic features. J Nerv Ment Dis 1985; 173:488–494

Lipowski ZJ: Delirium update. Compr Psychiatry 1980; 21:190–196

Lipowski ZJ: Transient cognitive disorders (delirium, acute confusional states) in the elderly. Am J Psychiatry 1983; 140:1426–1436

Lowenthal MF: Lives in Distress. New York, Basic Books, 1964

Marneros A, Deister A: The psychopathology of "late schizophrenia." Psychopathology 1984; 17:264–274

Mayer-Gross W: Die Schizophrenie. Berlin, Springer, 1932

Meyers BS, Greenberg R: Late-life delusional depression. J Affective Disord 1986; 11:133–137

Mukherjee S, Rosen AM, Cardenas C, et al: Tardive dyskinesia in psychiatric outpatients. Arch Gen Psychiatry 1982; 39:466–472

Myers JK, Weissman MM, Tischler GL, et al: Six-month prevalence of psychiatric disorders in three communities. Arch Gen Psychiatry 1984; 41:959–967

Odegaard O: New data on marriage and mental disease: the incidence of psychoses in the widowed and the divorced. J Ment Sci 1953; 99:778–785

Post F: The Clinical Psychiatry of Late Life. New York, Pergamon Press, 1965

Post F: Persistent Persecutory States of the Elderly. Oxford, Pergamon Press, 1966

Post F: Paranoid disorders in the elderly. Postgrad Med 1973; 53(4):52–56

Rabins P, Pauker S, Thomas J: Can schizophrenia begin after age 44? Compr Psychiatry 1984; 25:290–293

Roth M: The natural history of mental disorder in old age. J Ment Sci 1955; 101:281–301

Schneider K: Clinical Psychopathology. Translated by Hamilton MW. New York, Grune & Stratton, 1959

Seeman MV: Gender and the onset of schizophrenia: neurohumoral influences. Psychiatr J Univ Ottawa 1981; 6:136–138

Simon A, Cahan RB: The acute brain syndrome in geriatric patients. Psychiatric Research Reports 1963; 16:8–21

Talbott JA: The National Plan for the Chronically Mentally Ill: a programmatic analysis. Hosp Community Psychiatry 1981; 32:699–704

Tsuang MT, Dempsey GM: Long-term outcome of major psychoses: II. Schizoaffective disorder compared with schizophrenia, affective disorders, and a surgical control group. Arch Gen Psychiatry 1979; 39:1302–1304

Volavka J: Late-onset schizophrenia: a review. Compr Psychiatry 1985; 26:148–156

Zarit SH: Aging and Mental Disorders: Psychological Approaches to Assessment and Treatment. New York, Free Press, 1980

Zigler E, Levine J: Age on first hospitalization of schizophrenics: a developmental approach. J Abnorm Psychol 1981; 90:458–467

Chapter 15

Anxiety in the Elderly

Andrew L. Brickman, Ph.D.
Carl Eisdorfer, Ph.D., M.D.

Among adults in the United States, phobic and anxiety states are the most commonly reported psychiatric disturbances, exceeding even depression in prevalence (Robins et al. 1984). Some combination of our genes and cultural legacy has intensified our awareness of fear-producing stimuli and its concomitant emotional and behavioral responses. Anxiety as a disorder or factor in psychopathology is firmly rooted in the lexicon of medicine and psychiatry. Of the 208 classifications in the *Diagnostic and Statistical Manual of Mental Disorders (Third Edition-Revised) (DSM-III-R)* (American Psychiatric Association 1987), 54 involve anxiety or fear in some way (Delprato and McGlynn 1984).

As a result of the dramatic changes in human mortality, the elderly are emerging as a group of special concern. One-fourth of the United States population will be over age 65 by the year 2050 (U.S. Bureau of the Census 1982). The finding that anxiety is pervasive in the population suggests that the problems confronting the aged, and reactions to these problems, are consistent with a process that remains relatively constant throughout the life span. Indeed, much of what has been written about geriatric anxiety appears to reflect content that although appearing to be unique to the aged, is often conceptually identical to processes that occur throughout life. However, it may be the case that there are etiologic elements unique to the aged or that factors that contribute to longevity have a differential effect on the prevalence of anxiety. This chapter will review the literature on anxiety in the aged and seek to present alternative approaches to the problem.

415

The Epidemiology of Anxiety in the Elderly

There have been relatively few major efforts to investigate the relationship between age and mental health through the use of community-based survey techniques. Some relatively early data on anxiety in the aged were collected as a by-product of other research. For example, Warheit et al. (1975) examined the relationship between race and mental illness using the Health Opinion Survey (MacMillan 1957). Although not a focus of their study, an anxiety symptom scale score and an anxiety function scale score were computed. The anxiety symptom and function scale scores roughly correspond to measures of state and trait anxiety, respectively. This configuration of state and trait anxiety has come to play a valued role in the research literature. State anxiety refers to a transitory anxiety response that is situationally determined and can vary from moment to moment (Endler and Okada 1975; Spielberger 1972). In contrast, trait anxiety refers to a general and stable disposition of the individual to become anxious (Spielberger 1972). These data are presented in Table 1. What is of interest is the increase in anxiety symptom scale scores, suggesting an age-related increase in state anxiety, in contrast to a curvilinear relationship between anxiety function scale scores (trait anxiety) and increasing age.

It has been suggested that anxiety in the aged is not a major public mental health problem (Jarvik and Russell 1979). Data for the national prevalence of anxiety disorder in the aged come from the Epidemiologic Catchment Area (ECA) program (Robins et al. 1984; Myers et al. 1984). Both lifetime and 6-month prevalancy rates were obtained.

Lifetime prevalence rates for anxiety as a disorder were determined by household samples obtained in three large metropolitan areas. Lifetime prevalence is the proportion of persons who have ever experienced an anxiety disorder up to the date of assessment. Because there can be a first occurrence of anxiety at any time throughout the life span, it would be reasonable to predict that lifetime prevalence would increase with age. Paradoxically, this was not the case: age was inversely related to rate. The older the individuals, the less likely they reported experiencing a clinical anxiety disorder during their lifetime. This suggests differential survival rate, differential forgetting, or perhaps that older persons at greater temporal distance from the period of anxiety are more likely to have forgotten; or possibly that the aged are less willing or able to discuss mental and emotional symptoms.

Similar findings were found in the 6-month prevalence rates. Rates for panic disorder and somatization disorder were lower in the over-65 age groups than in younger age groups. In fact, somatization disorder was not found. However, this is not surprising in light of the realistic symptoms presented by the elderly (Table 2). Phobias, although more evenly distributed across the age span than other disorders, also had the lowest rates for persons

Table 1. Anxiety as a Function of Age

Age (years)	Anxiety Symptom Scale Scores			Anxiety Function Scale Scores		
	N	Mean	*SD*	*N*	Mean	*SD*
≤19	81	5.185	5.390	81	3.025	4.772
20–29	498	5.042	5.209	498	2.633	4.644
30–39	272	5.331	6.215	272	2.316	4.607
40–49	245	6.376	6.987	245	2.608	5.259
50–59	220	7.741	8.017	220	7.718	5.514
60–69	179	8.106	8.360	179	2.084	4.526
70–79	103	10.689	9.163	103	1.728	3.689
80–89	33	12.939	8.093	33	1.636	3.296
Analysis of variance:	$F = 17.08; df = 7,1623; p < .005$			$F = 1.06; df = 7,1623;$ NS		

Note. Reproduced with permission from Warheit GJ, Holzer CE, Arey SA: Race and mental illness: an epidemiologic update. J Health Soc Behav 1975; 16:243–256.

Table 2. Symptoms Most Frequently Mentioned During Physician Office Visits, by Patients Age 75 or Older

Symptom	No. of Mentions/100 Visits
Dizziness	3.8
Vision dysfunctions	3.4
Back pain	3.2
Leg pain	3.1
Cough	2.8
Chest pain	2.7
Shortness of breath	2.6
General weakness	2.6
Knee pain	2.0
Skin lesion	2.0
Abdominal pain	1.9
Headache	1.8
Foot and toe pain	1.7
Tiredness, exhaustion	1.5
Hip pain	1.5
Abnormal sensations, eye	1.4
Head cold	1.2
Shoulder pain	1.2
Anxiety, nervousness	1.2
Palpitations, abnormal pulsations	1.1
Nausea	1.0
Urinary frequency/urgency	1.0
Pain, generalized or unspecified	1.0
Fluid abnormalities	1.0
Skin irritations	0.9

Note. Adapted from National Center for Health Statistics (1985). Reproduced with permission from White LR, Cartwright WS, Cornoni-Huntley J, et al: Geriatric epidemiology. Annual Review of Gerontology and Geriatrics 1986; 6:215–311.

age 65 years and older, although the decline past 65 was not substantial. Only cognitive impairment and major episodes of depression associated with bereavement were more common in the over-65 age group.

Convergent validity for the 6-month prevalence data can be found by examining a list of the drugs most commonly prescribed for patients aged 75 and older in office visits (see Table 3; White et al. 1986). Conspicuously absent from this list are commonly prescribed anxiolytic medications. Although there are medications present that have psychoactive effects, good medical practice would not suggest their use in the treatment of anxiety. Therefore, we may assume that for this age group, few individuals are presenting with anxiety symptoms that are readily identified by the general medical community—unless there exists a hitherto unreported tendency to limit antianxiety medication in this older group.

Table 3. Drugs Most Commonly Prescribed During Physician Office Visits, by Patients Age 75 or Older

Drug	No. of Times Ordered or Provided/100 Visits
Hydrochlorothiazide	12.6
Digoxin	10.9
Furosemide	6.9
Triamterene	4.6
Aspirin	4.3
Propranolol	4.2
Methyldopa	3.6
Potassium replacements	3.5
Vitamin B_{12}	3.2
Nitroglycerin	3.2
Isosorbide	2.9
Reserpine	2.7
Multivitamins	2.5
Acetaminophen	2.3
Chlorthalidone	2.3
Dihydroergotamine	2.0
Ibuprofen	2.0
Meclizine	1.9
Theophylline	1.8
Iron preparations	1.7
Phenobarbital	1.7
Chlorpropamide	1.7
Papaverine	1.6
Spironolactone	1.5
Tetracycline	1.5

Note. Adapted from National Center for Health Statistics (1985). Reproduced with permission from White LR, Cartwright WS, Cornoni-Huntley J, et al: Geriatric epidemiology. Annual Review of Gerontology and Geriatrics 1986; 6:215–311.

Preliminary reports based exclusively on elderly subjects residing in the community are beginning to appear in the literature as part of the ECA program. The data from the ECA program are based on interviews with more than 9,000 community-residing adults using the Diagnostic Interview Schedule (DIS) to arrive at a *DSM-III* (American Psychiatric Association 1980) diagnosis. Kramer et al. (1985) reported on prevalence rates contrasted by age across the 18 and older population for cognitive impairment and other diagnoses in the Baltimore, Maryland, site of the ECA program. Differences in prevalence rates by age were striking. The general trend of decreasing psychopathology with increasing age is again evident in the data. For conditions with rates over 1 percent, those younger than age 64 had eight conditions: phobia (13.8 percent), alcohol use disorder (6.5 percent), obsessive–

compulsive disorder (2.2 percent), schizophrenia (1.4 percent), and panic disorder (1.2 percent). For the young elderly, 65 to 74 years, only five conditions had prevalence rates over 1 percent: phobic disorder (12.1 percent), severe cognitive impairment (3.0 percent), obsessive–compulsive disorder (2.2 percent), alcohol use disorder (2.1 percent), and dysthymia (1.0 percent). Finally, for the oldest group, those over 75 years, only four conditions had rates of 1 percent or more: phobic disorders (10.1 percent), severe cognitive impairment (9.3 percent), major depression (1.3 percent), and dysthymia (1.1 percent). Interestingly, not only did cognitive impairment increase with age, as would be expected, but the investigators found that the highest rates occurred in those who were never married or who were separated, divorced, or widowed. Some of the more salient aspects of these data for the purposes of this chapter have been summarized in Table 4.

Similar findings have been reported from the ECA sample living in the area of New Haven, Connecticut, and 12 surrounding towns in south central Connecticut. On the basis of the DIS, 6.7 percent of the respondents age 65 and older had a psychiatric diagnosis, and 3.4 percent had severe cognitive impairment during the past 6-month period. As found at the other ECA sites, these rates were lower than those found in the population under 65 years of age. Anxiety and affective disorders were among the most common psychiatric problems detected.

The validity of data at one of the sites of the ECA program, and indeed the entire ECA program, have been questioned by recent studies of the DIS. Psychiatric diagnoses of community-dwelling subjects previously given a diagnosis derived from the DIS differed significantly from psychiatric-based diagnoses (Anthony et al. 1985; Folstein et al. 1985). The most obvious cause

Table 4.　Selected 6-Month Prevalence Rates of 1 Percent or More: Psychiatric Disorders per 100 Population

Disorder	Age (years)		
	18–64	65–75	75+
Phobic disorders	13.8	12.1	10.1
Panic disorder	1.2	—	—
Obsessive–compulsive disorder	2.2	1.3	—
Somatization disorder	—	—	—
Major depression	2.5	—	1.3
Dysthymia	2.3	1.0	1.1
Alcohol use disorder	6.5	2.1	—
Severe cognitive impairment	—	3.0	9.3

Note.　Adapted from Kramer M, German PS, Anthony JC, et al: Patterns of mental disorders among the elderly residents of eastern Baltimore. J Am Geriatr Soc 1985; 33:236–245.

for this discrepancy appears to be the unreliability of either the DIS or psychiatric diagnoses. The authors suggest several other potential sources of disagreement, including (1) insufficient or inadequate information (on which to base a diagnosis), (2) recency of the disorder, (3) incomplete criterion coverage, (4) overinclusive DIS questions, and (5) degree of reliance on subject symptom reports. No analysis of differences was made based on diagnosis and age. A similar analysis was made of the St. Louis ECA by Helzer et al. 1985). They found that lay results (DIS) showed a bias for only two diagnoses: Major depression was significantly underdiagnosed, and obsessive illness was overdiagnosed.

It is significant that this was a non-institutionalized, community-residing elderly population. Barring methodologic bias, these findings may be explained by three alternative hypotheses. The first is that there is a cohort effect such that older persons in the three areas sampled have actually experienced less past and present anxiety than have younger cohorts. This hypothesis of differential environmental assault is interesting to contemplate but seems unlikely. A second explanation might be that persons 65 and older experienced the same number of anxiety disorders during their lifetime, but *perceive* them differently from their current perspective. That is, their present context in some way reframes their present and past life experience. A third is that there is a selective bias leading to differential survivorship. In other words, those individuals with a lifetime of less perceived anxiety survive longer and are thus relatively more represented in an elderly cohort.

It is unlikely that reframing of anxiety is due to fluctuations in personality, which has been found to be stable across adulthood (Costa et al. 1986). Nor is it likely that older adults perceive symptoms of psychopathology as part of the normal aging process (Hochman 1986). When anxiety concerns *are* present in the elderly, they are related to perceived changes in physical health (Himmelfarb and Murrell 1984). Older individuals are perhaps hypervigilant about their health. In contrast, cognitive concerns do not appear to have the same saliency for this group. Although the lifetime prevalence of cognitive impairment is highest for those over age 65 (Robins et al. 1984) and is the most common psychiatric impairment for men over age 65 (Himmelfarb and Murrell 1984), significant anxiety is an infrequent occurrence in the cognitively impaired elderly patient (Eisdorfer et al. 1981). The issue of selective survivorship has yet to be evaluated, however plausible it may seem.

The community data presented thus far do not pertain to the status of anxiety in the institutionalized elderly. In 1977, this rapidly growing segment of the population represented 1.5 percent of the U.S. population aged 65 to 74, 6.8 percent of those aged 75 to 84, and 21.6 percent of those aged 85 and older (Brody and Foley 1985). These data create a substantial bias in comparing older with younger subjects since the aged at high risk for psychopathology may be differentially housed in institutions for concurrent medical and psychiatric problems. Robins et al. (1984) have also suggested that the aged may be more likely to associate their symptoms with physical problems that occur more frequently among the aged or that there is a historic trend toward increasing psychopathology, therefore leading to relatively more mental illness among the young. This aged population has received little attention with respect to the spectrum of psychopathology, in part because of the high incidence of dementia.

Some Tentative Models and Hypotheses

The manner of presentation of anxiety may also differ between older and younger persons. Further, misclassification of anxiety symptoms may also come from confusion between anxiety and stress (Jarvik and Russell 1979). Stress is the precipitating stimulus to anxiety, but is a separate construct. There is altered ability to deal with stress as aging progresses (Eisdorfer and Wilkie 1977), although there do not appear to be age differences in stress-related adrenomedullary activation (Barnes et al. 1982). Jarvik and Russell (1979) suggest that in addition to the classical fight-or-flight reaction to chronic stress, the aged respond in a way that is more adaptive. They term this third emergency reaction as "freeze." The freezing response would not necessarily produce anxiety, but may result in the development of psychosomatic disease. Thus, when this reaction occurs in response to an emotionally challenging situation, but in the absence of significant sympathetic discharge, it may explain the lack of severe acute anxiety reactions in the aged. The elderly would be more likely to focus on their somatic state.

A distinction has been made between state and trait anxiety (Cattell and Scheier 1961; Spielberger 1972). State anxiety is a transitory condition characterized by feelings of tension, apprehension, and autonomic arousal. In contrast, trait anxiety is stable and characterized by individual variation in response to situations that produce anxiety. Persons with high trait anxiety are more likely to experience anxiety but may not be subjectively anxious at any given point in time.

The work of Eisdorfer and his colleagues has suggested that older men may perform in a learning situation as if they were anxious, although they may not experience anxiety per se. The greater likelihood of autonomic nervous system arousal in older men has been reported, but no studies have related autonomic nervous system changes to subjective state.

The hypothesis that anxiety may not be perceived as such but is reflected in other contexts is raised by a number of psychophysiologic studies (Eisdorfer 1978). Perceived loss of control may be one such mitigating variable. Recent research strongly suggests that mastery or perceived loss of control may affect emotional and physical health. Although there is no clear evidence that perceived control decreases as a function of chronologic age per se (Rodin 1986), the aged are more likely to be frail, institutionalized, and deprived of control over their lives. However, studies also suggest that healthy older subjects actually showed the greatest feelings of personal efficacy (Rodin et al. 1985). Holahan et al. (1984) studied a community sample between the ages of 65 and 75 years and found that higher levels of self-efficacy were associated with lower levels of psychologic distress for women and with fewer psychosomatic complaints for men. Similar findings have been obtained in institutionalized aged when an increased opportunity for control is presented (Rodin and Langer 1977).

Some of the most graphic descriptions of the effects of the association between control and health come from concentration camps during World War II. Bettelheim (1943) describes the "Muselmanner," walking corpses of the concentration camp who had given up all hope once they had decided that they could exercise no influence on their own lives whatsoever. Of special note, however, is the observation by Kral (1951) of an almost total lack of clinical anxiety in the Theresienstadt concentration camp. Unlike most other camps, in the face of terrible privations, the prisoners at Theresienstadt were allowed to establish a degree of autonomy, administered by a council of elders. Kral, a psychiatrist internee, recognized an absense of anxiety-related neuroses in prisoners with prior histories. Returning home after the war, anxiety-related symptoms reappeared in these same individuals.

The hypothesis that stems from these concentration camp data may be that those elderly who feel fully in control will be subject to signs of anxiety only in relation to uncontrollable problems such as their health. In such instances, the anxiety may be masked by medical problems. Where the individual perceives a total loss of control, as in an institution, manifest anxiety may also appear to be minimal. The implication then is that those individuals who are struggling for control (i.e., mastery over their situation) are the ones most likely to exhibit anxiety.

Assuming that the elderly are exposed to their fair share of stressful stimuli, Kastenbaum (1980, 1984) has offered a creative proposal. He has used the concept of habituation to develop a life span developmental approach to aging. "Aging begins when novel events and situations are treated as though repetitions of the familiar" (Kastenbaum 1984, p. 105). The implications of Kastenbaum's model for anxiety among the aged are obvious. If novel stimuli lose salience in old age, so, too, is lost the potential for stimuli to produce anxiety. His hypothetical developmental sequence progresses in nine steps. First, habituation begins in early infancy as a valuable adaptational process. Second, habituation is channeled by social pressures. Third, a concurrent loss of receptivity to internal stimuli takes place. Fourth, new generalization gradients appear, increasing the likelihood of hyperhabituation. Fifth, habituation continues to develop at individual rates as an energy-saving strategy. "It is easier and also quicker to treat new stimuli, situations, people, and events as though they were essentially repetitions of those already experienced, coded, and assigned a response orientation," according to Kastenbaum (1984, p. 110). Sixth, hyperhabituation becomes a liability as "development is sacrificed for the illusion of stability" (p. 111). (Note the need for the individual to maintain a sense of control.) Hyperhabituation is the "well-entrenched tendency to assimilate the novel to the familiar, to devour the stimulus" (p.111). Seventh, novaphobia (fear of the new) develops as habituation is augmented by fatigue, inability to discriminate between stimuli, and a disposition to cling to the past. Eighth, cognition becomes crystallized as the individual becomes proficient at ignoring internal and external stimuli. Ninth, the hyperhabituated individual is no longer able to call on inner resources and is feeling, thinking, and acting old. Kastenbaum concludes that "what we recognize as 'aging' or 'oldness' is the emerging tendency to overadapt to one's own routines and expectations rather than to adapt flexibly and resourcefully to the world at large" (p. 113). Unfortunately, Kastenbaum's conjectures are simply that. There has been no systematic attempt to quantify habituation in the elderly.

Hyperhabituation may extend to the elder's vigilance with regard to health. McCrae et al. (1976) found that anxious men age 64 and older reported no differences from controls in their self-report of symptoms. These findings were in marked contrast to those for young and middle-age groups, in which differences were reported between the two groups. Or, as stated earlier, elder controls may already be reporting symptoms at a high rate.

Conclusion

We have presented recent epidemiologic data that suggest that anxiety decreases in prevalence as individuals age. Although clearly present in the over-65 population, anxiety disorders are apparently less prevalent relative to younger groups. As was clearly reported in the ECA studies, cognitive impairment increases dramatically at age 65 and continues to do so for the next two decades of life. Thus, one possible explanation for the drop in anxiety prevalence may be that cognitive impairment is incompatible with (or at least masks) anxiety. This suggestion may be defended on two grounds. First, cognitive deficits in the elderly most often manifest themselves as an impairment in recent memory. Clearly, if the ability to remember stressful stimuli is diminished or lost, there will be a concomitant diminution in anxiety. Although this argument is largely intuitive, there is a second, and more substantial argument: A *DSM-III* diagnosis of anxiety disorder is incompatible with cognitive impairment. (*Note. DSM-III-R* does not have the hierarchic role of DSM-III; i.e., anxiety disorder is not preempted by a diagnosis of another mental disorder.) Thus, part of the variance can be accounted for by the age-related increase in cognitive impairment.

Presuming that a lower prevalence is a developmental rather than cohort-specific finding, it may be attributable to longer survival for those individuals who have not suffered from anxiety disorder during their lifetime. Because chronic stress and anxiety may have cardiovascular sequelae, it is possible that individuals with more trait anxiety may have either died or become institutionalized prior to age 65. A survival bias would act to skew the prevalence distribution in favor of those older persons with no lifetime history.

In conclusion, we are faced with several alternative interpretations of the data base indicating less anxiety among the aged in the community. One is that there is a systematic bias resulting from a failure to sample cognitively impaired and/or institutionalized elderly. The aged are many times more likely to be so impaired and living in institutional settings than the young. A second interpretation is that the data are misleading because the elderly are more prone to exhibit and interpret the signs and symptoms of anxiety as related to physical disorders. Third, there may indeed be an important developmental process, however poorly understood, in which selective survivorship may have occurred as a result of an adaptive configuration that includes personality and the pattern of traumatic life experiences. Finally, there is the possibility that denial and the forgetting of anxious experiences are adaptive.

The data base is scanty and clearly there is much to be learned by investigating these issues.

References

American Psychiatric Association: Diagnostic and Statistical Manual of Mental Disorders (Third Edition). Washington, DC, American Psychiatric Association, 1980

American Psychiatric Association: Diagnostic and Statistical Manual of Mental Disorders (Third Edition-Revised). Washington, DC, American Psychiatric Association, 1987

Anthony JC, Folstein M, Romanski AJ, et al: Comparison of the lay Diagnostic Interview Schedule and a standardized psychiatric diagnosis: experience in eastern Baltimore. Arch Gen Psychiatry 1985; 42:667–675

Barnes RF, Raskind M, Gumbrecht G, et al: The effects of age on the plasma catecholamine response to mental stress in man. J Clin Endocrinol Metab 1982; 54:64–69

Bettelheim B: Individual and mass behavior in extreme situations. Abnorm Soc Psychol 1943; 38:417–452

Brody JA, Foley DJ: Epidemiologic considerations, in The Teaching Nursing Home. Edited by Schneider EL. New York, Raven Press, 1983

Cattell, Scheier. The Meaning and Measurement of Neuroticism and Anxiety. New York, Ronald Press, 1961

Costa, PT, McCrae RR, Zonderman AE: Cross-sectional studies of personality in a national sample: 2. Stability and neuroticism, extroversion, and openness. Psychology and Aging 1986; 1:144–149

Delprato DJ, McGlynn FD: Behavioral theories of anxiety disorders, in Behavior Theories and Treatment of Anxiety. Edited by Turner SM. New York, Plenum Press, 1984

Eisdorfer C: Psychophysiologic and cognitive studies in the aged, in Aging: The Process and the People. Edited by Usdin G, Hofling CD. New York, Brunner/Mazel, 1978

Eisdorfer C, Wilkie F: Stress, disease, aging and behavior, in Handbook of the Psychology of Aging. Edited by Birren JE, Schaie KW. New York, Van Nostrand Reinhold, 1977

Eisdorfer C, Cohen D, Keckich W: Depression and anxiety in the cognitively impaired aged, in Anxiety: New Research and Changing Concepts. Edited by Klein DF, Rabkin J. New York, Raven Press, 1981

Endler NS, Okada M: A multidimensional measure of trait anxiety: the S-R Inventory of General Trait Anxiousness. Consult Clin Psychol 1975; 43:319–329

Fostein MF, Romanoski AJ, Nestadt G, et al: Brief report on the clinical reappraisal of the Diagnostic Interview Schedule carried out at the Johns Hopkins site of the Epidemiological Catchment Area Program of the NIMH. Psychol Med 1985; 15:809–814

Helzer JE, Robins LN, McEvoy LT, et al: A comparison of clinical and diagnostic interview schedule diagnoses. Arch Gen Psychiatry 1985; 42:657–666

Himmelfarb S, Murrell SA: The prevalence and correlates of anxiety symptoms in older adults. J Psychol 1984; 116:159–167

Hochman LO, Storandt M, Rosenberg AM: Age and its effects on perceptions of psychopathology. Psychology and Aging 1986; 1:337–338

Holahan CK, Holahan CJ, Belk SS: Adjustment in aging: the roles of life stress, hassles, and self-efficacy. Health Psychol 1984; 3:315–328

Jarvik LF, Russell D: Anxiety, aging and the third emergency reaction. J Gerontol 1979; 34:197–200

Kastenbaum RJ: Habituation as a model of human aging. Int J Aging Human Dev 1980–1981; 12:159–170

Kastenbaum RJ: When aging begins: a lifespan developmental approach. Research on Aging 1984; 6:105–117

Kral VA: Psychiatric observations under severe chronic stress. Am J Psychiatry 1951; 108:185

Kramer M, German PS, Anthony JC, et al: Patterns of mental disorders among the elderly residents of eastern Baltimore. J Am Geriat Soc 1985; 33:236–245

MacMillan A: The health opinion survey: technique for estimating prevalence of psychoneurotic and related types of disorders in communities. Psychol Rep 1957; 3:325–339

McCrae RR, Bartone PT, Costa PT: Age, anxiety, and self-reported health. Int J Aging Human Dev 1976; 7:49–58

Myers JK, Weissman MM, Tischler GL, et al: Six month prevalence of psychiatric disorders in three communities. Arch Gen Psychiatry 1984; 41:959–967

National Center for Health Statistics: Office-based ambulatory care for patients 75 years old and over: national ambulatory medical care survey, 1980 and 1981, in NCHS Advanced Data (No. 110) (DHHS Publication No. (PHS) 85–1250. Edited by Koch H, Smith MC. Washington, DC, U.S. Government Printing Office, 1985

Robins N, Helzer JE, Weissman MM, et al: Lifetime prevalence of specific psychiatric disorders in three sites. Arch Gen Psychiatry 1984; 41:949–958

Rodin J: Aging and health: effects of sense of control. Science 1986; 23:1271–1276

Rodin J, Langer EJ: Long-term effects of a control-relevant intervention with the institutionalized aged. J Pers Soc Psychol 1977; 35:897–902

Rodin J, Timko C, Harris S: Annual Review of Gerontology and Geriatrics 1985; 5(1)

Spielberger CD: Anxiety as an emotional state, in Anxiety: Current Trends in Theory and Research (Volume 1). Edited by Spielberger CD. New York, Academic Press, 1972

U.S. Bureau of the Census: Series P-25, No. 922, Washington, DC, U.S. Government Printing Office, 1982

Warheit GJ, Holzer CE, Arey SA: Race and mental illness: an epidemiologic update. J Health Soc Behav 1975; 16:243–256

White LR, Cartwright WS, Cornoni-Huntley J, et al: Geriatric epidemiology. Annual Review of Gerontology and Geriatrics 1986; 6:215–311

Chapter 16

Somatoform and Psychosexual Disorders

Ewald W. Busse, M.D.

Somatoform Disorders

Hypochondriasis is one of the seven somatoform disorders included in the *Diagnostic and Statistical Manual of Mental Disorders (Third Edition-Revised) (DSM-III-R)* (American Psychiatric Association 1987). Of the seven somatoform *DSM-III-R* categories, two are closely associated with hypochondriasis. These are idiopathic pain disorder and undifferentiated somatoform disorder. The former is associated with severe and prolonged complaint of pain that is the major or sole concern of the patient. No organic pathology or pathophysiologic mechanism can be found to account for the pain, and psychologic factors appear to be etiologically involved. Further, if organic pathology exists, it appears the complaint is often exaggerated and interferes with occupational and other daily activities. Vague, persistent complaints of at least 6 months' duration characterize undifferentiated somatoform disorder. The other *DSM-III-R* categories include somatization disorder (a kaleidoscope array of symptoms, onset before age 30, sometimes referred to as Briquet's syndrome) (Haberkern et al. 1985), conversion disorder, dysmorphic somatoform disorder (an imagined defect in one's physical appearance), and a residual category (somatoform disorder not otherwise specified).

The diagnostic term "hypochondriasis," not unlike some other psychiatric diagnostic terms, has been frequently redefined and has been omitted from and restored to official classifications of mental diseases. Regardless of this uncertainty regarding definition and accuracy of the diagnosis, the practicing physician is aware that hypochondriasis is a common and often frustrating clinical problem. The certainty of diagnosis in an elderly person is complicated by the existence of physical disabilities and diseases and the increase of social stress factors that accompany the aging process.

This discussion of the etiology of hypochondriasis and therapeutic intervention is based on the conviction that hypochondriasis in the elderly is frequently a biologic/psychosocial phenomenon. The psychotherapeutic rationale and techniques can be understood and used by any interested and motivated physician. The primary care physician carries a major burden for the care of the elderly, including the hypochondriacs, and it is held that many elderly hypochondriacs will respond favorably to a combined medical-psychotherapeutic approach. Treatment of the elderly hypochondriac is best accomplished by a psychiatrist working in a general medical clinic or by an adequately trained primary care physician.

The disorder of idiopathic pain is discussed elsewhere in this chapter. The two categories "hypochondriasis" and "undifferentiated somatoform disorder" overlap. In this discussion the disorder of hypochondriasis is considered to be an anxious preoccupation with the body or a portion of the body that is believed to be diseased or functioning improperly. The complaint can lack a discernible organic explanation or it may be an exaggeration of existing pathology. In the longitudinal research associated with this presentation, the subjects were identified as having "high bodily concern."

Hypochondriasis

Diagnostic Criteria

The *DSM-III-R* cites the following diagnostic criteria for hypochondriasis (Copyright © 1987 American Psychiatric Association. Reprinted with permission.):

A. The predominant disturbance is preoccupation with the fear of having or the belief that one has a serious disease based on the individual's interpretation of physical signs or sensations as evidence of physical illness (do not include misinterpretation of physical symptoms of panic attack).

B. Appropriate physical evaluation does not support the diagnosis of any physical disorder that can account for the physical signs or sensations or the individual's unwarranted interpretation of them, and the symptoms in A. are not only symptoms of panic attacks.

C. The fear of having or the belief that one has a disease persists despite medical reassurance.

D. The duration of the disturbance is at least 6 months.

E. The belief in A. is not a fixed delusion, as in delusional disorder somatic type.

It is acknowledged that hypochondriasis is commonly associated with a depressive mood (American Psychiatric Association 1987). Depressive symptoms, although present, rarely are of sufficient severity that the use of antidepressive agents is needed (Gallagher and Thompson 1983).

According to *DSM-III-R*, a panic attack is characterized by numerous anxiety symptoms such as shortness of breath, palpitation, sweating, dizziness, and *a fear of dying*. This is one of the symptoms that should not be confused with hypochondriasis. Although the symptoms of both hypochondriasis and the delusion associated with a psychosis can be considered false beliefs, a *delusion* is a fixed belief that some external source is maliciously attempting to control or harass the victim (American Psychiatric Association 1988).

Psychodynamics

Although each individual presents different psychosocial stress and responses, there are four psychologic defense mechanisms that often, but not exclusively, play an important role in the dynamics of hypochondriasis in the elderly.

1. The symptoms may be used as an explanation for failure to meet personal and social expectations and to avoid or excuse recurrent failure.
2. The patient may be experiencing increasing isolation and hence is withdrawing psychic interests from other persons or objects and redirecting his or her interests on the self, the body, and its functions.
3. The patient may be shifting anxiety from a specific psychiatric conflict to a less threatening bodily function.
4. The symptoms may be a means of self-punishment and atonement for unacceptable hostile feelings toward persons close to the individual.

The primary mental mechanisms are reinforced by secondary gain. Secondary gain is the increased attention and sympathy from friends and health care providers that is originally generated by the symptoms. It is important that the clinician keep the mechanisms in mind, since doing so will make the patient's complaints more understandable and provide a logical basis for the therapeutic approach.

Risk Factors

Stressful life events are often precipitating factors of hypochondriacal reactions in late middle life and early late life. These often include exposure to a work or social situation in which the individual suffers prolonged criticism and lacks escape opportunities (Busse 1982).

The older person is likely to experience other stresses such as a reduction in their economic status and/or loss of spouse and friends, both of which contribute to social isolation. A deterioration in marital satisfactions can result from chronic disability affecting one of the marital partners.

Remission and Course

The longitudinal studies of "normal" aging people conducted at Duke University Center for the Study of Aging and Human Development have uncovered some important observations relevant to the problem of hypochondriasis (Busse 1986). Observation of subjects over time found that hypochondriacal reactions are often transient, lasting from a few months to several years. Depressive signs and symptoms are not an unusual concomitant of hypochondriasis. The hypochondriacal reaction is often an adaptive response to an unfamiliar serious social stress. Hence, improvement is related to the fortuitous disappearance of the stress, such as the moving away of an adult child who has been a persistent critic of the older person.

The subjects observed in the Duke Longitudinal Study I that were classified as having "high bodily concern," that is, hypochondriasis, frequently did *not* seek medical attention but in fact resisted the urging of family or friends to seek medical relief for their multiple symptoms. Many of the hypochondriacal subjects used home remedies and excessive over-the-counter medication. Some additional observations suggested that if such hypochondriacal persons are forced to see a physician, particularly at the insistence of family or friends, their pattern of maintaining social adjustment and self-esteem is threatened and the hypochondriacal pattern may become solidified.

These longitudinal observations are consistent with those of Barsky and Klerman (1983). Barsky and Klerman explain that hypochondriasis is a learned social behavior. It is a type of social communication appealing for sympathy and support. The hypochondriacal person has learned that the illness behavior is a way to obtain support and attention. Furthermore, chronic illness behavior is also reinforced by the successful avoidance of adverse consequences such as unpleasant duties and obligations. Similar observations were made in the longitudinal studies: The individuals were using somatization as a way to deal with an adverse social situation and as a way of maintaining their self-esteem.

A particular caution should be expressed about diagnostic or exploratory surgical procedures in hypochondriacal patients. It never helps the patient to have a surgical scar that testifies to the fact that a competent physician believed that the patient had something wrong with his or her body. In addition, the operative scar can become a focus of new symptoms that are then attributed to "complications" or "adhesions" following the surgical procedure.

Forms of Brief Psychotherapy

A recent report claims that there are at least 250 "brands of therapy that are advocated for the treatment of mental, emotional, and behavioral problems" (Meredith and Turner 1986, p. 132). Each brand of therapy claims to have special features that make it more effective and are often said to be particularly useful in certain disorders. A number of brief psychotherapies have been described for the treatment of depression (not hypochondriasis) in the elderly. Some of the better known ones include cognitive therapy (Beck et al. 1979; Emery 1981), behavioral therapy (Lewinsohn et al. 1976; Gallagher et al. 1981), interpersonal therapy (Klerman and Weissman 1982), and brief psychodynamic psychotherapy (Bellak and Small 1965). These brief forms of psychotherapy (up to 20 visits) are useful, but are designed for those patients who are actively seeking psychiatric help. In contrast, the therapeutic approach described in this chapter applies to patients who are resistant or unwilling to be referred for psychiatric help.

Brown and Valient (1981) reported a study of severe hypochondriacal patients. Currently these would probably be considered somatization disorder. These clinical investigators reached the conclusion that this type of hypochondriasis can best be defined as "the transformation of reproach toward others arising from bereavement, loneliness, or unacceptable aggressive impulses into self reproach initially and then into complaints of other pain or somatic illness" (p. 725). They note that encounters with this type of hypochondriacal patient tend to elicit five responses that adversely influence therapeutic approaches. These include the ignoring of the patient's social history, the covert anger of the patient that may escape the physician's awareness, the hidden anger of the patient toward the physician, the physician's frustration and resentment that disrupt the doctor-patient relationship, the attempts to offer care that are misdirected and malfunction, and unexpected shifts in the patient's behavior that surprise and distract the physician. Brown and Valiant conclude that to treat hypochondriacs successfully, the physician needs to combine both an intellectual and an emotional understanding of the patient's predicament. The physician must appreciate the traumatic psychosocial history of the patient.

Therapeutic Techniques

The therapeutic techniques described herein are designed to assist the primary care physician and the psychiatrist practicing in a general medical setting in dealing with the hypochondriacal patient whose symptoms are of relatively recent onset (less than 2 years) on an outpatient basis (Busse and Blazer 1980). The techniques are basic to, but not sufficient for, the handling of the other six somatoform disorders described in *DSM-III-R* and for hospitalized patients. Furthermore, these techniques may be of limited usefulness in dealing with multiple physical complaints associated with an early-onset somatization disorder, schizophrenia, or severe depression.

Additional Information

This review of a therapeutic approach contains "basic" information. Additional relevant material can be found in various publications (Busse and Blazer 1980; Busse 1982, 1986).

Treatment—Ineffective Techniques

Limits of revelations. It seems logical that if the patient is given a full explanation of his or her medical condition, that is, the absence of any organic explanation, this would serve as reassurance.

Furthermore, consistent with the patient's "right to know" and "normal" thinking, the patient should be informed of physical and laboratory studies that are negative. For example, if the physician says "The results of my careful workup indicate that you are physically in good health," many hypochondriacs may react adversely. Such an abrupt revelation implies that the person's symptomatology must be of mental origin. The failure to find an organic explanation for the complaints seems to rob the patient of an unconscious defense mechanism, the disrupting of which further reduces self-esteem. Often following such an abrupt revelation, the patient's complaints will increase and the patient may terminate contact with the physician. Such hypochondriacs become medical shoppers. Even less specific explanations of how emotional upsets can sometimes cause physical symptoms are likely to be unsuccessful. These patients may agree that this can happen to some people, but they are sure that a mental or emotional explanation is not applicable to their symptoms. To balance the right to know with a measure of reassurance, it is suggested that the physician include in his remarks a supportive statement and manner. For example, "The results of this workup indicate there is no adequate explanation for your symptoms. It is obvious that you are having problems and I will be pleased to work with you to improve your situation."

Specific diagnosis. Another technique that is unlikely to be successful is to respond to the patient's demand to know "what's wrong with me?" by giving him or her a specific, but false, diagnosis. Often these patients respond by saying they are relieved to know what is wrong with them, but since their symptoms persist and may even increase, they will question the diagnosis and disrupt the relationship with the physician.

Many patients will demand to know "exactly what's wrong with me." A specific or fictitious diagnosis should be avoided because eventually such misinformation will come to light. Rather, the physician should say, "I'm sure it would be reassuring if I had a specific diagnosis. I will be willing to follow you carefully and attempt to find some way to improve your health and well-being."

The examples of statements in response to patients should be recognized as only suggestions since a physician must respond in a way that is consistent with his or her personal style. However, it is important for the physician to keep in mind the necessity to include supporting remarks—indicating a commitment to helping the patient while not threatening the patient's needed hypochondriacal defense.

Effective Techniques

For hypochondriacal persons to continue to live comfortably with their family and in society, their psychologic defense of hypochondriasis must be maintained until adequate coping mechanisms are put in place. The physician must understand this need, must listen to the patient's "organ recital" until a positive relationship between the patient and physician has been established, should use this relationship to provide the basis for a discussion of areas of emotional conflict, and must help the patient to seek new methods of coping. An important point in this relationship is that the physician should make it clear to the patient that he or she is aware that the patient is experiencing discomfort and unhappiness and is willing to help.

Use and limitation of medication. A patient–physician relationship is assisted by the use of prescribed medication or a placebo. The physician must be careful to avoid prescribing any medication that is likely to produce side effects since the signs and symptoms would only complicate an already confused clinical picture. Addictive drugs should be avoided. Also, drugs that have been used previously by the patient without success should not be repeated. Although placebos are rarely used by physicians (2.4 percent) caring for hypochondriacs, placebos have value in practice and research (Busse and Maddox 1985; Poe and Holloway 1980).

The use of prescribed "medication" may be criticized in that it implies to the hypochondriacal patient that he or she actually has an organic illness. This criticism is not without merit, but it should be pointed out that many hypochondriacal elderly patients actually do have changes in their physiologic functioning such as sleep disturbances. They can respond to improved medical surveillance. In fact, in this example it would be wise to eliminate the use of hypnotic drugs. Again, the physician must remember that medications and placebos do have symbolic value. A hypochondriacal complaint is a distress signal and patients' anxiety may be reduced and self-esteem increased by knowing that a reputable, professional person is "taking care" of them.

The roles of relatives. The handling of relatives is an important part of treatment. Relatives or friends, particularly those who begin to suspect that the patient's symptoms are of emotional origin rather than physical, may request an interview with the physician to confirm their suspicions. Under these circumstances, the physician should avoid saying that the patient's symptoms are of psychologic origin. Rather, physicians should communicate that they consider the patient ill and worried, that the patient needs help, and that they will do whatever they can to be of value. One of the surest ways for a patient to lose confidence in the physician is to be told by a relative or friend that in a conversation with the physician, the physician confirmed the belief that the patient's complaints are imaginary.

Frequency of visits. It is generally wise to see a hypochondriacal patient once a week for at least 8 to 10 weeks. Later the time between appointments can be lengthened. Appointments should be at a definite time. When a definite appointment is given to hypochondriacal patients, it is interesting how many will respond by saying that the time suggested is inconvenient and ask for another time to be arranged. The frequency of this pattern leads to the conclusion that it is a way of testing physicians to determine the extent of their interest in the patient. Generally the physician should insist that the patient adhere to a selected time for appointments and adhere to the therapeutic regimen. Firmness gives the patient new confidence that the physician is making a determined effort to be of help.

Length of interview. It is desirable to adhere to an appointment schedule. Although the first contact may require considerable time, return visits can be reduced to 15 to 20 minutes. The patient should be told when and how long the next appointment will be. This will discourage hypochondrical patients from making bids for additional time. Not infrequently when the duration of the interview has not been specified, the patient, sensing that the interview is about to be concluded, may "suddenly" remember something very important, thereby seeking to extend the period of contact with the physician. Generally, the physician should suggest to the patient that, since it is very important, it should be given more time and should be taken up at the next visit.

Hostility. In the second or third interviews, it is not unusual for the patient to express hostility against a previous physician. The treating physician must refrain from defending the colleague and must confine remarks to recognition that the patient's experiences have been both upsetting and disappointing. Occasionally the physician should mention that perhaps the patient is concerned whether the physician will maintain an interest in the patient and continue to seek for ways of helping. This understanding and acceptance of the patient's views can be very constructive.

Resistance. Psychiatrists working with an elderly hypochondriacal person must recognize that it is highly likely they will encounter more resistance and more expressions of hostility from the patients than are ordinarily directed toward the nonpsychiatrist physician. Many patients believe that the role of the physician is to determine or demonstrate that their physical symptoms are of mental origin. It is not unusual for the patients to confront the psychiatrist by asserting that imagination or nervousness plays no role in their symptoms. Such resistances can be dealt with in a number of ways including recognizing that other individuals may have indicated the symptoms were of mental or emotional origin and that this is understandably upsetting to the patient. Also, the psychiatrist's therapeutic role is not limited to psychiatry, but involves the total health and well-being of the individual.

Content of Follow-Up Visits

Interpersonal events. As return visits continue, the physician should encourage the patient to give details regarding the interpersonal events that occurred between interviews. Gradually the patient shifts away from physical complaints to a greater emphasis on psychosocial conflicts related to the family, work, and friends. When this change develops, treatment can follow two paths. Patients may gradually lose the intensity of their preoccupation with their imaginary illness as a result of confidence and improved self-esteem gained in the physician–patient relationship. Patients may become aware that exacerbations of symptoms occur as the result of certain events, but in the intervening period they can return to a more active and more efficient participation in their interpersonal relationships.

Insight. A still brighter outlook can be anticipated if the patient begins to develop some insight into the situation. The patient may notice that the symptoms become worse after an argument or after being criticized and, as a result, will begin to discuss ways of handling such stressful situations. As defense mechanisms become more effective, the patient will often begin to abandon the physical complaints.

Organic illness. With older hypochondriacal patients physicians must remain alert to the possibility that true organic illness can exist or develop. Included in this high cost of being neurotic is the distinct possibility that physical illness can be overlooked because the multiple symptoms make it difficult to separate functional from organic signs or symptoms.

Depression and Hypochondriasis

A number of observers have reported that in the Far East, particularly in the People's Republic of China, depression as we now recognize it is relatively rare. However, the conflicts are expressed in terms of somatic equivalents. This is explained in a number of ways including the observation that guilt feelings and depressive affect are rarely or poorly verbalized (Grauer 1984). It is also reported that the diagnosis neurasthenia is popular in China and often these patients represent the somatization of a depressive status. The existence of depression is denied by the patients (Kleinman 1982).

Affective disorders in late life may present with exaggerated fears and worries about the body. Depression is the most common affective condition to be masked by physical symptoms. Because depression is more common in the elderly, one might expect to see an increased prevalence of hypochondriacal symptoms. An added advantage of such symptoms is that the depressed patient may receive secondary gain in the form of attention, comfort, touching, and interest that are associated with the interactions between physicians, family members, and the patient regarding the pain (Busse and Blazer 1980).

Most studies indicate that the prevalence of "hypochondriasis" is quite high among the depressed elderly. In one study, hypochondriacal symptoms were found in 65.7 percent of men and 62 percent of women among 152 depressed patients over the age of 60. The most common presenting symptom was constipation. Hypochondriacal symptoms may be associated with overt symptoms of anxiety or depression. Of those individuals with hypochondriacal symptoms 24.8 percent attempted suicide, while among those free of such symptoms only 7.3 percent attempted suicide. The presence of hypochondriacal symptoms in the older patient with significant depression may present a potentially critical situation to the clinician (Alarcon 1964).

A community survey in Durham, North Carolina (Maddox 1964), revealed that approximately 10 percent of the elderly assess their physical health to be poorer than their health status actually was rated on an objective basis. These individuals were more depressed and had decreased life satisfaction. Though their physical health status was normal, their activities of daily living were decreased and they had an increased number of doctors visits compared with a control group. They also reported a greater number of symptoms when asked objectively. One surprising finding was that these individuals were actually more willing to see a mental health counselor (if they demonstrated some impairment in their mental health) than the control population. This finding is in contrast to the general belief that the hypochondriacal patient avoids mental health services and gravitates to individuals who they feel will take interest in their physical health only. A separate study found 53.6 percent of the elderly surveyed who felt themselves in better health than others. Thirty-one percent reported that they felt their own health about the same as others, and 9.8 percent considered their health to be poorer than those of other persons their age (U.S. Department of Health, Education and Welfare 1977).

Maddox and Douglass (1973), in another study of the elderly in Durham

County, reported that two of three elderly subjects displayed a reality orientation in their subjective evaluation of health status. Seventeen percent (17 percent) assessed their health as subjectively poor when it was objectively good and 13 percent assessed their health as subjectively good when it was objectively poor.

Together, these studies indicate that between 10 and 20 percent of the elderly who are in the community consider their health to be poor compared with persons their own age and view their health to be subjectively worse than it is demonstrated on objective examination. These individuals may not all deserve the label "hypochondriacal," but the factors contributing to the development of this negative assessment of health status may form a predictable pattern. This turning attention to the body may (1) facilitate communication and interaction with others (via symptom communication), (2) displace anxiety, (3) form an identification with a deceased or absent loved one, (4) provide punishment for unresolved guilt feelings, and (5) control the behavior of individuals within the immediate environment. Regardless of the etiology, these individuals are quite difficult for the physician to treat.

Idiopathic Pain Disorder

The *DSM-III-R* defines idiopathic pain disorder as follows (Copyright © 1987 American Psychiatric Association. Reprinted with permission.):

A. The predominant disturbance is at least six months of preoccupation with pain.
B. Either (1) or (2):
   (1) after appropriate evaluation, no organic pathology or pathophysiological mechanism (e.g., a physical disorder or the effects of injury) has been found to account for the pain
   (2) when there is related organic pathology, the complaint of pain or resulting social or occupational impairment is grossly in excess of what would be expected from the physical findings

Comparing the definitions of idiopathic pain disorder and hypochondriasis, the distinction is not clear. Idiopathic pain disorder is associated with "pain" while hypochondriasis is based on "physical signs and sensations."

The psychophysiology of pain is discussed in Chapter 3.

Clinical Implications of Pain

Although age affects many perceptions, including vision, hearing, taste, and smell, it is not clear what, if any, pain changes are associated with aging. Age does not influence pain thresholds for such diverse stimuli as tooth shock or forearm heat (Harkins et al. 1986). When psychophysiologic procedures are designed as a response to a noxious stimulus, changes may be detected, but this may be attributed to difficulties in the response rather than in differences in pain perception (nociception).

The clinician is justifiably concerned that age-associated pain changes may influence the diagnostic criteria that are customarily employed. A recent survey found that while 30 percent of those over age 70 did not experience pain as a major presenting symptom with myocardial infarction, an almost comparable percentage (i.e., 23 percent) of younger persons had the same painless experience (MacDonald et al. 1983). It is debatable if age-related changes affect referred pain, but this is not mentioned in the major medical textbooks.

Pain associated with appendicitis presents in a similar fashion regardless of the patient's age. Generally the symptoms are comparable to those in younger people, mainly pain of a generalized abdominal nature, localized to the right lower quadrant and associated with nausea and vomiting. What may be lacking in the elderly person is the associated elevation of temperature and leukocytosis. The lack of these manifestations may account for the diagnostic difficulties that are sometimes encountered in the elderly (Glenn 1978; Albano et al. 1975).

It is true that persistent or frequently recurring pain is associated with physical disorders that are common in late life. These include osteoarthritis, rheumatic arthritis, angina of effort, herpes zoster, and gout. There are other conditions that more likely produce chronic pain in younger adults. These include arthralgia, pleuritic pain, headaches, and backaches. It is highly likely that the presence of persistent pain does have significant effect on psychologic functioning, but this is true in middle-aged as well as elderly persons (Harkins and Nowlin 1983).

Pain Clinics

Pain clinics exist in many medical centers. The staff is usually multidisciplinary and often a psychiatrist plays a critical role in evaluating and devising a therapeutic plan. The therapeutic plan must take into account the estimate of the degree that the patient is aggravating or exaggerating the persistent pain, the patient's personal characteristics, and the environment in which the patient exists.

Although elderly people frequently report recurrent or persistent pain, they are underrepresented in the patient population of a multidisciplinary pain clinic. This suggests that either the elderly person tolerates chronic pain as an accepted part of the aging process or the referring physician is pessimistic as to what the clinic may offer an older person.

Pain and Depression

The symptom overlap between pain and depression is of great clinical importance. Lindsay and Wycoff (1981) observed that 59 percent of patients requesting treatment for depression also have recurrent benign pain. In contrast, 87 percent of patients in chronic pain clinics have depression. Often patients with chronic pain report insomnia, eating disturbances, and loss of interest in social activities as well as in sex (Lindsay and Wycoff 1981). Patients with chronic pain complaints deny depression, but their other symptomatology suggests the existence of a depression. Such symptoms include loss of energy, poor concentration, and inappropriate guilt, as well as such symptoms as sleep disturbances, early morning awakening, and psychomotor retardation.

Because of this overlap, the use of antidepressants has proved to be of value. Interestingly, such antidepressant medication may have a more rapid effect on pain than on the other manifestations of the depression. Therefore, it is important for the patient to remain on the medication despite the reduction in pain. Kwentus et al. (1985) report that some elderly patients who complain of chronic pain have long-standing personality disorders. The pain behaviors that are associated with such individuals may be particularly troublesome. Pain complaints may serve to manipulate friends, relatives, and physicians. In many respects this is not unlike the secondary gain found in hypochondriasis.

Obviously the psychiatrist must assist in a therapeutic approach by designing a multidisciplinary effort that avoids reinforcing such behavior and discouraging pain behaviors. Some of these techniques may include set-dose analgesic drug therapy, not the use of as-needed dosage, reinforcing involvement in activities unrelated to pain, the selective inattention to pain complaints, and the avoidance of prolonged discussion of pain.

A warning is important in dealing with pain in the elderly: Many elderly people are receiving multiple medications and drug interactions may seriously complicate the clinical picture.

Relief of Pain

For several thousand years before Christ, the Egyptians knew that extracts from the white poppy would relieve pain. Furthermore, from stone carvings in tombs from the fifth dynasty, about 2500 B.C., the Egyptians used an electric fish found in the Nile River to treat different pain conditions.

Acupuncture has been used in the Orient, particularly in China, for thousands of years. The classical textbook of Oriental medicine, *Nei Ching*, refers to the relief of pain by techniques of stimulation of tissue at special sites with sharp objects such as fish bones, stones, or bamboo sticks. An alternative method was to warm these points by pouring small urns of burning moxa (herbs) on the skin. Although acupuncture was used for relief of pain, it was not until 1955 that the unique technique of acupuncture anesthesia was developed in China. In the late 1950s, Chinese medical workers became aware that acupuncture reduced the pain of toothache, sore throat, tooth extraction, and tonsillectomy. This formed a basis for expanding the technique to more extensive surgical procedures. Early in the technique, many needles were used, but over the years this has been reduced so that currently in many important procedures only one to four needles are actually used. The needle insertions, however, are now supplemented by the use of electrical stimulation, eliminating the old procedure of rotating the needles by hand to maintain an input of sensation (Busse and Busse 1979).

Although most patients insist that they feel no pain when the needle is inserted, in order to achieve effective anesthesia with acupuncture, the patient must feel sore, distended, heavy, and numb over the site of the needle placement. The needle is usually inserted to a depth of one-fourth of an inch to one inch depending on the patient's body build, location of needle, and so forth. Needle insertion is carried out with care to avoid blood vessels and any disruption of vital organs. Ear points are frequently used. With ear points, some patients do report experiencing pain when being punctured. Acupuncture is usually employed as an anesthesia for surgical procedures after several days of trial and education of the patient. Occasionally in China supplementary drugs are used, but they are usually of relatively low dosage. The most plausible explanation for the effectiveness of acupuncture is consistent with the Melzack and Wall theory of gate control of pain. This theory holds that certain types of stimuli will flood gates in the nervous system and prevent other types of stimuli from going through the gate. It is also very likely that there is considerable individual variation as to those who respond to acupuncture.

Swedish advocates use a technique derived from acupuncture (Sjolund and Eriksson 1985). This technique is called transcutaneous electrical nerve stimulation (TENS). Other methods have been developed to stimulate nervous tissue with devices implanted in the body. Two that have come into clinical use are the spinal cord stimulation and the dorsal column stimulation. These techniques are used after other measures such as TENS have failed.

Treatment and Chronic Pain

Chronic pain, by definition, has persisted for a long time and its underlying cause may or may not be identified with a disease process. As mentioned in Chapter 3, chronic pain serves no useful biologic function. Further, the recognized pain pathways may not be involved in the perception of chronic pain and interruption of these pathways ordinarily results in only transient relief. Furthermore, Gildenberg and DeVaul (1985) believe that cutting pain pathways and usual analgesics are ineffective against chronic pain and may actually potentiate it. These authors observe that although there are similarities between patients with chronic pain they must be considered as individuals and the physician must be alert to the possibility that the pain is overevaluated. In such patients, pain plays a central role in how the patients relate to themselves and to others. Social factors may be present that reinforce the pain behavior and the physician must be careful, because often such patients have succeeded in maneuvering physicians into attempting ill-advised medical or surgical procedures. These authors concluded, "Little in the way of pain management can be accomplished unless and until both patient and treating physician exchange the goal of pain relief for that of rehabilitation" (p. 17).

Caution must be observed since these authors point out that pain from malignancies is quite different and contains characteristics of both chronic and acute pain and that cancer pain can often benefit by interrupting pain pathways.

Medications are used to reduce peripheral pain. The analgesic action of acetylsalicylic acid (aspirin) can be explained by the inhibition of cyclooxygenase. This enzyme controls the synthesis of prostaglandins, prostacyclins, and thromboxanes from arachindonic acid, all of which appear to be associated with pain generation. Many other drugs also inhibit cyclooxygenase. Ibuprofen, which is now commonly used, seems to have both an analgesic and an antiinflammatory effect. The corticosteroids have a somewhat similar antiinflammatory analgesic effect.

Herpes Zoster and Postherpetic Neuralgia

For many years, one of the most serious and common complaints associated with pain in the elderly is that caused by herpes zoster and postherpetic neuralgia (Bonica 1953).

The epidemiologic aspects of the zoster virus are of considerable interest to aging since the occurrence of the first attack increases rapidly after the age of 45, with the majority occurring between the age of 60 and 80. A second attack occurs between the ages of 60 and 80 years (Weller 1983). Postherpetic neuralgia occurs after the vesicles of herpes zoster have cleared. The pain is of a burning quality, is unrelenting, and follows the distribution of the peripheral nerve that was originally involved. Herpes zoster progresses to postherpetic neuralgia in 14 percent of men and 25 percent of women. This progression rarely occurs before the age of 65 and the majority are over 70 years of age. The chronicity of the pain produces a variety of psychologic problems. They are believed to be pain related and not age related (Graff-Radford et al. 1986). Acyclovir is a selective antiviral agent that is effective against herpes viruses (Wikman 1985).

Treatment. Acyclovir is an acyclic nucleoside analog of guanosine. There are five human herpesviruses; these include herpes simplex virus (types 1 and 2), varicella-zoster virus, the Epstein-Barr virus, and the cytomegalovirus. A few studies have attempted to treat herpes zoster. The acyclovir treatment of acute herpes zoster and postherpetic neuralgia is encouraging; however, further experience is required. Other attempts of treatment include the use of sympathetic blocks, the intravenous infusion of lidocaine, the infiltration of the painful area with long-lasting cortisone compounds, and the use of phenothiazines and tricyclic antidepressants (Bonica 1984).

Psychosexual Changes

Studies in aging in the mammalian reproductive system show that its functional decline typically occurs at a time when the animal is in good health and other systems appear to be operating normally. The onset of female menopause and male changes is obviously tied to the passage of time and indicates that aging processes can be initiated at various points throughout the life span (Goldman et al. 1985).

The Menopause: An Aging Phenomenon

The age of menarche in the human female has decreased with time. There are conflicting data as to whether there has been any change in age at the menopause. Many studies indicate that menopause now occurs at 48 to 51 years of age in a wide variety of populations. Births after the age of 50 are extremely rare.

The menopause involves the ovaries, the anterior lobe of the pituitary gland, and the hypothalamus. The anterior lobe of the pituitary gland undergoes marked histologic changes in postmenopausal women. The most prominent structural changes occur in the gonadotropin-secreting basophilic cells.

A fundamental question concerning aging within the female reproductive system is whether alterations in the brain–pituitary–ovarian axis and associated reproductive organs occur simultaneously as a general aging phenomenon or whether they are initiated in one particular organ and then spread to other components of the neuroendocrine system (Cooper 1983).

There are some fundamental differences between the causes of reproductive senescence in rats and in humans (Smith and Conn 1983). This is particularly important because much of the experimental work has been done in rats and some in mice. In human females, as in rats, irregular cycling reduces frequency of ovulation and the formation of cystic follicles is commonly observed prior to the complete loss of cyclic ovarian activity. In women, in contrast to experimental rats, the hormonal changes suggest that ovarian failure is of primary importance in the loss of the reproductive cycles in women.

Age-related changes in reproductive function are more similar in male rats and human males than in females of both species. In the human male, as in rats, there is a gradual reproductive decline with spermatogenesis continuing well past middle age. As to hormonal levels in human males during senescence, some males show a decline in circulating testosterone. This is not observed in rats; men, like rats, show a slight increase in gonadotropin levels. In the male the importance of the role of testicular alterations with aging is unknown. It is likely that the hypothalamus plays a critical role in males.

In studying aging in the hypothalamic–pituitary–ovarian axis, interest has been focused on which is the site of the first cause. Results suggest that simple ovarian age is unable to account for the cessation of ovulation.

Numerous studies indicate that estradiol has damaging effects on the human hypothalamus and the pituitary. This is a major reason that the controversy remains over the use of sex steroids as a contraceptive and replacement procedure.

Prolactin is a pituitary hormone that is prevalent in all vertebrates from fish to man (Ben-Jonathan 1985). It is involved with numerous reproductive and nonreproductive processes and is an essential hormone for the initiation and maintenance of lactation in humans. Hypersecretion of prolactin is one of the major causes of neuroendocrine-related infertility in women and impotence in men.

In the last decade, there has been an explosion in the number of publications dealing with the relationship of dopamine to prolactin. There are interactions that affect the whole body or various organs and/or have effects at cellular levels.

Sexual Behavior and Disorders

The *DSM-III-R* lists and defines 11 sexual disorders and 12 sexual dysfunctions. The psychopathology of sexual disorders is primarily that of a distorted sex object and an aberration of sexual expression and enjoyment. Sexual dysfunctions are manifested by physiologic disturbances that are linked etiologically to mental and emotional disorders. Although not classified as somatoform disorders, they not only are held to be physical manifestations of presumed psychologic factors, but are also without satisfactory explanation based on organic pathology or pathophysiology. Only a few of these 23 sexual dysfunctions and disorders are of major concern to the geriatric psychiatrist.

Sexual Activity in Late Life

Over the last 25 years sexuality in late life has been given increasing attention by investigators and gradual acceptance in society. This fact of research has done much to dispel a variety of myths surrounding the topic of sexuality in late adulthood. Although young and middle-aged adults have clearly become sexually more permissive in regard to their own generations, many adult children have difficulty accepting elderly persons who, by their behavior, indicate a continuing sexual interest. An adult child, observing the flirtatious behavior of an elderly parent, often becomes disturbed and questions the mental and emotional soundness of the parent. In turn, many elderly persons are aware that this type of behavior bothers their adult children and deliberately avoid such anxiety-producing behavior when in their presence.

Butler and Lewis (1976) observed that sexual activity of an elderly male is more likely to be sanctioned than that of a woman of comparable age. Furthermore, it is possible for the elderly male to marry a younger woman. In contrast, women who show an interest in sexuality are seen as depraved or "grasping for lost youth." Sexual interest by an older female involving a younger male is unlikely to be socially condoned.

Contributing to these differences in the attitudes toward men and women is the discrepancy of the male-to-female ratio in the general population. Since older women outnumber older men, it is obvious that the surviving male has the opportunity to expand his sexual choices while the elderly woman is being restricted by the reality of the male/female imbalance within the population.

The aging male and female undergo important anatomic and physiologic sex changes. The pioneer investigations of Masters and Johnson can be divided into two categories. The first category consists of laboratory observations related to the anatomic and physiologic changes in old age; the second category is composed of data derived from interviews with a larger but self-selected group of aged subjects. Laboratory observations were conducted on 35 men whose ages ranged from 51 to 89 years. Sociosexual interviews were carried out with 212 men beyond the age of 50 years. As to the study of females, 61 menopausal and postmenopausal subjects were included. In this grouping the youngest was 41 and the oldest 78. Thirty-four of the participants were considered to be postmenopausal.

In aging men, with the passage of time, the usual nipple erection that accompanies the act of ejaculation declines so that the majority, if not all, of males after the age of 60 do not demonstrate nipple erection at the time of ejaculation. Under the age of 60, the correlation of these two events is expected. It is evident that most, if not all, physiologic processes are slowed with the passing of time. Consequently, it takes the aging male a longer period of time to achieve erection. For the male age 60 or older full penile erection is frequently not attained until just before ejaculatory experience. However, the maintenance of penile erection over long periods of time without ejaculation is often an achievement of old age. The slowing of the sexual arousal process is inevitable and this slowing should be recognized as normal by both the male and his female partner. Probably the most important change in the male sexual function associated with the aging process is the reduction in both the frequency of ejaculation and the need to ejaculate. A male in his middle or late 60s often finds that his demand for ejaculatory release of sexual tension levels out to about once a week, while he may enjoy sexual intercourse twice a week or more. Again, the reduced demand for ejaculatory release should be accepted without reservation by both husband and wife.

The majority of aging men lose their ability to become erect at the sight of an attractive woman or a sexual thought or fantasy. Because of this psychologic change, men often are fearful that they are losing their potency. The change is really based on tactile stimulation since this becomes the most important means of obtaining an erection. Also auditory stimulation plays a role.

The aging process also has obvious physiologic influences on the sexual response cycle of the female. Production of vaginal lubrication is the exact physiologic counterpart of the male erection. Consequently, vaginal lubrication may be delayed in onset and in full development. These changes develop relatively rapidly in the postmenopausal woman. In addition to the delay in the response, there is also a reduction in the amount of lubrication. Not infrequently, the postmenopausal woman reports that she is more easily distracted from the sexual response cycle, and the lubricating process may be slowed or even terminated in situations in which previously stimuli may not have interfered with the response.

After the menopause the mucosal lining of the vagina usually becomes very thin and atrophic; hence the vaginal wall is vulnerable to the trauma associated with the sexual act. Local irritation and bleeding may occur. Aging usually brings a loss of some of the fatty integument of the external genitalia with the constriction of the vaginal outlet. Hence, there are other factors that may contribute to distress or pain during intercourse.

Few postmenopausal women experience painful tonic contractions of the uterus accompanying orgasm. In younger women the uterus contracts rhythmically with orgasm. This pattern is not dissimilar to the contractions observed during the first stage of labor. However, in advanced years the rhythm of the contractions may be lost and a spasm can occur that is experienced as a severe lower abdominal pain. This type of spastic uterus response accompanying orgasm reflects a state of sex steroid starvation. Consequently, sex steroid replacement is particularly useful in such cases.

The existence or absence of the male climacteric (similar to the female menopause) continues to be a subject of debate. The testes of the aging male show little change in normal structure. If one elects a trial hormone replacement for the elderly male, one must exercise considerable caution, since prostatic hypertrophy is common in elderly men, and testosterone frequently accentuates this condition. Furthermore, testosterone is definitely contraindicated if a neoplasm of the prostate is suspected, because this hormone accelerates the development of a carcinoma. Another complication in males is the possible development of polycythemia. Therefore, if testosterone is given to a male, regular hemoglobin and red cell determinations are important and attention must be given to the possibility of prostatic changes.

Several reports related to sexual behavior and attitudes based on data derived from the Duke Longitudinal Studies have appeared in journals (Verweort et al. 1969; Pfeiffer and Davis 1972). The reports concerned with the frequency of sexual activity have remained relatively consistent over two decades. The sexual changes that do occur provide useful information to clinicians but may reflect cohort differences rather than age changes. A publication (Busse et al. 1954) that was actually based on a cross-sectional analysis reported that the amount of sexual activity was correlated with socioeconomic status—the better the socioeconomic status of the subjects, the more likely was the continuation of sexual activity. Since then it is evident that the important variable of physical health must be given primary attention, since physical health is an important determinant regardless of socioeconomic status. Individuals who live in poverty or near poverty are not as likely to be in good health as those who are better off. Consequently, there are several interacting factors that influence the continuation or termination of sexual activity.

Sexual activity between marital partners tends to be maintained until after the age of 75. Approximately 60 percent of married couples between the ages of 60 to 74 years remain sexually active. After the age of 75 coitus declines to less than 30 percent of married couples. The continuation of sexual activity depends on several interrelated factors, including the availability of a sexual partner. Among the married, the physical and mental health of the partner is important, as are the patterns of sexual interest and activity that have been established in early adulthood. Only 7 percent of the elderly subjects without a wife or husband continued to have sexual relations in old age. This small percentage drops rapidly with advancing age. A larger number of men in good health, four out of five, express a continuing interest in sexual activity. Verbalized interest in sex is found in about one-third of elderly women—this loss of interest by the female may be a direct result of the lack of stimuli, since the older woman lives in a predominantly women's world.

Sexual activity in middle and late life is enhanced by distinguishing cohort effects as well as age and gender. George and Weiler (1981) reported that cross-sectional studies can be misleading and that longitudinal studies of multiple cohorts ranging in age from 46 to 71 years show that sexual intercourse remains relatively stable over a span of 6 years. These investigators identified several patterns of sexual activity within the sample. Over a 6-year span that included four test dates, they found that 58.27 percent of the sample, a majority, reported exactly the same level of sexual activity. No sexual activity at all at any of the four test dates was reported by 7.9 percent of the subjects. About 5 percent of the sample reported an increase in sexual activity. Approximately one-half of this group resumed sexual activity after a period of cessation. About 20 percent reported a decrease in sexual activity. The remaining 10+ percent showed fluctuation of patterns of sexual activity. Consistent with other reports, men reported higher levels of sexual interest and activity than women. Both men and women attributed the responsibility for cessation of sexual activity to the male partner. Their findings suggest that, as the number of intact couples surviving to old age increases (as is currently transpiring), there will be a concomitant increase in the number of older people reporting continuity in sexual behavior.

Two-thirds of men 65 years and older live with wives, but only one-third of women over 65 have husbands. Most older men are married, while most older women are widows. There are almost four times as many widows as widowers. It should be noted that about two-fifths of the older married men have wives under 65 years of age. There are at least 45,000 marriages a year in which the groom and/or the bride is 65 years of age or over. The number of marriages among elderly people has been steadily increasing.

Gavzer (1987) claims that in recent years there has appeared a trend for older women to marry younger men. In 1983 there were 151,000 marriages in which the bride was at least 5 years older than the bridegroom. This represented 6.2 percent of all marriages in 1983. By comparison, in 1970, only 3.7 percent of brides were 5 years or more older than their husbands. This trend is believed to be widespread, but is led by celebrities "who turn the tables on convention." Data are presented (Wilson 1983) claiming that 37.1 percent of brides age 65 and older are marrying younger men. This trend is compatible with the variation of life expectancy at age 65; for males it is approximately 14+ years and for females 18+ years.

The marital status of the aged group—that is, 75+ years—reflects the social tradition for many men to marry younger women. Twice as many aged men as women are married, and only one-third of the men have wives over age 75. About one-half have wives between 65 and 74 years of age, and one-fifth have wives under 65 years of age.

Of men 75 years or older, 33.9 percent are living with their wives. In contrast, of women age 75 or older, only 17.8 percent are living with their husbands. Of these women, 3 percent have husbands under 65 years of age, roughly 20 percent have younger husbands between the ages of 65 and 74, and the remainder have husbands their own age or older. Each year approximately 2,000 women age 75 or older marry, and 6,000 men 75 years or older go to the altar. Both of these groups are usually moving out of widowhood. Of these 8,000 marriages, more than 4,000 are involved with partners under age 75.

Impotency and Ejaculation

Although episodic impotence occurs in most men, persistent impotency is a devastating condition for most men. The masculine component of a self-image is largely attributable to sexual potency. Although organic impotence is rarely life threatening, it has far-reaching consequences producing serious anxiety and depression. Estimates of the incidence of biologic causes of impotency fluctuate from 10 to 70 percent. This biologically caused incidence is age related. One estimate is that 70 percent of those cases of impotence over the age of 70 are attributable to organic etiology (Crenshaw 1985).

Nocturnal penile tumescence is regularly associated with rapid eye movement (REM) during sleep. The total tumescence time occurring during a stage of REM sleep decreases from age 13 through late life (age 79). Non-REM-related penile tumescence also occurs, but it is not a dominant feature. A procedure can easily be conducted at home to determine the absence or presence of erections and their quality during sleep. Such tests are a significant contribution to evaluating any organic factors, including drug-induced impotence (Karacani et al. 1985).

The absence of an ejaculation does not preclude a man from having a satisfactory orgasm-like experience. Drugs such as thioridazine can both inhibit ejaculation and produce impotency. Since individuals respond differently to a wide spectrum of medications, no physician should dismiss the patient's complaint that impotency is a side effect of a medication. Furthermore, some medications have a long half-life and the withdrawal of medication often will not have a prompt positive response.

With aging there is a diminished volume of ejaculate as well as the force with which the ejaculate is expelled.

Men are capable of ejaculating with a completely flaccid penis. Consequently, they can experience an orgasm without having an erection. This particular condition is usually the result of anxiety. The phenomenon can be explained by the existence of different neuronal mechanisms, erection, and arousal. A problem in one area need not affect another mechanism.

Female Problems

As a woman ages there is very little orgasmic change. There is some decreasing intensity of orgasmic response and the woman is slower to achieve orgasm. However, many elderly women discover for the first time that they are capable of multiple orgasms. Because of the thinning of the vaginal wall as well as a decrease in vaginal lubrication, use of a water-soluble jelly is advised. Furthermore, if a woman has been sexually inactive for a long period, her vagina may atrophy and adhesions develop. A sexually inactive woman in her late 60s or 70s should not resume intercourse without adequate preparation. Mechanical dilatation supplemented with estrogen will permit the elderly woman to return to sexual functioning without discomfort.

Painful sexual intercourse can occur in elderly women and can be traced to an estrogen deficiency. However, a retroverted uterus that is diseased can also be a source of pain (Leiblums et al. 1983).

Illness and Disability

Cardiovascular disease, especially if a person has had a myocardial infarction, has led many older people, particularly men, to give up sex altogether for fear of causing another attack. Yet the risk of death during sexual intercourse is very low. Although a person who has suffered a heart attack should seek medical advice, sex usually can and should be resumed after a period of 12 to 16 weeks. A rehabilitation program of activity including sexual experiences may decrease the risk of a future attack (National Institute of Aging 1985).

Diabetes in late life is not infrequently associated with impotence. However, if the diabetes is under adequate control, particularly by means of diet and exercise, improvement can occur. Unfortunately, even in some cases of well-controlled diabetes, impotence persists.

Stroke rarely damages the physical aspects of sexual function, but residual incapacities may require that different positions and support systems may be necessary to complete the sexual act.

Arthritis is a very common problem in late life and the pain that results from activity may limit sexual responses. The painful experience can be reduced by the use of medication, exercise, and attention to position and the timing of sexual activity.

A hysterectomy or a mastectomy does not alter the capability of sexual responsiveness, but psychologic and emotional factors may impair sexual activity. In recent years the prompt reconstructive surgery following breast removal seems to have had a positive effect on these women.

Prostatectomy rarely affects potency of the male. There is often a lack of or reduction in seminal fluid, but sexual capacity and enjoyment after prostatectomy should return to the presurgical level. Those males who have cancer and require a perineal surgical approach are likely to become impotent. Excessive use of alcohol reduces potency in men and delays orgasm in women. Many elderly persons carefully control their alcoholic intake, as a small amount may produce a positive effect, while a larger amount may eliminate the pleasurable response.

Reports have shown that intracavernous injection of papaverine or a papaverine–phentolamine mixture can produce penile erection of satisfactory quality for sexual intercourse (Trapp 1987). Unfortunately, this report does not give the age distribution of the 700+ patients who were evaluated for sexual dysfunction. Seven hundred of these patients had impotency as their primary complaint. A series of 136 patients were treated for their impotency by pharmacologic erection techniques. Of this group, 61 percent were believed to have vascular pathology, 18 percent were diabetic, less than 1 percent of the cases were neurologic in origin, and 15 percent were considered to be of psychologic origin. The age range in this particular sample was 27 to 74 years. The only complication that has been identified is the appearance of an erection lasting for 8 hours and requiring reversal. This occurred in 2.3 percent of the patients. However, it is anticipated that some long-term side effects might develop, probably due to sclerosis or scarring. Although no clear outcome evaluations are presented in the article by Trapp, the results of this procedure are sufficiently encouraging to warrant very careful further research.

Aging and Homosexuality

A Consumers Union report published in 1984 (Brecher 1984), entitled *Love, Sex, and Aging,* was based on an in-depth survey of 4,246 women and men aged 50 to 93 (2,402 men and 1,844 women). The study included 324 women aged 70 or older and 498 men aged 70 or older. In accord with the general population, the men were much more likely to be married than the women. Of this large sample, only 56 of the men considered themselves homosexuals and only 9 of the women considered themselves lesbians. However, the report notes that many of the sample reported casual homosexual experiences, usually during adolescence or earlier. Casual homosexual experiences do occur in the lives of older men and women, even though they have usually considered themselves heterosexual; a few consider themselves bisexual. Although the title of this report is *Love, Sex, and Aging,* actually no data are presented regarding homosexuality and coping with aging. The attitudes and reactions of a few subjects are reported, and it is noted that as homosexual males grow older they are aware that fewer persons are interested in having sex with them.

In a report a number of years prior to the Consumers Union report, a conclusion was reached that homosexuals, particularly males, are likely to accept aging better than heterosexuals since the homosexual has learned to be more independent and the aging homosexual male experiences fewer role disruptions than the man with a wife and family (Kimmel 1977).

Intimacy in Late Life

Intimacy can be defined in many ways including objectionable familiarity (*Webster's Seventh New Collegiate Dictionary*). Intimacy as a positive relationship is accepted by most behavioral scientists as somewhat vague, but a definite human need. According to Weg (1987), intimacy may remain present throughout the life span although it can wax and wane. It is often suggested that intimacy in the latter part of the life span increases in importance as other sources of self-esteem are diminished. The decline in sexual capacity may be one of those alterations that is compensated for by increased need for intimacy. Calderone and Johnson, in a discussion of sex and aging, view intimacy as "when people delight each other and delight in each other in an atmosphere of security based upon mutuality, reciprocity, and total trust in each other" and that "this is surely the kind of relationship that every human being seeks, even if it does not involve physical sex" (Calderone and Johnson 1981). Although sexual behavior is considered to be a type of intimacy, it is not a totally favorable one when it is devoid of mutual caring, responsibility, and open communication. However, the need for physical intimacy clearly occurs in older people as many older persons appear to be "touch hungry" (Renshaw 1984). This need can be satisfied by physical contact with other adults, but particularly grandchildren and pets. Intimacy does include various components such as physical, social, intellectual, spiritual, and emotional. Each may occur relatively independently and have a cyclic aspect.

Intimacy in late life is particularly important since it can effectively serve as an intervening, mediating, or buffering factor in adaptation to stress (Weiss 1983).

Marital success in late life does seem to be tied to intimacy. According to Weg (1987), older men and women have described the most rewarding aspects of marriage as companionship and being able to express true feelings to each other. Marriages get into trouble when it is apparent that there are different values and that there is a lack of mutual interest. All older couples do not improve their intimacy, and the realization of the lack of intimacy may become very apparent early in retirement. The continuation of physical sexual activity is linked to general intimacy. In late life it is unlikely that one will occur without the other.

Passion and romance continue into old age. Observers of the behavior of older people in social situations, such as senior centers, often observe the festive dress and flirtatious behavior that emerge during certain social activity, especially dancing and singing. Playing games also provides this opportunity. The flirtatious behavior includes verbal remarks, changes in facial behavior, body movements, and touching. Such behavior rarely becomes objectionable and it is obviously important in providing an opportunity to pursue one form of increasing intimacy (Bulcroft and O'Conner-Roden 1986).

Institutionalized Elderly and Sexuality

Sexual problems are considered among the most disturbing of those encountered in skilled nursing facilities. Staff attitudes and beliefs do not seem to take into account the realization that sexuality has been an important part of self-image and that it remains important. Staff attitudes and beliefs may contribute to this problem.

There are a variety of behavioral disturbances that occur among the elderly in nursing homes. In a survey of a large number of patients in 42 skilled nursing facilities, 64.2 percent of the patients were reported to have significant behavioral problems. Of these, 23.6 percent had "serious problems" (Zimmer et al. 1984). These seriously disturbing problems included exposure of genitalia and masturbation. The staff was obviously horrified by such acts. These authors report another survey in which, among residents who were asked if patients should have sex, 39 percent of the men and 53 percent of the women said no. If asked if old people should be allowed sex, 81 percent of the men and 75 percent of the women said "yes" (Wasow and Loeb 1979).

Consistent with other studies of sexual behavior in late life, it appears that the concept of sexual activity in the institutionalized aged is related to these elders' interests and attitudes toward sexuality in the past and their prior level of frequency of sexual activity. If physical intimacy has been important in the past, it remains so. Although nursing home residents have physical and mental disabilities, some have a capacity for sexual pleasure.

Sexual problems of nursing home residents may involve an individual (open masturbation) while other problems (sexual advances to other people) may involve other residents, staff and/or family. Sexual behavior between two residents seemed to mobilize "the paternalistic tendencies of the staff" (McCartney et al. 1987, p. 332). A serious staff reaction can be anticipated when a mildly demented or nondemented resident pursues a resident who is more demented. This produces a situation between a perpetrator and a victim. In order to resolve the staff/resident conflict, it is important that there be staff meetings in which staff members can express their uncomfortable sexual feelings and be helped to understand that a resident's activity is not to be limited by someone else's moral values. Although of course it is necessary to avoid sexual abuse of a resident, a regressing adult should not be any more condemned or made to feel shame or guilt than a developing child (McCartney et al. 1987).

References

Alarcon R: Hypochondriasis and depression in the aged. Gerontologia Clinica 1964; 6:266

Albano WA, Zietinstic CM, Organ CH: Is appendicitis in the aged really different? Geriatrics 1975; 30:81–88

American Psychiatric Association: Diagnostic and Statistical Manual of Mental Disorders (Third Edition-Revised) Washington, DC, American Psychiatric Association, 1987

American Psychiatric Association: Psychiatric Glossary (sixth edition). Washington, DC, American Psychiatric Press, 1988

Barsky AJ, Klerman GL: Overview: hypochondriasis, bodily complaints, and somatic styles. Am J Psychiatry 1983; 140:273–283

Beck AT, Rush AJ, Shaw B, et al: Cognitive Therapy of Depression. New York, Guilford Press, 1979

Bellak L, Small L: Emergency Psychotherapy and Brief Psychotherapy. New York, Grune & Stratton, 1965

Ben-Jonathan N: Dopamine: a prolactin-inhibiting hormone. Endocr Rev 1985; 6:564–589

Bonica JJ: Herpes zoster and post-herpetic neuralgia, in Management of Pain. Philadelphia, Lea and Febiger, 1953

Bonica JJ: Herpes zoster and postherpetic neuralgia, in Sympathetic Nerve Blocks for Pain and Diagnosis in Therapy (Volume 1). Edited by Bonica JJ. New York, Winthrop-Breon, 1984

Brecher EM: Love, Sex, and Aging: A Consumers Union Report. Mount Vernon, NY, Consumers Union, 1984

Brown, HN, Valient GE: Hypochondriasis. Arch Intern Med 1981; 141:723–726

Bulcroft K, O'Conner-Roden M: Never too late. Psychology Today 1986; 20(6):66–69

Busse EW: Hypochondriasis in the elderly. Am Fam Phys 1982; 25:199–202

Busse EW: Treating hypochondriasis in the elderly. Generations 1986; 10(3):30–33

Busse EW, Blazer DG: Disorders related to biological functioning, in Handbook of Geriatric Psychiatry. Edited by Busse EW, Blazer DG. New York, Van Nostrand Reinhold, 1980

Busse EW, Busse OS: Medical care and education: impressions of China 1979. Center Reports on Advances in Research (Duke University Center for the Study of Aging and Human Development), December 1979, pp. 1–6

Busse EW, Maddox GL: Duke Longitudinal Studies of Normal Aging, 1955–1980. New York, Springer, 1985

Busse EW, Barnes RH, Silverman AJ, et al: Studies of processes of aging: VI. Factors that influence the psyche of elderly persons. Am J Psychiatry 1954; 110:897–903

Butler RN, Lewis MI: Sex After Sixty. New York, Harper & Row, 1976

Calderone MS, Johnson EW: The human response systems: how they develop and how they work, in The Family Book About Sexuality. Edited by Calderone MS, Johnson EW. New York, Harper & Row, 1981

Cooper RL: Pharmacological and dietary manipulations of reproductive aging in the rat: significance to central nervous system aging, in Experimental and Clinical Interventions in Aging. Edited by Walker RF, Cooper RL. New York, Marcel Dekker, 1983

Crenshaw TL: Age-related changes in sexual function. Geriatric Consultant 1985; 3(5):26–29

Emery G: Cognitive therapy with the elderly, in New Directions in Cognitive Therapy. Edited by Emery G, Hollon S, Bedrosian R. New York, Guilford Press, 1981

Gallagher DE, Thompson LW: Effectiveness of psychotherapy for both endogenous and nonendogenous depression in older adult outpatients. J Gerontol 1983; 38:707–712

Gallagher DE, Thompson LW: Depression in the Elderly: A Behavioral Treatment Manual. Los Angeles, University of Southern California Press, 1981

Gavzer B: Why more older women are marrying younger men. Parade Magazine 1987; 12–13

George LK, Weiler SJ: Sexuality in middle and late life. Arch Gen Psychiatry 1981; 38:919–923

Gildenberg PL, DeVaul RA: The chronic pain patient: evaluation and management (Pain and Headache Series Volume 7). New York, Karger, 1985

Glenn F: Surgical principles for the aged patient, in Clinical Aspects of Aging. Edited by Reichel W. Baltimore, Williams & Wilkins, 1978

Goldman JM, Walker RF, Cooper RL: Aging in the rat hypothalamic-pituitary-ovarian axis: the involvement of biogenic amines in the loss of reproductive cyclicity, in

Progress in Neuroendocrinology (Volume 1). Edited by Parvez H, Parvee S, Gupta D. Utrecht, The Netherlands, VNU Science Press, 1985

Graff-Radford SB, Kames LD, Naliboff BD: Measures of psychological adjustment and perception of pain in postherpetic neuralgia and trigeminal neuralgia. Clin J Pain 1986; 2:55–58

Grauer H: Geriatric depression in the West and the Far East. Psychiatr J Univ of Ottawa 1984; 9:118–120

Harkins SW, Nowlin JB: Persistent pain in the elderly. Paper presented at annual meeting of the American Psychological Association, Los Angeles, 1985

Harkins S, Price D, Martelli M: Effects of age in pain perception. J Gerontol 1986; 41:56–63

Karacani I, Williams R, Thornby J, et al: Nocturnal penile tumescence and REM sleep. Am J Psychiatry 1975; 132:932–937

Kimmel D: The aging gay male. Behavior Today, January 10, 1977, p. 4

Kleinman AM: Neurasthenia and depression: a study of somatization and culture in China. Cult Med Psychiatry 1982; 6:117–190

Klerman GL, Weissman MM: Interpersonal psychotherapy: theory and research, in Short-Term Psychotherapies for Depression. Edited by Rush AJ. New York, Guilford Press, 1982

Kwentus JA, Harkins SW, Lignon N, et al: Current concepts of geriatric pain and its treatment. Geriatrics 1985; 40(4):48–54

Leiblums S, Bachmann G, Kemmann E, et al: Vaginal atrophy in the postmenopausal woman: the importance of sexual activity and hormones. JAMA 1983; 249:2195–2198

Lewinsohn PM, Biglan A, Zeiss A: A behavioral treatment of depression, in Behavioral Management of Anxiety, Depression and Pain. Edited by Davidson P. New York, Brunner/Mazel, 1976

Lindsay PG, Wycoff FM: The depression syndrome and its response to antidepressants. Psychosomatics 1981; 22:571–577.

MacDonald J, Ballie J, Williams B, et al: Coronary care in the elderly. Age and Aging 1983; 12:17–20

Maddox GL: Self-assessment of health status. J Chronic Dis 1964; 17:449–460

Maddox GL, Douglass EB: Self- ssessment of health: a longitudinal study of elderly subjects. J Health Soc Behav 1973; 14:87

McCartney JR, Henry I, Rogers D, et al: Sexuality and the institutionalized elderly. J Am Geriatr Soc 1987; 35:331–333

Meredith N, Turner P: Therapy under analysis. Science 86; 29–52

National Institute of Aging: Sexuality in Late Life. 1985

Pfeiffer E, Davis GD: Determinants of sexual behavior in middle and old age. J Am Geriatr Soc 1972; 20:141–148

Poe WD, Holloway DA: Drugs and the Aged. New York, McGraw-Hill, 1980

Renshaw DC: Touch hunger—a common marital problem. Medical Aspects of Human Sexuality 1984; 18(5):63–70

Sjolund B, Eriksson M: Relief of Pain by TENS. Chichester, England, Wiley, 1985

Smith WA, Conn PM: Causes and consequences of altered gonadotropin secretion in the aging rat, in Experimental and Clinical Interventions in Aging. Edited by Walker RF, Cooper RL. New York, Marcel Dekker, 1983

Trapp JD: Pharmacologic erection program for the treatment of male impotence. South Med J 1987; 80:426–427

U.S. Department of Health, Education and Welfare: NIDA Services Research Report: A

Study of Legal Drug Use by Older Americans (Publication No. 77–495). Washington, DC, U.S. Department of Health, Education and Welfare, 1977

Verwoert AE, Pfeiffer E, Wang HS: Sexual behavior in senescence: changes in sexual activity and interest of aging men and women. Geriatrics 1969; 24:136

Wasow M, Loeb M: Sexuality in nursing homes. J Am Geriatr Soc 1979; 27:73–79

Weg RB: Intimacy in the later years, in Handbook of Applied Gerontology. Edited by Lesnoff-Caravaglia G. New York, Human Sciences Press, 1987

Weiss LJ. Intimacy in adaptation, in Sexuality in the Later Years: Roles and Behavior. Edited by Weg RB. New York, Academic Press, 1983

Weller TH: Varicella [chicken pox] and herpes zoster. New Engl J. Med 1983; 309:1362–1370

Wikman J: Acyclovir. Drug Information Bulletin, Duke University Medical Center 1985; 1(3)

Wilson BF: Hyattsville, MD, National Center for Health Statistics, 1983

Zimmer JG, Watson N, Treat A: Behavioral problems among patients in skilled nursing homes. Am J Public Health 1984; 74:1118–1121

Chapter 17

Bereavement and Adjustment Disorders

Dolores Gallagher, Ph.D.
Larry W. Thompson, Ph.D.

Phases of Normal Bereavement

The predominant symptoms of normal bereavement occur with such regularity that many writers speak of clearly defined phases of the grief process (Parkes 1972; Lopata 1973, 1979; Parkes and Weiss 1983). These seem to occur regardless of the age of the survivor, his or her relationship to the deceased, and mode of death, although several studies have reported that older persons may have a more difficult time with bereavement (Ball 1976–1977; Sanders 1980–1981); that death of a child may be more traumatic than death of a spouse or other relative or friend, particularly if the parent is elderly at the time of the death (Miles 1985; Rando 1984, 1986; Sanders 1979–1980); and that more traumatic modes of death (such as accidents, suicide, or homicide) may result in more complex grief reactions (Ball 1976–1977; Bugen 1979; Osterweis et al. 1984). However, in general, the phases of a normal grief reaction are predictable irrespective of age (although they will vary in intensity and duration according to other factors noted), and have been described in the following terms. The first phase begins at the death of a loved one and tends to persist for several weeks. Shock and disbelief combined with coldness, emotional numbness, emptiness, and cognitive confusion characterize this period. Intense "free-floating" anxiety is also seen, which often leads to

This chapter was partially supported by grants R01-MH37196 from the National Institute of Mental Health and RO1-AG01959 from the National Institute on Aging to Larry W. Thompson, Principal Investigator.

459

dramatic fluctuations in emotional state, ranging from feeling very little to feeling highly anxious for no apparent reason. Specific somatic symptoms including sleeplessness, loss of appetite and vague muscular aches and pains are quite common. These in turn lead to frequent visits to physicians and increased requests for medication. While the physician must pay careful attention to the patient's symptoms, for the most part clinicians who have worked extensively with the bereaved recommend that medications be used conservatively at this time so that the bereavement process can progress without unnecessary interruption. In the final analysis, patients must learn to cope with this event as best they can, and unless it is absolutely necessary, heavy medication usage may serve only to forego this process.

The second phase generally begins as the numbness and anxiety decrease somewhat. This usually occurs in about 4 to 6 weeks. Early on in this period friends and family often become less available and/or helpful, and with increased times of being alone, the finality of the loss becomes more prominent. Symptoms such as crying, chronic sleep disturbance, episodes of low mood, poor appetite, low energy and feelings of fatigue, loss of interest in many daily activities and problems with concentration and memory occur with alarming regularity, especially during the first half of this phase (Clayton 1982). Parkes (1972) refers to this period as a time of "yearning and protest." There is a yearning to be united with the loved one, while at the same time there is anger directed toward the deceased for leaving. It is quite common for the bereaved to actually search for the deceased; this has both behavioral and cognitive components. A typical example of behavioral searching would be a return to places frequented by the deceased. Such endeavors bring momentary comfort, while also paradoxically intensifying the feelings of grief. In such instances there often is the wish that the loved one would suddenly come in the door, or come around the corner, or appear there in the crowd. Often, someone so similar is seen that for a moment, the survivor is certain it must be the deceased. Cognitively, bereaved persons often report auditory or visual hallucinations of the deceased, and/or a strong "sense of presence" of the dead person (Hoyt 1980–1981; Rees 1971, 1975). They may see the deceased sitting in his or her favorite chair or hear their name being called, or receive a reassuring message that all is well. Despite the vividness of such phenomena, they are quite common and considered to be normal when they are transitory and limited in scope to the deceased (Rees 1975). In fact, the majority of bereaved who report these experiences find them helpful and comforting, once they receive reassurance that they are not "going crazy" and that these will pass in time.

Another common occurrence in the second phase of normal grief is a search, by the bereaved, for an explanation of why the death occurred and what meaning it may have had. This process often has religious or philosophic overtones, and may also include blaming self or others for things done or not done that might have contributed to the death, as well as dwelling on how the death could have been prevented. A final cognitive component involves the obsessional review of memories and scenes associated with the death. Often this makes survivors seem almost unbearable to family and friends because they seem to be able to talk of little else during this period. While this process can be extremely frustrating for those around the bereaved, it is usually very helpful for a gradual resolution and acceptance of the loss, and it does seem to be time limited in most people. If family and friends can be encouraged to "bear with it" for a period of time, their patient listening and assistance in reality testing will facilitate movement through the bereavement process to a point at which less psychic energy is bound up with the deceased. At that point, the survivor can redirect attention to a pragmatic reorganization of his or her life situation.

This second phase of the bereavement process seems to diminish substantially at about 1 year following the death of the significant other, although many bereaved begin to report noticeable changes around the 6-month mark. In our own study, for example, in which we followed elderly spousally bereaved respondents over a 30-month period, we found that a majority of the bereaved (as well as the interviewers who completed their repeated evaluations) reported a noticeable improvement in outlook and a reduction in symptoms as early as 6 months after the loss. There appears to be a very strong cognitive component in this transition into the third phase in that many report a realization that it is time to get on with the rest of life and stop focusing so intensely on matters of the past. Many religious and cultural groups have developed rituals to assist the individual through this anniversary time. It is of interest that the 1-year anniversary period may be a time of heightened grief for some. There are suggestions that this is particularly true for individuals who are having a difficult time adapting to the loss or who do not participate in any ritual providing a formal conclusion to the grief process.

Lopata (1973, 1975) has described the third phase of bereavement as the "identity reconstruction" process. This process will often take an additional year—more or less, depending on the centrality of roles that were lost as a result of the death, and the amount and kind of learning that must take place for a new sense of self to become firmly established. Most somatic symptoms have disappeared by this time, although sleep problems are still common (Clayton 1982). Recognition and acceptance of the finality of the loss are nearly achieved, and the person begins to think about developing an identity as being separate from the deceased. This involves cognitive changes in terms of modifying the self-concept and coping with loneliness, and concomitant behavioral changes, including the acceptance of new roles and the acquisition of skills required to function in these roles (Balkwell 1981). For others, the direction is not to seek new roles or relationships, but rather to strengthen other roles they maintained prior to the death. In either case, there is a clear indication of serious attempts to revamp situations and relationships in ways that will facilitate constructive adaptations that evidence an independence from the deceased. At the same time, however, there often is a continued sense of emotional involvement with the deceased, which need not be viewed as pathologic, even if maintained for years (Rubin 1984).

We may summarize the above by conceptualizing the bereavement process as involving three distinct tasks: first, that the loss be intellectually accepted; second, that the loss be accepted emotionally; and third, that the person's model of self and outer world be changed to match the new reality (Parkes and Weiss 1983). We can also state that, in general, this process ought to be near completion in about 2 years, irrespective of the kind of death, nature of the relationship, and age of the survivor. While there may be some pitfalls to viewing this stressful period as occurring in distinct phases, it does emphasize the lawfulness of the process and is very helpful in communicating with individuals who are undergoing bereavement. In our work, many widows and widowers who have been experiencing severe distress readily identify with the feelings and behaviors described in this time course, and view it as a credible explanation of a predictable series of events. Thus, although they may be in great anguish at any given moment, they can take comfort in the fact that what they are experiencing is part of a normal process that has a predictable endpoint.

Abnormal or Unresolved Grief and Its Impact

Although the course of bereavement will always be somewhat variable across individuals, it is generally thought that grief reactions will abate without significant professional assistance. However, if for some reason the grief process is inhibited, interrupted, or delayed or becomes chronic, then professional help may be needed to mitigate serious negative consequences. For example, Lazare (1979) has described several common reasons for failure to grieve adequately, including excessive guilt, present loss causing a reawakening of an incompletely grieved prior loss, the experience of multiple losses (causing what Kastenbaum, 1969, calls "bereavement overload"), and societal factors such as repression of grief following an "unspeakable" loss (e.g., death of an illicit lover or a suicide death). According to Lazare (1979) and others (Lindemann 1944; Worden 1982), certain symptoms or behaviors signal unresolved or "complicated" grief: acquisition of symptoms belonging to the last illness of the deceased; significant hostility toward persons connected with the death (e.g., physicians or nurses); acts detrimental to the bereaved's social or economic existence (e.g., giving away belongings or making foolish economic decisions); agitated depression including feelings of worthlessness, bitter self-accusation, and obvious need for punishment; feeling that the death occurred yesterday even though it took place months ago; false euphoria subsequent to the death; self-destructive impulses; overidentification with the deceased; failure to progress through the usual phases (as outlined above);

and a known history of delayed, prolonged, or absent grief reactions in the past.

It is important to recognize pathologic grief reactions because there are numerous studies that report serious consequences to the survivor's physical and mental health unless the problem is identified and treated. For example, grief (presumably unresolved) has been strongly associated with increased mortality (Jacobs and Ostfeld 1977; Shepherd and Barraclough 1974; Rees and Lutkins 1967), particularly in males. Stroebe and Stroebe (1983) reviewed then-extant studies on this issue and concluded that there is a greater likelihood of mortality (from suicide and/or natural causes) for bereaved men versus bereaved women. Also, widowers seem to be most vulnerable in the first year after bereavement, whereas the peak period of risk for widows appears during the second or third year of bereavement. In our own work (Thompson 1986), we observed that 12.1 percent of our widowers (mean age of 69.9, *SD* of 8.5 years at time of enrollment into the study) died within the first year. This increased to 16.1 percent by 30 months postloss, whereas the death rate for our male age-matched nonbereaved (control) sample (mean age of 71.1, *SD* of 7.9 years at enrollment) was 1.2 percent for the first year and rose to only a total of 4.8 percent by 30 months. For the widows, less than 1 percent died within the first year and only 2.6 percent by 2½ years. In contrast, none of the control females died within this interval. Their average ages were 66.6 (*SD* = 6.9) and 68.4 (*SD* = 6.9) years, respectively. These data are in strong agreement with previous findings regarding sex differences in mortality following a spouse's death. Further study of some of the demographic and psychosocial factors that characterized the men who died revealed that they were more emotionally isolated after their wife's death than their bereaved (but still living) counterparts, had apparently lost their main confidant and were unwilling or unable to replace that relationship, and seemed to somaticize their distress (with frequent physician's visits and poorer self-rated health). Taken together with aforementioned signs of abnormal grief, these may be significant indicators for identification of older widowers at risk for their own mortality subsequent to a spouse's death.

Additional negative consequences for survivor's physical and mental health have been reported in the bereavement literature for some time. Reviews by Gallagher (1986), Osterweis et al. (1984), Stroebe and Stroebe (1983), and Windholz et al. (1985) indicate that, in general, bereaved women experience more mental health problems (particularly depression and anxiety disorders) and report more somatic complaints, whereas bereaved men experience more actual physical health problems (in particular, cardiovascular disease) and have significantly less social support, than married counterparts. However, a recent study by Lund et al. (1986) that followed a sample of older individuals for 2 years after their spouse's death, failed to find sex differences among the bereaved on such measures as depression, life satisfaction, and grief resolution, suggesting that the adaptation process of older men and women may follow more of a similar course over the first 2 years than had been realized. Further research on this issue is needed.

Other research has focused on predictors of good versus poor outcome. Given that about 15 to 25 percent of bereaved persons have experienced significant psychopathology (particularly clinical depression) when assessed 1 to 2 years after the loss (cf. Clayton 1982; Lazare 1979; Parkes 1972; Vachon et al. 1982; Zisook and DeVaul 1983; Zisook et al. 1985), it may be important to identify those variables most associated with poor outcome so that appropriate prevention and/or intervention programs can be initiated with those at risk. Overall, these studies have found that adaptation at 1 or 2 months after the loss is one of the best predictors of later adjustment; persons who are highly distressed at that point tend to remain so over time (Clayton 1982; Vachon et al. 1982). Some other significant predictors, identified on empirical or theoretical bases, include the presence of multiple stressors before or after bereavement, such as low socioeconomic status and poor prior physical or mental health; absence of at least one confidant with whom to share feelings and experiences as grief proceeds (Lopata 1979; Lowenthal and Haven 1968); inadequacy of other aspects of the survivor's social support network; lack of an adequate repertoire of adaptive coping skills; mode of death; and whether or not the death was prepared for or anticipated. The last factor is controversial, with some studies reporting a salutory effect of anticipation on subsequent grief (e.g., Aldrich 1974; Weisman 1974) and others reporting that anticipatory grieving had either no apparent effect or a negative one (Clayton et al. 1973; Gerber et al. 1975b; Hill et al. in press). Taken together, these data suggest that profiles may be constructed of elders at risk for morbid bereavement; these then can be empirically evaluated through future research on prevention and intervention strategies.

Attitudes Toward Death

Providing a balance to the above material on correlates of poor adjustment is the growing literature on positive aspects of grief. Grief has been described by poets and mental health professionals as providing significant opportunity for personal growth, despite the pain involved (Kastenbaum 1981; Lewis 1961; Peterson and Briley 1977). This makes sense when we realize that for most adults, expected life events (including death of one's spouse) are not crises; rather they are "normal punctuation marks along the lifeline" according to Neugarten (1984). When death occurs "on schedule" or "on time" a psychiatric crisis need not ensue; rather, most adults will adapt successfully, as a result of years of practice in making similar psychologic adaptations throughout life. Attitudinal factors and expectations are an important part of this process. In addition to greater acceptance of the loss of others, research has shown that older individuals, despite their own nearness to death, do not fear their personal death more than younger people (Edinberg 1985; Kalish 1977). They seem to have developed an acceptance of death over time, although they are more likely to think about and talk about death than younger adults (Kalish 1985). Kalish notes that while death is highly salient to the elderly, it is not as frightening to contemplate as it was in middle life. He attributes this to several factors including degree of religious feeling, individual temperament or personality (especially the absence of neuroticism), and the sense that one has accomplished one's goals and that one's life had a definite purpose or meaning.

Still, there are two meanings of death that have clear relevance for the elderly: death as a limit and organizer of time, and death as a cause of significant loss for others in one's life (Kalish 1977). Knowledge of one's own impending death often brings about a reorganization of time and priorities to include leaving a legacy of some sort and putting things in order psychologically, financially, and in other ways. It may be that a morbid fear of death in later life reflects a sense of despair (to use Erikson's 1959 term) related to inability to resolve the various tasks and dilemmas of adulthood, which in turn causes "death anxiety." If this is so, then death anxiety is not a normal manifestation of aging but rather a mental health problem to be treated by professionals sensitive to both dying and developmental issues (Shneidman 1983).

Prevention and Intervention Strategies with the Bereaved

Preventive mental health approaches have been advocated for some time by such practitioners as Silverman (1969) who described the development of a self-help program called the Widow-to-Widow program, which has gained immense popularity throughout the country, and Worden (1982) who has described a comprehensive program for grief counseling to help facilitate the completion of normal grief work and assist those who might be at risk for pathologic grief by intervening early in the process. In Silverman's program (Silverman and Cooperband 1975), mutual help from others who have been through the process is emphasized, while in Worden's program (1982), mental health professionals are used in order to help the survivor complete any unfinished business with the deceased and be able to say a final good-bye. These goals are reached through application of cognitive, behavioral, and affective strategies (e.g. visiting the grave, encouraging expression of a wide range of feelings, and the like). Other programs involving group counseling with a psychoeducational focus have also been described as successful with nonpathologic mourners (DeBor et al. 1983).

In contrast, other types of treatment would be recommended for persons who are already experiencing abnormal grief reactions and/or severe depression following bereavement. These include grief therapy (Worden 1982), psychodynamic psychotherapy (Horowitz et al. 1984), cognitive–behavioral psychotherapy (Abrahms 1981; Averill and Wisocki 1981), and re-grief therapy

(Volkan 1975). In addition, judicious use of psychotropic medications may be indicated for some patients (Parkes 1972). Although it is beyond the scope of this chapter to review each of these methods in detail, it may be pointed out that while each approach is theoretically and technically distinct, each treatment method shares certain elements with the others. All stress the importance of affective expression of a wide range of feelings (including, for example, anger and resentment as well as sadness) and the need to eventually detach from the deceased so that life can go on; however, each person goes about reaching these goals in very different ways ranging from an almost implosive involvement in grief work (Volkan 1975) to an emphasis on cognitive reappraisal and restructuring of distorted fantasies and memories about the deceased (Abrahms 1981). While few of these approaches have been subjected to the methodologic rigor of controlled outcome research, each has been reported clinically to have been very effective in achieving the desired goals (see Gallagher, 1986, for more detail about these methods of treatment and existing efficacy data; see also Osterweis et al. 1984 and Rando 1984, 1986, each of which contains excellent review chapters on these and other types of bereavement interventions).

What can be stated from review of the current literature on bereavement interventions is that there are no data to suggest that elders benefit less from these treatment methods compared with younger persons. While none were developed specifically for the elderly, all have been used with this group and have been reported to be acceptable and efficacious to old as well as young. One promising type of intervention that may be particularly suited to the needs of elders involves regular telephone and/or in-home therapy for grief, which reduces medical morbidity in the treated versus nontreated elder bereaved sample (Gerber et al. 1975a). Number of office visits to physicians, minor illnesses reported, and medications taken regularly were all reduced significantly over time, although these positive effects were not reported until approximately 3 months after the intervention began. Clearly, much more remains to be learned about the best methods of psychiatric and psychologic treatments for the ever-increasing population of elder bereaved.

Adjustment Disorder

The *Diagnostic and Statistical Manual of Mental Disorders (Third Edition-Revised) (DSM-III-R)* (American Psychiatric Association 1987) portrays adjustment disorder as a "maladaptive reaction to an identifiable psychosocial stressor, or stressors, that occurs within three months after the onset of the stressor" (p. 329). Evidence of impairment in social or occupational functioning should be apparent during the reaction, or there should be symptoms above and beyond what might be expected as a normal reaction to a given stressor. This diagnosis is not applied if the symptom picture meets criteria for another specific disorder or if the reaction appears to be an exacerbation of another mental disorder. If the stressor has a discrete beginning and ending, it is assumed that this reaction will subside within a brief time after the stressor disappears. If the stressor is maintained for a long period, it is assumed that the individual will develop a more adaptive pattern of responding after a short time elapses. A time limit of 6 months has been set for the duration of the reaction, after which another diagnosis should be applied. The specific type of adjustment disorder is coded according to the predominant symptom pattern (e.g., adjustment disorder with anxious or depressed mood).

The diagnosis of adjustment disorder is also not used in instances of uncomplicated bereavement, which refers to a normal reaction to death of a loved one. According to the *DSM-III-R*, a depressive syndrome can be considered a normal reaction in bereavement, including dysphoria and other related symptoms such as poor appetite, weight loss, and insomnia. However, morbid preoccupation with worthlessness, severe functional impairment, and psychomotor retardation are seldom seen and suggest that the bereavement may be complicated by an episode of major depression. Guilt evidenced during bereavement is usually focused on things done or not done regarding the deceased. Any thoughts of death are usually limited to thinking that the individual would be better off dead. Often persons with uncomplicated bereavement will view their dysphoria as normal, but may seek professional help for relief of other symptoms, such as insomnia or eating difficulties. On the other hand, those who are clinically depressed in addition to being bereaved typically seek treatment for their affective distress. Gallagher (1986) discusses ways to distinguish between normal grief and clinical depression in bereaved elders.

The *DSM-III-R* reports that adjustment disorders are very common. However, very little attention has been focused on this disturbance in the literature. Out of 10 psychiatry texts reviewed, only 2 listed adjustment disorder in the index, and it was mentioned within the texts only slightly more often. Virtually no specific data could be found in recent publications concerning prevalence, whether or not there are age or sex differences, or other possible correlates. There has been little interest in this disorder shown in the geropsychiatry literature as well, which is somewhat surprising. Given the increase in losses experienced by the elderly, one might expect a greater incidence of adjustment disorders in this group. One reason for the lack of emphasis in the clinical literature may be that many of the individuals suffering with this disturbance may never have contact with the mental health system. Remedial assistance within the family or from other institutions not connected with the health system may facilitate quick recovery. Age stereotypes regarding emotional illness (Butler and Lewis 1982) may also discourage use of health care resources, or simply delay any help-seeking efforts until the disturbance becomes unbearably severe. This delay in seeking help would in turn increase the likelihood that the arbitrary 6 months may have elapsed, thereby excluding the individual from this diagnostic category.

Blazer (1983) called attention to the possible importance of this diagnostic category in a recent analysis of available literature on the epidemiology of depression. He noted that the prevalence of depressive symptoms in community samples ranged from 10 percent to 45 percent as reflected in self-report scales, but the actual rate of clinical depression was substantially lower, ranging around 2 percent to 5 percent, when more stringent interview techniques of assessment were employed. He concluded that the discrepancy between these two percentages could be accounted for in part by transient episodes of depressive symptoms accompanying bereavement or an adjustment reaction to other psychosocial stressors. More recent epidemiologic studies by Blazer et al. (1987) identified a clinical subtype, referred to as the "symptomatic depression" subgroup, which they suggested may be representative of elderly individuals in the community who are suffering from adjustment disorder. However, they acknowledged that a definitive diagnosis could not be made on the basis of their data. This subgroup constituted 4 percent of their community sample, but it is likely that even this proportion is an underestimate of the prevalence of the disorder.

In 1980 Gaitz and Varner provided compelling arguments for the utility of the diagnosis of adjustment disorder in working with the elderly, and lamented that it was not being used as often as it should. Application of this diagnosis, they reasoned, places the focus squarely on the importance of external stressors and the psychologic and social resources the patient has available to cope with whatever unfortunate events might have occurred. Since, as mentioned below, age-related changes are likely in both of these domains, there may be many instances with the elderly in which this classification would provide a useful working guide for assessment and subsequent treatment efforts.

Research findings indicate that while older people experience fewer negative events overall, they experience substantially more serious losses (Chiriboga and Cutler 1980; Dekker and Webb 1974; Goldberg and Comstock 1980; Holmes and Masuda 1974; Lazarus and DeLongis 1983). For example, retirement often leads to loss of the work role; declining health can lead to a host of losses in physical and social functioning; and loss of loved ones and friends can occur not only through death, but also by virtue of a move into a new environment, such as a retirement home. While it is true that some of these losses cannot be avoided, many of them are not in this category. In our own work with psychologically distressed elders, for example, we continue to be impressed with how often they have underestimated the importance of their social network when making decisions about moving to a new situation during a time of transition. In many instances had the significance of old friends and the difficulty of making new ones in a strange setting been given its proper due, the impact of loss of positive life events might have been mitigated. A similar story has been repeated many times for retirement. With proper preparation, individuals can make retirement a transition from one work role to another rather than a loss of role, but all too often the potential hazard of this change is ignored.

The stress of such losses, however, may not be of primary importance, but rather how individuals cope with them may be the critical feature affecting health and well-being in elderly individuals (Billings and Moos 1981; Folkman et al. 1986). Greater acceptance of this position in the field has stimulated considerable interest in possible age differences in coping processes. Some have argued that older individuals show negative changes in their coping abilities (Pfeiffer 1977; Gutman 1974), while others have emphasized increased maturity with age in handling stressful situations (Vaillant 1977). Still others have argued that age changes in coping behavior may be minimal, but the kinds of stressors encountered by the elderly and their severity are more problematic, thus requiring different types of coping responses (Folkman et al. 1987; McCrae 1982).

Although the explanation for differences in coping behavior is not yet established, there are clear indications that older individuals tend to use different coping strategies from those used by younger individuals. Folkman et al. (1987) reported that younger persons used proportionately more active, interpersonal, problem-focused forms of coping, whereas the elderly used intrapersonal, emotion-focused forms of coping involving distancing, acceptance of responsibility, and positive reappraisal. McCrae (1982) found that age differences in coping seemed to be due to the different kinds of stressors, but did find that older individuals were generally less hostile in reaction to negative events and less likely to rely on escapist fantasy. Foster and Gallagher (1986) compared elderly depressed patients with nondepressed community volunteers matched for sex, age, and education and found that depressed patients were more likely to use emotional discharge than were nondepressed. While there were no differences between the two groups on appraisal-focused and problem-focused coping, depressed patients rated all of their strategies as significantly less helpful than did the community participants. The extent to which such differences might account for age differences in adjustment reactions remains fertile territory for continued research.

However, the conceptual backdrop emanating from this line of research can provide clear direction for effective treatments of adjustment disorders. A logical first step would involve a collaborative effort with patients to determine ways of neutralizing the stressful agents. Helping patients learn how to cope with negative events can also be immensely helpful, particularly with those stressors that are not easily removed, such as chronic physical illness or drastic reductions in income. Such efforts will decrease the likelihood that a prolonged reaction to stress might lead to a more persistent and complicated psychiatric disorder. Particularly in the elderly, if the stressors are left unchecked, the high frequency of losses and other negative events is likely to render successful adaptation much more difficult. The end result of this process could be a more severe disorder, requiring hospitalization and the initiation of medical treatment. A frequent endpoint in this reaction to losses and negative events is a depressive episode.

The points advanced by Gaitz and Varner (1980) may be even more relevant now. Recent research trends showing increased emphasis on the search for biologic factors underlying psychiatric disorders may eventually serve to undermine the importance of external stressors in the development of some types of maladaptive behavior. Increased attention to adjustment reactions both in the clinical setting and in research can provide a healthy correction to any such trends by keeping the significance of negative events in the foreground. For example, despite recent successes in identifying biologic correlates of depression, considerable variance remains unexplained by such markers. This is understandable given that depression is likely the final common pathway of several different causes. However, continued attempts to identify unique symptom patterns occurring in response to external stressors, in the final analysis, should aid in improving the precision of differential diagnostic categories that emphasize specific etiologic agents and treatment programs.

References

Abrahms JL: Depression versus normal grief following the death of a significant other, in New Directions in Cognitive Therapy. Edited by Emery G, Hollon S, Bedrosian RC. New York, Guilford Press, 1981

Aldrich CK: Some dynamics of anticipatory grief, in Anticipatory Grief. Edited by Schoenberg B, Carr AC, Kutscher AH, et al. New York, Columbia University Press, 1974

American Psychiatric Association: Diagnostic and Statistical Manual of Mental Disorders (Third Edition-Revised). Washington, DC, American Psychiatric Association, 1987

Averill J, Wisocki P: Some observations on behavioral approaches to the treatment of grief among the elderly, in Behavioral Therapy and Terminal Care: A Humanistic Approach. Edited by Sobel HJ. Cambridge, MA, Ballinger, 1981

Balkwell C: Transition to widowhood: a review of the literature. Family Relations 1981; 30:117–127

Ball JF: Widow's grief: The impact of age and mode of death. Omega 1976–1977; 7:307–333

Billings AG, Moos RH: The role of coping responses and social resources in attenuating the impact of stressful life events. J Behav Med 1981; 4:139–157

Blazer D: The epidemiology of depression in late life, in Depression and Aging: Causes, Care and Consequences. Edited by Breslau L, Haug, MR. New York, Springer, 1983

Blazer D, Hughes DC, George LK: The epidemiology of depression in an elderly community population. Gerontologist 1987; 27:281–287

Bugen LA: Death and Dying: Theory/Research/Practice. Dubuque, IA, William C. Brown Publishers, 1979

Butler RN, Lewis MI: Aging and Mental Health (third edition). St. Louis, C.V. Mosby, 1982

Chiriboga DA, Cutler L: Stress and adaptation: life span perspectives, in Aging in the 1980s. Edited by Poon L. Washington, DC, American Psychological Association 1980

Clayton PJ: Bereavement, in Handbook of Affective Disorders. Edited by Paykel ES. New York, Guilford Press, 1982

Clayton PJ Halikas JA, Maurice WL, et al: Anticipatory grief and widowhood. Br J Psychiatry 1973; 122:47–51

DeBor L, Gallagher D, Lesher E: Group counseling with bereaving elderly. Clin Gerontol 1983; 1:81–90

Dekker D, Webb: Relationships of the social readjustment rating scale to psychiatric status, anxiety, and social desirability. J Psychosom Res 1974; 18:125–130

Edinberg MA: Mental Health Practice with the Elderly. Englewood Cliffs, NJ, Prentice Hall, 1985

Erikson EH: Identity and the Life Cycle. New York, International Universities Press, 1959 (reissued by Norton in 1980)

Folkman S, Lazarus RS, Gruen R, et al: Appraisal, coping, health status, and psychological symptoms. J Pers Soc Psychol 1986; 50:571–579

Folkman S, Lazarus RS, Pimley S, et al: Age differences in stress and coping processes. Psychology and Aging 1987; 2:171–184

Foster J, Gallagher D: An exploratory study comparing depressed and nondepressed elders' coping strategies. J Gerontol 1986; 41:91–93

Gaitz CM, Varner RV: Adjustment disorders of late life: stress disorders, in Handbook of Geriatric Psychiatry. Edited by Busse EW, Blazer D. New York, Van Nostrand Reinhold, 1980

Gallagher D: Therapeutic issues in the treatment of spousal bereavement reactions in the elderly, in Assessment and Treatment of the Elderly Neuropsychiatric Patient. Edited by Pirozzolo FJ, Maletta GJ. New York, Praeger, 1986

Gerber I, Wiener A, Battin D, et al: Brief therapy to the aged bereaved, in Bereavement: Its Psychosocial Aspects. Edited by Schoenberg B, Gerber I, Wiener A, et al. New York, Columbia Univesity Press, 1975a

Gerber I, Rusalem R, Hannon N, et al: Anticipatory grief and aged widows and widowers. J Gerontol 1975b; 30:225–229

Goldberg EG, Comstock GW: Epidemiology of life events: frequency in general populations. Am J Epidemiol 1980; 111:736–752

Gutmann DL: The country of old men: cross-cultural studies in the psychology of later life, in Culture and Personality: Contemporary Readings. Edited by LeVine RL. Chicago, Aldine, 1974

Hill CD, Thompson LW, Gallagher D: The role of anticipatory bereavement in older women's adjustment to widowhood. The Gerontologist, in press

Holmes TH, Masuda M: Life changes and illness susceptibility, in Stressful Life Events: Their Nature and Effects. Edited by Dohrenwend BS, Dohrenwend BP. New York, Wiley, 1974

Horowitz MJ, Marmar C, Weiss DS, et al: Brief psychotherapy of bereavement reactions. Arch Gen Psychiatry 1984; 41:438–448

Hoyt MF: Clinical notes regarding the experience of "presences" in mourning. Omega 1980–1981; 11:105–108

Jacobs S, Ostfeld A: An epidemiological review of the mortality of bereavement. Psychosom Med 1977; 39:344–357

Kalish RA: Death and dying in a social context, in Handbook of Aging and the Social Sciences. Edited by Binstock RH, Shanas E. New York, Van Nostrand Reinhold, 1977

Kalish RA: The social context of death and dying, in Handbook of Aging and the Social Sciences (second edition). Edited by Binstock RH, Shanas E. New York, Van Nostrand Reinhold, 1985

Kastenbaum RJ: Death and bereavement in later life, in Death and Bereavement. Edited by Kutscher AH. Springfield, IL, Charles C. Thomas, 1969

Kastenbaum RJ: Death, Society, and Human Experience (second edition). St. Louis, C.V. Mosby, 1981

Lazare A: Unresolved grief, in Outpatient Psychiatry: Diagnosis and Treatment. Edited by Lazare A. Baltimore, Williams & Wilkins, 1979

Lazarus RS, DeLongis A: Psychological stress and coping in aging. Am Psychol 1983; 38:245–254

Lewis CS: A Grief Observed. London, Faber & Faber, 1961

Lindemann E: Symptomatology and management of acute grief. Am J Psychiatry 1944; 101:141–148

Lopata HZ: Widowhood in an American City. Cambridge, MA, Schenkman Publishing, 1973

Lopata HZ: On widowhood: Grief work and identity reconstruction. J Geriatr Psychiatry 1975; 8:41–55

Lopata HZ: Women as Widows: Support Systems. New York, Elsevier, 1979

Lowenthal MF, Haven C: Interaction and adaptation: intimacy as a critical variable. Am Socio/ Rev 1968; 33:20–30

Lund D, Caserta M, Dimond M: Gender differences through two years of bereavement among the elderly. Gerontologist 1986; 26:314–320

McCrae RR: Age differences in the use of coping mechanisms. J Gerontol 1982; 37:454–460

Miles MS: Emotional symptoms and physical health in bereaved parents. Nurs Res 1985; 34:76–81

Neugarten B: Psychological aspects of aging and illness. Psychosomatics 1984; 25:123–125

Osterweis M, Solomon F, Green M (eds): Bereavement: Reactions, Consequences, and Care. Washington, DC, National Academy Press, 1984

Parkes CM: Bereavement: Studies of Grief in Adult Life. New York, International Universities Press, 1972

Parkes CM, Weiss RS: Recovery from Bereavement. New York, Basic Books, 1983

Peterson J, Briley MP: Widows and Widowhood: A Creative Approach to Being Alone. New York, Association Press, 1977

Pfeiffer E: Psychopathology and social pathology, in Handbook of the Psychology of Aging. Edited by Birren JE, Schaie KW. New York, Van Nostrand Reinhold, 1977

Rando TA: Grief, Dying, and Death. Champaign, IL, Research Press, 1984

Rando TA (ed): Parental Loss of a Child. Champaign, IL, Research Press, 1986

Rees WD: The hallucinations of widowhood. Br Med J 1971; 4:37–41

Rees WD: The bereaved and their hallucinations, in Bereavement: Its Psychosocial Aspects. Edited by Schoenberg B, Gerber I, Wiener A, et al. New York, Columbia University Press, 1975

Rees WD, Lutkins SG: Mortality of bereavement. Br Med J 1967; 4:13–16

Rubin SS: Mourning distinct from melancholia: the resolution of bereavement. Br J Med Psychol 1984; 57:339–345

Sanders CM: Comparison of younger and older spouses in bereavement outcomes. Omega 1980–1981; 11:217–232

Sanders CM: A comparison of adult bereavement in the death of a spouse, child, and parent. Omega 1979–1980; 10:303–322

Shepherd D, Barraclough BM: The aftermath of suicide. Br Med J 1974; 2:600–603

Shneidman ES: Deaths of Man. New York, Jason Aronson, 1983

Silverman PR: The widow-to-widow program: an experiment in preventive intervention. Mental Hygiene 1969; 53:333–337

Silverman PR, Cooperband A: On widowhood: mutual help and the elderly widow. J Geriatr Psychiatry 1975; 8:9–40

Stroebe MS, Stroebe W: Who suffers more? Sex differences in health risks of the widowed. Psychol Bull 1983; 93:279–301

Thompson LW: Multiple factors in coping with grief in the elderly (final technical report, grant AGO1959). Washington, DC, National Institute on Aging, 1986

Vachon ML, Rogers J, Lyall WA, et al: Predictors and correlates of adaptation to conjugal bereavement. Am J Psychiatry 1982; 139:998–1002

Vaillant GE: Adaptation to Life. Boston, Little, Brown, 1977

Volkan V: "Re-grief" therapy, in Bereavement: Its Psychosocial Aspects. Edited by Schoenberg B, Gerber I, Wiener A, et al. New York, Columbia University Press, 1975

Weisman AD: Is mourning necessary? in Anticipatory Grief. Edited by Schoenberg B, Carr AC, Kutscher AH, et al. New York, Columbia University Press, 1974

Windholz MJ, Marmar CR, Horowitz MJ: A review of the research on conjugal bereavement: impact on health and efficacy of intervention. Compr Psychiatry 1985; 26:433–447

Worden JW: Grief Counseling and Grief Therapy. New York, Springer, 1982

Zisook S, DeVaul RA: Grief, unresolved grief, and depression. Psychosomatics 1983; 24:247–256

Zisook S, Schuchter S, Schuckit M: Factors in the persistence of unresolved grief among psychiatric patients. Psychosomatics 1985; 26:497–503

Chapter 18

Sleep and Chronobiologic Disturbances in Late Life

Charles F. Reynolds III, M.D.
Carolyn C. Hoch, Ph.D.
Timothy H. Monk, Ph.D.

From a practical standpoint, the study of sleep (and of circadian rhythms in general) in late life is vitally important for two reasons. First there is an impetus from the changing demographics of the United States: It is estimated that by the year 2000 there will be more than 5 million persons in the 85+ year age group (15 percent of the elderly population). The elderly, both "young old" and "old old," are currently consuming more than 83 billion dollars in health care costs, averaging 20 percent of their annual income, with the figure expected to rise dramatically over the next few years (Rabin 1985). In this context, the elderly comprise the age group most severely affected by disorders associated with insomnia, consuming disproportionate quantities of sleeping pills and tranquilizers. Very often, nighttime insomnia (and/or the medication used to "relieve" it) leads to significant deterioration in daytime alertness and functioning (Carskadon and Dement 1981; Carskadon et al. 1982), and a significant degree of distress is caused. However, even when disorders other than those connected directly with sleep are considered, interactions with the aging circadian timekeeping system are observable.

This work was supported in part by National Institute of Mental Health grants 37869 and 00295 (Dr. Reynolds), by NIA grant AG06836 (Dr. Monk and Dr. Reynolds), and by a grant from the John D. and Catherine T. MacArthur Foundation Research Network for the Psychobiology of Depression.

475

The second reason for studying sleep and circadian rhythms in the elderly is that they provide an "extreme sample" that can be used to study aging effects in general, effects that are likely to be most clear-cut in the old old, and that are more likely to provide clues to improving the health and quality of life of all late-life age groups. In this context, the two most common neuropsychiatric disorders of late life, depression and dementia of the Alzheimer type, are both associated with profound disturbances in sleep and often with impaired alertness during the day (Feinberg et al. 1967; Prinz et al. 1982; Reynolds et al. 1985a). Further, many of the ills that old age is heir to (or their treatment) have a negative impact on the ability to achieve long uninterrupted periods of sleep and adequate depth of sleep, thus compounding the distress associated with chronic medical diseases.

Recent studies (Sanford 1975; Rabins et al. 1982) have suggested that sleep-related behaviors very often precipitate a family's decision to institutionalize an elderly relative. Any understanding that would help reduce the institutionalization rate, even by a single percentage point, would pay for itself many times over. Thus, the benefits that would accrue from an understanding of how the aging circadian system might be mediating some of the deterioration observed in sleep, health, and well-being of the elderly would have an impact not only on the elderly themselves, but on society as a whole.

Psychobiology of Sleep Disturbances in Late Life

The nocturnal sleep of older people is brittle and shallow; that is, it is characterized by numerous transient arousals (3 to 15 seconds) and by a loss of the deepest levels of non-rapid eye movement (NREM) sleep (slow-wave sleep). (For a review, see Miles and Dement 1980.) In addition, the sleep of older persons is often redistributed around the clock, as evidenced by both the fragmentation of nighttime sleep and the occurrence of daytime naps. The extent of nighttime sleep fragmentation (for example, the number of transient arousals) predicts the degree of physiologic daytime sleepiness (Carskadon et al. 1982).

If the ability to have slow-wave sleep and long, uninterrupted sleep periods declines with age, nonetheless, the issue of ability to sleep versus need for sleep is not entirely settled. That is, do older people sleep less because they need less sleep or because they cannot sleep as well as younger people? The weight of evidence currently favors the view that older people have less ability to sleep, rather than less need. For example, an important manifestation of unmet sleep need may be the occurrence of daytime sleepiness in many older people. At the same time, recent studies also suggest that some aspects of age-related sleep decay are reversible. Thus, following sleep deprivation or sleep restriction, older people show an ability to have recovery sleep with increased amounts of slow-wave sleep and improved sleep continuity (Reynolds et al. 1986; Spielman et al. 1983; Hoch et al. 1987a).

Previous reports of sleep in the healthy elderly have also noted large gender-related differences in sleep continuity and slow-wave sleep, with elderly men showing more impaired sleep maintenance and less slow-wave sleep than elderly women (Williams et al. 1974; Reynolds et al. 1985b). These studies have suggested that the ability of older women to achieve slow-wave sleep and to have long interrupted sleep periods is better preserved than that of men.

Older women, though, are more likely than men to *complain* of sleep disturbance and to receive sleeping pills (Miles and Dement 1980). A possible explanation of this paradox may lie in the different behavior of older men and women in reporting their sleep accurately and reliably, as well as the differential effects of sleep disruption on mood in men and women. We have found that elderly women show higher and more stable correlations between estimates of sleep quality and objective laboratory measures of sleep (Hoch et al. 1987b) and that older women find sleep deprivation to be a more mood-disturbing experience than do elderly men (Reynolds et al. 1986). Possibly, therefore, older women may be more sensitive to sleep quality and sleep loss than old men.

In this same clinical context, numerous studies have now shown that sleep-disordered breathing increases with advancing age, but more so in men than in women. (The best epidemiologic work in this area is exemplified by Ancoli-Israel et al. 1984.) Reports of sleep apnea prevalence have ranged from 27 percent to 76 percent in men 60 years of age and older, and from 0 percent to 32 percent in aged women. (For review, see Smallwood et al. 1983.) In addition, we have reported that the prevalence of sleep apnea may be higher in patients with probable Alzheimer's dementia than in age-, sex-, and health-matched controls and that the severity of sleep-disordered breathing is correlated significantly with the severity of dementia (Reynolds et al. 1985c; Hoch et al. 1986). The interrelations of nighttime sleep fragmentation (some of it due to sleep apnea), daytime sleepiness, mood, and vigilance in the elderly are all salient to the clinical understanding and management of late-life sleep disturbances. Also, sleep patterns in the healthy aged show strong relationships with preservation of intellectual function (Prinz 1977).

From a biologic rhythms perspective, temperature exerts powerful effects on the regulation of sleep, and conversely, sleep abnormalities are associated with changes in body temperature regulation (for a review, see Szymusiak and Satinoff 1985.) The endogenous component of the body temperature cycle is the generally accepted marker of the output of the circadian pacemaker, which also drives the daily cycles in cortisol release, rapid eye movement (REM) sleep propensity, alertness, and vigilance performance. One parsimonious explanation of at least some of the age-related sleep changes described above is that the circadian pacemaker itself is changing (Webb 1982; Kupfer and Reynolds 1983). It is now generally accepted that, like animal circadian temperature rhythms (Brock 1985), human temperature rhythms tend to flatten with age (Sasaki 1972; Weitzman et al. 1982). This reduction in amplitude appears to result from an increase in the nadir temperature level (Weitzman et al. 1982; Vitiello et al. 1986). In normal diurnal situations, this results in less a nighttime drop in temperature in the old than in the young (Zepelin 1983), and such a difference is also apparent between "poor" and "good" young sleepers (Monroe 1967).

There is also a change with age in "circadian type." Thus older people tend to prefer earlier timings of bedtime and wake-up time than their younger counterparts, and tend to be rated as "morning larks" rather than "night owls" in questionnaires such as that of Horne and Ostberg (1976). Since the timing of sleep changes with age, one might expect the timing (or phase) of the temperature rhythm to also change with age. Here, however, the evidence is not strong, with a suggestion of a phase advance in the elderly in some studies (Sasaki 1972; Zepelin 1983), but no phase difference found in another (Vitiello et al. 1986). Also, in other circadian rhythms thought to be driven by the same circadian oscillator as the temperature rhythm, no age-related phase advance was found (Touitou 1982).

One of the many interesting aspects of REM sleep is the cessation of physiologic thermoregulation. The suppression of thermoregulation during REM sleep leads to the body's temperature becoming a function of environmental temperature, thus decreasing at low ambient temperature (with a subsequent increase during NREM sleep) and increasing at neutral or high ambient temperature (with a subsequent decrease during NREM sleep). To date, little is known quantitatively about the degree of suppression of REM-sleep-related thermoregulation in humans or its sensitivity to basic variables such as developmental age. In other words, given that sleep is associated with lower body temperature and that REM sleep is associated with a loss of thermoregulation, we need to know more about how thermoregulation during sleep is affected by aging. Is sleep a special time of risk during environmental heat or cold stress? Do the elderly have less ability to respond to thermoregulatory challenges, particularly during sleep? These issues are central to the psychobiology of sleep disturbance in old age and, as we shall suggest below, have implications for the development of new treatment strategies. We will now examine, from a clinical standpoint, the etiologies of sleep disturbances in old age.

Etiology of Sleep Disturbances in Late Life

Almost 90 percent of persons aged 60 to 90 complain of insomnia at one time or another (Miles and Dement 1980). Although the elderly comprise only about 10 percent of the U.S. population, they take 25 to 40 percent of the nation's prescription drugs, including sleeping pills (Miles and Dement 1980); among the institutionalized elderly, survey evidence indicates that more than 90 percent are prescribed sedative-hypnotic drugs (U.S. Public

Health Service 1976). What are the clinically salient causes of sleep disturbances in old age?

Age-dependent changes in sleep composition, amount of sleep, and distribution of sleep across the 24-hour day interact with medical and neuropsychiatric disorders and their treatments, as well as with psychosocial and environmental changes, to produce an array of sleep-related complaints in the elderly. These complaints are usually of insomnia, excessive daytime sleepiness, disturbed behaviors associated with sleep, or a shifting of the major sleep period (generally to an earlier time of the night—so-called advanced sleep phase syndrome).

Sleep disturbances in late life, regardless of clinical presentation, generally reflect the following factors: (1) age-dependent decreases in the ability to sleep; (2) increased prevalence of sleep-disordered breathing and nocturnal myoclonic activity; (3) sleep phase alterations, particularly advancement of the major sleep period to an earlier time of day; (4) neuropsychiatric disorders (particularly depression and dementia); (5) pain and limitation of mobility, with excessive time in bed with resultant decay in sleep/wake rhythm amplitudes; (6) poor sleep habits and/or negative conditioning; (7) gastroesophageal reflux associated with hiatal hernia; (8) iatrogenic factors; and (9) adverse environmental factors, such as excessive noise or temperatures outside of the thermoneutral zone. These factors determine the overall strategy of clinical and laboratory assessment.

Clinical and Laboratory Assessment of Sleep Disturbances in Late Life

The initial aim of clinical assessment is to determine the duration of the patient's complaint and its probable causes. Transient disturbances (e.g., insomnia), lasting less than 3 to 4 weeks, are often situationally determined, while persistent disturbance (lasting longer than a month) indicates evaluation for a variety of disorders. Sources of diagnostic information should include interviews with both the patient and bedpartner and a sleep/wake diary, kept over a 14-day period, to determine the distribution and quality of the patient's sleep during the 24-hour day. A physical examination and portable screening (for example, a cassette tape of the patient's breathing patterns during sleep, monitoring for cardiac arrhythmia, or body temperature measurements to document circadian rhythm abnormalities) may also prove necessary.

Keeping in mind age-dependent decreases in the ability to sleep, the clinician should investigate the following possibilities: (1) poor sleep habit practices (for example, irregular sleep/wake scheduling, excessive environmental noise, temperature outside the thermoneutral zone, or evening self-medication with nicotine, alcohol, or caffeinated beverages); (2) obsessive worry about sleep or the use of the sleep setting for activities not conducive to sleep (i.e., adverse conditioning factors); (3) dependency on sleeping pills and other central nervous system depressant drugs; (4) temporal redistribution of the major sleep period, such as phase advancement or excessive daytime napping; (5) heavy snoring or obstructive breathing during sleep, which may indicate sleep apnea; (6) feelings of restlessness in the legs at sleep onset, which may indicate nocturnal myoclonus; (7) neuropsychiatric disorders, particularly depression, dementia, and anxiety disorders; (8) medical causes of pain, such as nocturnal angina and arthritis; and (9) gastroesophageal reflux, possibly leading to laryngospasm. Finally, but of great importance, the use of sedating medication (not only sleeping pills, but also antihypertensives, antihistamines, and anxiolytics),their timing, and dosage should be reviewed for potential adverse effects on sleep and on daytime alertness (Table 1).

To thoroughly understand an older person's sleep complaint, it is also necessary to place it within the context of his or her daily schedule of activities or that of the institution in which he or she resides. Very often, many of the preceding factors operate concurrently in an older person to produce a complaint of insomnia, daytime sleepiness, shifting of the major sleep period, or disturbed behavior during sleep. As is well known, if the patient is a nursing home resident, wakefulness, wandering, or nighttime confusion may be major management problems that, unfortunately, often lead to excessive sedation, falls, deterioration of mental status during the day, and accidents. The physiologic basis of nocturnal confusion, particularly in demented patients, is not well understood. In some instances, these episodes may be related to partial arousals from REM sleep (Feinberg et al. 1967); or, like other overnight changes in mental status, they may be temporally linked to episodes of sleep-disordered breathing and attendant cerebral hypoxia (Moldofsky et al. 1983). Some of the episodes may also be iatrogenic, reflecting the impact of sleeping pills or other nonpsychotropic drugs (Table 1).

Sleep laboratory evaluation can be helpful in the elderly person with a sleep disturbance and is indicated if the physician suspects sleep apnea (suggested particularly by the presence of heavy snoring and excessive daytime sleepiness), nocturnal myoclonus (suggested by a complaint of restless legs or akathisia-like sensations in the legs interfering with sleep onset), or sleep phase disturbance of irregularity (for example, prominent advancement of the major sleep period or extremely fragmented sleep/wake scheduling, with loss of sleep/wake consolidation). Laboratory evaluation should also be strongly considered if routine treatment measures for persistent insomnia have not been effective. In this context, "routine" treatment includes (1) consistent attention to regulation of sleep/wake schedule and a comfortable sleep environment, with diminution of noise and assurance of temperature in the thermoneutral zone; (2) reduction or omission of nicotine, alcohol, or excessive liquid ingestion in the evening, including caffeine; (3) use of the bedroom for sleep only and avoidance of activities in the

Table 1. Nonpsychotropic drugs with significant effects on sleep, wake, and mood

Antihypertensives	**Corticosteroids**
Reserpine	Cortisone
Methyldopa	**Hormones**
Propranolol	Progesterone
Guanethidine	Estrogen
Hydralazine	**Antiinflammatory drugs**
Clonidine	Indomethacin
Antiparkinsonian drugs	
Levodopa	
Levodopa and carbidopa	

bedroom that are not conducive to sleep; (4) careful attention to the timing of activity, meals, medication, and sleep periods; (5) detoxification from depressant or stimulant drugs; (6) appropriate nonpharmacologic treatment when indicated, such as chronotherapy or behavioral therapy (see below); and (7) antidepressant medication for the treatment of an affective disorder.

We will now briefly review pharmacologic and nonpharmacologic approaches to treating sleep disturbances in older persons.

Guidelines for Pharmacologic Approaches to Late-Life Sleep Disturbance

Diagnosis is the most salient of all clinical considerations involved in the decision to prescribe medication for a late-life sleep disturbance. Sleeping pills have some place in the management of transient or situational insomnia, persistent sleep loss associated with negative conditioning or bad habits, or persistent insomnia associated with nonpsychotic psychiatric disorders. Additional considerations involved in prescribing sleeping pills for the elderly include (1) a review of the relative indications and contraindications for using low-dose sedating tricyclic antidepressant drugs, benzodiazepines, or sedating antipsychotic compounds; (2) changes in rate of metabolism; (3) effects on daytime alertness and performance; (4) other concurrent medications that might potentiate the sedative effects of sleeping pills; and (5) the potential effects on borderline or full-blown sleep apnea syndrome.

With respect to the class of compound, it should be noted that there is a paucity of data from controlled pharmacotherapeutic trials on well-diagnosed samples of geriatric patients. For example, we found six studies of sleeping pill use in elderly patients with "dementia" or "organic brain syndrome," published during the past 15 years (Stotsky et al. 1971; Linnoila et al. 1976, 1980a, 1980b; Viukari et al. 1978; Schubert 1984). These studies involved a total of 134 inpatients, some with mild to moderate dementia and others diagnosed to have "organic brain syndrome" with agitation. None of the studies employed sleep laboratory or objective methods to assess drug effects. With the exception of the Schubert (1984) study, all studies employed a placebo control and were double blind. The major dependent measures in the studies reviewed were nursing observations of sleep-onset time, sleep duration, and number and duration of arousals during the night. The studies investigated the effects of several different psychoactive agents on sleep in institutionalized demented patients, including butabarbital (50 to 100 mg), nitrazepam (10 mg), thioridazine (25 mg), flurazepam (15 mg), chloral hydrate (500 mg), lorazepam (2 mg), oxazepam (30 mg), temazepam (15 mg), and hydroxyzine (50 to 200 mg).

In general, the studies reported that compared with placebo, the use of active compounds was associated with nursing observations of increased sleep time, via reduction in sleep onset and in the number of intermittent awakenings. The 1980b study by Linnoila et al. reported, however, that the use of lorazepam (2 mg), oxazepam (30 mg), and temazepam (15 mg) was not associated with a reduction in sleep latency but did result in improved sleep maintenance. In the 1976 study by Linnoila et al., low-dose thioridazine was reported to be superior to nitrazepam, with use of the latter leading to increased daytime memory impairment, incontinence, diminished activities of daily living, and daytime sleepiness. Viukari et al. (1978) likewise reported decreased motor performance following the use of flurazepam and nitrazepam, as well as rebound insomnia following the use of nitrazepam. Similarly, Linnoila et al. (1980a) also observed significant withdrawal insomnia with chloral hydrate when used in elderly patients with dementia. Finally, Schubert (1984) observed the development of tolerance to the sedating effects of hydroxyzine.

At this writing, we are reluctant to recommend the use of benzodiazepines to manage sleep disturbance associated with dementia. From the published studies, it is not clear that the use of benzodiazepines represents a viable long-term strategy for successful maintenance of sleep disturbance in dementia; moreover, the studies suggest the development of withdrawal effects, tolerance, or unacceptable side effects including daytime sleepiness. Moreover, given the finding that sleep apnea occurs significantly more often in dementia than in other types of late-life mental disorder, there might result an interaction between sleep-disordered breathing and cognitive deterioration in dementia, an interaction that could become more pernicious with the use of sleeping pills or central nervous system depressants. In this context of uncertainty, therefore, we generally recommend the use of sedating antipsychotic compounds (e.g., 25 to 75 mg of thioridazine at bedtime) for patients with marked behavioral disturbances at night who have dementia (generally of the Alzheimer's type) associated with psychosis and/or delirium. Essentially, we are reluctant to recommend the use of benzodiazepines in such patients, because sleep-disordered breathing might be worsened, and the depressive effects of such compounds could cause further deterioration in the patient's mental status.

In other older patients with chronic insomnia who cannot function without maintenance sleep-promoting medication, we generally suggest the use of a low-dose sedating tricyclic antidepressant, rather than a benzodiazepine. Our hypothesis (still to be adequately tested) is that antidepressants may retain their sedating effects longer than benzodiazepines, without the development of tolerance, daytime sequelae, or withdrawal syndromes. Moreover, such patients often have diagnosable affective disorders; they frequently also have low-grade sleep apnea that might be diminished by a tricyclic compound but exacerbated by a benzodiazepine. We would consider a benzodiazepine as maintenance therapy in chronic insomnia associated with a diagnosable anxiety disorder, if there is no sleep apnea.

When using benzodiazepines in the elderly, the key pharmacokinetic consideration is the half-life of the compound. (For a review, see Greenblatt et al. 1981.) It is well known that long-lasting sleeping pills are more likely to produce daytime sedation, the desirability of which will vary for specific patients. Related to this, relative contraindications to sleeping pill use in the elderly include heavy snoring (which suggests sleep apnea), systemic illnesses that diminish the patient's ability to eliminate these compounds, the use of other medications (including alcohol) with potentially dangerous interactions, a history of drug abuse, jobs requiring alertness, and suicidal risk. If the physician determines that a benzodiazepine is indicated in an elderly patient, the physician should establish the smallest effective dose (often one-third to one-half that prescribed in younger patients); tell the patient to take the medication about 30 minutes before bedtime; monitor daytime consequences (especially daytime sleepiness); follow the patient regularly; try to limit the use of a benzodiazepine to less than 20 doses per month and for not more than 3 months total; and encourage the patient to increase reliance on nonpharmacologic approaches to sleep disturbance.

With respect to the use of tricyclic antidepressants to treat sleep disturbances in late life associated with depression, we have recently reviewed our experience with the tricyclic drug nortriptyline (Reynolds et al. 1987). We have found the use of this agent, in doses ranging from 20 to 75 mg at bedtime, to be helpful in reducing depressive symptoms, including sleep disturbance, in late-life depression with or without associated cognitive impairment (Reynolds et al. 1987). In general, we recommend avoiding tertiary amine tricyclic antidepressants in the elderly (e.g., amitriptyline or imipramine) because of unacceptable side effects (e.g., orthostasis, anticholinergic delirium, and peripheral atropinic effects). Our clinical experience at the Benedum Geriatric Center of the University of Pittsburgh has been more favorable with low-dose trimipramine (25 to 75 mg at bedtime) or low-dose trazodone (50 to 100 mg at bedtime) as maintenance therapy in geriatric insomnia related to depression.

Guidelines for Nonpharmacologic Approaches to Late-Life Sleep Disturbances

Elderly persons and their families need to be told that some sleep disturbance may be an unavoidable consequence of aging; not that they need less sleep, but rather that their ability to sleep seems to diminish with age. Reinforcement of the sleep/wake rhythm becomes extremely important in order to combat the age-related tendency to lose the consolidation of sleep and to develop a polyphasic sleep/wake cycle. The use of strong and consistent external time cues might achieve this without side effects associated with sleeping pills. In practical terms, the elderly person should be encouraged to maintain temporal control by going to bed only when sleepy, by getting up at the same time each morning, and by reducing or eliminating naps. The elder should also be instructed to maintain stimulus control by avoidance of using the bedroom for activities other than sleep. The latter will serve to keep the bed as a powerful stimulus to sleep. We emphasize the importance of strengthening temporal and stimulus control, together with education and reassurance, to give the elderly person a sense of increased control and to diminish the perceived need for sleeping pills.

In our studies of healthy older sleepers, we have also noted that elderly persons who habitually restrict themselves to $6\frac{1}{2}$ or 7 hours in bed a night tend to have sleep continuity superior to that observed in persons who remain in bed 8 hours and whose lives are generally less active and structured (Hoch et al. 1987a). Our observation is consistent with Spielman et al.'s earlier claim (1983) that sleep restriction may be appropriate treatment in some types of insomnia (notably, conditional or "psychophysiologic" insomnias).

The development of nonpharmacologic treatment approaches for sleep disturbances in the elderly certainly remains a high priority in clinical investigation. In this context, and related to our earlier discussion of the psychobiology of sleep disturbances in late life, we would like to remind the reader that temperature affects major aspects of sleep state control and that, conversely, some or many sleep abnormalities are likely to be associated with abnormalities in body temperature regulation, especially with increasing age. As reviewed by Szymusiak and Satinoff (1985), total sleep time is greatest during minimal thermal stress and declines in heat and cold. Further, sleep-enhancing and thermoregulatory mechanisms with the basal forebrain appear to be closely related, both functionally and anatomically. It may therefore be asked (Szymusiak and Satinoff 1985) whether the thermosensitivity of sleep is due to a convergence of sleep-promoting and thermosensing functions within the same population of basal forebrain neurons. Similarly, the sleep disturbance in Alzheimer's disease, including diminished REM sleep, may be compared to that seen in cold-exposed humans. In both instances, diminished function of basal forebrain hypnogenic neurons has been invoked as a mechanism. These observations have led Szymusiak and Satinoff (1985) to predict that sleep in

Alzheimer's disease should improve when residual activity of basal forebrain neurons is enhanced by a higher than normal ambient temperature. Alternatively, since increases in core body temperature (by either active or passive means) seem to increase slow-wave sleep and slow-wave incidence during subsequent sleep (Horne and Reid 1985), it is a researchable question whether increases in body temperature (for example, by passive heating in the afternoon) might lead to a correction of the sleep continuity and slow-wave sleep abnormalities of late-life neuropsychiatric disorders.

The existence of putatively chronobiologic sleep abnormalities in the elderly (advanced sleep phase syndrome) and in young adults (delayed sleep phase syndrome) suggests the possibility of an age-related continuum of sleep schedule disturbances (for a review of biologic research in aging, see Brock 1985). This age-related continuum of chronobiologic sleep disturbances may in turn be related to a shortening of the circadian temperature rhythm period seen with advancing age. Since the external light/dark cycle provides important time cues for the body's endogenous oscillator (whose major output is the circadian temperature rhythm); and since this "oscillator," or clock, governs the internal organization and spontaneous duration of sleep; then it should be possible to use bright light exposure as a way of treating chronobiologic sleep disturbances. For example, if advanced sleep phase syndromes in the elderly are associated with an advancement of the circadian temperature rhythm, then bright light exposure in the evening may serve to reset the phase of the temperature rhythm with respect to external clock time, thereby resulting in a redistribution of sleep to a more appropriate time.

Research in nonpharmacologic approaches to the treatment of sleep disturbances in late life, involving (for example) the manipulation of ambient temperature or the external light/dark cycle, is based on a recognition that sleep regulation depends on both homeostatic and circadian principles. Thus, sleep is viewed as a self-regulated process contingent upon the duration of prior waking. At the same time, the underlying circadian oscillator allows sleeping and waking to occur at predictable intervals in synchrony with the environmental day/night cycle. These two aspects of regulation meet the requirements of flexibility and stability (for further discussion of homeostatic and circadian principles in sleep regulation, the reader is referred to Borbely and Tobler 1985).

Conclusion

In conclusion, we are suggesting a more thoughtful approach to the management of late-life sleep disturbances, with the fundamental aim of enhancing daytime alertness and quality of life. The conceptual approach that we suggest for the clinician is grounded within a psychobiology of aging and of late-life sleep disturbances. First, specific etiologic factors should be identified. Often, multiple factors are operating in the patient to produce sleep/wake disturbances. Second, it is important to recognize and educate the patient about age-dependent changes in the ability to sleep. Third, given the apparent fragility and brittleness of the older person's circadian timekeeping system, it is important to reinforce sleep/wake rhythms by strengthening time cues and by enhancing stimulus control. Often, modest habitual sleep restriction to $6\frac{1}{2}$ or $7\frac{1}{2}$ hours will help improve sleep continuity. At the same time, mild daytime sleepiness may be alleviated by a regularly scheduled brief nap. Fourth, chronopharmacologic issues must be addressed, particularly the timing of both psychotropic and nonpsychotropic drugs with respect to adverse effects on sleep and wake periods. Finally, pharmacotherapy should be used for specific indications only, for limited periods of time, and with attention to possible adverse effects on breathing during sleep.

References

Ancoli-Israel S, Kripke DF, Mason W, et al: Obstructive sleep apnea in a senior population. Sleep Research 1984; 14:130

Borbely AA, Tobler I: Homeostatic and circadian principles of sleep regulation in the rat, in Brain Mechanisms of Sleep. Edited by McGinty, DJ, Drucker–Colin R, Morrison A, et al. New York, Raven Press, 1985

Brock MA: Biological clock and aging. Review of Biological Research in Aging 1985; 2:445–462

Carskadon MA, Dement WC: Cumulative effects of sleep restriction on daytime sleepiness. Psychophysiology 1981; 18:107–113

Carskadon MA, Brown ED, Dement WC: Sleep fragmentation in the elderly: relationship to daytime sleep tendency. Neurobiol Aging 1982; 3:321–327

Feinberg I, Koresko RL, Heller N: EEG sleep patterns as a function of normal and pathological aging in men. J Psychiatr Res 1967; 5:107–144

Greenblatt DJ, Shader RI, Divoll M: Benzodiazepines: a summary of pharmacokinetic properties. J Am Geriatr Soc 1981; 11:11S–16S

Hoch CC, Reynolds CF, Kupfer DJ, et al: Sleep disordered breathing in normal and pathologic aging. J Clin Psychiatry 1986; 47:498–503

Hoch CC, Reynolds CF, Kupfer DJ, et al: The superior sleep of healthy elderly nuns. Int J Aging Human Dev, 1987a; 25:1–8

Hoch CC, Reynolds CF, Kupfer DJ, et al: Empirical note: self–report versus recorded sleep in healthy seniors. Psychophysiology 1987b; 24:293–299

Horne JA, Ostberg O: A self–assessment questionnaire to determine morningness–eveningness in human circadian rhythms. International Journal of Chronobiology 1976; 4:97–110

Horne JA, Reid AJ: Nighttime sleep EEG changes following body heating in a warm bath. Electroencephalogr Clin Neurophysiol 1985; 60:154–157

Kupfer DJ, Reynolds CF: A critical review of sleep and its disorders from a developmental perspective. Psychiatr Dev 1983; 4:367–386

Linnoila M, Viukari M: Efficacy and side effects of nitrazepam and thioridazine as sleeping aides in psychogeriatric inpatients. Br J Psychiatr 1976; 128:566–569

Linnoila M, Viukari M, Numminen A, et al: Efficacy and side effects of chloral hydrate and tryptophan as sleeping aids in psychogeriatric patients. International Pharmacopsychiatry 1980a; 15:124–128

Linnoila M, Viukari M, Lamminsivu U, et al: Efficacy and side effects of lorazepam, oxazepam, and temazepam as sleeping aids in psychogeriatric inpatients. International Pharmacopsychiatry 1980b; 15:129–135

Miles LE, Dement WC: Sleep and aging. Sleep 1980; 3:119–220

Moldofsky H, Goldstein R, McNicholas WT, et al: Disordered breathing during sleep and overnight intellectual deterioration in patients with pathological aging, in Sleep/Wake Disorders: Natural History, Epidemiology, and Long–Term Evolution. Edited by Guilleminault C, Lugaresi E. New York, Raven Press, 1983

Monroe LJ: Psychological and physiological differences between good and poor sleepers. J Abnorm Psychol 1967; 72:255–264

Prinz P: Sleep patterns in the healthy aged: relationship with intellectual functions. J Gerontol 1977; 32:179–180

Prinz P, Peskind ER, Vitaliano PP, et al: Changes in the sleep and waking EEGs of nondemented and demented elderly subjects. J Am Geriatr Soc 1982; 30(2):86–93

Rabin DI: Waxing of the gray, waning of the green, in America's Aging—Health in an Older Society. Washington, DC, National Academy Press 1985

Rabins PV, Mace NL, Lucas MJ: The impact of dementia on the family. JAMA 1982; 248:333–335

Reynolds CF, Kupfer DJ, Taska LS, et al: EEG sleep in healthy elderly, depressed, and demented subjects. Biol Psychiatry 1985a; 20:431–442

Reynolds CF, Kupfer DJ, Taska LS, et al: Sleep of healthy seniors: a revisit. Sleep 1985b; 8:20–29

Reynolds CF, Kupfer DJ, Taska LS, et al: Sleep apnea in Alzheimer's dementia: correlation with mental deterioration. J Clin Psychiatry 1985c; 46:257–261

Reynolds CF, Kupfer DJ, Hoch CC, et al: Sleep deprivation in healthy elderly men and women: effects on mood and on sleep during recovery. Sleep 1986; 9:492–501

Reynolds CF, Perel JM, Kupfer DJ, et al: Open-trial response to antidepressant treatment in elderly patients with mixed depression and cognitive impairment. Psychiatry Res 1987; 21:111–122

Sanford JRA: Tolerance of debility in elderly dependents by supports at home: significance for hospital practice. Br Med J 1975; 3:471–473

Sasaki T: Circadian rhythm in body temperature, in Advances in Climatic Physiology. Edited by Itoh S, Ogata K, Yoshimura H. Tokyo, Igaku Shoin, 1972

Schubert DSP: Hydroxyzine for acute treatment of agitation and insomnia in organic mental disorder. Psychiatr J Univ Ottawa 1984; 9:59–60

Smallwood RG, Vitiello MV, Giblin EC, et al: Sleep apnea: relationship to age, sex and Alzheimer's dementia. Sleep 1983; 6:16–22

Spielman A, Saskin P, Thorpy MJ: Sleep restriction treatment for insomnia. Sleep Research 1983; 12:286

Stotsky BA, Cole JO, Tang YT, et al: Sodium butabarbital as an hypnotic agent for age to psychiatric patients with sleep disorders. J Am Geriatr Soc 1971; 19:860–870

Szymusiak R, Satinoff E: Thermal influences on basal forebrain hypnogenic mechanisms, in Brain Mechanisms of Sleep. Edited by McGinty DJ, Drucker–Colin R, Morrison A, et al. New York, Raven Press, 1985

Touitou Y: Some aspects of circadian time structure in the elderly. Gerontology 1982; 28(suppl 1):53–67

U.S. Public Health Service: Physicians' drug prescribing patterns in skilled nursing facilities (Publication No. 76–50050). Bethesda, MD, U.S. Department of Health, Education and Welfare, 1976

Vitiello MV, Smallwood RG, Avery DH, et al: Circadian temperature rhythms in young adults and aged men. Neurobiol Aging 1986; 7:97–100

Viukari M, Linnoila M, Aalto U: Efficacy and side effects of flurazepam, fosazepam, and nitrazepam and sleeping aides in psychogeriatric patients. Acta Psychiatr Scand 1978; 57:27–35

Webb WB: Biological rhythms, sleep and performance. New York, Wiley, 1982

Weitzman ED, Moline ML, Czeisler CA, et al: Chronobiology of aging: temperature, sleep/wake rhythms, and entrainment. Neurobiol Aging 1982; 3:299–309

Williams RL, Karacan I, Hursch CJ: EEG of human sleep: clinical applications. New York, Wiley, 1974

Zepelin H: Normal age–related change in sleep, in Sleep Disorders: Basic and Clinical Research. Edited by Chase M, Weitzman E. New York, Spectrum, 1983

Chapter 19

Alcohol and Drug Problems in the Elderly

Dan G. Blazer, M.D., Ph.D.

The problems of elderly alcohol abuse and inappropriate elderly drug use are closely related. Of the two, alcohol abuse is the more publicized but not necessarily the more prevalent. Misuse of both alcohol and drugs derives from the context of Western society. Primary care physicians and geriatric psychiatrists cannot diagnose or treat these disorders without appreciating the milieu from which they emerge and the factors that reinforce the behaviors.

Use of alcohol has a long and complex history in human societies (Maddox and Blazer 1985). Among the ancients, alcohol was described as "the water of life" and given magical, symbolic significance in religious and social ceremonies that marked transitions over the life course from birth to death. In other words, alcohol is such a domesticated drug (the recreational beverage of choice) that it is difficult even to discuss alcohol as a potentially addictive substance like those "other drugs," such as cocaine. Yet clinicians are ambivalent about alcohol (with good reason). Alcohol is associated with a wide range of personal and social problems across the life cycle. For example, intoxication is involved in an estimated 50 percent of all traffic fatalities.

Drug abuse must also be considered within the context of its culture. Neither illegal nor prescription drugs are perceived as recreational by the vast majority of older adults. Admitted drug abuse is a rare phenomenon in the older adult. Yet 25 percent of drugs and drug sundries consumed in this country are consumed by those 65 years of age and older (2.5 times the proportion for the entire population). Older adults frequently suffer from one or more chronic illnesses. Most will receive prescription medications in any

489

given year. Elders are comfortable taking medications and frequently skilled at detecting the optimal dose for certain types of subjective effects. They also recognize the nuances of side effects from one medication to the other. The veritable pharmacy within the medicine chest provides older persons with a wide selection of prescription and over-the-counter agents for treating a given malady. Coupled with the decreased availability of primary medical care in some communities and the increased cost of this care, self-medication for physical and mental health problems is common. An inevitable outcome for older persons from an individualistic society with multiple barriers to appropriate medical and psychiatric care is the abuse of prescription and over-the-counter medications.

Both alcohol and drug problems confront clinicians treating older adults. Occasionally, medication and alcohol misuse or abuse are the primary problems encountered. More often, however, these problems accompany other disorders and thus complicate therapy. In this chapter, alcohol and drug problems will be reviewed separately. Though the disorders undoubtedly overlap, the unique characteristics of each deserve separate attention.

Alcohol Abuse and Dependence

Investigation of alcohol abuse and dependence among older adults has increased in recent years. The reason for this attention is not a dramatic or even persistent increase in rates of alcohol problems in the elderly. As reviewed in Chapter 9 on epidemiology, the current prevalence of alcohol abuse/dependence for persons 65+ years of age ranges from 1.9 to 4.6 percent for males and 0.1 to 0.7 for females (Myers et al. 1984). Even the lifetime prevalence of alcohol problems in older adults is lower than for younger persons in the population. This may partially be explained by cohort differences in drinking experience and selective survival of more moderate drinkers. The risk factors for alcohol abuse in the elderly are similar to those for the general population—male sex, poor education, low income, and a history of other psychiatric disorders, especially depression.

One explanation for increased interest by clinicians and the public is that late life is perceived as a time of stressful events such as retirement, widowhood, illness, and isolation. Alcohol use has traditionally been a culturally accepted strategy for stress reduction. With increased stress, older individuals may increase their alcohol intake and their risk for problems from alcohol. Decreased ability of the older adult to metabolize alcohol, coupled with concomitant medical problems, increases the risk of accidents, side effects, and overt toxicity. Alcohol abuse may first be noticed as elders become less capable of living alone, especially by family. Discovery that a parent has a long history of alcohol intake may offend the social sensibilities of middle-aged children and grandchildren (Maddox and Blazer 1985). The potential for alcohol problems to emerge in individuals who have maintained a relatively constant intake of alcohol over the majority of the adult life cycle will increase as more older adults reach their 80s and even 90s.

Despite the scenario above, the problem of alcohol abuse and dependence in late life, albeit serious, is not as severe as among young adults. Though the population at risk for alcohol problems increases with each successive cohort (the graying of the Western world), the rate of increase has not been dramatic. In fact, most older persons living today were raised in a culture that included a strong tradition of temperance. In a national survey by Armor et al. (1977), 52 percent of elderly men and 68 percent of elderly women were abstainers. These percentages, however, will drop with those cohorts entering late life in the 21st century. The increased percentage of users does not necessarily suggest an increased percentage of those who abuse alcohol, though increased per capita consumption is usually associated with an increase in the magnitude of abuse (Faris 1974).

Longitudinal studies of risk factors for alcohol problems in the elderly are virtually nonexistent. Nevertheless, suggestive data from cross-sectional research may inform regarding potential etiologic agents. For example, Glatt (1978) identifies three precipitating factors in late-onset alcoholism; a habitual drinking pattern prior to late life, personality factors, and environmental factors. Personality characteristics that predispose to late-life drinking problems include anxiety and worry about one's social environment, such as loss of a loved one and loneliness. Personality factors appear less related to late-onset alcoholism than at earlier stages of the life cycle. Alcohol problems in the elderly, in contrast, may precipitate stressful events such as marital discord and social isolation (especially from family). Rathbone-McCuan et al. (1976) report on 695 persons 55 years of age and older in Baltimore. They found older alcoholics drank primarily to alleviate depression and to escape existing social problems. The older problem drinkers generally reported poorer health and had more physical problems than did the elderly normal drinkers. In addition, they had more problems with finances and social isolation. Warheit and Auth (1984) found that among those 50 years of age and older (compared with persons earlier in the life cycle), the older high-risk alcohol group was less likely to report difficulties in marital status and life satisfaction, though the trend was in a similar direction to younger persons.

Risk factor studies of alcohol intake over time are relatively rare in the literature. Longitudinal studies for drinking patterns, however, are more common and provide insight into changing patterns of alcohol intake through adult life. For example, more than 1,800 men aged 28 to 87 were studied for more than 10 years in the Veterans Administration's normative study of aging (Glynn et al. 1984). In this panel there was almost no change in mean alcohol consumption during the follow-up. Rates of problems with drinking did not decline over time within age groups. These data do not support findings from previous cross-sectional studies that aging modifies drinking behaviors. Men in their 40s and 50s in 1973 were especially persistent in their alcohol intake over time. In an earlier investigation, Gordon and Kannel (1983) found that participants in the Framingham heart study increased their consumed alcohol by more than 63 percent over a 20-year follow-up (1952–1972). An increase in consumption from 1952 to 1972 is consistent with the stability in consumption reported from the normative aging study if one recognizes that both cohorts were influenced by a national trend to increase alcohol use. For example, the tendency to decrease alcohol consumption with aging may have been counterbalanced by social forces encouraging greater consumption.

In a follow-up of nearly 1,300 adults treated for moderately severe to severe alcohol problems, Helzer et al. (1984) found few age differences to predict outcome. There was some evidence that among the survivors, older alcoholics are less likely to suffer persistent severe problems. At the same time, the all-cause mortality rate was higher for older adults, and the alcohol-related mortality rate was similar for both the young and the elderly. Among the predictors of continued alcoholism, social isolation was a stronger correlate in the older group. Organic brain syndrome was not associated with outcome for the younger sample, but its absence was associated with good outcome for the older group. In summary, this sample of treated alcoholics followed for 6 to 10 years revealed good outcome in a large proportion of the older subjects. The higher mortality rate in the older group may have balanced the difference in outcome when comparing the young and the elderly, however.

Pharmacologic Properties

Ethyl alcohol is absorbed easily through the mucous membranes of the stomach, small intestines, and colon. Though peak blood levels are generally reached 30 to 90 minutes following alcohol intake, it may take from 2 to 6 hours for complete absorption. Many factors alter the rate of absorption, some of which are age related. In general, alcohol absorption is as rapid in late life as it is at earlier stages of the life cycle. Most foods in the stomach retard absorption, especially milk and milk products. In contrast, because absorption from the small intestine is extremely rapid, patients who have undergone gastrectomy frequently complain that they quickly become intoxicated by small amounts of alcohol that would not have been a problem prior to the operation (Garver 1984; Muehlberger 1958; Ritchie 1981).

Once absorbed, ethanol is distributed throughout the body, but not evenly. Alcohol does not distribute to fatty tissues (Garver 1984). Older adults, as described previously, have less total body water per unit mass, less extracellular fluid, and higher body fat. The net result is that a standard ingested dose of ethanol will result in a higher blood level in an older adult than in a younger adult because of the lower effective fluid volume for distribution (Wiberg et al. 1977) in the older adult. Since most older adults have a relative increase in lipid tissue with aging, higher plasma ethanol concentrations are especially more likely.

More than 90 percent of the alcohol that enters the body is completely oxidized. This process takes place in the liver primarily under the influence of the hepatic enzyme alcohol dehydrogenase. There is no evidence that the activity of this enzyme decreases as a function of aging in humans (Garver 1984). At all ages, the metabolism of alcohol is slow and constant. Therefore, a definite limit must be placed on the amount of alcohol that is consumed in a given period of time; otherwise, intoxication or more serious consequences may result secondary to an accumulation of alcohol. The small amount of alcohol not oxidized may be either excreted in the urine (or other body fluids) or diffused into the alveolar air and exhaled. In other words, the body must process virtually all the alcohol ingested.

The process of alcohol metabolism can lead to secondary problems for the older adult. Gastric secretions are mediated psychically by alcohol, for alcohol is a very strong stimulus if enjoyed by the individual. The presence of alcohol in the stomach in concentrations of around 10 percent results in gastric secretions rich in acid, but poor in pepsin (in contrast to the reflex secretion which is rich in both). Alcohol at stronger concentrations (such as 40 percent or over) is directly irritating to the mucosa and may cause congestive hyperemia and inflammation. Plasma protein may be lost into the gastrointestinal lumen. Alcohol, therefore, produces an erosive gastritis (Ritchie 1982; Chowdhury et al. 1977). Alcohol may also facilitate constipation if taken habitually in moderate amounts. The mechanism is probably secondary to an inadequate food intake and insufficient bulk. Diarrhea, on the other hand, may result from the irritant action of alcohol.

The oxidation of alcohol in the liver leads to a change in the ratio of nicotinamide-adenine dinucleotide (NAD) to the reduced form of NAD (NADH). This change, in turn, apparently enhances lipid synthesis by the liver. Alcohol may also promote the accumulation of fatty tissue in the liver indirectly. Acetylglycerophosphate increases in concentration with an accompanying stimulation of the esterification of fatty acids, which leads to a collection of fat in the liver (Ritchie 1981; Kalant et al. 1980). Accumulation of fat and an accompanying accumulation of protein may initially cause no difficulties, but eventually the process cannot be reversed and progresses to various stages of liver disease, especially cirrhosis.

Alcohol also exerts a diuretic effect on the kidneys. This effect appears to be above and beyond the large amounts of fluids usually ingested with alcoholic beverages among the chronic alcohol abusers. The origin of this diuresis may be secondary to a decrease in the release of antidiuretic hormone from the posterior pituitary. The relative increase in urine formation can especially be a problem for elderly males whose urine flow is compromised by prostatic difficulties (Garver 1984; Ritchie 1981).

Although alcohol is popularly thought to be a sexual stimulant, in humans chronic ingestion of alcohol may result in decreased sexual interest, if not impotence. The mechanism by which this occurs is a decrease in the release of luteinizing hormone from the anterior pituitary. The older adult who already believes his or her sexual functioning is compromised may enter a vicious cycle by drinking to avoid the anxiety of decreased sexual performance yet enhancing the disability through alcohol intake.

The Physical Consequences of Alcoholism in Later Life

When evaluating alcohol intake through time, the clinician must attend to the interaction between alcohol use and chronic or periodic illness in the elderly. Though alcohol directly affects organ systems (e.g., alcohol increases cardiac rate and output secondary to its effect on cardiac muscle), the primary impact is cumulative. For example, the chronic alcoholic develops compromised hepatic functioning, which may exacerbate osteomalacia secondary to decreased hepatic metabolism of vitamin D_3 to its more active 25-hydroxylated form. Undernutrition that results from chronic alcohol intake, especially among those who use heavy amounts of alcohol over long periods (the "skid-row alcoholics"), commonly resulted in cirrhosis. Cirrhosis is one of the eight leading causes of death in the 65 and older population.

Alcohol can damage the heart, such as the alcohol-induced cardiomyopathies. In contrast, some investigators report an actual reduction in coronary artery disease in subjects who drink moderate quantities of alcohol over time (Yano et al. 1977).

Chronic effects of alcohol intake on the gastrointestinal tract are well known to clinicians working with older adults. In general, chronic alcoholics have a lower gastric basal acid output, maximal acid output, and an increased likelihood of developing chronic atrophic gastritis. The preexisting atrophic gastritis that is common in the elderly may facilitate the formation of gastric mucosal lesions leading to upper gastrointestinal bleeding. Both folic acid and B_{12} absorption declines with chronic alcohol use. Since these dietary supplements are essential to cognitive functioning, their loss in the diet may lead to cognitive and psychologic impairment.

Nutritional requirements do not change dramatically with aging, though older persons may require more protein (Gersovitz et al. 1982). Chronic alcohol ingestion reduces intake of a number of nutrients, including protein. Protein malnutrition is manifested in alcoholics as muscle wasting, hypoproteinemia, and edema. Iron deficiency, however, is generally due to gastrointestinal blood loss (as opposed to decreased dietary intake or malabsorption). As noted above, older adults may be more subject to gastric lesions, which in turn may lead to chronic occult bleeding.

A concern of equal importance with the medical consequences of late-life alcohol use is the interaction of aging, alcohol, and dementia. Many investigators report chronic alcoholism to be associated with a variety of neuropsychologic and cognitive deficits. Though chronic alcoholism does not appear to disrupt cognitive and neuropsychologic functioning diffusely, specific clusters of function are affected in the older alcoholic. Most investigators agree that intelligence remains relatively unaffected compared with deficits in subtle memory and information processing. These deficits are similar to the impairment of patients suffering from Wernicke-Korsakoff's disease. Specifically, deficits most frequently found in alcoholics are impaired performance in tasks involving visual spatial analysis, tactual spatial analysis, nonverbal abstraction, and set flexibility. Though recovery of many of these functions may occur with abstinence from alcohol, recovery rarely leads to complete remission of symptomatology.

Alcohol produces a range of impairment, from the subtle cognitive difficulties experienced in nonalcoholic heavy drinkers through progressively greater impairment in older adults who drink heavily over short periods of time to long-term alcoholics with the "worst case," alcoholic amnestic dementia (Wernicke-Korsakoff's disease). This chronic end-stage dementia is caused by thiamine deficiency as well as direct toxic effects of alcohol on brain tissues. The dementia, at autopsy, is characterized by widespread neuronal loss, especially in the frontal regions. Alcoholics also experience more rapid rates of cerebral atrophy and degeneration of the mammillary bodies. Clinically, the end stage of alcoholic dementia is characterized by relatively intact intellectual functioning associated with severe anterograde and retrograde amnesia.

To understand the scope of alcohol problems in the elderly, potential mortality from alcohol use should be explored. In the 8-year outcome study described by Helzer et al. (1984), 24 percent of the 234 subjects who were age 60 or older at the interview (midpoint of the field period) were dead at completion of the study, compared with 9 percent of the 1,048 subjects under the age of 60. The proportion of subjects reported to have died of alcohol-related causes was similar for both younger and older alcoholics. Death certificate data will tend to underestimate deaths due to alcohol, but that bias should not be differential across age groups. The relative increased mortality for alcoholics compared with nonalcoholics, however, may be underestimated.

In another study by Nashold and Naor (1981), reports of alcohol as the cause of death in Wisconsin increased markedly between 1963 and 1977. In the older age group, the majority of alcohol-related deaths were due to an underlying cause involving alcohol, for example, cirrhosis. In a further study, Edwards et al. (1983) followed 99 married men diagnosed as having alcoholism over a 10-year period. The increase in risk over the expected deaths in this group was 2.68. Five patients died by suicide or circumstances suggesting suicide. In summary, alcohol leads to an increased risk of mortality both in middle life—thus limiting the number of alcoholics who survive to late life—and in late life. The causes of death among these individuals who drink chronically vary across suicide, accidents, cardiovascular disease, and even cancer. Chronic heavy drinking throughout adult life unquestionably leads to increased mortality.

There are a number of parallels between sleep characteristics of normal aging and those of the chronic alcoholic who is abstinent. For example, the sleep of chronic alcoholics who have withdrawn from alcohol is characterized by decreased slow-wave sleep, interruptions of sleep, and decreased or interrupted periods of rapid eye movement sleep (Adamson and Burdick 1973). Prolonged abstinence from alcohol in middle life, however, will lead to improved sleep over time. In other words, the central nervous system abnormalities produced by alcohol apparently reverse. The older person who uses alcohol as a sedative experiences an additional sleep problem. The relatively rapid metabolism of alcohol, in contrast to most sedative–hypnotics, may produce a rebound awakening 3 to 4 hours into sleep. Even though the older adult using alcohol may fall asleep without difficulty, the sleep is disrupted in the middle of the night.

Given the relatively large number of prescription and nonprescription drugs used by older adults, the interaction of alcohol with these drugs is of special importance in the elderly. The impairments produced by alcohol are augmented by drugs such as sedatives, anticonvulsants, antidepressants, major and minor tranquilizers, and analgesics (especially the opiates). Poor muscle coordination, impaired judgment, and slurred speech are common when these agents are used together. Other side effects are less frequent but can be equally serious. Older adults using oral hypoglycemic agents to treat adult-onset (type II) diabetes can experience unpleasant symptoms (such as nausea and flushing), as do patients who combine disulfiram and alcohol use. Unpredictable fluctuations of plasma glucose concentrations are another potential adverse effect. Some drugs, such as coumarin-type anticoagulants, are blocked in their effectiveness by alcohol, because alcohol increases the metabolism of these drugs (Ritchie 1981). In contrast, plasma concentrations of alcohol are usually not changed by the use of other medications (Garver 1984).

Addiction, Tolerance, and Withdrawal

The most significant clinical problem faced by the clinician treating the older alcoholic is the potential for addiction and tolerance to the agent, with the concomitant problem of alcohol withdrawal. Since alcohol is the only easily available addictive agent in Western society, it is usually the drug of choice for individuals wishing to block unpleasant emotions via drugs. Chronic use of high concentrations of alcohol will lead to addiction. Jaffe (1980) suggests that addiction can operationally be defined as "a behavioral pattern of drug use, characterized by overwhelming involvement with the use of a drug (compulsive use), the securing of its supply, and a high tendency to relapse after withdrawal" (p. 536). Older adults manifest their addiction when placed in a situation in which alcohol is not readily available. They may demonstrate increased anxiety and pursue alcohol in order to decrease this anxiety. In addition, they experience sleep disturbance, nausea, and weakness that are concomitants of a lowered blood-alcohol level. Addiction is a major problem for older adults for at least two reasons. First, patterns of drinking have continued for many years (often dating from early or middle life). In addition, the relatively "quiet" use of alcohol over the years desensitizes both the older adult and the family to the problems with alcohol (Pascarelli 1974; Schuckit 1977).

Akin to addiction is the potential for tolerance with chronic use of alcohol. Not only can older adults become tolerant to alcohol, but they may also in turn become cross-tolerant to a number of drugs similar to alcohol. Despite the potential for relatively normal function among alcoholics (even with ethanol blood levels relatively high), the heavy use of alcohol associated with tolerance continues to create irreversible changes in the liver, the gastrointestinal tract, and the central nervous system (Bosmann 1984). Cross-tolerance, especially with benzodiazepines, is a major clinical concern. Given that older adults are more likely to take benzodiazepines than younger adults, the potential for abuse of both agents separately or in combination increases dramatically (Mellinger et al. 1978).

The symptoms following alcohol withdrawal are not appreciably different across the life cycle. Nevertheless, the older adult may manifest these symptoms, especially the more severe ones, for a longer period following acute cessation of alcohol intake. Initial symptoms include tremors, anxiety, nausea, vomiting, and perspiration. If the withdrawal syndrome is allowed to continue without intervention with either a cross-tolerant drug (such as diazepam) or reinstitution of alcohol, the tremulous state will peak 1 to 2 days following the onset of the withdrawal syndrome. This tremulous peak is accompanied by hallucinations and, in severe cases, withdrawal seizures. Confusion, agitation, and disorientation mark the level of consciousness of the individual. In the older adult with compromised health, the severity of this withdrawal syndrome naturally is greater (Bosmann 1984; Mello and Mendelson 1977).

Diagnostic Workup

The diagnostic workup of the older adult, when alcohol problems are suspected, hinges on a compehensive history. Detailed information should be obtained from the patient first regarding specifics of the drinking behavior. Yet this information must be supplemented by the family, preferably from family members of two generations. Unfortunately, some alcoholic older adults have little or no social network (such as the skid-row alcoholic), and historical information is therefore limited. First, information should be obtained on what the individual drinks and how often he or she drinks in order to make an estimate of alcohol consumption. Does the patient drink constantly? Is there a pattern of binge drinking? Elders who suffer from chronic problems with alcohol are usually regular drinkers. Tolerance for binges decreases with age. A lifetime history of patterns of alcohol use provides a background for present patterns of use. Once again, family members are critical for obtaining such information.

The *CAGE* questions for screening alcohol problems are not as applicable in late life. These questions are as follows:

[C] "... felt the need to *c*ut down on your drinking?"
[A] "... ever felt *a*nnoyed by criticism of your drinking?"
[G] "... had *g*uilty feelings about drinking?"
[E] "... *e*ver take a morning 'eye opener'?"

Since older alcoholics tend to have problems with emergent physical and psychologic symptoms given a persistent drinking pattern over time, personal guilt or concern about drinking is less common. In fact, the older adult may not recognize the connection between new symptoms and drinking habits that have continued for decades.

Additional data to identify drinking problems in the elderly should be derived from the following categories: personal health, family health problems, interpersonal difficulties, and work difficulties (Ewing 1985). The patients should be asked about gastrointestinal symptoms such as nausea, vomiting, diarrhea, abdominal pain, and unexplained gastrointestinal hemorrhages. Neurologic problems should be reviewed, including episodes of amnesia, headaches, and especially peripheral neuropathy. Evidence of falls and lack of attention to personal health, such as bruises, cuts, sprains, cigarette burns, or skin diseases, result from neglect secondary to alcohol.

A thorough review of psychiatric symptoms is essential, including a detailed evaluation of cognitive status, history of major depression, generalized anxiety, and psychotic symptoms (delusions and hallucinations). Paranoid ideation regarding relatives or friends is not uncommon in the severe elderly alcoholic. Suicidal ideation is critical to document, given the elevated risk for suicide in both the elderly and the alcoholic.

Although a genetic predisposition to alcohol problems is less likely in the elderly (especially if the onset of significant drinking problems occurs later in life), obtaining a history of alcohol abuse in the family of the older adult is also biased by other factors. Historical information is less complete for parents and siblings with the elderly. A documented family history of psychiatric disorder (especially major depression and schizophrenia) or alcohol abuse/dependence is important nonetheless.

An indicant of emerging alcohol problems among older persons is concomitant problems in interpersonal relations. Though most often occurring in the marriage, these problems can present between the older adult and children or occasionally with friends. Family problems may be the result of the drinking behavior (such as arguments over an appropriate amount to drink), or they may result from symptoms of the alcohol abuse (such as paranoid ideation or cognitive difficulties).

The physical examination of the older alcoholic is especially important. Not only must the clinician screen for medical problems that may exacerbate alcohol problems (or that may be exacerbated by chronic alcohol use), but overt evidence of alcohol abuse, such as signs of personal neglect of hygiene, provides valuable supplementary information to the history. The neurologic examination should be performed in detail, with attention directed to the evaluation of peripheral neuropathy. Traditional signs of chronic alcohol abuse, such as flushing of the face, injected conjunctiva, tremors, and malnutrition, may merge with normal signs of aging or poor health status.

If evidence of cognitive abnormalities emerges during the mental status examination, further cognitive workup is indicated. The clinician should make every effort to keep the alcoholic older adult abstinent for 2 to 3 weeks prior to detailed psychologic evaluation. These tests may be threatening to the older adult because deficits will frequently appear that have been previously undetected. Baseline cognitive scores, however, can be especially important in monitoring the longitudinal progress of the patient as well as providing additional force to the clinical admonition to abstain from further alcohol use. For example, Parker et al. (1982) suggest that alcohol use above usual consumption increases problems with abstraction significantly in formal testing.

Laboratory evaluation of the alcoholic older adult should include thorough liver-function evaluation (lactate dehydrogenase, serum glutamic-oxaloacetic transaminase, serum glutamic-pyruvic transaminase, and alkaline phosphatase). Given the potential for an electrolyte imbalance, a screening chemistry is essential (with special attention to glucose). Low blood magnesium suggests a magnesium deficiency may occur with alcohol use. Elevated serum and urine amylase suggests chronic pancreatitis. A thyroid panel is also of value, as well as routine evaluation of the pulmonary and cardiovascular system. The electrocardiogram in alcoholic cardiomyopathy will reveal frequent arrhythmias, especially atrial fibrillation.

Once the history, physical, and laboratory examination have been completed, the clinician should assign a diagnosis. Schuckit et al. (1985) have recently reviewed the clinical implications of the diagnoses of alcohol abuse and dependence on the basis of *Diagnostic and Statistical Manual of Mental Disorders (Third Edition) (DSM-III)* (American Psychiatric Association 1980). Ideally, a diagnostic system should provide etiologic information, prognostic information, and information regarding response to treatment. Since etiologic information is difficult to integrate into a diagnostic system (as evidenced by the move away from etiology in *DSM-III* that is continued in the revised edition, *DSM-III-R* [American Psychiatric Association 1987]), more emphasis has been placed on prognosis. When the authors reviewed the clinical significance of the *DSM-III* distinction between a group of males who were diagnosed as suffering from either alcohol abuse or alcohol dependence, they found the two groups were virtually identical. Subjects with alcohol dependence, however, took more drinks per drinking day and had more alcohol-related medical problems and past hospitalizations. During the 1-year follow-up, those diagnosed as suffering from alcohol dependence were somewhat more likely to visit a public detoxification facility. Nevertheless, the authors did not support prognostic implications for the differentiation between alcohol abuse and alcohol dependence in alcoholic patients. These data should be considered within the context of more dependent patterns of alcohol intake emerging in late life.

Schuckit et al. (1985) also propose that the criteria for alcohol dependence should be changed to include not just the accumulation of symptoms gathered retrospectively over the lifetime of the alcoholic's drinking behavior. Specifically, they suggest more objective criteria for tolerance and withdrawal. Their definition of tolerance requires a history of being able to function despite relatively high alcohol concentration, for example, walking or talking coherently in the presence of high blood-alcohol levels. Withdrawal must hamper the ability to work or interact with peers or necessitate medical intervention to qualify. In summary, the clinician may need to adapt the symptom presentations of alcohol abuse/dependence in the elderly from *DSM-III-R* in order for them to be more relevant to clinical management. Documentation of these symptoms and signs, however, is critical regardless of the nomenclature.

Treatment

The treatment of the older patient suffering from alcohol abuse/dependence must include biologic, psychologic, and psychotherapeutic intervention within the social milieu of the patient, especially the family. If the older adult suffers from acute intoxication that leads to a stuporous or comatose state, hospitalization must be instituted for withdrawal from alcohol and institution of the therapeutic program (pharmacologic initially). In milder cases of alcohol dependence, in which withdrawal is the first step, treatment may proceed in the outpatient setting. Outpatient withdrawal is possible only if the patient is highly motivated and willing to allow open monitoring of the withdrawal program by the family, with frequent (often daily) contact with the clinician. Regardless, the initial step in the treatment of alcoholism is to stop alcohol intake. Attempts to work over longer periods of time with the alcoholic who continues to drink are generally doomed to failure.

During the initial phase of withdrawal, restoring fluid and electrolyte balance is essential for the treatment of the severe older alcoholic. Yet the clinician must beware of complaints of thirst and dry mucous membranes. These symptoms and signs may delude the clinician into accepting a diagnosis of dehydration when in fact drying results from alcohol expired through the lungs. To avoid iatrogenic overhydration, the clinician should begin 500 to 1000 ml of a 5 percent normal saline solution while waiting for the results of the blood chemistry. Use of glucose solutions should be avoided, since the older alcoholic may subsist on a diet high in carbohydrates in addition to the alcohol's being metabolized almost entirely as a carbohydrate. Because of poor dietary intake, fluids should be supplemented with parenteral B vitamins. Chronic alcoholics, as noted above, may suffer from magnesium deficiency. A deep intramuscular injection of magnesium at a dose of 0.10 to 0.15 ml/kg added to the initial therapeutic treatment is an important adjunct to therapy (Blazer and Siegler 1984).

The next step in treatment is the institution of medications cross-tolerant with alcohol. Chlordiazepoxide has in the past been the drug of choice for withdrawal because of its relatively extended half-life and clear cross-tolerance. Initial doses obviously depend on the patient's age, weight, and the amount of alcohol consumed over the week prior to admission. Even with these data, however, doses must be carefully titrated during the first 24 to 48 hours of withdrawal. The usual starting dose of the drug is between 50 and 200 mg every 6 to 12 hours until the delirium, agitation, and/or hallucinations appear improved. The older adult may not require as much of the drug. If this therapy proceeds on an outpatient basis, careful monitoring is necessary to ensure that alcohol is not added to the regimen of the benzodiazepine. Chlordiazepoxide, after the first day, can usually be decreased at a rate of approximately 20 percent per day.

When an overt delirium emerges with seizures and hallucinations, diazepam may be a better anticonvulsant because of its more rapid onset. If memory problems increase, dysarthria emerges, and ataxia presents in the elderly patient, drug intoxication has developed secondary to excessive medication (or synergistic effects of the drug with alcohol). When drug intoxication occurs, the drug should be discontinued for 24 to 36 hours and the patient carefully observed for a recurrence of the withdrawal symptoms. Then the drug can be reinstituted. If persistent signs and symptoms of withdrawal are seen beyond 3 days after the last known drink, the clinician should consider dependence on minor tranquilizers or hypnotics as well as alcohol.

Some withdrawal programs in communities encourage withdrawal within a social setting (a detoxification center) based on social support in the absence of drug use. Though some rehabilitation centers in hospitals may overuse medication, the severe effects of withdrawal, such as delirium tremens, should dissuade the clinician from routinely using such withdrawal settings, especially in the older adult.

Following detoxification, the long-term goals of treatment become paramount in the treatment process. First, the clinician should consider prophylaxis with disulfiram (Antabuse). If the drug is used, a contract must be established between the physician, the patient, and at least one family member. A family member (or possibly a local emergency room) should have responsibility for administering the daily dose of disulfiram to the alcoholic. The older alcoholic, in turn, must take the tablet when offered. Both the patient and family members are to be warned of potential effects of disulfiram if alcohol is ingested. The acetaldehyde that increases in the blood when ethanol and disulfiram are present concurrently can lead to the "acetaldehyde syndrome"—a flushing of the face, tense throbbing in the head and neck (which may develop into a pulsating headache), difficulty breathing, nausea, vomiting, sweating, thirst, chest pains, hypertension, vertigo, blurred vision, and confusion. These can be easily reviewed from the package insert provided by the manufacturer. There is no evidence that disulfiram is contraindicated in late life. Nevertheless, if medical status is compromised, the clinician must carefully weigh the benefits versus potential problems of prescribing disulfiram.

Therapeutic intervention with the family is essential. First, they should be warned of the severe and potentially irreversible problems that alcohol can create in the older adult, specifically, memory problems. Most families are more concerned with the immediate effects of intoxication. If the older family member drinks silently without overt signs of alcohol abuse, this may be tolerated without being accepted. The threshold for concern in the family must therefore be lowered through the process of education. Patient, family, and clinician become a team as they seek to correct the problem of concern to all.

Self-help groups are essential in the long-term support of the abstinent alcoholic. Alcoholics Anonymous has proved over many years to be effective in encouraging abstinence for individuals throughout the life cycle. Support groups provide social support coupled with appropriate pressure from peers who have suffered from similar problems. They are complementary to the authority of the clinician and must not be considered a threat to medical authority. Alcoholics Anonymous may be especially beneficial to the older alcoholic who is discouraged and lonely secondary to isolation and feelings of uselessness. Involvement in the group setting, coupled with a sense of helping others and interaction with individuals at other stages of the life cycle, may reintegrate such individuals into society.

Many older persons, however, resist the suggestion to join one of these self-help groups. One reason is that the elder continues to deny the problem or believes him- or herself perfectly capable of correcting the problem alone. One reason such beliefs are so persistent in the elderly is the self-sufficient attitude of many in the current elderly cohort. More commonly, the older adult feels no fit with the environment of such self-help groups. The cohort of elderly alcoholics in the latter part of the 20th century have not had the experience with recovery groups and the self-help phenomena that older adults will have had who reach late life in the early years of the 21st century. Clinicians should encourage participation in such self-help groups (given their frequent success) but not force the older adult to participate. Support from family members and the clinician and integration into more traditional social environments may accomplish the same purpose (Butler and Lewis 1977). In mobilizing coping resources, the environmental system (acute and chronic stressors, social network resources), the health care system (availability of health care services such as medical intervention, behavioral therapy, and educational programs), and coping strategies of the older patient can be woven into a unique matrix for a given elder. Such an integrated approach not only enables a more comprehensive evaluation of the diagnostic profile, it also provides a framework from which treatment outcomes can be derived. Successful approaches to intervention should target specific points within the system for change while maintaining a recognition that the entire system is interdependent.

Drug Abuse

Drug abuse is usually associated with adolescents and young adults. Certainly the abuse of illicit drugs is uncommon in older adults. Nevertheless, the problem must not be overlooked. The propensity of older adults to use prescription drugs inappropriately suggests that late life is a period of high risk for the side effects of this misuse. Glantz (1981) suggests that the motivation for drug abuse among the elderly may have many similarities to the motivation among adolescents. Both must negotiate a period of uncertain and changing roles as well as changes in self-concept. Older persons face step-downs on the economic ladder and disadvantages in the employment market. Friends and relatives may not be as available through distances or may be removed by death. Though self-sufficiency continues to be a means of coping (adolescents and the elderly both strive for control), the ability of the impaired older adult to maintain self-reliance and independence is compromised. Drugs are easily available to both groups. The adolescent seeks illegal drugs on the street; the older adult obtains addictive drugs from local physicians. For example, Capel et al. (1972) discovered that the majority of addicts who survive to late life continue their drug use via concealed habits and using substitute narcotics such as hydromorphone hydrochloride (Dilaudid). Alcohol and barbiturates may be added to the lower dosed narcotic.

Even the progress from milder to more powerful drugs, frequently seen in the movement to addiction among adolescents, may have parallels among the elderly (Glantz 1981). Older persons begin taking mild analgesics and sedative–hypnotic agents but fail to obtain the relief they desire. Without realizing the danger of addiction, they progress to the use of narcotic analgesics for chronic pain problems and higher doses of tranquilizing and sedative–hypnotic agents. Once addiction and tolerance are established, the older adult exhibits little initiative to reverse the problem. Obtaining medications from multiple physicians and borrowing medicines from family members feed the habit over time. Frequently, hospitalization uncovers the addiction, since withdrawal symptoms appear 3 to 4 days after admission.

Problems deriving from excessive and inappropriate prescription and over-the-counter drug use are well documented in the geriatric literature. Eighty-five percent of older persons living in the community and 95 percent in long-term care facilities receive prescription drugs (Law and Chalmers 1976). In 1976, more than 12 prescriptions were written per person each year for those 65 and older (Lamy and Vestal 1976). Undoubtedly, these estimates are even higher today.

The Scope of the Problem

The frequency of excessive drug use in the elderly, especially the use of psychoactive drugs, is well documented in the literature. Mellinger et al. (1978) reported from a household survey of more than 2,000 people that among those persons over 60 years of age, 20 percent of women and 17 percent of men regularly used psychoactive drugs during the year preceding the survey (higher than any other age group). Eleven percent of the men and 25 percent of the women had used a minor tranquilizer and/or sedative at least once during the year prior to the survey in the 60+ age group (again higher than for any other age group).

A more recent report from the National Medical Care Expenditure Survey (Rossiter 1983) documents that persons 65 years of age and older are more likely to use pain relievers (25.9 percent) and psychoactive drugs (23.4 percent) prescribed by a physician during the past year. Except for cardiovascular medications, analgesic and psychotherapeutic drugs were used the most by older adults. In a review of nursing home prescribing habits, Ray et al. (1980) found that in 173 Tennessee nursing homes, 43 percent of the patients had received antipsychotic medications during the year prior to the survey and 9 percent were chronic recipients; that is, they received at least 365 daily doses during the preceding year.

Christopher et al. (1978), reporting on 873 hospitalized persons in Dundee, Scotland, concluded that prescribing in this inpatient population was not excessive, an average of three medications being received at any given time. Patients on the geriatric ward were receiving the highest number of drugs. However, certain drug groups, especially the sedative–hypnotics, were prescribed excessively with few attempts to reduce the dose with increasing age. The prevalence of hypnotic use ranged from more than 40 percent among the medical patients to more than 70 percent on the geriatric wards. Salzman and van der Kolk (1980) found, in 195 hospitalized persons over the age of 60, that one-third received at least one psychotropic drug the day of the survey. Hypnotics were the most frequently prescribed drugs, with flurazepam being the drug of choice. The authors noted that each of the psychoactive drugs prescribed had potentially dangerous side effects and dosing of these drugs did not reflect attention paid to the aging population by the clinicians treating these patients.

In the community, however, the evidence of significant abuse of illicit drugs in the elderly is remarkably absent. The best data available are those derived from the Epidemiologic Catchment Area (ECA) studies. Myers et al. (1984) found no evidence of drug abuse in the 65+ age group at two of the three ECA sites surveyed and a prevalence of 0.2 percent at the third site. More than 3,000 persons age 65 and older were interviewed during this survey. Regarding the lifetime prevalence of drug abuse or dependence, fewer than 0.1 percent of these subjects at the three ECA sites reported any history (Robins et al. 1984). These studies are subject to bias, given the difficulty in recalling information regarding drug abuse and/or denial of this use. Nevertheless, denial and selective recall are probably no more a problem for the elderly than any other stage of life. What is more likely to contribute to the relatively low prevalence of current and lifetime drug abuse among the elderly, compared with younger persons, is a cohort effect (older persons in the 1980s were never heavy users of drugs) and selective mortality (persons from the present generation of older adults who did use medications did not survive to late life). However, community surveys that rely on household data may underestimate drug abuse, especially by failure to include the homeless and transients.

Behavioral and Social Correlates of Drug Abuse in Older Adults

Many psychosocial factors contribute to the potential toxicity and addictive potential of both prescription and illicit drugs among the elderly (Blazer 1983). Certain character traits of older adults contribute to increased drug use (Baldessarini 1977). The more passive older adult may use drugs prescribed by a number of physicians without question. Even "double prescribing," the prescription of the same drug by two or more physicians, goes unchallenged by the dependent elder. Addiction accrues over time without being noticed by the patient, family, or physician. Only when admitted to the hospital for possibly an unrelated disorder will the symptoms of an addiction become apparent. Once hospitalized, passive older adults often fail to report a change in medications from the outpatient to the hospital setting, expecting the physician to "know" how to manage their problems. Those patients who appear most compliant could be the most prone to drug abuse in an outpatient medical or psychiatric practice.

In addition to character traits, the social setting surrounding the prescription of medications affects the patient's potential for abusing medications. Many psychosocial factors determine the pattern of therapeutic drug use. Noncompliance, a most important factor in treating psychiatric disorders, usually does not contribute to drug abuse. Rather, older adults are more inclined not to take prescribed medications on schedule than to use prescribed drugs excessively. Blackwell (1973) estimated that up to 50 percent of patients do not take prescribed medications. The potential for addiction may be actualized, however, if the milieu for prescribing medications discourages communication between the older adult and the physician (Lamy 1980). In the distracting and hurried environment of the physician's office, proper use of medication frequently is not communicated to the older adult. Because older persons are hesitant to ask questions, they leave the office without understanding how a drug is to be used. To please the physician, they take the medication, but not at the dose required. As a result of older persons' frequently carrying all of their medications in one container, the potential for confusion regarding when a particular drug should be taken is exacerbated. Intoxication from excessive use of the benzodiazepines is not uncommon under these circumstances.

Sharing and swapping medications among older adults are a not infrequent precipitant of abuse or dependence. Friends, roommates, or spouses are treated by different physicians for similar problems. Through informal communication with one another regarding the effectiveness of individual drug therapies, the elder may mistakenly determine that a friend's physician has prescribed a better treatment than his or her own. Because limited finances frequently preclude obtaining a second opinion (or even in investing in a new prescription), medications are informally shared. Through the additive effects of drugs, such as the sedative–hypnotics, evidence of addiction or abuse appears, often unexplained to the primary care physician. The diagnosis of the problem is further complicated because older adults are hesitant to reveal that they have obtained medications from another source.

Another contributor to problems of abuse is over-the-counter drug use. In Western societies, over-the-counter drugs are used even more often than prescription drugs. Chaiton et al. (1976) estimated that more than 50 percent of one group of elders surveyed had used at least one over-the-counter drug during the 48 hours preceding the community survey. Most of these elders had not consulted a physician regarding the use of the drug or potential interaction with prescription drugs. The most commonly used of the over-the-counter drugs are agents to improve sleep, to improve gastrointestinal symptoms (such as constipation), and to relieve pain. The combination of nonprescription drugs with anticholinergic effects (such as diphenhydramine) with prescribed antidepressants and/or phenothiazine agents can lead to significant anticholinergic toxicity or even a full-blown central anticholinergic syndrome.

"Do something" prescribing is an iatrogenic contributor to drug abuse in the elderly. If the older adult pays for a doctor's consultation, he or she expects a result—the result usually being a prescription. Physicians also gain some assurance that they have contributed their part to the patient–physician contract when they write a prescription. Drugs prescribed under these circumstances are often not prescribed to treat specific target symptoms. Benzo-diazepines, sedative–hypnotic agents, tricyclic antidepressants, and even neuroleptics become the drugs of choice because of the mistaken view that the drugs promote the general well-being of the patient. Not only does such a prescribing practice reinforce a pattern of medical care that discourages the physician from talking with the older adult, it also increases the likelihood of polypharmacy.

A variation on the theme of "do something" prescribing that may contribute to drug addiction and/or abuse in the elderly is defensive prescribing. Those physicians who serve as medical directors or have large consulting practices in long-term care facilities are frequently called by nursing staff and even family members about disturbing and uncontrollable physical or behavioral symptoms. Agitation and sleep problems are among the most common encountered by a stressed nursing staff. Against his or her better judgment, a physician may prescribe medications not so much to alleviate a specific symptom in an older adult as to reassure staff and family members. Defensive prescribing is not an indictment of the lack of care by a physician, nursing staff, or family. Rather, it is a symptom of a difficult situation—the management of an acutely agitated and frequently cognitively impaired older adult in a facility with limited personnel. Nevertheless, such prescribing practices are major contributors to addiction and abuse in older adults.

Diagnostic Workup

The diagnostic workup of the older adult when drug abuse or dependence is suspected is similar to that described for the workup of alcohol abuse and dependence. Many of the symptoms described earlier apply to prescription and nonprescription drug abuse as well. Though older adults may present to the clinician as having overdosed on a sedative, narcotic, or other agent, the most common presentations of drug misuse/abuse are symptoms of toxicity and/or withdrawal.

The benzodiazepines (both anxiolytic and sedative–hypnotics) are the most commonly prescribed drugs and therefore the most likely to be abused. Symptoms characteristic of benzodiazepine toxicity include sedation, confusional states, and "sundowning" (heightened agitation or frank delirium at night), ataxia, and even stupor or coma. The potential for a fatal overdose is low with these agents alone, but when benzodiazepines are combined with other agents, such as alcohol, the potential increases dramatically. Withdrawal symptoms, in contrast, may mimic the psychiatric disorder for which the drugs were originally prescribed. Anxiety and agitation, sleep problems, muscle cramps (especially in the legs), tremors, and perceptual distortions may emerge upon withdrawal. The most serious symptom, however, is the onset of seizures.

Tricyclic antidepressants are frequently prescribed and may contribute to increased problems with memory, confusion, and sedation. Confusion and even fugue states are described in the morning following an excessive nighttime dose of the tricyclic antidepressants, frequently accompanied by postural hypotension and excessive lethargy. In a bipolar patient, successful use of a tricyclic to reverse depressive symptoms may later trigger an elevation in mood and an increase in activity. Even a frank manic episode with delusions and hallucinations can be precipitated by these drugs.

Lithium carbonate, a most effective drug in the treatment of manic–depressive illness, can be especially problematic for older adults. Symptoms including dizziness, ataxia, drowsiness, and especially confusion may occur on serum levels below 1.0 mEq/l. Older persons do not tolerate lithium therapy as well as persons in middle life, and therefore the drug must be prescribed with extreme caution. Self-abuse with lithium is uncommon, but the desire of the clinician to obtain therapeutic effect in a patient who suffers from rapid-cycling bipolar disorder or unipolar recurrent depression augments the potential for lithium toxicity.

When these or other symptoms emerge, a thorough history from the patient and family (similar to that described above for alcohol problems) is the next clinical step of importance. If the clinician questions the history, many laboratories provide a toxic drug screen. Most of these laboratories can return results within 6 hours to the clinician. Specimens can be from either urine or blood. Toxic screens must be interpreted cautiously, for drugs are often cross-reactive to the probes used in the screen. Other ancillary laboratory procedures, such as electrophysiologic tracing, cardiac monitoring, and radiologic examination (for problems deriving from drug use), can be obtained as well.

Treatment of Drug Abuse/Dependence in Older Adults

Treatment approaches for drug abuse/dependence in the older adult are similar to those at other stages of the life cycle. Given that the older adult is frail, however, the clinician must be careful to err on the side of conservatism. Specifically, early hospitalization is especially indicated when evidence of abuse is presented. For example, the older adult who chronically takes benzodiazepines and is found to be excessively lethargic should be hospitalized (despite the clinician's recognition of the cause of the problem and the family's insistence that the problem can be managed at home).

The immediate goal upon hospitalization is to remove the potential for acute toxicity from the medication. If drug ingestion is recent, gastric evacuation is indicated. In the elderly, however, special care must be taken to avoid aspiration. Activated charcoal (30 g) has been recommended along with the lavage to absorb barbiturates, alcohol, and propoxyphene (Ellinwood et al. 1985). Once the clinician is convinced that the potential for acute toxicity has been removed, the patient should be transferred to a ward where close monitoring is possible. Electrocardiographic monitoring is often indicated for the first 24 to 48 hours. Monitoring of respirations, however, is of most importance (especially if evidence of slow, rapid, or shallow breathing presents). When improvement does not ensue, peritoneal dialysis or hemodialysis may be indicated.

Once the patient has survived the immediate problems of overdose, the next challenge presented to the clinician is to avoid the emergence of withdrawal. Depending on the half-life of a given agent, withdrawal may last from 6 hours to 8 to 10 days (for example, the half-life of flurazepam may exceed 200 hours in an older adult). Support with the medication or a substitute drug is indicated during this period. At the same time, the clinician must begin educating the patient and family regarding the cause of the hospitalization and the need to change the outpatient drug therapy significantly in order to avoid the recurrence of such a problem. With most elders, such education and intervention, in the course of an acute hospitalization for drug problems, are effective. Older adults are often unaware of the potential problems from drug use and therefore are most happy to be free of the potential of future addiction or toxic reactions secondary to a medication.

In some cases, however, the older adult will continue to seek medications, especially analgesics and benzodiazepine-like compounds. In such cases, careful monitoring as outpatients and much work with the family provide the best means for successfully achieving a long-term abstinence from drugs of potential abuse. Because elders tend to use the same pharmacy despite multiple physicians, contact with the pharmacist to monitor drug use can be especially helpful.

References

Adamson J, Burdick JA: Sleep of dry alcoholics. Arch Gen Psychiatry 1973; 28:146–149

American Psychiatric Association: Diagnostic and Statistical Manual of Mental Disorders (Third Edition). Washington, DC, American Psychiatric Association, 1980

American Psychiatric Association: Diagnostic and Statistical Manual of Mental Disorders (Third Edition-Revised). Washington, DC, American Psychiatric Association, 1987

Armor D, Johnston D, Pollich S, et al: Trends in U.S. Adult Drinking Practices. Santa Monica, CA, Rand Corporation, 1977

Baldessarini RJ: Chemotherapy in Psychiatry. Cambridge, MA, Harvard University Press, 1977

Blackwell B: Patient compliance. N Engl J Med 1973; 289:249

Blazer D: Drug management in the elderly, in Experimental and Clinical Interventions in Aging. Edited by Walker RF, Cooper RL. New York, Marcel Dekker, 1983

Blazer D, Siegler IC: A Family Approach to Health Care in the Elderly. Menlo Park, CA, Addison-Wesley, 1984

Bosmann HB: Pharmacology of alcoholism in aging, in Alcoholism in the Elderly. Edited by Hartford JT, Samorajski T. New York, Raven Press, 1984

Butler RN, Lewis MI: Aging and Mental Health (Second Edition). St. Louis, C.V. Mosby, 1977

Capel WC, Goldsmith BM, Waddell KJ, et al: The aging narcotic addict: an increasing problem for the next decades. J Gerontol 1972; 27:102–106

Chaiton A, Spitzer WO, Roberts RS, et al: Patterns of medical drug use—a community focus. Can Med Assoc J 1976; 114:33–37

Chowdhury AR, Malmud LS, Dinoso VP: Gastrointestinal plasma protein loss during ethanol ingestion. Gastroenterology 1977; 72:37–40

Christopher LJ, Ballinger BR, Shepherd AMM, et al: Drug-prescribing patterns in the elderly: a cross-sectional study of in-patients. Age Ageing 1978; 7:74–82

Edwards G, Oppenheimer E, Duckitt A, et al: What happens to alcoholics? Lancet 1983; 2:269–271

Ellinwood EH, Woody G, Krishnan RR: Treatment for drug abuse, in Psychiatry (Volume 2). Edited by Michels R, Cavenar JO. Philadelphia, J. B. Lippincott, 1985

Ewing JA: Substance abuse: alcohol, in Psychiatry (Volume 2). Edited by Michels R, Cavenar JO. Philadelphia, J.B. Lippincott, 1985

Faris D: The prevention of alcoholism and economic alcoholism. Prev Med 1974; 3:36–48

Garver DL: Age effects on alcohol metabolism, in Alcoholism in the Elderly. Edited by Hartford JT, Samorajski T. New York, Raven Press, 1984

Gersovitz M, Motio K, Munro HN, et al: Human protein requirements: assessment of the adequacy of the current recommended dietary allowance for dietary protein in elderly men and women. Am J Clin Nutr 1982; 35:6–14

Glantz M: Predictions of elderly drug abuse. J Psychoactive Drugs 1981; 13:117–126

Glatt MM: Experiences with elderly alcoholics in England. Alcoholism 1978; 2:23–26

Glynn RJ, Bouchard GR, Locastro JS, et al: Changes in alcohol consumption behaviors among men in the normative aging study, in Nature and Extent of Alcohol Problems Among the Elderly (Research Monograph No. 14). Edited by Maddox G, Robins LN, Rosenberg N. Rockville, MD, National Institute on Alcohol Abuse and Alcoholism, 1984

Gordon T, Kannel WB: Drinking and its relation to smoking, blood pressure, blood lipids and uric acid: the Framingham study. Arch Intern Med 1983; 143:1366–1374

Helzer JE, Carey KE, Miller RH: Predictors and correlates of recovery in older vs younger alcoholics, in Nature and Extent of Alcohol Problems Among the Elderly (Research Monograph No. 14). Edited by Maddox G, Robins LN, Rosenberg N. Rockville, MD, National Institute on Alcohol Abuse and Alcoholism, 1984

Jaffe JH: Drug addiction and drug abuse, in The Pharmacological Basis of Therapeutics (Sixth Edition). Edited by Gilman AG, Goodman LS, Gilman A. New York, Macmillan, 1980

Kalant H, Kahnna JM, Israel Y: The alcohols, in Principles of Medical Pharmacology (Third Edition). Edited by Seemen P, Sellars VM, Roschlau WHE. Toronto, University of Toronto Press, 1980

Lamy PP: Prescribing for the Elderly. Littleton, MA, PSG Publishing, 1980

Lamy PP, Vestal RE: Drug prescribing for the elderly. Hosp Pract 1976; 11:111–118

Law R, Chalmers C: Medicines and elderly people: a general practice survey. Br Med J 1976; 1:565–568

Maddox GL, Blazer DG: Alcohol and aging. Center Reports on Advances in Research, (Duke University Center for the Study of Aging and Human Development) 1985; 8(4):1–6

Mellinger GD, Balter MB, Manheimer DI, et al: Psychic distress, life crisis, and use of psychotherapeutic medications. Arch Gen Psychiatry 1978; 35:1045–1052

Mello NK, Mendelson JH: Clinical aspects of alcohol dependence, in Drug Addiction: I. Morphine, Sedative/Hypnotic and Alcohol Dependence. Edited by Martin WR. Berlin, Springer-Verlag, 1977

Muehlberger CW: The physiologic action of alcohol. JAMA 1958; 167:1840–1845

Myers JK, Weissman MM, Tischler GL, et al: Six-month prevalence of psychiatric disorders in three communities. Arch Gen Psychiatry 1984; 41:959–970

Nashold RD, Naor EM: Alcohol-related deaths in Wisconsin: the impact of alcohol mortality. Am J Public Health 1981; 71:1237–1271

Parker ES, Parker DA, Brodie JA, et al: Cognitive patterns resembling premature aging in male social drinkers. Alcoholism 1982; 6:46–52

Pascarelli EF: Drug dependence: an age-old problem compounded by old age. Geriatrics 1974; 29(12):109–110

Rathbone-McCuan E, Lohn H, Levenson J, et al: Community Survey of Aged Alcoholics and Problem Drinkers. DHEW Grant No. 1R18 AAD 1734-01 Final Project Report to DHEW by Levindale Geriatric Research Center, June 1976

Ray WA, Federspiel CF, Schaffner W: A study of antipsychotic drug use in nursing homes: epidemiologic evidence suggesting misuse. Am J Public Health 1980; 70:485–491

Ritchie JN: The aliphatic alcoholics, in The Pharmacologic Basis of Therapeutics (Sixth Edition). Edited by Gilman AG, Goodman LS, Gilman A. New York, Macmillan, 1981

Robins LN, Helzer JE, Weissman MM, et al: Lifetime prevalence of specific psychiatric disorders in three sites. Arch Gen Psychiatry 1984; 41:949–958

Rossiter LF: Prescribed medications: findings from the National Medical Care Expenditure Survey. Am J Public Health 1983; 73:312–315

Salzman C, van der Kolk B: Psychotropc drug prescriptions for elderly patients in a general hospital. J Am Geriatr Soc 1980; 28:18–22

Schuckit MA: Geriatric alcoholism and drug abuse. Gerontologist 1977; 17:168–174

Schuckit MA, Zisook S, Mortola J: Clinical implications of *DSM-III* diagnoses of alcohol abuse and alcohol dependence. Am J Psychiatry 1985; 142:1403–1408

Warheit GJ, Auth JB: The mental health and social correlates of alcohol use among differing life cycle groups, in Nature and Extent of Alcohol Problems Among the Elderly (Research Monograph No. 14). Edited by Maddox G, Robins LN, Rosenberg N. Rockville, MD, National Institute on Alcohol Abuse and Alcoholism, 1984

Wiberg GS, Samson JM, Maxwell WB, et al: Further studies on the acute toxicity of ethanol in young and old rats: relative importance of pulmonary excretion and total body water. Toxicol Appl Pharmacol 1971; 20:22–29

Yano K, Rhoads GG, Kajan A: Coffee, alcohol, and risk of coronary artery disease among Japanese men living in Hawaii. N Engl J Med 1977; 297:405–409

Treatment of Psychiatric Disorders
in Late Life

Chapter 20

The Pharmacologic Treatment of Psychiatric Disorders in the Elderly

Jonathan Davidson, M.D.

The number of aging individuals in the U.S. population continues to grow. In 1950, approximately 8 percent of the population was above age 65, a figure that is expected to grow to 12 percent, or 32 million people, by the year 2000. There is a particular increase in the number of individuals above age 80, who are perhaps the most vulnerable group from the standpoint of health problems. Similar trends have occurred in other countries, such as Great Britain, where the number of people between ages 65 and 74 has increased one-third between 1950 and 1981, while those over 75 have increased by 40 percent. Older people are more likely to experience bereavement, which also serves as a risk factor for illness. For example, Mor et al. (1986) found an increased use of antianxiety medication and alcohol and more physician visits following bereavement; bereaved spouses are twice as likely to be hospitalized. An idea of the kinds of illness that are commonly seen in older patients can be obtained from the Epidemiological Catchment Area study (Weissman et al. 1984), which showed the following disorders to be most frequent in men over age 65: severe cognitive impairment, phobic anxiety, alcohol abuse, dysthymic disorder. Older women presented most often with phobic anxiety, severe cognitive impairment, dysthymic disorder, and major depression without bereavement. Treatment of psychiatric illness in the elderly is often difficult because of the greater likelihood on concomitant chronic physical illness, such as cardiovascular, cerebrovascular, and degenerative joint diseases, as well as malignant disease.

515

General Pharmacologic and Physiologic Considerations

In using phamacotherapy, it is important to recognize that physiologic changes in the elderly affect the pharmacokinetics and pharmacodynamics of drug activity. Patients often take multiple medications, which can lead to compliance problems, drug–drug interactions, and iatrogenic illness. In an elderly person, it is sometimes unnecessary to look further than the combination of drugs in order to explain the appearance of new symptoms. The physiologic changes will often mean that a drug that might be well tolerated in a younger patient will produce a heightened effect at the same dose in an older person. It is usually preferable to initiate treatment at a dose no more than one-half the recommended adult dose, and then build up the dose slowly. The four main processes involved in drug disposition are absorption, distribution, metabolism, and elimination.

Drug absorption can be delayed in older people, as a result of any of the following factors: reduction of motility, impaired epithelial transport mechanism, or reduced intestinal blood flow. In addition, there is reduced blood flow to the liver relative to brain and coronary arteries in old age. These considerations may be of more theoretical than actual importance, because drug effects are often enhanced in older persons. Thus, any reduction of absorption can be more than offset by changes in other processes that effect drug disposition.

Many drugs are lipophilic, being taken up for storage in fatty tissue. The fraction of fat to total body weight increases with age from 25 percent up to 45 percent. As a result there is a relatively larger volume of distribution available for antidepressant, antipsychotic, and benzodiazepine drugs, all of which are lipophilic. Conversely, a hydrophilic drug like lithium will have a small volume of distribution. Another important change with respect to drug distribution relates to the declining amount of albumin, which is reduced by as much as 25 percent between the ages of 40 and 60. Many drugs are protein bound, and only a small fraction are transported in the active, or free, state. Even a limited reduction of the protein-bound fraction will increase the free fraction by a substantial amount, thereby effectively raising the amount of active drug.

Drug metabolism usually takes place in the liver; with reduced perfusion, the process of metabolism and inactivation will be delayed and/or reduced. Drugs that are inactivated by glucuronidation are less affected than those that are oxidized. Drugs having a higher potential for hepatotoxicity (e.g., chlorpromazine and hydrazine monoamine oxidase inhibitors [MAOIs]) should be used more cautiously. As a general rule, it is preferable to choose the drug with the simplest metabolic profile. For example, haloperidol would be preferred over thioridazine, desipramine over imipramine, and oxazepam over diazepam, all other things being equal.

Other concomitant medication can affect drug metabolism. Methylphenidate, propranolol, and neuroleptics may all increase the plasma level of tricyclic drugs by competing for the same metabolizing enzymes. Other drugs, such as dilantin and barbiturates, can induce hepatic enzymes and thereby lower the plasma level of a tricyclic.

Elimination of drugs is related not only to liver function, but also to renal function. Renal function and perfusion decline with age, and drugs like lithium, dextroamphetamine, fluvoxamine and nortriptyline, in all of which renal excretion is a significant pathway, are likely to have a more prolonged effect in the elderly. Plasma levels of antidepressant drugs may increase in the elderly because of impaired renal excretion (Richey 1975). Drug pharmacodynamics alter with age, as a result of decreases in receptor number, neurotransmitter levels, and structural changes in the target organs. The catecholamine and indoleamine metabolizing enzyme, monoamine oxidase, increases above age 55, and this might partially account for the lowered concentration of norepinephrine and serotonin in old age.

Treatment of Psychotic States

Slater and Roth (1972) have described the development of first-onset schizophrenic-like psychosis in late life. Sometimes referred to as late paraphrenia, this term has not been sanctioned by *DSM-III-R*. Post (cited in Slater and Roth [1972]) believes that paraphrenia should be seen as a partial or incomplete form of schizophrenia, and he draws no distinction over drug responsiveness. However, there appears to be some evidence from human lymphocyte antigen studies that this condition differs genetically and biologically from schizophrenia (Naguib et al. 1985). It may account for 8 to 9 percent of all female first hospital admissions above age 65. The disorder occurs characteristically in single women, being accompanied by paranoid delusions or hallucinations, but with little or no evidence of dementia. As many as one-third have hearing impairment, and visual impairment is by no means rare. Five percent have cerebral disease, but lack organic features. The prognosis for survival is better than for the dementias, and the life expectancy is identical to that of the normal population (Kay 1959). In Post's (1962) study, 27 out of 35 cases responded to adequate doses of phenothiazines for an extended period, but showed a high relapse rate when medication was stopped. If the illness is not properly treated by pharmacotherapy, the remission rate is as low as 7 out of 23, and the illness can pursue a chronic course. Many patients with late-onset paraphrenic illness have exhibited suspiciousness and a long-standing tendency to isolate themselves from others; therefore it is often important to mobilize all available support systems to ensure compliance with medication and to detect signs of relapse at the earliest opportunity.

Schizophrenia of early onset tends to change its presentation with age: Rather than exhibiting florid positive signs and symptoms of the disorder, the older patient will more often manifest withdrawal.

Mania can occur in the older individual, and it has been estimated that between 6 and 19 percent of consecutively admitted older patients with affective disorder carry a diagnosis of mania (Post 1984). The coexistence of perplexity in the symptom picture may lead to the mistaken impression of an organic state. Treatment of mania in an older person follows the same psychopharmacologic principles that would apply to a younger patient, with due allowance being made for dose adjustment, greater likelihood of side effects, reduced renal clearance in the case of lithium, and reduced rate of inactivation of neuroleptics.

Organic psychoses are characteristically seen in elders. These can be produced by a number of pathologic states, for example, electrolyte imbalance; alcohol withdrawal or hallucinosis; tumor; infection; metabolic, endocrine, and iatrogenic causes (e.g., such drugs as anticholinergic compounds, including antihistamines, antidepressants, antiparkinsonian drugs, and antiarrhythmics); steroids, bronchodilators, digitalis, diuretics, and analgesics. It is important to establish possible etiology before embarking on a neuroleptic crusade. If there is some urgency to initiate treatment without knowledge of cause, then neuroleptic therapy should proceed with caution, and it is better to use a drug with minimal anticholinergic properties. Dementia may lead to psychotic symptoms, such as paranoid delusions, hallucinations, or behavioral and psychomotor changes that will respond to treatment with antipsychotic medication.

Antipsychotic Drugs

The same drugs that are used to treat psychosis in the younger adult are also used in the older patient, the primary drugs in this regard being the dopamine-receptor-blocking neuroleptics. Other potentially useful but less well researched drugs for treating psychosis in the elderly include lithium, benzodiazepines, and carbamazepine.

The major classes of neuroleptics are listed in Table 1. Aliphatic phenothiazines are of low potency and are nonspecific in their effect; that is, they have impact on a number of other systems besides dopaminergic pathways. They have marked anticholinergic, antiadrenergic, and sedative properties, and are more likely to produce organ toxicity than are other neuroleptics. The aliphatic drugs contain a three-ring nucleus and carbon atom side chain, similar to tricyclic antidepressants when viewed two-dimensionally, but differing from the antidepressants when viewed in a three-dimensional or configurational way. The following drugs belong to the aliphatic group: chlorpromazine (e.g., Thorazine) and promazine (e.g., Sparine). Piperidine phenothiazines also have low potency and resemble the aliphatic drugs in many ways. The piperidine phenothiazines include thiordiazine (e.g., Mellaril) and its metabolite, mesoridazine (e.g., Serentil).

The dose range of each drug is given in Table 1. Although they are

Table 1. Classes of Neuroleptics and Their Dose Ranges

Category	Drug Name	Dose Range (mg/day)[a]
Phenothiazines		
Aliphatic	Chlorpromazine	30–300
Piperidine	Thioridazine	30–300
Piperazine	Trifluoperazine	1–15
	Perphenazine	8–32
	Fluphenazine	1–10
Butyrophenones	Haloperiodol	2–20
Thioxanthenes	Thiothixene	2–20
	Chlorprothixene	30–300
Dibenzoxapines	Loxapine	
Dihydroindolones	Molindone	

[a]Although there is in reality a very wide dose range, and dose selection should be determined on the basis of individual response, these ranges are sufficient for most older patients.

generally not the drugs of first choice, and despite having more side effects than other neuroleptics, the aliphatic and piperidine phenothiazines are in many cases the most effective drugs for older patients. The initial dose will be determined by a number of factors besides the patient's age: Adequacy of hydration, degree of orthostatis, cardiac function, concomitant medications, and severity of psychotic symptoms are all important considerations. In almost all cases the starting dose will be lower than the starting dose for younger adults.

Other neuroleptic drug classes are of higher potency, and do not have such a wide spectrum of activity; that is, they are less sedating and have weaker effects on the peripheral autonomic nervous system, but they are more likely to induce extrapyramidal reactions. Tardive dyskinesia, however, is equally likely to arise in association with any neuroleptic. These other classes of neuroleptics include (1) piperazine phenothiazines—trifluoperazine, fluphenazine, perphenazine, acetophenazine, and prochlorperazine, although the latter two are rarely used and prochlorperazine has poor antipsychotic

effect; (2) thioxanthenes—thiothixene and chlorprothixene; (3) butyrophenones—haloperidol; (4) dibenzoxapines—loxapine; and (5) dihydroindo-
lones—molindone.

Side effects of antipsychotic drugs. Anticholinergic effects of the
aliphatic and piperidine phenothiazines include dry mouth, constipation,
erectile impairment, urinary delay, tachycardia, impaired sweating, aggravation of narrow-angle glaucoma, impaired memory, and varying levels of
delirium. If these are troublesome, the clinician has three options: lower the
dose, change medicine to a less anticholinergic kind, or leave the dose
unchanged and add urecholine.

Antiadrenergic effects consist of orthostatic hypotension and ejaculatory
impairment. The former can be managed by dose reduction or by medication
change to a higher potency drug. Very severe hypotension, which is more
likely to happen after parenteral administration, can be treated by use of
levarterenol or phenylephrine, but not with epinephrine, since the unop-
posed ß-adrenergic effects of this drug will lower the blood pressure even
further.

Extrapyramidal effects consist of dystonia, parkinsonian symptoms and
signs (including tremor, rigidity, and rabbit syndrome), akathisia, akinesia,
and the tardive symptoms of dyskinesia and dystonia. While acute dystonic
reactions occur more often in younger patients, other extrapyramidal reactions including tardive dyskinesia are common in older people. Akinesia,
parkinsonism, and acute dystonic reactions respond to the antiparkinson
drugs described later in this chapter. Akinesia can present as drowsiness,
lethargy, weakness, and fatigue and may be mistaken for psychosis or depression. The differential diagnosis is important, since treatment is different.
Akathisia manifests as restlessness, muscle cramps, jitteriness, pacing, inner
anxiety, or some combination of these. It is not always easy to recognize, and
should not be mistaken for being part of the illness. While it often responds to
the above-mentioned medication, it may prove to be distressingly unresponsive and give rise to noncompliance. Benzodiazepines and ß-blockers may be
of help, however. In using anticholinergic compounds to treat these side
effects, it should always be borne in mind they can induce many other side
effects, including psychotic symptoms and delirium.

Other neuroleptic side effects include an increased risk of seizures,
agranulocytosis, cholestatic jaundice, photosensitivity, alterations of cardiac
conduction, ocular damage, temperature disturbance, and the so-called neuroleptic malignant syndrome. Seizure threshold is lowered most of all by
chlorpromazine, but the overall risk is still rare. Agranulocytosis is a life-
threatening, but fortunately rare, complication of neuroleptic drugs, which is
most likely to occur in the first few months of treatment; 75 percent of all cases
have occurred in patients over age 50 (Holloway 1974). Cholestatic jaundice is
also rare, occurring mostly with low-potency drugs. Although a 1 percent

incidence figure has been given, it is generally held that this side effect has declined in frequency and that its appearance may have been related to the manufacturing process, rather than being intrinsic to the drug. Thioridazine is limited to an upper dose of 800 mg, because of the greater risk of causing retinal damage at doses above this level. In neuroleptic malignant syndrome, which carries a 20 percent mortality rate, there is hyperthermia, hypertension, sweating, muscular rigidity, and alteration in level of awareness. Elevation of white cell count and creatinine phosphokinase levels are found. Dantrolene and bromocriptine are both effective in this condition. Should it be necessary to reinstitute a neuroleptic, it is prudent to pick a low-potency drug, since this reaction seems to be more likely with a high-potency compound. Catatonia can develop as a result of neuroleptics and presents with rigidity, immobility, and waxy flexibility. This can lead to serious medical complications, and the reaction may be prolonged. Antiparkinson drug therapy is ineffective. While most of these are rare reactions, they are among the more serious side effects. Conduction changes are more likely with the low-potency drugs, and there have been some reports of serious ventricular arrhythmias, including Torsade de Pointes, with thioridazine: High-potency drugs are safer in this regard.

Forms of Administration

Although tablets or capsules will serve adequately in most cases, there are special circumstances in which liquid or injectable administration is preferable. Liquid medication is advantageous when the patient's compliance is questioned or if swallowing presents a problem, and it can be given under supervision, thereby ensuring that the patient does in fact ingest the medication. All neuroleptics come either in concentrate or elixir form. Injectable preparations are formulated for all drugs except molindone and thioridazine. Depot-release long-acting injectable haloperidol and fluphenazine are also available. Injectables are also useful in situations of noncompliance, and when there is an urgent need to bring an acutely psychotic patient under control. Intramuscular administration is adequate in all except the most unusual situations, but intravenous haloperidol has been espoused in the very agitated intensive care patient. A suggested approach to managing an acutely psychotic, debilitated older patient, or one with organic brain syndrome, is to inject 0.5 mg of haloperidol two or three times a day. A graduated insulin syringe will facilitate the use of such small doses (Granacher 1979). The dose can then be adjusted as necessary.

Once in vogue, the so-called rapid tranquilization approach is probably of no greater benefit than simply using conventional doses. In rapid tranquilization, the patient receives higher than usual intramuscular and/or oral doses of drug over a 24 to 48-hour period.

Intramuscular doses of a neuroleptic can be supplemented by parenteral use of a benzodiazepine, such as lorazepam, to control an acutely agitated, psychotic patient. Another indication for the use of intramuscular therapy is when oral therapy has been ineffective. It is possible to tell this way if nonresponse to oral therapy is related to poor absorption through the gut or a high first-pass effect. Generally, it may be assumed that a comparable intramuscular dose is one-half to one-third of the oral dose. Before embarking on a full dose of long-acting injectable neuroleptic, it is prudent to administer a test dose of 2.5 mg (0.1 cc) fluphenazine decanoate, or 5 mg haloperidol decanoate, as appropriate. The use of small doses of fluphenazine (e.g., 2.5 to 5.0 mg) every 1 or 2 weeks is preferred to monthly injections in older patients. Some elderly patients with paranoid psychosis can respond to doses of depot fluphenazine as low as 5 mg and may need only a small number of injections.

Antidepressant Drug Treatments

Depression is common in older persons, who are more likely to experience bereavement, other personal loss, and decline in physical health. It has been estimated that the suicide rate at age 65 exceeds by fivefold the rate for younger age groups, and it continues to increase for males in their 70s. The majority of suicides in the elderly are related to problems associated with physical illness (Goodstein 1985). Deaths from reasons other than suicide are also increased in the depressed elderly; therefore, effective treatment of depression has a number of implications besides the short-term impact. Differential diagnosis is often required before embarking on a course of drug therapy, and it may be necessary to rule out endocrine, metabolic, cardiac, hematologic, infective, drug-induced, and other physical causes of the symptoms. Distinction must sometimes be made from other psychiatric states, such as grief, dementia, and delirium. Atypical presentations should also be recognized, such as alcohol abuse, violations of the law, and so forth.

In choosing antidepressant medication, some general principles should be observed. (1) The clinician should inquire about previous treatments, paying close attention to degree of response, type and magnitude of side effects, and whether the medication was adequately tolerated. The word "allergy" is sometimes used without clear meaning, and the exact nature of the reaction should be identified, since it sometimes turns out that the reaction was not allergic in nature and was dose related. (2) If a family member has been treated with antidepressants, the response should be noted. This will give useful information as to which drug may help the patient. (3) It is important to identify what other medication a patient may be taking. This is not always an easy task, since older individuals may be on a variety of different drugs and may be unable to tell their names without help. It is advisable for them to bring all medicines to their appointment; the availability of a family member will be helpful for this. Besides the need to inquire about prescribed medicines, the physician should also ask about nonprescription medicines, since the patient and relative may not think of these as medications. Questions should also be posed as to the use of unapproved substances such as alcohol. (4) In older people, depression is more often nonresponsive, or is only partially responsive, to a single antidepressant, and there is greater likelihood that a combination of drugs will be needed to bring about the desired improvement. Familiarity is therefore needed with the types of combinations, how to apply them, and the problems that might arise.

The principal drug groups are tricyclics, tetracyclics, triazolopyrridines, lithium, MAOIs, stimulants, and triazolobenzodiazepines. All have their place, even though some are used only infrequently. Conventional doses and drug categories are listed in Table 2.

Tricyclic and Tetracyclic Antidepressants

The tricyclics can be subdivided into secondary and tertiary amines, according to the number of methyl groups on the side chain. Secondary amines are demethylated products of the parent, tertiary, drug. These are shown in Table 2, along with customary dose ranges. In older patients, the secondary drugs are often better tolerated because of their lower side effect potential, although some patients complain that they do not sleep as well as with the tertiary drugs. There is only one currently marketed tetracyclic drug, maprotiline, and in action it resembles more the secondary amine than tertiary amine tricyclics. These drugs have widely varied effects on different receptor systems, as described by Richelson (1985), including antihistaminic, anticholinergic, antiadrenergic, and antidopaminergic effects.

Amitriptyline, doxepin, trimipramine, and maprotiline all have marked antihistaminic effects and as a result may produce sedation and weight gain. The extent to which marked weight gain occurs in older patients on these drugs needs further clarification, however, and it is this writer's opinion that such a side effect is less common among the elderly.

The tertiary drugs imipramine, amitriptyline, and doxepin have marked anticholinergic properties, whereas the secondary amine drugs, and also maprotiline, are relatively weak in this regard. Anticholinergic effects, which have been described earlier, can pose major problems in older patients, most notably confusion, delirium, urinary retention, erectile impairment, constipation, paralytic ileus, and tachycardia. It is generally preferable to avoid a tertiary amine tricyclic as the first-line treatment in patients who are vulnerable to these complications.

Antiadrenergic effects are thought to be related to the induction of orthostatic hypotension, although this is by no means the only factor. The degree of orthostasis present at baseline, the use of other concomitant hypotensive medication, and the dose of drug may all influence degree of orthostasis. Nortriptyline is the least likely of the tricyclics to produce orthostatic drop. Roose et al. (1987) have shown 7 percent and 0 percent incidences, respectively, of orthostatic hypotension for imipramine and nortripty-

Table 2.   Classes of Antidepressants and Stimulants and Their Dose Ranges

Category	Drug Name	Dose Range (mg/day)[a]
Tricyclics	Imipramine	25–300
	Desipramine	10–300
	Amitriptyline	25–300
	Nortriptyline	10–150
	Doxepin	10–300
	Trimipramine	25–300
	Amoxapine	50–300
	Protriptyline	10–40
	Carbamazepine	Poorly defined
Tetracyclics	Maprotiline	25–150
Monoamine oxidase inhibitors	Phenelzine	15–90
	Isocarboxazid	10–60
	Tranylcypromine	10–60
	Pargyline	25–150
Triazolopyridine	Trazodone	50–600
Stimulants	Dextroamphetamine	2.5–30
	Methylphenidate	5–40

[a]It is uncommon for high doses to be required, and they should be attained only very gradually in keeping with patient tolerance.

line in patients with normal electrocardiograms (ECGs), compared with frequencies of 32 percent and 5 percent, respectively, in patients with either conduction disease or cardiac failure. Orthostasis can be potentially serious in older patients, because of the risk of falling and sustaining fracture or other injury. Measures that can be taken to reduce the risk of orthostasis include ensuring adequacy of hydration, instruction to change position slowly, ingestion of caffeine, or use of triiodothyronine or ephedrine. Administration of medicine three or four times a day is preferred, on the grounds that blood-pressure-altering effects of antidepressants are partly related to the peak plasma level attained. Administration of the full dose at bedtime may increase the chance of a patient getting out of bed in the night and falling. Although orthostatic hypotension is viewed as an unwanted effect of therapy, at least two studies have shown that in elderly depressives, the presence of marked pretreatment systolic orthostatis predicts a high likelihood of recovery to tricyclic therapy.

Antidopaminergic effects of antidepressants are rarely a source of concern, with the exception of amoxapine, which has a dopamine-receptor-blocking metabolite and can give rise to extrapyramidal side effects.

There is a small risk of seizures with tricyclic antidepressants, amounting to about 1 in 1,000 if there are no other predisposing factors. With maprotiline, the risk is about 2 in 1,000 and is somewhat higher for clomipramine. In overdose, amoxapine, maprotiline, and desipramine are all more likely to cause seizures.

Cardiac conduction changes will occur in some older patients, and it should be remembered that drugs in this class act as type 1 quinidine-like antiarrhythmics. Increased PR, QRS, and QT intervals appear on the ECG. In patients with normal cardiac function, imipramine and nortriptyline carry a 0.7 percent incidence of 2:1 atrioventricular block. When bundle branch block is already present, as many as 18 percent of patients treated with imipramine may develop significant QRS prolongation or 2:1 atrioventricular block. Patients already on quinidine or procainamide will need to have their dose reassessed: Sometimes it is possible to discontinue the medication and replace it with the antidepressant. The degree of drug-induced intraventricular conduction delay is related to plasma levels in the case of nortriptyline. As a procedural guide, it is recommended that all elderly patients receive an ECG before starting on antidepressant drugs.

Skin rash, liver toxicity, hematologic changes, tinnitus, and myoclonus are all seen with the tricyclics. Rash is more commonly seen with maprotiline than with other drugs. Hematologic changes are a particular problem with carbamazepine. Myoclonus is more common with drugs that have a serotonergic action, and it can be treated with quinine or with a benzodiazepine, by dose reduction, or by changing medication.

Measurement of plasma levels. There is much interest in the use of plasma levels in patients undergoing antidepressant therapy. Therapeutic ranges have not been defined for most drugs, but measuring plasma levels is nonetheless useful; it does not yet form part of routine management, however. The American Psychiatric Association Task Force (1985) concludes that it is worthwhile obtaining imipramine and nortriptyline levels in any patient who receives these drugs. The existence of a therapeutic window between 50 and 140 ng/ml for nortriptyline in endogenous/major depression is well documented. At levels below or above, clinical response is less satisfactory. If the dose is pushed too high, then deterioration may set in and the appropriate course would be to lower the dose. A minimum combined imipramine and desiprimine level of 180 to 200 ng/ml is associated with a high probability of success with imipramine therapy in major depression. A minimum level of 120 ng/ml has been advanced in the case of desipramine. With respect to amitriptyline, the literature is contradictory, but in general it more convincingly argues against, rather than for, any consistent relationship. There are few data for doxepin, trimipramine, protriptyline, amoxapine, and maprotiline.

Situations in which knowledge of the plasma level would be useful include (1) nonresponse at a "reasonable" dose; (2) if unusually high doses are about to be or are being used; (3) if noncompliance is suspected; (4) when there is drug toxicity or overdose; (5) in the presence of side effects that may be related to plasma level, such as conduction defects with nortriptyline; (6) prior to introducing another drug that is known to affect plasma levels or metabolism of the tricyclic antidepressant; and (7) change in clinical state after switching to a generic brand of the same drug.

Procedurally, the optimum time for collecting samples to determine steady state levels is 10 to 14 hours postdose when this is given once a day, and just before the morning dose when given in divided doses. The collection tube should not contain trisbutoxyethyl in the stopper, since this elutes drug into the red cells and spuriously lowers plasma level. The dark blue Becton-Dickinson stoppered tube, and the Venoject Kimble-Terumo tubes are suitable.

Dose initiation. Low starting doses are advisable—25 mg of the tricyclics and maprotiline, or 5 mg protriptyline. In some cases, e.g. patients above age 75, those who are in poor physical health, or those with a known history of sensitivity to the side-effects of drugs, starting doses as low as 10 mg of a tricyclic drug are indicated. Frequent monitoring is required as the dose is slowly raised every 2 to 3 days. Lying and standing pulse rate and blood pressure, sensorium, and urinary and bowel function should all be checked. Dose increase should continue until there is evidence of improvement or side effect. It may take several weeks for full response to set in, and the physician should not give in to impatience. Patient and family should be instructed on this delay and at the same time told that side effects may precede improvement. Despite advertised claims, there is no solid evidence that any particular tricyclic acts more rapidly than any other. Some sign of response by 2 weeks is thought to predict good ultimate outcome, and if there is absolutely no improvement after 3 weeks, then little is to be gained by persisting any longer. In depressed patients as a whole (i.e., not specifically in the elderly), improvement of the following symptoms at the end of 1 week distinguished responders from nonresponders: depressed mood, anxiety, hostility, and depressed appearance (Bowden 1984). Initial signs of improvement are often more apparent to staff and family members than they are to the patient. Such observations, when made by others, can be shared with the patient who may still be doubting whether improvement can occur.

Some symptoms are viewed as having predictive value for successful outcome with tricyclic therapy. These include the "endogenous" symptoms such as greater initial severity of psychomotor retardation, anhedonia, weight loss, and early waking. However, it should be noted that in its pure form, endogenous depression is uncommon, and the prominence it has received in textbooks echoes a bygone era in psychiatry when the concept of depression was narrower. Marked hypochondriasis, delusions, and "hysterical" symptoms are thought to predict a poor response. However, a tricyclic in combination with a neuroleptic is more likely to be successful in psychotic depression (Spiker et al. 1985). Poststroke depression is responsive to tricyclics, such as nortriptyline.

Duration of drug therapy is longer in older patients, since depression pursues a more protracted course. Between the ages of 31 and 50, the natural length of depression varies from 9 to 18 months, whereas after age 50, its cycle lasts for an average of 3 to 5 years (Ayd 1983). Premature discontinuation of therapy or overenthusiastic dose reduction carries the chance of depressive relapse.

Tricyclic drugs may need to be combined with other drugs in order to overcome nonresponse or partial response. The addition of lithium at full doses can translate partial response into full response, especially in patients with melancholic presentations (Price et al. 1986). It may be necessary to persist with additional lithium for 3 or 4 weeks until improvement sets in. Although there are few guidelines in the literature, perhaps because it is not easy to study a large number of such patients, there is some evidence that lithium add-on therapy is more likely to be effective in older depressives. An advantage of this treatment approach is its relative safety.

Triiodothyronine, 25 µg daily, can be added, although this may not be as effective as lithium. L-tryptophan at doses of 1 to 4 g daily can also be tried, although there is little to help the clinician as to selection of appropriate patients. Addition of methylphenidate, which results in an increased blood tricyclic level, can be useful, but there is the risk of agitation and insomnia. Addition of a MAOI can be tried; however, even though the dangers of this combination have been disproportionately exaggerated, such treatment should nonetheless be left to an experienced psychopharmacologist. Suggestions as to how this treatment can be given are available elsewhere (Davidson 1985). Certainly the clinician should not accept that a patient is treatment refractory until one or more antidepressant combinations have been tried. There is no reason to think that a patient with major depression cannot potentially be restored to his or her premorbid level of adjustment.

Monoamine Oxidase Inhibitors

The MAOIs form a valuable second or third line of treatment in the older person. Offsetting their undoubted benefit in previously nonresponsive depressives, is the knowledge that they are potentially more dangerous and have a lower safety margin than the tricyclic drugs. The efficacy of phenelzine compared with that of nortriptyline and placebo has been demonstrated in older depressives (Georgatas et al. 1987).

The MAOIs can be grouped into the hydrazine and nonhydrazine types. Phenelzine and isocarboxazid belong to the first category, and tranylcypromine and pargyline belong to the second. Hydrazines are purportedly more hepatotoxic but the risks appear to be exceedingly low. There is no overall difference in efficacy of the two groups, but individual patients sometimes respond better to one than to another drug. Sometimes the side effects of one drug are tolerated less well than those of another. The MAOIs inhibit monoamine oxidase, an enzyme that is an important regulator of biogenic amine activity. The drugs are irreversible inhibitors. They permanently inactivate the available enzyme supply, and new enzyme must be synthesized once the drug is stopped before its effect has worn off. This may take 10 to 14 days, although by the end of 1 week the supply of monoamine oxidase may be back to 50 percent of the baseline level as a result of new synthesis. These considerations are important from the safety perspective, since dietary and medication restrictions will need to remain in force for this time period.

Side effects of monoamine oxidase inhibitors. The anticholinergic effects that often bedevil tricyclic therapy are of lesser concern with MAOIs, except at high doses. Therefore MAOI therapy is sometimes indicated when a tricyclic drug has failed on account of anticholinergic properties. Impaired sexual arousal, constipation, and urinary delay do occur at higher doses of MAOIs, however. Anticholinergic effects are much more pronounced when a MAOI is used in conjunction with tricyclics, antihistamines, and antiparkinson drugs.

Blood pressure changes are problematic with MAOIs: Both the lying systolic and the orthostatic blood pressures may drop. This can present as dizziness, weakness, or inability to stand up. Sometimes it may be asymptomatic, and for that reason it is important to check blood pressure at each visit in the older person on a MAOI. I have found that isocarboxazid-induced hypotension is dose related, although this is not the case for orthostatic drop. These changes do not occur at first and may not become apparent until after 3 weeks. Sodium chloride supplement, 2 to 3 g/day, can help, although this treatment is contraindicated if there is evidence of heart or kidney disease or if the patient must restrict sodium intake. Other measures that can be taken are those described above for tricyclic drugs, although great caution should be used with regard to ephedrine since this can lead to a hypertensive reaction. As with the tricyclics, pretreatment systolic orthostasis is related to outcome at least for isocarboxazid.

Increased blood pressure from pressor agents, such as tyramine, phenylephrine, phenylpropanolamine, pseudoephedrine, and amphetamine, can lead to a hypertensive crisis in patients undergoing MAOI therapy. The incidence may be as high as 8 percent (Rabkin et al. 1984), although in my experience it is far lower. The fatality rate is estimated at 1 in 100,000 patients treated with tranylcypromine. A hypertensive reaction may be treated with 5 mg of the α blocker phentolamine intravenously, 300 mg of diazoxide intravenously, or sodium nitroprusside infusion. The practice of carrying around 50 mg chlorpromazine "just in case" is not advisable. The risk of hypertensive crisis cannot be eliminated altogether, but it can be substantially lowered through proper counseling, patient selection, and family involvement. Nifedipine (10 mg) can be chewed and taken sublingually.

Impaired sleep, weight gain, myoclonus, memory impairment, headache, restlessness, and anorexia may all occur as side effects with MAOIs. Tranylcypromine is more likely than the hydrazine drugs to cause weight loss, anorexia, agitation, headache, and insomnia. Dietary and drug instructions and contraindicated medications for patients on MAOIs are described by Davidson et al. (1984); issues of compliance and patient education are described by Walker et al. (1984). Before any elective operative procedure, MAOIs should be discontinued for at least 2 weeks. In an emergency, however, a patient can undergo surgery, with due precaution being taken by the anesthesiologist. Further suggestions as to patient management are given elsewhere (Churchill-Davidson 1965).

Extrapyramidal symptoms from MAOIs are rare, but these drugs do potentiate the extrapyramidal effects of neuroleptics.

Monitoring of platelet monoamine oxidase activity is not routinely indicated, and there is little evidence for a relationship between enzyme inhibition and clinical response to a MAOI, other than for phenelzine in younger patients with atypical depression. In the case of tranylcypromine, it appears that full monoamine oxidase inhibition occurs at doses below those needed for an antidepressant effect.

Dose is a critical determinant of outcome with MAOI therapy, in that an increase of 15 mg phenelzine, 5 mg isocarboxazid, or 10 mg tranylcypromine may be pivotal. In patients who are unable to tolerate the side effects, but who relapse when the dose is lowered by one tablet, a half-tablet can be sufficient. Isocarboxazid has an advantage in this case, since it is the only scored MAOI tablet: Coated tablets are more difficult to break. Recommended doses are given in Table 2, and the importance of reaching the maximum tolerated dose is stressed. It is recommended that the initial dose be low—10 mg of isocarboxazid of tranylcypromine, 25 mg of pargyline or 15 mg of phenelzine; it can then be increased every few days one tablet at a time up to four or five tablets a day. If side effects become a problem, the dose can be lowered, but if there is neither response nor side effect, then further dose increases can be undertaken. Duration of therapy is similar to that of the tricyclics; however, since many patients only receive a MAOI because they have a chronic depression that has been resistant to other drugs, they may need a longer period of maintenance therapy.

Features that invite the use of an MAOI in the elderly include phobic anxiety, nonpsychotic agitation, somatic anxiety, anergia, reserpine-induced depression, or a previous history of panic attacks or chronic anxiety. A number of older depressives have been noted to develop psychotic symptoms, such as paranoid delusions, or to stop eating and become mute or withdrawn within 2 weeks of beginning treatment, usually at high doses of the drug (50 to 60 mg of isocarboxazid, 75 to 90 mg of phenelzine). There has been a history of previous psychotic depression, or the patient may have presented with psychomotor retardation. The degree to which each of these features contributes to overall variance in outcome may be relatively small, and in general an MAOI should be thought of as potentially helpful in practically any form of major depression. Some hold the opinion that tranylcypromine is the most effective MAOI in older depressives.

Other Antidepressants

Trazodone has a definite role in the treatment of older depressives. Its freedom from anticholinergic effect gives it a major advantage over tricyclic and tetracyclic drugs. Side effects include sedation, hypotension, and dizziness; priapism is a rare, but serious, risk. A low starting dose of 50 mg is recommended, with progressive increase up to a maximum of 600 mg, which would correspond roughly to a tricyclic dose of 225 mg. With trazodone, the hypnotic dose is often below the antidepressant dose, an important point since there may be a tendency to rest content with a suboptimal antidepressant dose once the patient starts to sleep better.

Alprazolam has been documented to have antidepressant effects equivalent to those of tricyclics, and greater than those of placebo treatment. However, it may be that the drug is less effective in melancholia or in cases of marked vegetative change. Its lack of autonomic and cardiovascular properties confers a potential advantage over other antidepressants. Chief drawbacks are sedation, interference with memory, and possible withdrawal effects. Although the recommended dose range is 0.5 to 4 mg, the upper range has not been fully explored, and there are anecdotal reports indicating that substantially higher doses may be needed. The long-term effects of alprazolam need to be better understood. Withdrawal of the drug must always be approached with caution, and the patient and family should be warned about the possibility of withdrawal seizure upon abrupt discontinuation.

Carbamazepine is being used in treatment-refractory depression (Post et al. 1986). Use of the drug should be preceded by a complete blood count and differential, liver function tests, electrolyte levels, and an ECG. The starting dose of 200 mg twice daily may be gradually raised by 200 mg increments up to as high as 1,200 mg/day. Blood level monitoring is recommended, more for safety than for efficacy reasons. Regular blood counts should be performed, and the drug discontinued if red cells fall below 4,000,000/mm^3, if hematocrit falls below 32 percent, if leukocytes fall below 4,000/mm^3, if platelets are less than 100,000/mm^3, or if reticulocytes are below 0.3 percent. An alert should also be sounded if the patient develops fever, sore throat, mouth ulcers, bleeding, or any infection; further hematologic assessment should be undertaken and the drug stopped until the basis for the cause has been established.

Stimulants

Almost consigned to the scrap heap of psychopharmacology, stimulants can have a useful role in treating depression in old age that is not sufficiently realized. The main reservations have traditionally centered around risks of abuse, dependency, and assumed inefficacy. In medically ill depressives, in withdrawn postoperative states, and in poststroke depression, stimulant drug therapy is often beneficial. Another indication is when tricyclic or other drugs produce unacceptable side effects. Response to drugs in this class is characteristically rapid, with improvement being noted within 48 hours. In fact, if there is no response to a sufficient dose within 3 days, the drug trial can be considered as having been adequate. There is an impression that methylphenidate is preferable in adjustment disorder, while dextroamphetamine is more effective in major depression, but these contentions require more rigorous testing.

Double-blind studies do not, in general, conclusively show efficacy for stimulant drugs, but this question still remains little studied. Recommended starting doses are 5 mg of dextroamphetamine and 10 mg of methylphenidate. Dextroamphetamine has a longer half-life than methylphenidate, and can be given in the morning, while methylphenidate is best given on a twice-daily basis. The total daily doses range from 2.5 to 30 mg for dextroamphetamine and from 5 to 40 mg for methylphenidate. In one survey (Woods et al. 1986), the mean maximal daily doses were 12 mg and 13.5 mg for dextroamphetamine and methylphenidate, respectively. Mood, motivation, psychomotor state, sleep, and appetite all improved, and the overall improvement often permitted gains in the underlying medical disorder, once the patient's depressed state had lifted.

It is best to administer the last dose of methylphenidate in the afternoon, since insomnia can be a side effect, but in general the psychostimulants are remarkably free of unwanted effects in older patients. At high doses there is a risk of agitation. It is stated that therapy can be discontinued shortly after the patient has become asymptomatic.

Psychostimulant therapy may also be indicated for potentiating the effect of a tricyclic drug or to counteract the hypotensive effects of antidepressants. This can lead to potentially dangerous hypertension in conjunction with an MAOI, but it is nonetheless noted that such therapy may have a place in carefully selected treatment-refractory patients (Feighner et al. 1986).

Lithium

Lithium is indicated to treat acute mania, hypomania, and some schizoaffective states; it is also indicated for regulation and prophylaxis is recurrent unipolar and bipolar disorders. Lithium is excreted through the kidney; therefore in older patients, whose renal clearance of lithium will be reduced, the half-life will be longer, averaging 36 hours.

Before starting a patient on lithium, a prelithium workup should be performed, including complete blood count and differential, urinalysis, thyroxine and triiodothyronine uptake, free thyroxine index, thyroid-stimulating hormone, electrolytes, creatinine, and ECG. If renal function is thought to be impaired, a 24-hour creatinine clearance test may be performed.

It is recommended that lithium be started at a low dose and slowly increased as tolerated. In an acutely manic elderly patient, 300 mg is usually well tolerated and this can be increased up to 900 mg in most cases. Because of the 36-hour half-life, it can take as long as 180 hours before steady state has been reached and therefore for a blood level to be meaningful. In older and/or medically compromised patients, a small initial dose of 75 mg or 150 mg can be used. In mania, the desired blood lithium level will be in the range of 1.0 to 1.4 mmol/l. In acute mania, the effect of lithium will take several days to appear, and concomitant neuroleptic therapy is usually needed. In hypomania, lithium alone is sufficient. If lithium is being administered for prophylaxis to a patient who is not acutely symptomatic, then plasma levels of 0.4 to 0.7 mmol/l may be adequate. In spite of the fact that plasma levels are invariably recommended in managing a person on lithium, there is some doubt as to what ranges are most closely associated with successful outcome. Monthly or bimonthly lithium levels are suggested for older patients. In order to properly interpret a lithium level, the blood sample should be drawn 12 hours after the last dose. Debate exists as to whether lithium is best given on a divided dose or single daily dose basis; there is some evidence that once-a-day dosing is associated with less polyuria and less structural damage to the kidney.

Side effects of lithium. Benign side effects may appear early in lithium therapy, such as fine tremor, nausea, headache, tiredness, and polyuria. Other side effects include memory impairment, weight gain, thyroid enlargement, hypothyroidism, diabetes insipidus, psoriasis, skin infection, and sinus arrhythmia.

At blood lithium levels in excess of 1.5 mmol/l, toxic effects are likely to supervene. These consist of coarse tremor, slurred speech, ataxia, nystagmus, hyperreflexia, weakness, drowsiness, muscle fasciculations, and vomiting. If unchecked, they can progress to impaired consciousness, clonus, seizures, electroencephalograph slowing, coma, electrolyte imbalance, and death. Prompt recognition and management are most important. In such a situation lithium should be stopped, the patient monitored on a daily basis for EKG, lithium and electrolyte measured, and fluid intake be increased to 5 to 6 l/day. 20G urea given intravenously bid, or mannitol 50–100 G iv daily, will increase lithium diuresis. Aminophylline given slowly iv increases tubular blood flow and decreases tubular reabsorption of lithium. Sodium lactate increases lithium excretion. Hemodialysis may be indicated in refractory lithium toxicity.

Lithium interacts with a number of drugs, resulting in either a decrease or an increase of lithium level. Drugs that can raise the plasma lithium level and/or reduce renal excretion include thiazide diuretics, spironolactone, triamterene, nonsteroidal antiinflammatory drugs (except aspirin), and possibly tetracycline. Any of these drugs can therefore lead to a state of lithium toxicity. Theophylline drugs have been reported to lower lithium levels.

Other drugs that do not directly alter the disposition of lithium can still lead to a state of toxicity. A lithium-neuroleptic interaction may lead to confusion, extrapyramidal side effects, and cerebellar signs; this is rare, however, and should not deter the clinician from using such combinations. Increased neurotoxicity can result from lithium and phenytoin, and from lithium and carbamazepine. High-dose combinations of a MAOI and lithium can produce a serotonin syndrome, with muscular overactivity and temperature increase.

It is sometimes necessary to combine lithium and a diuretic in the elderly. If the patient is already on lithium, then it is best to check the level and lower the dose by half. Lithium levels and electrolytes should then be monitored at least twice weekly at first, and the dose adjusted according to side effects and blood indices. Potassium supplementation is generally advisable with thiazides. Loop diuretics such as furosemide and ethacrynic acid cause less retention of lithium than do the thiazides.

Patient and family education is an important part of lithium management. Reliability and possession of the requisite information are needed in order to obtain the maximum benefit and avoid potentially serious side effects. One consideration is that manic patients are not always willing to accept the need for lithium, and a good doctor-patient relationship will go some way toward forestalling this problem. Family support, good dietary habits, supervision of other medications, and adequate care of coexisting physical pathology are also major considerations. Any gastrointestinal upset, change in salt intake, or change in dietary plan should signal the need to consult with a physician or temporarily curtail medication, in a geriatric patient on lithium.

Antianxiety and Hypnotic Medications

The benzodiazepines have almost entirely supplanted barbiturates and pro-panediols for treating anxiety, although today there are still some older patients who have been well stabilized on a barbiturate for many decades, and in whom there is little to be gained by tampering; indeed such patients may rightly resist any attempt at this. Other drug groups have a place in treating older individuals with anxiety disorder, among which are the antidepressants, antihistamines, neuroleptics, and the ß-blockers. The new azaspirodecane-dione drug, buspirone, may also be especially useful in the older patient.

Benzodiazepines

It is always important to rule out other causes of anxiety, which can be the presenting symptom of numerous physical and psychiatric disorders. Precipitating factors should be looked for, identified, and dealt with as appropriate. The first-line choice of drug therapy will be a benzodiazepine, and while all benzodiazepines are equally effective, there are important differences in metabolism and side-effect profiles. It is also possible that the triazolobenzodiazepines differ from other benzodiazepines with respect to cross-tolerance, which would have practical importance in managing with-drawal reactions.

Triazolam is a short-acting drug, with a half-life of 2 to 4 hours. Short- to intermediate-acting drugs include alprazolam, lorazepam, oxazepam, and temazepam. Long-acting drugs include flurazepam, diazepam, chlordiazepox-ide, chlorazepate, and prazepam. Oxazepam and lorazepam, which are metabolized by conjugation, do not yield active metabolites and are less likely to produce cumulative side effects. While short-acting benzodiazepines pro-vide an advantage over long-acting drugs in this regard, they have some disadvantages, such as the potential for withdrawal effects and rebound insomnia, and the need to administer the drug in divided doses.

Side effects of benzodiazepines consist of sedation, drowsiness, lethargy, memory and cognitive impairment, ataxia, paradoxical hostility, aggravation of noctural breathing difficulty (e.g., sleep apnea), nightmares, hallucinations, dysarthria, diplopia, nystagmus, weakness, and depression. Anxiety may be intensified if the drugs interfere with respiration. Their effects will be poten-tiated by alcohol, other sedatives, anticonvulsants, MAOIs, sedating tricyclics, sedating neuroleptics, and antihypertensives.

Clinical indications for benzodiazepines include insomnia (see below), generalized anxiety disorder, post-traumatic stress disorder, panic disorder, acute states of anxiety or agitation, and alcohol withdrawal. They are some-times useful as an adjunct to antidepressant therapy in anxious or agitated depressives or in a depressive who requires treatment with a secondary amine tricyclic but who is not sleeping adequately. Insomnia induced by a

MAOI may also respond to a benzodiazepine. In controlling panic attacks, alprazolam and clonazepam may be particularly beneficial.

Starting doses in the elderly will be one-half to one-third those used in younger individuals. Illustrative starting doses are 2 to 5 mg of diazepam, 10 mg of oxazepam, 0.25 to 0.5 mg of alprazolam, and 2 mg of lorazepam. The dose can be raised every few days until the desired effect is obtained or side effects appear. It is recommended that attempts be made to reduce the dose or discontinue medication after a few weeks and to present the treatment as either a short-term measure or, if the patient has a chronic anxiety state, as an intermittent treatment to be used in conjunction with other approaches. It is questionable whether daily long-term benzodiazepine therapy is either effective or indicated, except in rare cases, and there is a real risk in the elderly of producing cumulative toxicity. There is a chance of withdrawal symptoms, psychosis, or other major decompensation in a significant number of patients who have taken long-term benzodiazepines at standard doses (Tyrer et al. 1983). A daily dose reduction at the rate of 10 percent per day is recommended for drug withdrawal.

Other Drugs

Buspirone is a new anxiolytic drug that differs in many respects from the benzodiazepines. It is nonsedating, does not interact with alcohol, and has no abuse liability; it may take somewhat longer to relieve symptoms, at least as far as patient perception is concerned. The starting dose is 5 mg twice a day, to be increased as needed up to 60 mg/day. Some patients who have become used to and responded well to benzodiazepines do not feel buspirone to be as helpful.

Because the full implications of long-term benzodiazepine use are unknown, consideration should be given to the advantages of low doses of tricyclic antidepressants, such as doxepin, trimipramine, or nortriptyline, which frequently provide adequate anxiety relief.

ß-blockers can be useful for managing somatic anxiety, although side effects to be concerned about in older patients include dizziness, hypotension, depression, aggravation or respiratory distress, diabetes, bradycardia, and heart failure. However, some individuals are receiving ß-blockers for other reasons, yet still complain of anxiety: Their role as anxiolytics appears to be limited in this age group.

Patients with organic brain disease, who exhibit nonpsychotic anxiety or agitation, may respond better to a neuroleptic. High-potency, nonsedating drugs such as haloperidol 0.5 mg, and thiothixene 1 mg, are well tolerated and unlikely to produce troublesome extrapyramidal effects. Low-potency drugs are more likely to affect autonomic function.

An alternative approach is available with the antihistamines, which may be indicated in patients with chronic obstructive pulmonary disease. Daily doses of 25 to 100 mg hydroxyzine or diphenhydramine can be used. Side effects include those associated with all anticholinergics, as described in earlier sections of this chapter.

Pharmacologic Management of Insomnia

When deciding whether to use a hypnotic drug, and how long to use it for, the following points should be addressed. (1) Has the cause been adequately identified? If polysomnography is available, has it been used? (2) Is the patient taking other medications that might interact with a hypnotic? Could medication be the cause of insomnia? (3) Is a sleep apnea syndrome present? (4) What side effects may the hypnotic produce, and what is the drug's metabolic profile? What is known of the patient's physical state that might have impact on drug effects? (5) The following are relative contraindications to benzodiazepine therapy in older patients: previous substance abuse; lack of adequate support systems; heavy snoring; impaired renal, liver, and pulmonary function; and suicide potential (Reynolds et al. 1985).

For short-term management, a benzodiazepine is indicated, and it may also be useful in chronic insomnia which is clearly part of a generalized anxiety disorder. Maintenance dose of benzodiazepines in older persons should be kept at lower levels than in younger people. The medication should be taken 30–60 minutes before bedtime, and instructions can be given to omit doses at least one or two night per week. It is important to provide information as to possible daytime complications, such as hangover, sedation, forgetfulness, etc.

Other approaches to sleep hygiene should be used, such as instructing the patient not to use the bed for activities which are antithetical to sleep, e.g., paying the bills, preparing the grocery list, etc. Other nonpharmacological approaches are outlined (Reynolds et al. 1985).

Antiparkinson Medication

Opinion is divided about whether medication should be given routinely to prevent neuroleptic-induced extrapyramidal side effects (EPS). With low-potency agents the frequency of EPS is not appreciably different as a result of prophylaxis (Stramek et al. 1986), but with high-potency drugs, such as haloperiodol, the frequency of EPS is reduced threefold by routine prophylaxis (Winslow et al. 1986). Whether a patient develops EPS will be affected by age, physical and central nervous system conditon, and dose and selection of drug, to name only a few factors. In general, about 20 to 40 percent will experience EPS.

Most antiparkinsonian agents carry anticholinergic side effects, although amantadine is an exception in this regard. Anticholinergic, antihistamine, ß-blocker, and benzodiazepine drugs all effectively treat EPS.

The following drugs are classified as anticholinergic (daily doses are given in parentheses): benztropine (1 to 4 mg), biperiden (2 to 6 mg), ethopropazine (50 to 600 mg), procyclidine (5 to 15 mg), and trihexyphenidyl (2 to 15 mg). Two antihistamine drugs are diphenhydramine (25 to 150 mg) and orphenadrine (50 to 200 mg). Any one of these drugs is likely to be effective in most EPS.

Second-line antiparkinsonian agents are propranolol (10 to 40 mg) and diazepam (2 to 10 mg) for akathisia that has not responded to other drugs. Akathisia can sometimes be difficult to recognize. Amantadine (100 to 300 mg) is a nonanticholinergic drug that has dopaminergic effects and is a useful, if expensive, alternative treatment.

Injectable forms of benztropine, diphenhydramine, and orphenadrine are available for severe EPS. Also in acute dystonia, intramuscular lorazepam or intravenous diazepam can be used.

Dementia: Brain Stimulants and Vasodilators

Loss of brain tissue functioning results in organic brain syndrome, character-ized by a decrease in intellectual ability, memory loss, disorientation, and impaired judgment. In contrast to acute organic brain syndrome, which is reversible when the precipitating cause is removed, chronic brain syndrome is insidious and its treatment empirical and less successful.

Poor nutrition contributes to impaired cognition in the elderly. The plasma lipids play a major role in developing organic brain syndrome second-ary to atherosclerosis, so that serum cholesterol should not exceed 220 mg%, and the triglyceride level should remain below 150 mg% (Frederickson 1974). A low-cholesterol diet containing no more than 30 percent of the daily calories as fat is beneficial. Saturated animal fats should be eliminated as far as possible, and steady exercise, cessation of smoking, and control of blood pressure are all important (Walker and Brodie 1980). A majority of elderly hospitalized patients were found in one study (Whanger and Wang 1974) to have inadequate diets, low folate, and low vitamin B_{12}. Daily vitamins have been recommended for all patients over age 65 (Verwoerdt 1976).

Vasodilators may have some limited effect in early/mild dementia of vascular origin but have no impact in more severe forms of the disorder. Cyclandelate (800 to 1200 mg/day) and papaverine (150 mg/day) are smooth muscle vasodilators, which can cause flushing, hypotension, and headaches. Nicotinic acid (0.5 to 3 mg daily) dilates cutaneous blood vessels. Nylidrin (9 to 48 mg/day) and isoxsuprine (30-60 mg/day) are ß-agonists, which increase blood flow. Although they are indicated as being possibly effective for symp-toms associated with cerebral vascular insufficiency, there is no conclusive evidence that these drugs are useful in Alzheimer's disease.

Ergoloid mesylates (Hydergine) appear to be somewhat more effective than other vasodilators. This drug represents a mix of four ergot alkaloids, and was originally marketed as an α-adrenergic antagonist vasodilator, but possesses other attributes, including agonist activity at serotonin and dopamine receptor sites. When given for 12 weeks at doses of up to 7.5 mg/day, ergoloid mesylates have been found to reduce confusion, recent memory impairment, depression, and emotional lability (Dysken 1987). Even further improvement compared with placebo takes place over 6 months, and in that period, no patient on ergoloid mesylates deteriorated, while many placebo patients do so. The drug is currently being tested further in Alzheimer's disease. Although the recommended dose range is 1 mg three times a day, this may not be adequate for all cases, and higher doses of 9 mg may be more effective.

Side effects are rarely troublesome. Sublingual irritation can occur with the sublingual preparation, and nausea and gastrointestinal disturbances can also result at times. The medication comes in tablet, liquid capsule, liquid, and sublingual tablet forms.

Other treatments have been used in dementia, all of which must still be considered as experimental and of unproved efficacy. These include physostigmine, choline, lecithin, and tetrahydroaminoacridine. Each of these therapies is discussed in Chapter 12 in the section on cognitive acting drugs in Alzheimer's disease. Still other therapies including opioid antagonists and hyperbaric oxygen have not been demonstrated to be successful.

Gerovital is an interesting compound that is no longer available, but did show some promise for improving memory, attention span, and concentration. Piracetam, a cyclic γ-aminobutyric acid derivative, has resulted in some overall general improvement in patients diagnosed as having organic brain syndromes.

Special Considerations

It is important for the physician to understand those factors that determine compliance and drug-taking behavior, as outlined by Salzman (1982).

The issue of medication cost is inadequately appreciated by many physicians, and it is not always easy for either the patient or the doctor to obtain comparative prices. This was recently studied by Weiner et al. (1983). Some principles can be laid out nonetheless:

- Generic products are less expensive than the original brand;
- New drugs cost more than older ones;
- Newer drugs that are the sole representatives of their chemical class are usually sold at premium prices, since high development costs have to be recouped;
- Preparations containing larger doses cost less per milligram than those containing lower doses;
- Prescriptions containing orders for large quantities of medication can often

be filled in the pharmacy at a less expensive rate than can prescriptions written for a smaller amount.

Some drugs, such as chlorpromazine and lithium, are remarkably inexpensive, while L-tryptophan, whose indications are less clear, is highly priced. A down side to the use of generics is that on occasion they are not bioequivalent for a particular patient who had previously been well stabilized on the brand product.

Older patients are often on multiple medications, prescription and nonprescription. Most common are digoxin, hydrochlorothiazide, hydrochlorothiazide-triamterene, propranolol, diazepam, aspirin, and multiple vitamins (Stewart 1986).

Compliance is probably higher in older patients, but this can be adversely affected by the appearance of side effects and also by the fact that many patients are on multiple medications, since compliance is inversely related to the number of medications a person takes. Poor vision can make it difficult to read the label and can lead to a patient mistaking one pill for another that may visually resemble the first one. Arthritic changes can make it hard to open the safety-capped bottle, to cut the pill in half, or to measure out liquid.

The following example of an outpatient's medication profile, taken from this author's clinical practice, illustrates the issues and problems surrounding the question of compliance. A 66-year-old man was receiving the following medications: aspirin 325 mg 1 to 2 qid prn; cerumenix 1 drop as needed; potassium chloride 10 percent $1\frac{1}{2}$ teaspoons in the morning; nitroglycerin 0.4 mg 1 sublingually prn; diltiazem 30 mg qid; tetracycline 250 mg 1 q12hr; sulfamethoxazole 2 twice a day; Xylocaine 5 percent prn; oxybutynin 5 mg tid prn; L-tryptophan 500 mg 3 qhs; phenelzine 15 mg 2 bid; trifluoperazine 2 mg 2 bid; and chlordiazepoxide 10 mg 1 qid prn. It is clear that a substantial amount of time at each visit needed to be given to medication management. The patient was married, but his wife was unable to play an important role in helping him to keep his medication organized, since she too was being treated with medication for depression and had health problems of her own, which meant that the patient had to care for her over a protracted period of time. A significant other can definitely assist with medication compliance, but at times this can give rise to difficulty relinquishing control to another person in the matter of taking medication. A look at this list also illustrates the problems faced by a patient in having to judge whether and when to take some as-needed medications, having to take medicines according to many different schedules, and having to maintain constant awareness as to MAOI diet and medication precautions. The use of a written list and instructions were of great help in managing this case. It has been observed that verbal instructions alone are associated with lower compliance as compared with written guidelines (Wandless and Davie 1977).

In prescribing for the elderly, it is necessary to begin with low doses, as was described for each of the main drug groups in this chapter, and to increase the dose slowly, paying frequent attention to the symptom picture, to physiologic state, and to the emergence of side effects. Under careful control, many older patients can in fact be led up to full therapeutic drug doses. In patients over age 70, however, dose requirements may be less than those of younger patients. An example of this is the finding that therapeutic levels of nortriptyline can be achieved with doses of only 30 mg/day (Dawling et al. 1981). It may often be necessary to adjust the dose of other medications or even discontinue them as part of psychotropic management. Coordination with other physicians is sometimes important and should not be overlooked. Frequent review is needed, and it is appropriate to periodically reaffirm with patients and/or their relatives that they understand any special conditions and restrictions about their medicine. Although one strives to give medication for the shortest time, it has to be recognized that very often older patients require long-term medication. To get the best results from pharmacotherapy in older patients, more than usual care and skill are generally needed: When these are applied, even the most difficult challenges can give rewarding results.

References

Ayd F: Continuation and maintenance antidepressant drug therapy, in Affective Disorders Reassessed 1983. Edited by Ayd FJ, Taylor I, Taylor B. Baltimore, Ayd Medical Communications, 1983

Bowden CL: Early signs of response to antidepressants. International Drug Therapy Newsletter 1984; 10:5–6

Churchill–Davidson HC: Anesthesia and monoamine oxidase inhibitors. Br Med J 1965; 1:520

Davidson JRT: Non–response to TCA and MAOI drugs. What comes next? in Depression in Multidisciplinary Perspective. Edited by Dean A. New York, Brunner/Mazel, 1985

Davidson JRT, Zung WWK, Walker JI: Practical aspects of MAO inhibitor therapy. J Clin Psychiatry 1984; 45(7, Sec 2):78–80

Dawling S, Crome P, Braithwaite RA, et al: Nortriptyline therapy in elderly patients: dosage prediction from plasma concentrations at 24 hours after a single 50 mg dose. Br J Psychiatry 1981; 139:413–416

Dysken M: A review of recent clinical trials in the treatment of Alzheimer's dementia. Psychiatric Annals 1987; 17:179–196

Feighner JP, Herbstein J, Damlooji N: Combined MAOI, TCA and direct stimulant therapy of treatment resistant depression. J Clin Psychiatry 1985; 46:206–209

Frederickson D: Atherosclerosis and other forms of arteriosclerosis, in Principles of Internal Medicine (Seventh Edition). Edited by Wintrope MW, Thorn GW, Adams RD, et al. New York, McGraw Hill, 1974

Georgatas A, McCue RE, Hapworth W, et al: Comparative efficacy and safety of MAOIs versus TCAs in treating depression in the elderly. Biol Psychiatry 1986; 21:1155–1166

Goodstein RK: Common clinical problems in the elderly. Psychiatric Annals 1985; 15:299–312

Granacher RP: Titrating intramuscular dosages for elderly patients. Am J Psychiatry, 1979; 136:997

Holloway D: Drug problems in the geriatric patient. Drug Intell Clin Pharm 1974; 8:632–642

Kay DWK: Observations on the natural history and genetics of old age psychoses: Stockholm material 1931–1937. Proc Roy Soc Med 1959; 52:791

Mor V, McHonrey C, Sherwood S: Secondary morbidity among the recently bereaved. Am J Psychiatry 1986; 143:158–163

Naguib M, McGriffin P, Levy R, et al: Genetic markers in late paraphrenia—study of HLA antigens. Presented at the meeting of the Royal College of Psychiatrists, London, 1985.

Post F: The impact of modern drug treatment on old age schizophrenia. Geront Clinica (Base 1) 1962; 4:137–141

Post F: Affective disorders in old age, in Handbook of Affective Disorders. Edited by Paykel ES. New York, Guilford Press, 1984

Post RM, Uhde TW, Roy–Burne P, et al: Antidepressant effects of carbamazepine. Am J Psychiatry 1986; 143:29–34

Price LH, Charney DS, Heninger GR: Variability of response to lithium augmentation in refractory depressions. Am J Psychiatry 1986; 143:1387–1392

Rabkin J, Quitkin FM, Harrison W, et al: Adverse reactions to monoamine oxidase inhibitors: I. A comparative study. J Clin Psychopharmacol 1984; 4:279–288

Reynolds CF, Kupfer DJ, Hoch CC, et al: Sleeping pills for the elderly: are they ever justified? J Clin Psychiatry 1985; 46(2, Sec 2):9–12

Richelson E: Pharmacology of antidepressants in use in the United States. J Clin Psychiatry 1982; 43(11 Sec 2):4–11

Richey DP: Effects of human aging on drug absorption and metabolism, in The Physiology and Pathology of Human Aging. Edited by Goldman R, Rockstein M, Sussman ML. New York, Academic Press, 1975

Roose SP, Glassman AH, Giardina EGV, et al: Tricyclic antidepressants in depressed patients with cardiac conduction disease. Arch Gen Psychiatry 1987; 44:273–280

Salzman C: Basic principles of psychiatric drug prescription for the elderly. Hosp Community Psychiatry 1982; 33:133–136

Slater E, Roth M (eds): Mental disorders of the aged, in Clinical Psychiatry. London, Balliere, Tindall and Cassell, 1972

Spiker DG, Weiss JC, Dealy RS, et al: The pharmacological treatment of delusional depression. Am J Psychiatry 1985; 142:430–436

Stewart RB: Applied phamacology in the elderly: an overview of the Dunedin program, in Dimensions of Aging. Edited by Bergener M, Ermini M, Staehlin HB. New York, Academic Press, 1986

Stramek JJ, Simpson GM, Morrison RL, et al: Anticholinergic agents for prophylaxis of neuroleptic–induced dystonic reactions: a prospective study. J Clin Psychiatry 1986; 47:305–309

Task Force on the Use of Laboratory Tests In Psychiatry: Tricyclic antidepressants—blood level measurements and clinical outcome: an APA Task Force Report. Am J Psychiatry 1985; 142:163–169

Tyrer PJ, Owen R, Dowling S: Gradual withdrawal of diazepam after long term therapy. Lancet 1983; 1:1402–1406

Verwoerdt A: Clinical Geropsychiatry. Baltimore, Williams & Wilkins, 1976

Walker JI, Brodie HKH: Neuropharmacology of aging, in Handbook of Geriatric Psychiatry. Edited by Busse EW, Blazer DG. New York, Van Nostrand Reinhold 1980

Walker JI, Davidson JRT, Zung WWK: Patient compliance with MAO inhibitor therapy. J Clin Psychiatry 1984; 45(8, Sec 2):78–80

Wandless I, Davie JW: Can drug compliance in the elderly be improved? Br Med J 1977; 1:359–361

Weiner RD, Coffey CE, Campbell CP, et al: The price of psychotropic drugs: a neglected factor. Hosp Community Psychiatry 1983; 34:531–535

Weissman MM, Tischler GL, Holzer CE, et al: Six month prevalence of psychiatric disorders in three communities. Arch Gen Psychiatry 1984; 41:959–971

Whanger AD, Wang HS: Vitamin B_{12} deficiency in normal aged and psychiatric patients, in Normal Aging (Volume 2). Edited by Palmore E. Durham, NC, Duke University Press, 1974

Winslow RS, Stillner V, Coors DJ, et al: Prevention of acute dystonic reactions in patients beginning high potency neuroleptics. Am J Psychiatry 1986; 143:706–710

Woods SW, Tesar GE, Murrary GB, et al: Psychostimulant treatment of depressive disorders secondary to medical illness. J Clin Psychiatry 1986; 47:12–15

Chapter 21

Diet, Nutrition, and Exercise

Robert J. Sullivan, Jr., M.D.

Simply by achieving old age, one can be assured that the diet consumed has been sufficiently nutritious to support an individual throughout life. This is no mean feat in a period when the longevity of human survival has reached limits previously unknown in the history of mankind. As age increases, lifelong eating habits need periodic reevaluation. Alterations in senses make prior patterns of food consumption less palatable. Changes in living conditions alter diet requirements. Illness creates special diet needs. Those responsible for the care of elderly persons must be aware of potential problems with nutrition and diet if they are to respond appropriately. What previously was taken for granted throughout life may need direct attention in old age.

Along with diet, exercise habits are commonly slighted by many elderly persons. Little time is spent considering how vigor declines with each hour of indolence. But decline it does, and it affects one's ability to manage the demands of daily life. With the reduction of activity, appetites can diminish, and food consumption declines. Since balance in nutrient intake depends on eating a variety of foods, subtle deprivation may follow if intake falters. This chapter explores how nutrition, diet, and exercise contribute to vigor in late life.

Nutrition

The science of nutrition involves the study of food intake to promote growth and replace worn or injured tissues. The elderly are vulnerable to nutrition problems as a result of health problems unique to their age. In this section, established standards of nutrition are explained, and results of assessments made using those standards are presented.

543

Documenting Nutritional Needs

National standards and studies of nutrition. The Food and Nutrition Board of the National Research Council publishes the Recommended Dietary Allowances (RDA), which has been continuously updated since the 1940s. The ninth edition (National Research Council 1980) describes the nutrition needs of persons over age 51 as similar to those of youth except for caloric intake, which is reduced from 40 kcal/kg at ages 20 to 37 to 30 kcal/kg at ages 75 to 90. On the basis of a consensus of experts, this publication provides a benchmark for nutrition studies (Schneider et al. 1986). Using RDA guidelines as a standard, two United States National Health and Nutrition Surveys (HANES) revealed that 50 percent of the population, especially the elderly, were deficient in one or more nutrients (Health and Nutrition Examination Survey 1974). A Ten State Nutrition Survey showed similar deficits (Ten State Nutrition Survey 1972). Such reports are unsettling and cause for concern.

Individual nutritional assessment. Nurtiture studies of large population groups such as the HANES and the Ten State study rely primarily upon *dietary histories* for data. This method is limited by the requirements that respondents have excellent recall of what they ate and that unbiased responses are given. Food quality, preparation technique, and portion size are difficult to assess. When nutrient levels are determined by chemical measurements on blood samples, frank deficiencies are rarely found. It appears that many people consume adequate amounts of nutrients even when reporting a suboptimal intake according to RDA guidelines. Because of these discrepancies, the assessment of individual nutritional status rarely rests on diet history alone.

The use of standard *height/weight* tables for nutrition status assessment in the elderly has limited utility because of a loss of height due to vertebra compression, kyphosis, and spinal disk collapse. Ideal weight recommendations for the elderly are in transition since a reanalysis of life insurance table data now suggests mild adiposity is not detrimental (Manson 1987).

Assessment of *body protein stores* is one alternative to height/weight determinations for documenting nutritional status. Measurement of somatic protein stores by creatinine/height index determination is inaccurate in the elderly because creatinine rises due to renal degeneration with age, and height falls due to spinal collapse. Knee-height measures, while of theoretical advantage, are not yet in wide use (Chumlea 1985). Mid-arm circumference to assess muscle mass is an accepted tool although often difficult to accomplish with accuracy (Grant 1981). Determination of visceral protein stores is accomplished by measuring serum levels of various marker substances. Serum transferrin levels, or related iron-binding proteins, are low in malnutrition. Regrettably, elevations in iron-rich states and reductions in chronic inflammation or anemia further cloud their accuracy. Serum retinol and prealbumin determinations are not well standardized for the elderly. The serum albumin level, in the absence of renal or intestinal disease, is the most widely used assessment tool for nutrition assessment despite evidence of limitations in the elderly.

Assessment of body *fat stores* permits determination of energy reserves. Water immersion studies are accurate but difficult and time consuming to accomplish. Skin-fold measurement by caliper is easily done at the bedside and is widely used to estimate fat stores. Sophisticated body composition assessment tools such as total body potassium determination and total body water measurement, while of interest for research, are not clinically useful for bedside nutrition assessment.

Tests of *immune system function* can detect malnutrition. Skin tests to ascertain lymphocyte T-cell activity are popular, but fresh antigens for injection must be available and the test takes time to interpret (Grant 1981). A total lymphocyte count below 1,500 is evidence of an inadequate diet and is quickly determined from routine blood counts.

For the majority of people, a diet history coupled with documentation of weight, triceps skin-fold thickness, mid-arm circumference, hemoglobin level, albumin level, and a total lymphocyte count will permit adequate evaluation of nutritional status. When applied to healthy elderly, these parameters are found to be in close agreement with national norms for all age groups (Burns et al. 1986), suggesting that when abnormal, they do present a true indication of malnutrition and not simply changes related to aging.

The clinical presentation of malnourished elderly persons may be quite subtle. Kwashiorkor; marasmus; specific vitamin deficits such as scurvy, pellagra, beriberi, and rickets; and similar extreme syndromes are virtually unknown in Western society. Where compromised dietary intake occurs, marginal deficits are likely with weight loss exceeding 10 percent, confusion, dehydration, flakey dermatitis, and glossitis. The presence of hypoalbuminemia, anemia, anergy, and lymphocytopenia provides documentation necessary to support the diagnosis. A bleeding tendency, slow wound healing, light sensitivity, hair loss, thin nails, imbalance, and depression are common in healthy elderly and thus provide little additional diagnostic information.

Caloric Intake Profile Over a Lifetime

A fascinating series of studies of rats done years ago suggested diet modification can prolong life (McCay et al. 1939). Spartan fare helped them live longer. Total calorie limitation was more important than fat or protein limitaton alone and there could be no deficit of essential nutrients. The ideal program began with limitation in youth and extended throughout the life of the laboratory animal. The precise reason for improved longevity is not yet clear. From recent analysis of longitudinal study data in humans, it is apparent that low weight in the elderly is not necessarily beneficial and that obesity is a significant problem (Andres 1980). Thus there is active interest in determining the ideal weight for humans throughout life (Andres 1985).

Variation of Nutritional Need with Age

On the basis of current data, one can assume that for most nutrients no special diet supplements are required for older persons. Caloric needs will vary widely with individual activity level and need adjustment accordingly. Regular weight checks are the best means to assess caloric intake adequacy.

Variation in Nutritional Needs with Level of Health

When illness strikes, nutritional demands can change dramatically. Most individuals compensate spontaneously or have sufficient reserves to tide themselves over acute situations. When chronic medical illness occurs, as often afflicts the elderly, specific attention will be needed to assure adequate nutrition.

Many older persons develop a reputation of being finicky or light eaters. In part this is a normal response to a reduction in energy expenditure and also to a reduction in lean body mass. Nutrition problems will evolve if different food types in adequate quantity are not regularly consumed. Immobilization will certainly lead to rapid loss of bone mass. A return to weight-bearing exercise whenever it can be tolerated is an excellent method to halt skeletal deterioration, stimulate appetite, and encourage better nutrition. Old age may be associated with a loss of appetite due to changes in opioid stimulation (Gosnell 1983). If true, this raises the possibility of producing an appetite stimulant or suppressant for administration to persons needing intake modification.

Nutrition is often compromised in the course of acute illness. Hospitalized patients have been found malnourished at rates of 17 to 44 percent for medical and 30 to 65 percent for surgical patients (Bienna 1982). Impaired wound healing (Irvin 1978) and reduced immunocompetence (Mullen 1980) have been attributed to malnutrition. Because of the ubiquity of nutrition problems among hospitalized patients, it is essential to record a weight on admission. Laboratory values needing documentation include a chemistry panel with albumin levels, a blood count for assessment of anemia, and a lymphocyte count. Nutrition deprivation will reach critical proportions whenever someone has been without substantial intake for a period of 10 days or suffers a weight loss exceeding 10 percent.

Heart failure, lung failure, renal failure, chronic infection, and depression all result in weight loss, sometimes of substantial proportions. Studies in cancer patients have implicated humoral substances as partially responsible for the anorexia that accompanies and often precedes overt clinical manifestation of neoplasia (Odell 1978). Dementia is accompanied by weight loss, but the etiology of this remains unknown. The underlying mechanisms for appetite modulation need further elucidation in order that we might exert a greater influence on this vital function.

Diet

Building on the preceding discussion of nutrition, diet recommendations can be made for daily food consumption to achieve specific health goals. Diet manipulation falls within the traditions of primary, secondary, and tertiary preventive medicine. Taken to a proper degree a diet can prevent the occurrence of malnutrition, obesity, or cachexia (primary prevention). In disease states such as iron lack, a diet supplement can cure an illness already present (secondary prevention). In diseases such as heart failure, dietary modification can control the course of an illness not otherwise curable by diet alone (tertiary prevention). The following discussion explores diet alternatives in sickness and in health.

Variation in Diet Is Infinite

People live to old age in many societies throughout the world despite dietary habits that vary widely. Studies of disease patterns show that dietary preferences affect the kinds of illness experienced by members of a population. Drawing from these "natural experiments" has led to specific diet recommendations to capture the beneficial aspects of a particular cuisine. Each new generation has access to dietary alternatives that their predecessors could not have imagined. Frozen foods, fast foods, irradiated foods, and hybrid foods, to mention only a few of the latest options on the grocer's shelves, were not available in the recent past. Population mobility has expanded the mingling of cultures with the result that foods from many corners of the earth are widely known and appreciated. These trends yield expanded opportunities to achieve a healthful diet.

Barriers to an Adequate Diet

Throughout their lives people seek to satisfy their basic needs of shelter, food, and security. At times, they encounter unforeseen difficulties in securing these necessities. In terms of diet, there are both major and minor events that pose potentially threatening problems.

Major factors. Often cited as exerting an important influence on the diet of the elderly are social barriers. Inadequate financial reserves, poor housing, and limitations in benefit programs make pursuit of a balanced diet difficult (Massachusetts Department of Public Health 1976). Safety of access and distance to food markets are problems for residents of cities. Those living in rural areas experience similar isolation when driving skills are lost or family members depart. The death of a spouse or housemate who prepared meals may be a devastating blow. Without the means for getting food to the table, no one can consume a balanced diet.

Elusive factors. When adequate food is available, one must be aware of discreet influences that can contravene adequate dietary intake. People who eat alone often fail to prepare sophisticated or varied fare, with a resultant decline in consumption volume and variety. Dental problems reduce the types of food that can be masticated (Wayler et al. 1984). Vision limitations due to cataracts or glaucoma make food preparation and consumption problematic. Fear of food-soiled clothes or a messy table will lead sensitive vision-impaired individuals to withdraw from congregate meals and valued social interactions.

With age, subtle shifts in gustatory senses occur. Disease or medication use can have a similar impact. Particularly distressing are the effects of dysosmia or dysgeusia (altered smell and taste) whereby common aromas or flavors are perceived as distinctly unpleasant (Schiffman 1983). Substantial changes in food preference are an inevitable consequence.

Medications can create the need for specific dietary supplements (Watkin 1983). Trimethoprim and dilantin are associated with increased need for vitamins D and K and folic acid. The use of barbiturates, cholestyramine, and aspirin calls for extra folic acid, iron, and vitamin C in the diet. Alcohol, neomycin, cholestyramine, and cholchicine influence fat-soluble vitamin absorption. The list goes on and on.

Altered anatomic function with age may introduce further subtle dietary requirements. Atrophic gastritis, often clinically undetected, affects the absorption of several nutritional factors, with both reductions and elevations documented (Krasinske et al. 1986). Altered intestinal transit time with aging is a factor of importance. Fortunately, in the absence of surgical removal or alteration of intestinal integrity, elderly persons usually absorb sufficient nutrients to remain healthy if their diet contains a reasonable blend of needed components.

Programs to Reduce Barriers to an Adequate Diet

There has been continuing social concern for the health status of the elderly in our country since early in this century. The greatest evidence of this concern is the Social Security legislation enacted in the mid-1930s to provide financial support for living in retirement. In 1960 the food stamp program provided further support for those elderly who qualify as recipients. The Older Americans Act of 1965 led to creation of the National Program for Older Americans (NPOA), which offers congregate feeding, health care, education, escort, transportation, and leisure services for the elderly (Lee 1984).

In theory, the NPOA programs aim directly at the major barriers to adequate diet cited previously. The Meals on Wheels program, for example, has been remarkably helpful in many communities. However, reliance on congregate feeding (which is how 83 percent of the NPOA meals are provided) requires mobility on behalf of the recipient. Studies show that 56 percent of program participants come only once a week, and 50 percent drop out yearly. Long-term dietary support of an individual is unlikely to be achieved by this approach. The major impact of the program is socialization. Some suggest that the food stamp program does a better job of placing food resources in the hands of those most in need and that congregate feeding monies should be diverted to that end (Schaefer 1982). The development of convenient, inexpensive, prepackaged, familiar foods from commercial purveyors suitable for consumption by elderly persons living alone may have the greatest potential for improving dietary intake among the elderly (Morley 1986).

Diet as Preventive Therapy

In numerous circumstances, diet modification is capable of disease alleviation, if not outright cure. With the passage of time, more health problems can be expected to join the list, of which a few examples follow.

Dehydration. The elderly lose sensitivity to dehydration (Phillips et al. 1984), especially if they become demented (Seymour et al. 1980) or if treated with diuretics. Therapy requires maintenance of sufficient water intake that the body can perform normal adjustments to maintain renal integrity and electrolyte balance. A fluid intake of 2,000 ml/day is recommended as a minimum. Juice, coffee, tea, milk, and other liquids constituting the daily diet are combined in calculating total consumption.

Atherosclerosis. The value of a normal serum cholesterol level in reducing cardiovascular disease risk is well established (Kuske and Feldman 1987). Diet modification can play a major role in reducing body cholesterol levels, yielding involution in atherosclerotic lesions (Kannel 1986). Stroke, myocardial infarction, claudication, renal failure, visual decline, and other degenerative processes are favorably influenced in the bargain. Alcohol will raise the high-density lipid ratio favorably if consumed in modest amounts of 2 ounces or less daily (Friedman and Lieber 1983). Highly unsaturated omega-3 fatty acids from fish oil also have received notoriety as a potentially valuable dietary supplement capable of shifting cholesterol levels toward a more favorable balance (Glomset 1985). Enthusiasm for this oil has been moderated by the possibility that it may alter the immune system or prove carcinogenic (Feinleib 1981). While concentrated fish oil is not yet of proved value as a diet supplement, fish per se remains an excellent protein source and should be encouraged as a regular diet component.

Diverticulosis. In the past, fiber was thought to irritate colons with diverticula. Intraluminal recording devices revealed that dietary fiber actually reduced pressure and therefore could contribute to a reduction in diverticula formation. Epidemiologic studies of populations known to consume high-fiber diets support this conclusion. For this, and for other reasons mentioned elsewhere in this chapter, dietary fiber now is being emphasized as a daily dietary constituent.

Cancer. A number of significant trends are emerging in the area of diet and cancer causation. An association has been observed between serum cholesterol level, beta lipoprotein, and the risk of developing colon cancer (Tornberg et al. 1986). High dietary fat intake over a prolonged period is thought to increase bile production with subsequent deoxycholic and litho-cholic acid deposition in the large intestine (Reddy 1981), which may encourage tumor development (Mannes et al. 1986). High dietary fat has also been correlated with breast cancer (Helmrich et al. 1983), perhaps because of the formation of estrogens synthesized by gut bacteria using fat in the diet (Hill et al. 1971). Caloric excess is associated with cancer (Lew and Garfinkel 1979), particularly endometrial and gallbladder cancer. Alterations in mitotic activity, hormonal levels, and immune competence are suggested as mechanisms.

Some diet components are outright carcinogens. Nitrosamines produced by fats dripping on hot coals and redeposited with smoke on barbecued or charred meat are considered examples. Salt-preserved foods are also suspect (Sugimura and Sato 1983). Stomach cancer is on the decline in the United States, where smoked or salted foods are infrequently consumed in comparison with food preserved by other methods. Other diet components mentioned as associated with cancer include alcohol, coffee, microbial contamination, food additives, environmental contamination, and effects of food processing and cooking (Willet and MacMahon 1984).

Cancer protective factors have also been identified in foods. Carotene may reduce cancer incidence throughout the body by favorably influencing host defenses or trapping free radicals and thus limiting cell damage (Krinsky and Deneke 1982). Vitamin C may be protective because of its influence on immune mechanisms, inhibition of nitrosamine formation in the stomach, and antioxidative effect (Willett and MacMahon 1984). Vitamin E and selenium are other intracellular antioxidants that are considered protective of cancer initiation (Bieri et al. 1983; Willett and MacMahon 1984).

Fiber in the diet may protect against cancer through several mechanisms. It speeds transit of fecal material through the body while it binds noxious elements such as deoxycholic acid and lithocholic acid, thus reducing gut contact (Hill et al. 1971). The relatively low colon cancer incidence in developing countries is explained in part by the high fiber content of primitive diets (Armstrong and Doll 1975). High fiber consumption can cause problems for some people. Minerals and drugs are bound by dietary fiber, reducing absorption, and gas production may be physically uncomfortable and socially inhibiting.

Despite scientific evidence regarding diet and cancer, there is no unanimity of opinion about specific dietary modifications for cancer reduction (Committee on Diet, Nutrition, and Cancer 1982). Factors such as smoking or environmental pollutants and carcinogens may wield a much greater influence (Pariza 1984).

Diet as Therapeutic Intervention

In disease states that incorporate discrete nutrient deficits, it is sometimes possible to achieve improvement by supplementing intake of the needed item.

Iron deficiency. Iron is found in red meat and certain vegetables. Most older persons easily maintain sufficient iron reserves through consumption of their normal diet. Blood loss through the gut is the most common cause of iron deficit. Whenever iron store depletion is found, it is mandatory to seek a reason for blood loss. Once a diagnosis is made, and effective treatment has returned the body to stability, iron lack is treated by dietary supplements. The usual course of therapy returns iron stores to normal within 3 to 6 months.

Osteoporosis. The cause of osteoporosis is unclear. It is related to a complex interaction within the body of vitamin D, calcium, and estrogens, coupled with weight-bearing activity. Kyphosis, hip fractures, and spinal vertebrae collapse are among the common sequellae of this disease, which is estimated to result in more than 70,000 fractures yearly. Very few people want to look old and bent. Thus the search for a control of osteoporosis is driven by both medical and cosmetic considerations.

Dietary calcium deficiency among older persons is commonly found in community surveys of eating habits. Since bones that are weak lack calcium, logic suggests that calcium supplements could reverse the trend, and they have become extremely popular on this basis. Regrettably, there may be adverse consequences of calcium supplementation. Intestinal irritation is common, with symptoms of bloating or stomach pain. Constipation may develop, sometimes of major proportions. Absorption of excessive calcium is likely to lead to renal stone formation. These side effects perhaps are acceptable if bone integrity is maintained in the bargain. However, it is unclear that supplemental calcium alone can halt osteoporosis.

Fluoride has been found to influence calcium balance favorably by creating an increase in bone density. Distribution of this mineral is widespread in soil and finds its way to us dissolved in the water we drink and through vegetables we eat. Many persons receive additional minute quantities of fluoride through public water supplies that have been supplemented to reduce tooth decay. High-dose fluoride supplementation to promote bone calcification is associated with toxicity to the stomach lining. Regrettably, new bone formed in response to supplemental fluoride intake is somewhat brittle and may fail to improve weight-bearing ability or resistance to fracture as much as originally hoped (Bernstein and Cohen 1967).

Lactase deficiency. Many adults gradually lose the ability to digest lactose, the milk sugar, as a result of the steady decline in intestinal lactase levels with each passing year. Lactase deficiency creates uncomfortable symptoms of gas production, diarrhea, and cramping within an hour or two of eating dairy products. The degree of lactase decline is variable and some people must avoid all foods containing lactose.

Alleviation of symptoms starts with total elimination of milk products for a period of 3 days. A reintroduction of foods will then delineate the level at which symptoms reappear. Acidophilus-treated milk and yogurt contain bacteria that digest the lactose molecule, thus bypassing the need for intestinal lactase. Some cheeses are also low in lactose. Many persons find specific dairy products that can be consumed with no discomfort.

Vascular volume modification. In heart failure and some forms of hypertension, an attempt is made to modify intravascular volume by limiting dietary sodium intake. Edema may be reduced and blood pressures normalized by this relatively simple intervention. Unfortunately, sodium intake is difficult to avoid and some persons cannot tolerate the food restriction. In such cases, diuretic therapy can help alter sodium balance.

In some diseases such as renal failure, sodium restriction may be detrimental if it creates a reduction in vascular volume with loss of renal perfusion. Such an illness requires skilled care with precise diet adjustment to optimize function.

Glucose regulation. Diabetics need multiple interventions to successfully control their disease, and one intervention is dietary. Limits on carbohydrate consumption have traditionally been imposed. Of greater importance is a limitation in total calories to achieve an ideal weight when obesity is a contributing factor in the disease.

Some individuals suffer from hypoglycemia, a condition in which serum glucose levels fall below that necessary to maintain normal body functions. After excluding serious causes such as an insulin-secreting tumor of the pancreas, it is reasonable to treat this problem with between-meal dietary supplements of carbohydrate and protein-rich foods throughout the day. A typical recommendation would be to eat crackers and cheese or a handful of peanuts and raisins between scheduled meals and at bedtime. Often this simple therapy will result in remarkable alleviation of symptoms.

Systemic illness. In the preceding examples, discrete dietary components have been supplemented or altered to manage specific deficits. Many illness conditions call for broad dietary intervention to stem a tide of adverse effects set in motion by the underlying pathologic process. Systemic infections will create metabolic demands at a time when the patient may not wish to eat. Stroke patients may be unable to eat because of paralysis, confusion, or unconsciousness. Comprehensive diet augmentation is necessary to offset the demands of illness in these settings. Fortunately, food supplements are widely available that contain a balanced array of nutrients and are suitable for consumption as a beverage or for instillation directly into the body if required.

Mention should be made of zinc supplementation, which has been touted for its role in wound healing and immune cell function (Sandstead et al. 1982), particularly in regard to decubitus ulcers. If overall intake is adequate, and especially when using commercial dietary formulas, zinc needs should be well achieved with no need for additional supplementation.

Specific Dietary Recommendations

Calories and water. Drawing on the preceding discussions, a number of dietary suggestions can be made. The total fluid intake should be more than 2,000 ml/day. Calories from all sources should be about 30 kcal/kg, with attention to weight change as an indication of success in management.

Protein. The daily protein intake should consist of approximately 12.5 percent of total calories. High protein consumption has been shown to lower body calcium by increasing renal exertion (Marsh et al. 1980) and may contribute to a gradual decline in renal function (Brenner et al. 1982).

Fat. Consumption of fats should be modest to keep weight within accepted limits and should emphasize the polyunsaturated forms when possible. A diet with about 10 percent of calories as monounsaturated fat, 10 percent as polyunsaturated fat, and 10 percent saturated fat, and with less than 300 mg/day of cholesterol is ideal.

Carbohydrates. Carbohydrates consisting of refined and processed sugars and complex carbohydrates, starches, and fiber fill out the remainder of a daily diet. The major role of sugar is to provide energy while the more complex carbohydrate molecules have other important values for the body.

Fiber. Dietary fiber includes cellules and fibrils of vegetable origin including cellulose, hemicelluloses, and pectins. Gums and mucilage from plant secretory cells represent another portion of the fiber spectrum. While not absorbed as nutrients, these carbohydrate molecules exert numerous beneficial effects previously mentioned. Figs, prunes, raisins, and fresh fruits and vegetables are particularly rich sources of fiber and are recommended for daily consumption. Vegetarians, who necessarily consume substantial fiber daily, have excellent lipid profiles (Fisher et al. 1986).

Minerals. Recommendations regarding the mineral content of the diet usually start with sodium. About 2 g daily is adequate for health, a level that can be found easily in the ordinary diet without adding salt. In bygone days, salt supplementation of food was rare, except among the wealthy. Nowadays, with wide availability to all, salt is overused. Fortunately, absent disease, the body is capable of discarding excess sodium in the urine where it does no harm.

Iron is found in abundance in a balanced diet and is readily absorbed. In the absence of iron-loss disease, no supplemental sources are required.

Calcium intake for older men and women should be in the neighborhood of 1,500 mg daily, primarily from natural foods. For most adults, this means consuming some dairy products daily. Calcium carbonate tablets are an alternative supplemental source for people unable to consume dairy products. Calcium citrate is used if achlorhydria is present. Fluoride supplements are not recommended because of toxicity and the absence of proved value (Riggs et al. 1980).

The zinc content of a regular diet is usually adequate to maintain skin integrity and immune function. If supplements are considered, 15 mg daily are recommended as a maximum. It will interfere with copper absorption if taken to excess.

Iodine is needed for normal thyroid function. Commonly found in soil, we consume adequate quantities with vegetables and fruits. Where the soil is iodine depleted, supplementation is necessary. Since iodized salt is widely available, iodine lack is now virtually nonexistent throughout the United States.

Trace elements including magnesium, copper, chromium, silicone, manganese, cobalt, and selenium are readily available in a mixed diet, and supplements are not currently recommended. For persons on tube feedings, these minerals may need specific supplementation. The role of these minerals in hypertension and heart disease is receiving close attention that may lead to dietary recommendations in the future (Kannel 1986).

Vitamins. Most vitamins necessary for maintenance of our metabolism are readily found in the food of a balanced diet. While vitamin supplements are often recommended to alleviate fatigue or malaise, after daily minimum requirements are met there is little likelihood that a significant improvement will be appreciated.

Vitamin A is the second most popular vitamin purchased as a specific supplement after vitamin C. It is often used in large quantities but has no proved value beyond recommended minimum levels. Sufficient quantities are present in yellow vegetables to meet our nutritional needs. Although excessive carotene consumption is free from toxic effects, the closely related vitamin A itself can cause many adverse effects.

Components of the B vitamin group are often sold in drug and nutrition stores in combination or individual formulations. B_{12} and folic acid are among the best known of this collection. A balanced diet has more than adequate resources to meet dietary minimums of all these drugs. Alcoholics may require folic acid supplements, particularly when their habit prevents adequate dietary intake. Persons deficient in B_{12} will need intramuscular shots to supplement their needs since absorption is often impaired.

Vitamin C has been in the headlines for years since Dr. Linus Pauling promoted its value as a cold remedy. Regrettably, overuse of this vitamin has toxic effects. It has the potential to create renal oxalate stones, diarrhea, and vitamin B_{12} absorption difficulties if used in excess (Chalmers 1975). Reliance on a balanced diet alone is sufficient for maintenance of needed tissue levels.

Vitamin D is synthesized in the body whenever sunlight is available. As little as 15 minutes of sun exposure twice weekly is enough to meet body demands. Where no sunlight is available, oral supplementation with 400 units daily is sufficient/ Amounts in excess of that level may lead to renal stone formation (Weisman et al. 1984)

Vitamin E is likewise found in adequate amounts in a regular diet. Supplements are of no proved value.

Summary

A balanced diet can be selected that meets nutritional needs quite well even late in life. Acute nutritive deficiencies are uncommon in the United States, although the incidence and impact of lifelong marginal deficiencies remain to be delineated. Cultural differences have provided insights regarding components of diets that yield the greatest benefit for disease prevention and therapy. Adoption of those specific components as part of our daily intake can be expected to pay long-term dividends in terms of our overall health.

Exercise

Along with diet, exercise receives insufficient attention in terms of its potential contribution to a healthy and active life. Exercise is a subcategory of physical activity that is planned, structured, repetitive, and purposive (Caspersen et al. 1985). If regularly employed, it will contribute to the development of physical fitness, defined as the ability to carry out daily tasks with vigor and alertness, without undue fatigue and with ample energy to enjoy leisure-time pursuits and to meet unforeseen emergencies (President's Council on Physical Fitness and Sports 1971). The following discussion explores the value of and the problems associated with an exercise program.

Correlation of Age and Inactivity

There is a remarkable similarity between growing old and being inactive (Bortz 1982). When forced to be immobile, the body of a youth will quickly lose vigor and begin to look old. Balance becomes unsteady, and strength declines in any adult who withdraws from an active life-style. The apparent correlation between aging and inactivity is remarkable. The value of such an observation lies in the opportunity to recover lost function (Posner et al. 1986). One can never reclaim lost years of age. But lost physical conditioning due to inactivity is capable of being redeveloped with remarkable benefits (Larson 1987).

Etiology of Inactivity

When the opportunity arises to participate in exercise programs, older persons are less likely than their more youthful counterparts to step forward (Ades 1987). Several possible reasons for this can be postulated, as outlined below.

Knowledge of exercise value or methods. In the past, exercise as an enjoyable activity was eclipsed by the perception of exercise as a painful exertion or a competitive endeavor. Recent changes in the understanding of physical conditioning have changed that image considerably. It is now appropriate for all ages and sexes to exercise. Sport and competition may be included if desired, but numerous noncompetitive options are also available. This new perception of exercise has not been adopted by many elderly people.

Fear of injury. The older person may justifiably fear falling or bone fracture if exuberant exercise is undertaken. There is also a possibility of sudden death from cardiac disease triggered by overexertion. The key to avoiding this risk is participation exclusively in fitness activities that stay within restrictions imposed by disease, disuse, or inherited conditions. Careful preexercise evaluation will delineate the precise limits a person should observe. Within those limits, regular participation will create steady growth in physical reserve yielding improved resources for participation in daily life.

Lack of time. A lack of time to participate in exercise activities is frequently cited as a critical factor by youthful persons eligible for fitness programs (Godin et al. 1985). Prior to retirement, work demands indeed may impose substantial limits on time availability. After retirement, even with involvement in numerous activities, most individuals have sufficient flexibility that they can establish their own priorities and place exercise among items considered essential should they choose to do so.

Access to resources. One problem that all individuals interested in a physical conditioning program encounter is access to suitable resources. The cost of membership at an exercise facility, the distance from home to the facility, the absence of exercise periods specifically dedicated to older members at the facility, and companionship while exercising are important considerations that affect participation.

As an alternative to facility-centered exercise, one should make use of resources close at hand to accomplish similar development. Rapid walking is an extremely effective, inexpensive, and enjoyable exercise that can be done in the immediate home environment. When coupled with stretching and upper body exercises, such a program can achieve and maintain a remarkable level of fitness.

Lack of interest in exercise. There is a large group of persons who simply lack the motivation to be active (Dishman et al. 1985). Physical inactivity among the elderly is not unique to modern Western society and may represent a cross-cultural phenomenon (Beall et al. 1985). Since exercise programs are voluntary, people who join are self-selected as perceiving significant value in the undertaking.

To minimize participant dropout and maximize attendance, emphasis is needed on companionship among the participants, with close attention to graded advancements. Inclusion of a strong education component, with attention to the special needs of smokers or obese patients, is also helpful (Moritznik et al. 1985).

Types of Activity

Exercise program components have evolved over a number of years and continue to change as research indicates special value for particular aspects. Flexibility and limbering, strength, and endurance are three elements around which any program is built.

Limbering and flexibility. First among the activities that any individual should do at the start of an exercise session are rapid limbering and warm-up movements followed by gentle stretching and flexing. The effect is to prepare ligaments and muscles for the strengthening and endurance activities to follow. Injuries are much less likely if a proper warm-up is undertaken.

Limbering and warm-up exercises can be done in any open space. Chair exercises are available for those who are incapable of standing because of balance problems or weakness. Floor mats are useful since many of the activities require lying on one's side or back. A pool with water at chest height is a great asset for flexibility training when available. The maintenance of flexibility has daily value for donning clothes, trimming toenails, and support of personal hygiene.

Strength. Physical conditioning programs traditionally emphasize development of specific muscle groups for a particular sport or event. The same concept applies to conditioning programs for life. A person must have sufficient strength to accomplish daily activities. Muscle cells developed in youth persist throughout life, representing banked reserves waiting to be used. Building muscle strength is accomplished by muscle contraction against resistance. Weight lifting is the traditional resistance method used for this purpose. Machines have been devised that permit every muscle fiber in the body to be selectively laden with precisely the ideal pull to extract maximum development. Resistance devices using hydraulic pistons are available where the load is adjusted by twisting a dial. Hydraulic devices can resist motion in two directions, thereby speeding reciprocal muscle development in one exercise effort.

Home-grown alternatives to professional weight equipment are legion. Sacks filled with sand, strips of rubber tubing, water-filled bags lifted by ropes on pulleys fastened to doors are but a few of the ingenious ways to provide resistance for muscle development. Vigorous walking or regular stair-climbing are remarkably effective, inexpensive, and available means to encourage musculoskeletal development.

Endurance. The third part of a fitness program involves enhancement of the cardiovascular system to improve endurance. "Aerobic conditioning" is the term commonly used to describe training that requires an individual to stay within limits that permit inhaled oxygen to fully supply the needs of the body during exercise. The body responds by increasing its efficiency of oxygen transport and use (VO_2 Max) from the lung to each individual cell component. Improved oxygen use permits extended periods of muscle activity without fatigue.

Endurance and strength aspects of conditioning are distinct. One has only to compare a football player and a long-distance runner to see the archetypes of these two concepts. Most elderly need the track-style development rather than a football approach. One can always get help to move the sofa, but no one can help you walk briskly down the sidewalk in order to catch the next bus.

Activity Initiation

Getting involved in exercise after years of inconsistent exertion calls for careful planning. Injuries to the musculoskeletal or cardiovascular system should be avoided while precariously balanced medical conditions are managed effectively. Physical limitations must be identified, specific exercises selected, monitoring parameters chosen, and exertion ranges established. Regular reassessment is then needed to upgrade the program in response to participant progress. The following shows how this can be accomplished.

Injury risk assessment. Medical review should seek occult problems such as diabetes, thyroid conditions, anemia, or electrolyte imbalance. The circulatory system, orthopedic questions, and physical deformity must receive particular attention because of the limits they impose on exertion. Lung disease and asthma may restrict needed ventilation, while neurologic disease can alter balance, muscle coordination, or muscle use. Dementia precluding understanding of exercise limits must disqualify an exercise applicant unless a sponsor will always be on hand to provide guidance. Medication review includes notation of those items likely to influence the physical evaluation or exercise success, for example, propranolol. Medication use occasionally signals the presence of disease not previously documented and provides an index of disease severity.

Fitness assessment. Initial evaluation should include flexibility assessment to assess the applicant's ability to participate in established workout routines and the need for special attention. Muscle strength can be measured accurately using devices developed for disability determination. While such baseline data will provide a satisfying measure of progress for the participant, they are rarely obtained in community programs. More commonly, strength is simply assessed for adequacy to accomplish daily tasks. If specific things cannot be done, such as rising from a chair, then strengthening of the involved muscle groups is undertaken.

Endurance assessment requires simultaneous performance by two interrelated body functions. First, the individual must have musculoskeletal strength and flexibility to do physical work. Second, the cardiovascular system must be able to respond to the oxygen transport challenge imposed by that work. Bicycle ergometry and treadmill testing are two standard means for assessing endurance that are valuable for establishing the limits of a safe exercise program.

The physical capacity for exercise is measured in terms of metabolic equivalents (METS). Sitting and doing nothing is the equivalent of one MET. Youthful persons vary from 1 to 24 (world-class athletes) in terms of MET capability. Older persons commonly enter exercise programs with 6 to 8

METS of reserves. Those in good condition may achieve a level of 12 METS on treadmill or bicycle ergometry testing.

Research studies usually assess physical condition in terms of maximal oxygen consumption capacity (VO_2 Max). This complex measurement is not required for preexercise assessment or program monitoring and need not be used in defining the parameters of a safe exercise program.

Program initiation. The value of group versus solo exercise programs is the subject of some debate (Miller et al. 1984). Exercising alone yields the maximum versatility in terms of scheduling and privacy, with remarkable improvement possible (DeBusk et al. 1985). Group exercise programs are widely available at fitness centers, community agencies such as the YMCA/YWCA, and recreation departments. The majority cater to persons with no known impediments. Some programs are tailored exclusively to special needs of those recovering from an illness such as myocardial infarction. All supervised programs incorporate many weeks of gradually increasing exertion with careful observation for untoward events. During this time, the participant is taught principles of safe and effective exercise that can be applied throughout the remainder of the participant's life.

Many people skip preevaluation and plunge into a self-designed exercise program without hesitation. Of course, the majority do very well with this approach, especially when they are prudent in listening to signals their bodies convey about exercise limits. An ideal program includes a 5- to 10-minute limbering and warm-up period, followed by a 20- to 30-minute exercise period where the heart rate is kept in a target training range previously determined as ideal. This is followed with a gradual cool-down period for an additional 10 minutes. Each part of this sequence is important for safe and effective exercise.

One aspect of exercise that is often misunderstood is the tremendous value that accrues at submaximal exertion levels (Badenhop et al. 1983). One need not punish the body to vastly improve physical performance (Sidney and Shephard 1978). A person should be comfortable at all times and easily able to converse while exercising. Most important of all, the person should be enjoying the process.

Potential Benefits

The benefits of exercise are thought to be marvelous. With time, scientific proof may be forthcoming to validate these expectations. Self-image and emotional stability, while reputed to improve (Taylor et al. 1985), may not change much (Blumenthal et al. 1982). Weight control, while facilitated by an increase in caloric consumption related to exercise, is ultimately determined by food intake (Blair et al. 1985). Nutrition can be improved by physical exertion, particularly calcium balance, provided an increased caloric intake is associated with improved food variety in the diet. Hypertension and diabetic control may be favorably affected as well (Siscovick et al. 1985). Oxygen use is improved and the circulatory system receives substantial benefit (deVries 1970; Cunningham et al. 1987). Serum lipid reduction, collateral development in the peripheral and coronary circulation, and cardiac muscle reserve all are noted to improve (Bortz 1980).

Virtually all who partake of regular exercise programs report an improved ability to manage their activities of daily living. They are less dependent on motorized resources such as elevators or automobiles and can participate in more activities without exhaustion than in the recent past. They are delighted to find that former vigor can be successfully recalled.

Hazards

The majority of older persons experience few problems as they undertake exercise as part of a fitness program. The benefits are assumed to outweigh the risks provided appropriate limits are set and cautious advance is undertaken (Koplan et al. 1985).

Of greatest concern is the possibility of sudden death induced by exercise. Provided a careful physical evaluation has been made in advance, and the patient cooperates by observing established limits, there is little likelihood that the exercise constitutes a significant risk (VanCamp and Peterson 1986). In the long run, there will be a risk reduction resulting from the program (Siscovick et al. 1985).

Musculoskeletal injuries can be kept to a minimum by attention to proper warm-up routines, use of good equipment during the workout, and avoidance of overexertion. Osteoarthritis flares are a constant concern that may limit or terminate the experiment. For many, exercise will strengthen supporting muscles and yield improved joint use. Pool exercises with motion against water resistance are remarkably effective and safe for arthritic patients. When arthritis flares do occur, rest and antiinflammatory medication are the only recourse. Restarting exercise later with altered routines may protect fragile joints.

Osteoporosis presents significant risks for the elderly patient. Falls of any nature can lead to fractures, particularly of the hip and wrist. Vertebral collapse can be terribly painful. When fractures occur, total cessation of exercise is required until healing is complete. In most cases, reinstitution of exercise is then appropriate. There is some comfort in knowing that weight-bearing activity will strengthen bone. Some particularly fragile persons must limit exercise to a pool, where falls are impossible and stress is greatly reduced.

Thermal condition during exercise needs attention since older persons fail to appreciate extremes of heat or cold. Avoiding outside exercise in freezing weather is essential. Warm clothing is needed whenever the temperature is below 60°. Temperatures above 80° are troublesome, especially if the humidity is high. Brisk walking in shopping malls has become popular because of stable temperatures year round, a social environment, solid footing, and the availability of help if problems occur.

Fatigue may be a complaint of the exercise program participant. This usually represents an overly vigorous approach to physical exertion. However, close watch must be kept for congestive heart failure or other medical conditions that have become unbalanced and are presenting as systemic complaints. Prior screening of the exercise candidate should exclude those whose medical status is too precarious to undertake an active fitness program. The risks are minimized by maintaining the target intensity of 60 to 70 percent of maximal heart rate (Larson 1987). Within this range, comfortable, safe and effective programs can be created to keep most of us feeling far younger than our chronologic years of age would suggest.

Conclusion

Intensive efforts are underway to find the optimum nutrition elements throughout life that will reduce the likelihood of developing disease. As of this time, there are a number of trends worth following, among which fat intake limitation and the regular consumption of fiber seem of greatest value. Provided we are able to eat a proper diet, our nutrition status should maintain itself with no need for supplementation. Supplements, if used at all, should include only calcium. With disease states, special attention to nutrition is essential for recovery or control. Numerous helpful diet modifications can be prescribed that may control illness with little or no need for medications.

Physical exertion, when enjoyed as part of an ongoing fitness program, can make older persons feel and act younger than their chronologic years. Care is necessary when initiating any activity change, but experience has shown that reserves from early life can be recalled to active service without undue hardship. The improvements in activities of daily living and the potential for expanding one's resources for dealing with stress or illness make exercise an attractive element in a program of health promotion or maintenance.

References

Ades PA, Hanson JS, Gunther PGS, et al: Exercise conditioning in the elderly coronary patient. J Am Geriatr Soc 1987; 35:121–124

Andres R: Influence of obesity on longevity in the aged. Adv Pathobiol 1980; 7:238–246

Andres R: Impact of age on weight goals. Ann Intern Med 1985; 103:1030–1033

Armstrong B, Doll R: Environmental factors and cancer incidence and mortality in different countries with special reference to dietary practices. Int J Cancer 1975; 15:617–631

Badenhop DT, Cleary PA, Schaal SF, et al: Physiological adjustments to higher- or lower-intensity exercise in elders. Med Sci Sports Exerc 1983; 15:496–502

Beall CM, Goldstein MC, Feldman ES: Social structure and intracohort variation in physicial fitness among elderly males in a traditional third world society. J Am Geriatr Soc 1985; 33:406–412

Bernstein DS, Cohen P: Use of sodium fluoride in the treatment of osteoporosis. J Clin Endocrinol Metab 1967; 27:197–210

Bienna R, Ratcliff S, Barbour GL, et al: Malnutrition in the hospitalized geriatric patient. J Am Geriatr Soc 1982; 30:433–437

Bieri JG, Coras L, Hubbard VS: Medical uses of vitamin E. N Engl J Med 1983; 308:1063–1071

Blair SN, Jacobs DR, Powell KE: Relationships between exercise or physical activity and other health behaviors. Public Health Rep 1985; 100:172–180

Blumenthal JA, Schocken DD, Needles TL, et al: Psychological and physiological effects of physical conditioning on the elderly. J Psychosom Res 1982; 26:505–510

Bortz WM: Effect of exercise on aging—effect of aging on exercise. J Am Geriatr Soc 1980; 28:49–51

Bortz WM: Disuse and aging. JAMA 1982; 248:1203–1208

Brenner BM, Meyer TW, Hostetter TH: Dietary protein intake and the progressive nature of kidney disease: the role of hemodynamically mediated glomerular injury in the pathogenesis of progressive glomerular sclerosis in aging, renal ablation and intrinsic renal disease. N Engl J Med 1982; 307:652–659

Burns R, Nichols L, Calkins E, et al: Nutritional assessment of community-living well elderly. J Am Geriatr Soc 1986; 34:781–786

Caspersen CJ, Powell KE, Christenson GM: Physical activity, exercise, and physical fitness: definitions and distinctions for health-related research. Public Health Rep 1985; 100:126–131

Chalmers TC: Effects of ascorbic acid on the common cold. An evaluation of the evidence. Am J Med 1975; 58:532–536

Chumlea WC, Roche AF, Steinbaugh ML: Estimating stature from knee height for persons 60 to 90 years of age. J Am Geriatr Soc 1985; 33:116–120

Committee on Diet, Nutrition and Cancer: Diet, Nutrition and Cancer. Washington, DC, National Academy Press, 1982

Cunningham DA, Rechnitzer PA, Howard JH, et al: Exercise training of men at retirement: a clinical trial. J Gerontol 1987; 42:17–23

DeBusk RF, Haskell WL, Miller NH, et al: Medically directed at-home rehabilitation soon after clinically uncomplicated acute myocardial infarction: a new model for patient care. Am J Cardiol 1985; 55:251–257

de Vries HA: Physiological effects of an exercise training regimen upon men aged 52 to 88. J Gerontol 1970; 25:325–336

Dishman RK, Sallis JF, Orenstein DR: The determinants of physical activity and exercise. Public Health Rep 1985; 100:158–171

Feinleib M: On a possible relationship between serum cholesterol and cancer mortality. Am J Epidemiol 1981; 114:5–8

Fisher M, Levine PH, Weiner B, et al: The effect of vegetarian diets on plasma lipid and platelet levels. Arch Intern Med 1986; 146:1193–1197

Friedman HS, Lieber CS: Alcohol and the heart, in Nutrition and Heart Disease. (Contemporary Issues in Clinical Nutrition, Volume 6). Edited by Feldman EB. New York, Churchill Livingstone, 1983

Glomset JA: Fish, fatty acids, and human health. N Engl J Med 1985; 312:1253–1256

Godin G, Shephard RJ, Colantonio A: The cognitive profile of those who intend to exercise but do not. Public Health Rep 1985; 100:521–526

Gosnell BA, Levine AS, Morley JE: The effects of aging on opioid modulation of feeding in rats. Life Sci 1983; 32:2793–2799

Grant JP, Custer PB, Thurlow J: Current techniques of nutritional assessment. Surg Clin North Am 1981; 61:437–463

Health and Nutrition Examination Survey 1971–1972 (HANES): Preliminary Findings— Dietary Intake and Biochemical Findings (publication no. (HRA) 74-1219-1). Washington, DC, Department of Health, Education, and Welfare, U.S. Government Printing Office, 1974

Helmrich SP, Shapiro S, Rosenberg L, et al: Risk factors for breast cancer. Am J Epidemiol 1983; 117:35–45

Hill MJ, Crowther JS, Drasar BS, et al: Bacteria and aetiology of cancer of large bowel. Lancet 1971; 1:95–100.

Irvin TT: Effects of malnutrition and hyperalimentation on wound healing. Surg Gynecol Obstet 1978; 146:33–36

Kannel WB: Nutritional contributors to cardiovascular disease in the elderly. J Am Geriatr Soc 1986; 34:27–36

Koplan JP, Siscovick DS, Goldbaum GM: The risks of exercise: a public health view of injuries and hazards. Public Health Rep 1985; 100:189–195

Krasinske SD, Russell RM, Samloff IM, et al: Fundic atrophic gastritis in an elderly population: effect on hemoglobin and several serum nutritional indicators. J Am Geriatr Soc 1986; 34:800–806

Krinsky NI, Deneke SM: The interaction of oxygen and oxyradicals with carotinoids. JNCI 1982; 69:205–210

Kuske TT, Feldman EB: Hyperlipoproteinemia, atherosclerosis risk, and dietary management. Arch Intern Med 1987; 147:357–360

Larson EB, Bruce RA: Health benefits of exercise in an aging society. Arch Intern Med 1987; 147:353–356

Lee SL: Nutrition services for adults and the elderly. Hum Nutr Clin Nutr 1984; 3:109–120

Lew EA, Garfinkel L: Variations in mortality by weight among 750,000 men and women. J Chron Dis 1979; 32:563–576

Mannes GA, Maier A, Thieme C, et al: Relationship between frequency of colorectal adenoma and serum cholesterol. N Engl J Med 1986; 315:1634–1638

Manson J, Stampfer MJ, Hennekens CH, et al: Body weight and longevity: a reassessment. JAMA 1987; 257:353–358

Marsh AG, Sanchez RB, Mickelsen O: Cortical bone density of adult lacto-ovo-vegetarian and omnivorous women. J Am Diet Assoc 1980; 76:148–151

Massachusetts Department of Public Health: Determining the needs of the elderly and chronically disabled. N Engl J Med 1976; 294:110–111

McCay L, Maynard L, Sperling G, et al: Retarded growth, life span, ultimate body size and age changes in the albino rat after feeding diets restricted in calories. J Nutr 1939; 18:1–13

Miller NH, Haskell WL, Berra K, et al: Home versus group exercise training for increasing functional capacity after myocardial infarction. Circulation 1984; 70:645–649

Moritznik J, Speedling E, Stein R, et al: Cardiovascular fitness program: factors associated with participation and adherence. Public Health Rep 1985; 100:13–18

Morley JE: Nutritional status of the elderly. Am J Med 1986; 81:679–695

Mullen JL: Reduction of operative morbidity and mortality by combined pre-operative and post operative nutritional support. Ann Surg 1980; 192:604–610

National Research Council, Food and Nutrition Board: Recommended Dietary Allowances (Ninth Edition). Washington, DC, National Academy of Sciences, 1980

Odell WD, Wolfson AR: Humoral syndromes associated with cancer. Annu Rev Med 1978; 29:379–406

Pariza MW: A perspective on diet, nutrition and cancer. JAMA 1984; 251:1455–1458

Phillips PA, Rolls BJ, Ledingham JGG, et al: Reduced thirst after water deprivation in healthy elderly men. N Engl J Med 1984; 311:753–759

Posner JD, Gorman KM, Klein HS, et al: Exercise capacity in the elderly. Am J Cardiol 1986; 57:52c–58c

President's Council on Physical Fitness and Sports: Physical Fitness Research Digest, Series 1, No. 1. Washington, DC, U.S. Government Printing Office, 1971

Reddy BA: Dietary fat and its relationship to large bowel cancer. Cancer Res 1981; 41:3700–3705

Riggs BL, Hodgsons F, Hoffman DL, et al: Treatment of primary osteoporosis with fluoride and calcium: clinical tolerance and fracture occurrence. JAMA 1980; 243:446–449

Sandstead HH, Henriksen LK, Greger JL, et al: Zinc nutriture in the elderly in relation to taste acuity, immune response and wound healing. Am J Clin Nutr 1982; 36:1046–1059

Schaefer AE: Nutrition policies for the elderly. Am J Clin Nutr 1982; 36:819–822

Schiffman S: Taste and smell in disease. N Engl J Med 1983; 308:1275–1279, 1337–1343

Schneider EL, Vining EM, Hadley EC, et al: Recommended dietary allowances and the health of the elderly. N Engl J Med 1986; 314:157–160

Seymour DG, Henschke PJ, Cape RDT, et al: Acute confusional states and dementia in the elderly; the role of dehydration/volume depletion, physical illness and age. Age Ageing 1980; 9:137–146

Sidney KH, Shephard RJ: Frequency and intensity of exercise training for elderly subjects. Med Sci Sports Exerc 1978; 10:125–131

Siscovick DS, LaPorte RE, Newman JM: The disease-specific benefits and risks of physical activity. Public Health Rep 1985; 100:180–188

Sugimura T, Sato S: Mutagens–carcinogens in food. Cancer Res 1983; 43(suppl):2415s–2421s

Taylor CB, Sallis JF, Needle R: The relation of physical activity and exercise to mental health. Public Health Rep 1985; 100:195–202

Ten State Nutrition Survey 1968–1970: Highlights (publication no. (HSM) 72-8131, 72-8132, 72-8133). Atlanta, United States Department of Health, Education, and Welfare, Centers for Disease Control, 1972

Tornberg SA, Holm LE, Carstensen JM, et al: Risks of cancer of the colon and rectum in relation to serum cholesterol and beta-lipoprotein. N Engl J Med 1986; 315:1629–1633

VanCamp SP, Peterson RA: Cardiovascular complications of outpatient cardiac rehabilitation programs. JAMA 1986; 256:1160–1163

Watkin DM: Handbook of Nutrition, Health and Aging. Park Ridge, NJ, Noyes Publications, 1983

Wayler AH, Muench ME, Kapur KK, et al: Masticatory performance and food acceptability in persons with removable partial dentures, full dentures and intact natural dentition. J Gerontol 1984; 39:284–289

Weisman Y, Schen RJ, Eisenberg Z, et al: Single oral high-dose vitamin D_3 prophylaxis in the elderly. J Am Geriatr Soc 1984; 34:515–518

Willet WC, MacMahon B: Diet and cancer. N Engl J Med 1984; 310:633–638, 697–703

Chapter 22

Psychotherapy with Geriatric Patients in the Ambulatory Care Setting

Lawrence W. Lazarus, M.D.

In recent years, psychiatric assessment and treatment of the elderly patient have moved more and more from the hospital or institutional setting to the community or ambulatory care setting. This shift was influenced, during the 1960s and 1970s, by the closure of many state mental hospitals, by the community mental health movement, and more recently by insurance and federal reimbursement policies that influence the elderly person's medical admission to, and length of stay in, the hospital. For example, shorter hospital stays restrict time available for a consulting psychiatrist to develop a therapeutic relationship to prepare elderly patients and their families for subsequent psychiatric treatment in the office setting.

America's rapidly changing health care system poses new stresses for elderly patients and their physicians, but also new challenges and opportunities for developing innovative programs for assessing and treating the elderly. In this increasingly complex health care system, psychiatrists and their physician colleagues find themselves being patient managers or coordinators, or delegating the responsibility to others, so that the patient's care can be carefully planned and carried out.

This chapter will focus on psychiatric treatment in the outpatient or office setting. Discussion of strategies for overcoming barriers that interfere with engaging elderly patients in psychiatric treatment will be followed by an elucidation of individual psychotherapy, including such specialized approaches as brief psychodynamic, cognitive, and life review therapy. Special issues and techniques of family and group therapy with the elderly will be followed by practical approaches to psychopharmacotherapy in the outpatient setting.

Barriers to Psychotherapy

Although citizens age 65 and older currently comprise about 11 percent of the U.S. population and are especially at risk for developing psychiatric illness, they comprise only about 2 to 4 percent of cases in psychiatric outpatient clinics (Eisdorfer and Stotsky 1977) and even less in most private psychiatric practices (Finkel 1978). Reasons for this low use of psychiatric outpatient services can be understood from the perspective of the elderly patient, the family, and the health care system and physician.

Patient-Related Barriers

Some elderly people believe that unhappiness, depression, and anxiety are expected concomitants of the later years and attribute these abnormal psychologic states to growing old. Thus, they either ignore them or assume a physical etiology and therefore seek out medical rather than psychiatric treatment. The elderly may shun psychiatric intervention because they were raised in an era when shame and embarrassment were associated with such treatment or because of beliefs about psychiatry common to their geographic locale. The psychiatric problems themselves, such as depression with its attendant hopelessness and apathy, may impede the elderly from seeking psychiatric treatment. Finally, such practical considerations as difficulty arranging transportation to the psychiatrist's office and reimbursement limitations of Medicare and other insurers for outpatient psychotherapy pose additional barriers to treatment (Gibson 1973).

Family-Related Barriers

Adult children of aging parents may minimize and attribute psychiatric symptoms in their parents to "growing old." The family may hesitate to suggest psychiatric assessment because of ambivalence about assuming a parenting, caregiving role and fear of the aging family member's disapproval and anger. In addition, adult children may have a psychologic need to maintain an idealized image of their aging family member. Conscious or unconscious ambivalence and resentment toward the aging parent may prevent needed medical and psychiatric intervention. Negative, stereotypic family attitudes toward psychiatry may be another deterrent to treatment.

Health Care System and Physician-Related Barriers

Primary care physicians may experience frustration and therapeutic nihilism when faced with chronic, debilitating illness and dying patients and may feel that psychiatric intervention for associated emotional problems is futile. Shortened hospital lengths of stay and reimbursement policies may influence decisions about psychiatric referral. Referral may be impeded because of the belief that the elderly person's shortened remaining life renders him or her unsuitable for psychotherapy.

Psychiatrists in general, have been resistant to work therapeutically with the elderly. Arnhoff and Kumbar (1970) found that 56 percent of psychiatrists surveyed spent no time with patients over age 65. More than 86 percent of the psychiatrists spent less than 10 percent of their working time with the elderly. An American Psychiatric Association report (Gurel 1973) indicated that only 50 percent of the psychiatric residency programs surveyed offered an opportunity for clinical experiences with the elderly. Residency programs in the past spent comparatively little curriculum time on the special problems of the geropsychiatric patient. Young psychiatrists may have difficulty empathizing with the problems of older patients. The therapist's unresolved conflicts with parents and grandparents may be reactivated and lead to countertransference difficulties. Physicians whose self-image and self-esteem are overly dependent on the success of their therapeutic efforts may experience frustration and disappointment when confronted by patients with serious physical as well as psychiatric disorders. Older psychiatrists may, because of overidentification, experience anxiety with patients who talk of loss, depletion, and depression.

Psychiatrists' previous reluctance to engage the elderly has changed considerably in the past decade, as exemplified by the expanding number of postresidency fellowship programs in geriatric psychiatry supported by the Mental Disorders of the Aging branch of the National Institute of Mental Health and the educational and patient advocacy activities of such psychiatric organizations as the American Association for Geriatric Psychiatry.

A number of innovative, model psychiatric programs were developed in the late 1960s to provide outpatient psychiatric treatment to elderly persons who may never have availed themselves of such services. At the Langley Porter Neuropsychiatric Institute (Feigenbaum 1973) a special psychiatric outpatient program was developed for geriatric patients and the availability of these services was then publicized. Before the initiation of this special program, the elderly comprised 2 percent of the psychiatric outpatient population. After 3 years, the proportion of elderly patients rose to more than 5 percent. Furthermore, the improvement rates of elderly patients was similar to that of patients in younger age groups. The San Francisco Geriatric Screening Project (Simon and Lowenthal 1970) demonstrated that early detection, evaluation, and treatment of emotionally impaired elderly in the community reduced the admission rate of elderly patients to state mental hospitals.

Overcoming Barriers to Psychotherapy

Given these formidable patient-, family-, health care system, and physician-related barriers, strategies have been developed to engage the resistant elderly patient in treatment. The literature regarding psychotherapy with the elderly (Butler and Lewis 1973; Kahana 1987; Meerloo 1961; Pfeiffer 1971) has suggested that the psychiatrist be active, engaging, and therapeutically flexible. Elderly patients usually respond positively to the therapist's listening, empathic, hopeful, and encouraging attitude. Since some elderly patients are accustomed to talking about their physical complaints when visiting a physician, the psychiatrist may decide to begin the initial interview in a medically oriented style before shifting into an inquiry about psychologic problems. Attention is paid to previously overlooked medical problems and medication side effects that may be contributing to current psychiatric symptoms. The initial interview may require more than 1 hour because of the patient's complex and extensive personal, medical, and family history. The "identified" elderly patient is usually interviewed first and alone because it denotes respect for the patient and may elicit information not otherwise obtainable. It is informative and facilitates the therapeutic alliance, if family members are also interviewed. Not only may other family members, or the entire family, require treatment, but also vital information may be obtained from them when interviewed both in the absence and the presence of the elderly patient.

With debilitated, frail elderly patients the therapist may need to speak slowly, loudly, and concretely, and demonstrate (by word and sometimes by touch) concern, respect, and hopefulness. Realistic treatment goals are negotiated with as much of the patient's participation as possible in order to avoid frustration and failure. It is especially helpful for the patient to feel as if he or she has obtained something from the initial interview (e.g., the therapist's empathic understanding) to ensure continued treatment. The therapist's treatment plan, with the patient's permission, is discussed with other health professionals involved in the patient's care.

Because of the complex problems and changing health care needs of elderly patients, as treatment progresses the therapist may need to assume different roles with the same patient, such as that of psychopharmacologist, individual and/or family therapist, and sometimes coordinator of the health care team.

Individual Psychotherapy

This section will focus on two principal psychotherapeutic approaches with the elderly—insight-oriented and supportive psychotherapy. Following discussion of some of the major issues or themes brought up by the elderly in psychotherapy and transference–countertransference issues will be a discussion of three specialized therapy techniques: brief (time-limited) psychodynamic psychotherapy, cognitive therapy, and reminiscence or life review therapy. Emphasis will be placed on what distinguishes psychotherapy with the elderly from that with adults, and clinical vignettes will illustrate major issues.

Common Themes and Issues

Loss is among the most prominent issues discussed by elderly patients. Many writers (Cath 1976; Meissner 1975) believe that a major developmental task of the aging individual is to find restitution for the inevitable biopsychosocial losses associated with this stage of the life cycle. Pfeiffer (1978) has called old age "a season of loss." Common examples of losses are death of spouse, loss of friends, loss of work and job identity, decline in health, decline in standard of living, and loss of mobility. For many elderly persons, it is the accumulative effect of multiple repeated losses, before sufficient time has passed for mourning and resolution, that is so devastating.

Another common theme is the older person's attempts to maintain self-esteem, ego integrity (Erickson 1968), and a sense of purpose in life at a phase of the life cycle characterized by diminishing ego resources, increasing self-doubt, and the onslaught of narcissistic traumas. Narcissistic traumas refer to those events that erode one's self-esteem, confidence, and positive self-image. Constantly threatened with extinction are those activities responsible for the maintenance of a person's positive self-image and self-esteem.

The psychology of the self, as theorized by psychoanalyst Heinz Kohut (1966, 1971, 1977) and others (Cath 1976; Meissner 1975) adds another dimension to our understanding of personality development across the life cycle that has particular relevance to aging. The self may be defined as a developmental psychologic structure responsible for the maintenance of one's self-image, self-esteem, feelings, and affects associated with bodily and psychologic integrity, and relative need for others to idealize and to regulate self-esteem. Kohut believes that personality development in the course of life can be viewed not only from the traditional perspective of the progression from infantile autoeroticism to object love, but also from a second line of development, one that begins with what he terms the "archaic nuclear self," progresses to the "cohesive self," and finally attains, in varying degrees, higher forms of the self including potential transformation of the self across the second half of life. On the basis of the more or less successful development of an integrated cohesive self, persons vary in their sense of cohesiveness and integration from sustained feelings of vitality, spontaneity, and vigor to feelings of enfeeblement, depletion, and, where functioning is seriously disrupted, a sense of inner fragmentation (Kohut and Wolf 1978). Cath (1976) has noted that psychologically healthy older people have the capacity to tolerate loss, to grieve, and to be depressed without losing basic self-respect or suffering irreparable damage to self-esteem.

From the perspective of self psychology, the magnitude of an elderly person's reactions to a loss is dependent, to some degree, on the amount of narcissistic investment in the lost function or object. For example, for aged persons whose intellectual achievements accounted for much of their pride and self-esteem, reminders of failing memory may provoke anger, rage, and depression. Kohut (1972) cites the example of the aging person who, because of brain injury, is unable to solve simple problems. He becomes enraged over the fact that "he is not in control of his own thought processes, of a function which people consider to be most intimately their own, i.e., as a part of the self" (p. 383).

Turning to a conceptualization of self-esteem maintenance from a sociologic perspective, Atchley (1982) believes that people who lose self-esteem in later life do so because (1) physical changes become so pronounced that the person is forced to accept a less desirable self-image, (2) self-esteem was too dependent on social or work roles, (3) loss of control over one's life and environment has occurred, and (4) problems with self-esteem regulation during earlier developmental periods still exist. Atchley believes that the elderly adaptively defend themselves against negative societal stereotypes of old age and the other potential eroders of self-esteem by (1) focusing on past successes, (2) discounting messages that do not fit with the older person's existing self-concept, (3) refusing to apply general myths and misconceptions about aging to themselves, (4) choosing to interact with people who provide an ego-syntonic experience, and (5) perceiving selectively what they are told.

In response to the threat of diminishment of self-esteem, regression within the self sector of the personality may serve adaptive functions by preserving one's self-esteem and warding off feelings of emptiness and depression. For example, the retired industrialist whose self-esteem rested on financial successes may brag exhibitionistically about past accomplishments as a way of compensating for current feelings of loss of self-esteem. The tendency of older persons to reminisce about the past may serve not only to stave off depression and preserve a sense of continuity with the past, but also to remind them of a time when they felt worthwhile, vital, and competent.

Another important issue in psychotherapy with the elderly is that of termination. Many patients, particularly those who are in supportive forms of psychotherapy, do not formally terminate therapy. The therapist usually indicates continued availability because of recognition that the stresses of advancing years and associated losses may precipitate further conflict and decompensation. The knowledge of the therapist's continued availability is very reassuring to the elderly patient.

The therapist conveys an understanding of these themes and developmental tasks and indicates, by word and by gesture, a willingness to assist the patient to work through the losses, to discover old and new sources of satisfaction and gratification, and to modify the goals to which the patient formerly aspired. In addition, the therapist accepts the elderly patient's limitations and repeatedly modifies the goals of therapy.

The therapist is sensitive to the patient's tendency to attribute his or her own feelings of hopelessness and futility to the therapist, thus believing the therapist to be rejecting and critical. The elderly patient, especially one who has problems with self-esteem, is exquisitely sensitive to subtle behavior indicating the therapist's annoyance or rejection. The therapist may also serve as a replacement for those important friends and relatives the patient has lost.

Insight and Supportive Psychotherapy

Although many elderly outpatients can benefit from a combination of insight-oriented and supportive approaches, for purposes of discussion a distinction will be made between the two. The indications, process, and techniques for these two approaches are similar for the elderly and for adults. What distinguishes psychotherapy with the elderly is discussion of age-related issues, specific transference–countertransference reactions, and modifications of supportive and specialized techniques especially applicable to the frail elderly.

Elderly patients who are suitable candidates for insight-oriented psychotherapy include those with motivation for change, the capacity to use insight and resolve transference, ability to mourn and work through losses, previous capacity for work and pleasure, and the ability to tolerate painful affects. Goals for patients able to undertake intensive psychoanalytically oriented psychotherapy aimed at structural or intrapsychic change include mourning of that which has passed; resolving interpersonal conflicts often stemming from the past that are now emotionally draining; working through of intensely private, conflicted, and shame-engendering past experiences; and establishing and working through conflicts in the transference. Principal therapeutic techniques include clarification, interpretation, and mobilization and resolution of the transference. It is important for therapists not to assume that all elderly patients are too physically and psychologically impaired to tolerate insight-oriented psychotherapy, because an overly supportive approach may reinforce the patient's regression and negative self-image. Meyers's (1984) excellent book about psychodynamic therapy with the elderly provides detailed case studies illustrating their potential for conflict resolution and change.

In contrast to insight-oriented psychotherapy, supportive techniques are used for the frail elderly, such as those with organic mental disorders and other chronic debilitating illnesses. Supportive therapy is more concrete, active, structured, and slower paced, with implicit acknowledgment of the patient's limitations (Lawton 1976; Lazarus and Newton 1986). It does not aim at conflict resolution. Instead, the therapist uses a psychodynamic understanding of the patient's conscious and unconscious needs to help increase the patient's realistic tolerance for incapacities and to explore means to ameliorate problems through environmental change (Yesavage and Karasu

1982). For example, the therapist may help the family to be more understanding and tolerant of the patient's behavioral problems and suggest constructive approaches to assist in the patient's management. Supportive therapeutic techniques include ventilation, reminiscence, reassurance, education, suggestions, and validation of the patient's self-worth.

A brief therapy technique has been described (Goldfarb and Turner 1953) for institutionalized, cognitively impaired patients that is applicable to debilitated elderly outpatients wherein the therapist fosters the illusion of being an omnipotent, benevolent, parental figure. The therapist tries to gratify one or more of the patient's requests, thereby enhancing the patient's self-esteem and feelings of control and mastery over the therapist.

Transference–Countertransference Reactions

The elderly patient develops parental or filial transference reactions to the therapist; the latter especially occurs when the therapist is similar in age to the patient's children. The patient may idealize the therapist. This may derive partly from belief in the physician's healing powers, projection onto the therapist of the patient's grandiosity, or from inner feelings of emptiness and despair associated with a corresponding overvaluation of a perceived helper. Depending on the particular patient and stage of therapy, it is sometimes therapeutically helpful to accept these idealized transference reactions without interpretation and without diminishment by the therapist of his or her healing powers under the guise of improving the patient's reality testing. The patient's diminished confidence, self-image, and self-esteem may derive considerable benefit from idealizing the therapist. The trust and security that the patient feels toward the therapist can also be used to encourage the patient to regain old and establish important new nurturing relationships.

Negative transference reactions also occur fairly often. If the patient feels angry, humiliated, and coerced into seeing a psychiatrist by his or her family and physician and has little understanding of its purpose, the patient may be understandably suspicious and uncooperative. Coping already with numerous losses and disappointments, the patient anticipates and fears that the therapist will likewise reject him or her. The patient's initial hostility may also serve to test the therapist's sincerity. The patient may perceive the therapist as an intrusive voyeur and express directly or indirectly envious feelings regarding the therapist's youthfulness and vitality.

Psychotherapy with the elderly may rekindle the therapist's unresolved conflicts with his or her own parents and grandparents. The frequent omission of a sexual history from psychiatric case reports of elderly patients may represent unconscious prohibitions against discussing sexual issues with one's elders (i.e., one's parents). Psychotherapy with the elderly may stimulate the therapist's own fears about aging and death. The inevitability and nearness of the older patient's death may make both patient and therapist shun a close, meaningful relationship. Meerloo (1955) believed that "treating a declining life hurts our medical narcissism and our expectations of magical cure" (p. 227).

Specialized Psychotherapy Approaches

Brief (Time-Limited) Psychodynamic Psychotherapy

A brief, or time-limited, psychodynamic therapy approach could be considered for elderly patients with circumscribed, clearly defined, age-related problems that can be expected to resolve within a brief period of time, such as an adjustment disorder, an unresolved grief reaction, or a traumatic stress disorder. Setting a time limit may reinforce the patient's confidence in his or her ability to resolve problems within a circumscribed period of time, focus and accelerate the therapeutic process, diminish the patient's fear of dependency, and accommodate to limited financial resources. Brief therapy uses the therapist's psychodynamic understanding of the patient and the anticipated transference to clarify and interpret the patient's emotional reactions to a current life stress.

A recent study of the process and outcome of brief, psychodynamic psychotherapy (Lazarus et al. 1987) found that the therapist was used by the patient for validation of competency and normalcy and for restoration of feelings of mastery and self-esteem. Symptomatic improvement occurred to a greater extent than the achievement of insight or self-understanding.

Cognitive Therapy

Cognitive psychotherapy, as developed by Beck et al. (1979), is a time-limited, brief therapy approach that attempts to correct, by using interpretations, explanations, and practical information, the depressed patient's stereotypic, self-defeating thinking patterns and dysfunctional attitudes in order to promote integration of positive perceptions and thinking patterns and thereby diminish depression. Techniques include confrontation, education, explanations and interpretations. Patients learn to reverse their negative cognitive sets by the following five processes: (1) learning to monitor negative thoughts; (2) recognizing connections between negative thoughts and feelings of depression; (3) examining the evidence for and against specific automatic thoughts; (4) learning to identify and alter dysfunctional beliefs that sustain these negative cognitions; and (5) developing more reality-oriented or adaptive strategies for coping with depression.

Gallagher and Thompson (1982a) suggest modifications of cognitive therapy to account for the special problems presented by elderly depressed patients. For example, if patients complain they are "too old to change," the therapist may respond, "Perhaps it is true that you cannot learn new ways of thinking about your problems, but how will you know this for certain unless you try?" The patient may complain that the therapist is "too young to help me," whereupon the therapist may encourage temporary suspension of this belief so that a trial of therapy can proceed. Other suggestions for modifying cognitive therapy include (1) acclimatizing patients for therapy (e.g., presenting therapy as a way to learn to adjust better to this phase of life, explaining what therapy can and cannot do, encouraging active participation); (2) enhancing learning capabilities (e.g., encouraging the recording of notes in a therapy journal, using age-relevant examples, understanding the patient's hesitancy to follow through with therapeutic suggestions); and (3) terminating therapy gradually (e.g., anticipating future problems, encouraging use of the newly learned cognitive skills, and leaving the door open for the patient to return to therapy in the future).

The limited number of controlled clinical studies and experience to date indicate that cognitive therapy may be especially efficacious for cognitively intact, motivated elderly patients with minor and major depressions (especially those without many endogenous features). Cognitive therapy supports higher level defense mechanisms, such as intellectualization and rationalization, encourages patients' active participation, and provides a highly structured treatment approach for depression.

A comparison of brief therapy approaches—cognitive, behavioral, and psychodynamic therapy—for elderly outpatients with major depression found that all three were equally efficacious at therapy's completion (the overall positive response rate for the three therapies was 70 percent), with a trend (not statistically significant) at follow-up for those treated with either cognitive or behavioral therapy to maintain their improvement more than those treated psychodynamically (Thompson et al. 1987). Advanced age did not affect treatment outcome. Very elderly patients responded as well as less elderly patients to all three treatment modalities. Patients with major depression who tended to be unresponsive to all three treatment modalities had many endogenous signs, a concomitant personality disorder, and/or low expectations of improvement.

Karasu (1986) recently discussed the shortcomings and positive aspects of cognitive therapy. Positive aspects include its time-limited nature, which reinforces the expectation of positive change within a circumscribed period of time; consideration of the patient's financial resources; support of higher level defense mechanisms such as intellectualization and rationalization; encouragement of patient's active participation; structured procedures for treatment of depression; and potential for integration with other treatment modalities (e.g., behavioral, psychodynamic). Potential shortcomings of cognitive therapy include its restricted application to depression and less severely impaired patients and the potential, when used as the sole treatment modality, to produce overintellectualization or to be applied mechanically to fend off feelings.

Reminiscence or Life Review Therapy

Butler (1963) has noted the universal tendency of the aging person to reflect on and reminisce about the past—a process that helps the person to conceptualize his or her life over time and to give it significance and meaning. The life review process is stimulated by the realization of one's mortality. Reminiscence is characterized by the progressive return of memories of past experiences, especially those that were meaningful and/or conflictual.

To varying degrees, most elderly patients in therapy reminisce about the past, search for some meaning for their life, and strive for some resolution of interpersonal and intrapsychic conflicts. The purpose of life review therapy is to enhance this process and make it more conscious and deliberate. This technique has been reported (Lewis and Butler 1974) to resolve old problems, increase tolerance of conflict, relieve guilt and fears, and enhance creativity, generosity, and acceptance of the present.

Life review therapy is facilitated by pilgrimages to places of earlier experiences, written or taped autobiographies, reunions with family and old friends, looking through memorabilia (scrapbooks, albums), and verbal or written summation of the patient's life's work.

Life review therapy may be contraindicated for patients who have realistic guilt about the past or who are overwhelmed by unmourned or unresolvable past disappointments and losses.

Family Therapy

Contrary to the widespread belief that the nuclear and extended family was eroded by America's change from an agricultural to an industrialized society and the increased mobility of family members, empirical studies have shown that family life continues to be a vitally important stabilizing influence in today's society. It is estimated that in 8 percent of families in the United States three generations live in the same household. About 80 percent of all older people have living children. Shanas (1963) found that 82 percent of all currently unmarried old persons in the United States who have children are less than 30 minutes distance from at least one of their children. Sussman (1965) emphasized the importance for the elderly of the "extended" family, which consists of a complex and integrated network of social relationships that operates along bilateral kin lines and vertically over several generations. Butler and Lewis (1973) stated, "When families do not offer to help their older members a whole range of personal, social, and economic forces are usually at work rather than an attitude of neglect and abandonment" (p. 107).

Some of the potential developmental tasks and social roles for elderly persons with regard to their family include accommodation—to the role of grandparent, to changing relationships with children, to a spouse's disability, to the possibility of widowhood, and to the inevitability of death.

The elderly derive self-esteem and enjoyment by contributing to the welfare of the family. For example, a grandparent may be called on to be a temporary or permanent parent surrogate. Grandparents are the repository of family myths and secrets and the reservoir of wisdom derived from lifelong experiences. Benedek (1970) views grandparenthood as a time that permits the elderly to "project the hope of the fulfillment of their narcissistic self-image to their grandchildren. Since they do not have the responsibility for raising the child toward that unconscious goal, their love is not as burdened by doubts and anxieties as it was when their own children were young" (p. 201).

Middle-aged children of aging parents face several developmental tasks of their own. As a result of their parents' increasing dependency and debility, adult children may be called on for emotional and financial support. Blenkner (1965) believes that one indication that the adult children of aging parents have achieved maturity with regard to their filial responsibility is their ability to help their parents, both emotionally and financially. Adult children may have difficulty responding to their parents' diminishing capacities, especially if they need to preserve a childhood idealized image of their parents as being all-powerful and omnipotent or if lifelong conflicts have existed. Adult children of aging parents may require psychotherapy to help them resolve their ambivalent feelings and accept some responsibility for their parents. Family undecisiveness about who will accept responsibility for an aging parent may stimulate unresolved sibling rivalry and other family conflicts. Sometimes it is the least loved adult daughter of aging parents who takes on this responsibility in a last attempt to try and gain the parents' love and acceptance before death and to rework earlier parent–child conflicts. Family conflict over aging family members may be expressed by family indecision and disagreement about placement in a long-term care facility, resentment toward the sibling with whom the parent decides to live, and disagreements about division of the family estate and debts.

Assessment of the family is a vitally important component of the comprehensive evaluation of elderly outpatients, for purposes of gathering history, confirming data about the family system, and creating a family treatment alliance that can facilitate, when necessary, family and individual therapy. Assessment generally involves evaluating stresses and strengths of a family system of three or more generations. Common family problems facing the primary care physician and psychiatrist include helping the family care for a relative afflicted with Alzheimer's disease or another degenerative dementia, educating them about depression, resolving intrafamily conflict that is interfering with the medical and psychiatric needs of the older person, helping the family decide about nursing home care, and assessing and treating suspected abuse of the elderly family member.

The Family with a Demented Relative

The psychologic and neurologic problems of the demented patient make the role of those in the patient's social support network, such as the family or surrogate family (e.g., friends), especially important. The therapist can be an important source of support and information to the family. Sometimes families place unrealistic expectations on the physician to whom they have turned for assistance. They may have difficulty accepting the diagnosis of dementia and endlessly seek additional medical opinions in the hope of refuting the diagnosis.

Family members often experience feelings of hopelessness and helplessness as they watch the patient's insidious deterioration. Former, unresolved family conflicts may dramatically resurface. The psychiatrist helps the family work through feelings of despair, ambivalence, guilt, and impending loss. He or she reassures family members as to the normality of these reactions and helps them come to realistic, comfortable decisions regarding such issues as home care versus institutionalization.

The psychiatrist provides the family with practical, specific suggestions regarding day-to-day management of the demented patient. These suggestions can be guided by the following five useful principles helpful in the psychologic management of the demented patient (Ripeckyj and Lazarus 1984). First, family members help the patient to preserve some measure of self-esteem by their empathic approval and positive responsiveness. They assist only in those activities that the patient can no longer manage alone. Family conflict may be expressed by an overprotective and overindulgent attitude toward the afflicted relative. This excessive gratification of the patient's dependency wishes may reinforce his or her already low self-esteem and regression. This leads to frustration, guilt and anger within the family. The psychiatrist can identify the underlying feelings and help the family break this cycle. Second, the demented patient is encouraged, whenever possible, to have some measure of control and influence over his or her own care and environment. Cognizant of the patient's limited ego resources, the family nevertheless defines and periodically redefines functional roles that will allow the patient to have some control over his or her environment. Third, the treatment plan for each patient realistically reflects the patient's available supply of energy and potential for rehabilitation. Otherwise, everyone involved will experience frustration, despair, and disappointment. Fourth, family members are helped to mourn the loss of the loved one as he or she once was and to remain involved, as much as possible, in the patient's care. Finally, the family is encouraged to realize that they may need outside help, such as hiring a companion, involving a social agency, and joining one of the many family support groups that have developed in cities and towns in the United States for support and guidance from the Alzheimer's Disease and Related Disorders Association.

Coping with Depression

The use of family therapy in appropriate cases of depression is supported by the view that depression can be assessed in the context of the social system in which it occurs. Depressed individuals will affect those around them and will in turn be affected by others. Bowlby's (1977) attachment theory provides a way of conceptualizing the elderly's susceptibility to loss of significant others. Many instances of depression relate to the breaking, or threatened breaking, of attachments or "affectional bonds" with family members. The family is involved in treatment both for the sake of the identified patient and to help other family members cope with the patient's altered mood and behavior. The therapist may serve as an empathic role model during the family sessions. Providing assistance to the significant "other" family members may enhance their ability to give to the afflicted one. The family helps the patient by providing empathy and support and by timely encouragement to renew activities that bolster self-esteem. Feelings of anger, guilt, frustration, and helplessness are confronted and resolved. If an antidepressant is necessary, the family is educated about its use and side effects.

Institutionalization of an Aging Parent

It is usually a combination of increasing debility of the elderly person and decreasing emotional and financial resources of the caretaking family members that raises the emotionally charged question of a long-term care facility. The prospect of any exchange, particularly a move from familiar to unknown surroundings, is usually experienced by the elderly person as a threat to his or her security. According to Sussman (1976), institutionalization may be seen as a final surrender to the recognition that the older person can no longer care for him- or herself and that the hope of regaining the activity lost due to illness or natural aging processes is permanently lost. To other elderly people, "nursing home" may connote safety and security. The elderly person may become increasingly aware of a need for more comprehensive care and the burden that his or her failing health imposes on the family. Nevertheless, this recognition may conflict with a wish to remain in his or her own home or the children's home. Although ostensibly agreeable about the move to a nursing home, the patient may nevertheless covertly sabotage it by provoking guilt and ambivalence in the family. The family's guilt may lead to procrastination and indecision. Having to consider a long-term care facility for their aging parent may force the family to recognize their parent's increasing debility, the task of mourning the image of the parent as he or she once was, and their own aging and mortality.

Following the elderly parent's admission to a long-term care facility, guilt over having disappointed and abandoned their elderly member may lead to difficulty in the family's adjustment to this new situation. The family may accuse staff of not caring adequately for their parent's needs. The family may behave toward their parent in an overprotective, solicitous manner. Rather than working cooperatively with nursing home staff, the family may find themselves on opposing sides. The elderly patient may instigate these disagreements about the care, only to end up confused and anxious about the disputes.

The physician or psychiatrist can help minimize such reactions in the following ways. He or she can assist the family in arriving at a realistic decision concerning nursing home care, help them to understand and work through conflicts that interfere with a realistic treatment plan, and encourage the elderly patient to participate, whenever possible, in decisions regarding his or her future. Whenever possible, trial visits can precede the transfer to a long-term care facility so that the elderly person is less subject to the trauma that sometimes accompanies relocation (Aldrich and Mendkoff 1963; Lieberman 1961). Personal possessions, such as photographs, books, and valued objects, can accompany the patient to the nursing home. These objects provide a sense of identity and continuity with the past. The family is encouraged to develop a close working relationship with the staff at the facility. Some families may need counseling before and after their elderly member's admission to a facility in order to better understand their feelings and behavior toward the parent and the nursing home.

Elder Abuse

Physical, psychosocial, and financial abuse of elderly people by their caretakers (family member or employed helper) has become an increasingly serious problem for dependent, debilitated elderly people. Factors contributing to the abuse of the elderly include the dramatic increase in life expectancy, concomitant increases in debilitative illnesses, conflict and stress within the family, psychopathology in the abuser, lack of financial and community resources to assist the caretaker, and problems in the prompt identification and treatment of elder abuse. According to the Elderly Abuse Reporting Act bill prepared by the American Medical Association Department of State Legislation (1985), " 'Abuse' shall mean an act or omission which results in harm or threatened harm to the health or welfare of an elderly person. Abuse includes intentional infliction of physical or mental injury; sexual abuse; or withholding of necessary food, clothing, and medical care to meet the physical and mental health needs of an elderly person by one having the care, custody, or responsibility of an elderly person" (p. 5).

Although difficult to quantify because both victim and abuser tend to deny its occurrence, elder abuse has been estimated to occur, in some type or combination of types, in 10 percent of Americans over age 65 (Clark 1984). About 4 percent of elderly Americans (1 in every 25) may be victims of moderate to severe abuse (U.S. Congress 1985). It is estimated that only one in five cases of elder abuse is ever reported. Rather than occurring as isolated instances, elder abuse is frequent and recurring in up to 80 percent of cases (O'Malley et al. 1983). The abuser is a relative in about 86 percent of cases and lives with the elderly person in 75 percent of cases (O'Malley et al. 1983). Approximately 50 percent of elder abusers are children or grandchildren of the victims and about 40 percent are spouses, thus implicating family stress and conflict as the most prevalent cause of elder abuse.

Although there are few scientific investigations into the causes of elder abuse, a combination of stress factors within the family is believed to play the major role. Frail elderly people at highest risk for family-mediated abuse are those (1) who live at home and whose needs exceed their family's ability to meet them, (2) whose primary caretakers evidence psychopathology (history of alcohol or drug abuse or episodes of loss of control) and/or are under severe external stress, (3) whose family has a history or tradition of family violence, and (4) whose caretakers have limited assistance from other family members, friends, and the health care community (O'Malley et al. 1983).

Given the complex array of etiologic factors contributing to elder abuse, it has been proposed (Council Report, 1987) that a multidisciplinary team of health professionals would be best suited for identifying, treating, and coordinating services for the abused and the abuser as well. For example, for the abused elderly person dependent on the abusive caregiver at home, the multidisciplinary team could consider alternative living arrangements, psychiatric assessment and treatment for the abusive caregiver and the abused, and increasing support services in the home to both maximize the patient's care and minimize caregiver stress. Psychotherapy for the abusive caregiver could include help in identifying the causes of frustration and loss of control, ways of responding constructively to their elderly family member's behavioral and other problems, and assistance in clarifying and meeting the caregiver's personal needs.

Management objectives for physicians involved in cases of elder abuse can include identifying the abused elder person; instituting measures to prevent further abuse; treating the physical and/or emotional injuries; maintaining a therapeutic alliance with the family; arranging necessary social, medical, psychiatric, legal, and other services for the distressed family; and reporting cases of elder abuse in accordance with local statutes (Council Report 1987).

Group Psychotherapy

Various group therapy approaches for the elderly have been used, such as psychoanalytically oriented, supportive, family, cognitive, and reminiscence group therapy. The type of therapy selected depends on the setting, the composition of the group, and the theoretical orientation and personality of the group leaders. All these approaches have in common the provision of a therapeutic and social setting for patients in which to reestablish feelings of self-esteem, provide information and conduct problem solving, encourage reality testing, reactivate former interests, and use the therapists as facilitators, patient advocates, and role models.

The early therapists in the 1950s such as Silver (1950), Linden (1953), Rechtschaffen (1954), and Wolff (1957) reported the therapeutic value of group psychotherapy with elderly regressed institutionalized patients. There have been fewer reports about group psychotherapy with elderly outpatients, in part because of the practical difficulties involved in assembling 6 to 10 elderly patients at one time. Schwartz and Goodman (1952) conducted outpatient group therapy with 19 obese elderly diabetics and found that 13 lost considerable weight and 2 were able to discontinue insulin. Butler and Lewis (1973) conducted "age-integrated, life crisis" group therapy. Their groups were composed of patients of different ages who were experiencing a life crisis. Elderly members made unique contributions to other group members by serving as role models for growing older, for dealing with loss and grief, and for their creative use of reminiscing. Butler and Lewis believe that psychotherapy groups should be composed of patients of varied ages because heterogeneity minimizes the elderly's sense of isolation and encourages discussion of issues pertinent to the whole range of the life cycle. Steuer et al. (1984) compared cognitive–behavioral with psychodynamic group therapy with elderly depressed outpatients and found that both types of therapy were equally efficacious. Pfeiffer (1978) advocated group psychotherapy for persons with depressive syndromes precipitated by object loss. A therapist's time is more efficiently used in group psychotherapy, but more important is the fact that other patients often provide excellent models of coping behaviors and as replacement for lost loved ones. Futhermore, the fact of belonging to a group is of itself an important therapeutic tool.

From the foregoing literature review, it appears that group psychotherapy for the elderly serves to:

1. Enhance self-esteem and self-worth;
2. Provide information and suggestions for problem solving;
3. Encourage socialization;
4. Provide contact with therapists who serve as role models for identification;
5. Encourage reality testing and orientation;
6. Increase motivation to renew former interests and relationships;
7. Supplement the goals of individual and other forms of psychotherapy;
8. Provide an opportunity for patients to share and help one another;
9. Clarify the patient's diagnosis and prognosis; and
10. Clarify and resolve intrapsychic and interpersonal conflicts.

A major problem in conducting group psychotherapy in an ambulatory care setting is inconsistent attendance because of patients' physical illnesses, depression, lack of interest, withdrawal, or social uneasiness. Poor attendance may arise because of interpersonal problems between group members and conflict between the cotherapists. There are several ways to address this problem. During the preparatory interview, before members are selected for the group, the patient's resistance to group therapy is explored and worked through. The importance of regular attendance is emphasized. If a patient is concurrently involved in individual psychotherapy, the individual therapist can be encouraged to support regular attendance at the group sessions and to work through patient resistances. Group pressure also deters absenteeism. Discontinuity of patient membership is compensated for by the permanency of the cotherapists.

Transference–Countertransference Issues

The types of transference reactions to the group therapists depend on patient and group psychodynamics and the personality of the therapists. In general, elderly patients transfer idealized or ambivalent feelings felt toward their own parents or children. The group setting acts as a catalyst that reactivates issues and conflicts pertinent to each patient's family life. For example, if sibling rivalry had been a problem for a patient, this may be expressed as competition with other patients for the therapists' attention, as the following vignette illustrates:

> Mrs. D., a cantankerous paranoid 70-year-old woman, constantly tried to leave the group when the cotherapists' attention was not on her. She was able to modify her behavior into more socially acceptable means for gaining attention after she understood how rivalrous feelings toward her siblings were reactivated in the group therapy.

Typical reactions on the part of the group therapists include overprotectiveness, competition between cotherapists for patients' affection, therapeutic overzealousness, and premature closure about such issues as death, dying, and sexuality. The therapists' anxiety about death and sexuality may lead to covert discouragement of such discussion. Some therapists tend to view the elderly as more impaired than they really are, resulting in attempts to gratify patients' inappropriate dependency wishes, which may inadvertently reinforce feelings of helplessness and dependency. It is sometimes more therapeutic to support the patient's own ability and resourcefulness to solve problems, as the following example illustrates.

> Mrs. H., a 70-year-old dependent, depressed woman with hemiplegia, concluded each session by asking the cotherapists to assist her into her walker. After complying with her request several times, the therapists encouraged

her to try this on her own. She responded angrily at first, but her later accomplishment of this act led to eventual mastery of other independent behaviors.

Linden (1954) reported the benefits of cotherapy group leadership. The cotherapy relationship facilitates sharing and clarification of each therapist's observations and interventions, promotes parental transference reactions, and provides the therapist with the support and assistance of a trusted colleague. In an outpatient setting, it is especially helpful if one cotherapist is a social worker or nurse who is knowledgable about community resources because coordination of medical, psychologic, social, and other services enhances continuity of patient care.

In summary, group psychotherapy is a valuable addition to the therapist's armamentarium. It provides both a social and therapeutic setting for elderly patients to reestablish old and develop new relationships. The problem of irregular attendance is countered by careful patient selection and preparation, group pressure, and working through of patient resistances. Cotherapy leadership helps to diffuse patients' dependency needs and to share and clarify the therapists' observations and interventions.

Outpatient Psychopharmacotherapy

The physician is faced with several challenges when considering the use of a psychotropic drug for an elderly outpatient. Elderly patients often have several chronic illnesses for which they visit different physicians, each of whom may prescribe various medications. Also, they may secretly abuse over-the-counter medication, alcohol, or other drugs. These, in combination with prescribed medication, may contribute to confusion, depression, and anxiety. The intricate interplay of medical, psychologic, pharmacologic, and sociocultural variables makes it challenging to determine the extent to which each variable contributes to the patient's symptomatology.

The following are suggested guidelines for prescribing psychotropic drugs in an outpatient or office setting. It is useful to have the elderly patient or the patient's family bring to the physician's office all currently used medications, because polypharmacy may be contributing to the patient's symptoms. If the patient is taking psychotropic drugs at the time of this comprehensive evaluation, it is helpful, if possible, to consider discontinuing those medications that may be contributing to symptoms and to reevaluate the patient during a drug-free, baseline period. Learoyd et al. (1972) found that the abnormal behavior of 16 percent of 236 patients who were receiving psychotropic drugs before admission to a psychogeriatric hospital unit was directly attributable to the drug's deleterious effects.

Drug selection and dosage are sometimes determined more by the presenting signs and symptoms than by the specific psychiatric syndrome.

One psychotropic drug, rather than a combination of such drugs, is used in order to minimize side effects and evaluate its effectiveness. There are advantages to selecting a medication with which the physician has the most knowledge and experience and that has withstood the test of time. Drug compliance is sometimes facilitated by attaching a positive value to the development of mild side effects, such as dry mouth. For example, when prescribing an antidepressant, the patient can be told to not only notify the physician about such anticholinergic symptoms, but also that these side effects are an indication that the medication is working.

The dosage of psychotropic medications is individualized. In general, with most psychotropic drugs one usually begins with one-fourth to one-third of the initial dose prescribed to healthy adults, with gradual increments based on clinical response and side effects. For debilitated patients, the initial dose may be even less.

Most psychotropic drugs are given in divided doses two or three times a day because elderly patients may be intolerant of a sudden rise in drug blood level resulting from one large daily dose. Changes in blood pressure, pulse, and other side effects are monitored. Liquid preparations are useful for elderly patients who cannot swallow tablets.

The patient is reassessed at frequent intervals to determine the need for maintenance medication, changes in dosage, and development of side effects. An antiparkinsonian drug to counteract extrapyramidal side effects of a major tranquilizer is used only as needed and not prophylactically. It may further aggravate the anticholinergic side effects of the neuroleptic and other medications. If an antiparkinsonian drug is used, Fann and Lake (1974) recommend that it be discontinued on a trial basis after 4 to 6 weeks since only 18 to 20 percent of patients whose antiparkinsonian drug is discontinued will have a recurrence of extrapyramidal side effects. Decreasing the dosage of the neuroleptic may circumvent the need for an antiparkinsonian drug.

If a major tranquilizer is indicated for such symptoms as agitation, delusions, or hallucinations, it is best to choose a drug that is least likely to further aggravate concurrent medical problems. For example, an elderly, withdrawn psychotic patient whose cardiovascular system is impaired may be particularly sensitive to the hypotensive side effect of a phenothiazine drug such as thioridazine. Haloperidol, because it produces less hypotension and sedation, may be preferable for this patient.

Elderly persons, particularly those who have an organic mental disorder, are especially susceptible to the side effects of major tranquilizers. A particularly distressing side effect of psychotropic drugs is a toxic confusional state resulting from the anticholinergic properties of a single psychotropic drug or a combination of psychotropics (Davis et al. 1973). Also referred to as the "central anticholinergic syndrome" or atropine psychosis, it is characterized by a marked disturbance in short-term memory, impaired attention, disorientation, anxiety, visual and auditory hallucinations, increased psychotic thinking, and peripheral anticholinergic side effects. The syndrome is sometimes difficult to recognize, particularly in patients who are psychotic, confused, and agitated before they develop this side effect. Its onset may be signaled by a worsening of the preexisting psychosis or by the above-described anticholinergic signs and symptoms. If the syndrome is attributed to a worsening of the psychosis, an increase in the offending medication may be instituted, resulting in a predictable increase of symptoms. The most efficacious treatment is to discontinue the offending medication. If the medications were contributing to the confusional state, the confusion and other anticholinergic symptoms will usually clear within 1 to 4 days.

The elderly patient with mild to moderate anxiety may be a candidate for antianxiety medication, such as alprazolam, 0.25 to 0.5 mg twice or three times daily, or lorazepam, 0.25 mg to 1 mg two or three times a day. Some antianxiety drugs can be addictive and can produce paradoxical excitement or confusion. It is usually best to prescribe those medications over short periods of time and consider trial reduction or discontinuation. Some patients with anxiety disorders may need long-term maintenance treatment.

In an ambulatory setting, the physician should be cautious in prescribing antidepressants to the frail elderly because of the risk of orthostatic hypotension and cardiotoxicity. The secondary amine tricyclics, such as nortriptyline and desipramine, have fewer anticholinergic and other side effects than the tertiary amines and appear to be better tolerated by the elderly. Nortriptyline has been found to produce less orthostasis than many other antidepressants. Some elderly patients require a trial of antidepressant for 3 to even 5 weeks before a therapeutic response occurs. For nonresponders to tricyclic antidepressants, checking antidepressant blood levels, adding a low dose of ritalin, or changing to a different class of antidepressant is sometimes effective. Electroconvulsant therapy, usually in the hospital setting, is especially effective for drug-resistant, suicidal, and delusionally depressed patients.

Ritalin has been found to be especially useful for withdrawn, apathetic, cognitively impaired geriatric patients (Kaplitz 1975) and for depression following stroke. The initial dose can be as low as 2.5 mg every morning and noon, up to a total of 25 to 40 mg/day with monitoring for hyperactivity, cardiac effects, and other side effects.

Conclusion

Psychiatric treatment of elderly patients and their families in the ambulatory care setting is a challenging and rewarding task for the primary physician and the psychiatrist. The carefully performed, comprehensive clinical evaluation serves as the cornerstone of this process.

The physician gathers information from and, with the patient's permission, shares information with various sources—the patient, family, other health professionals, and agencies—so that a comprehensive coordinated treatment plan can be effected. The physician's diagnostic skill and acumen are challenged as he or she attempts to unravel the intricate interplay of biologic, psychologic, and sociocultural variables that contribute to the patient's symptomatology.

A wide range of treatment approaches have been reported to be effective with the elderly, from the more intensive, insight-oriented therapies (psychoanalysis, insight-oriented psychotherapy), to time-limited psychotherapies (cognitive, brief psychodynamic psychotherapy), to more supportive approaches and various family and group therapies. For many elderly patients, insight-oriented psychotherapy provides the opportunity to meaningfully integrate a lifetime of experience while fostering self-understanding and resolution of old and new conflicts. This process can open new avenues for personal growth and development, even in the very last years of life. For many other elderly patients, supportive psychotherapy can shore up stressed defenses and coping mechanisms and reestablish a sense of self-worth and a measure of control over their environment.

A majority of elderly patients coming to the psychiatrist's office require more supportive forms of psychotherapy that require the therapist to be active, directive, and sometimes involved in arranging a supportive, nurturing environment. Some patients need to feel secure and protected by feeling some control over someone perceived to be benevolent and powerful.

Despite the optimism of case reports and some controlled studies of the efficacy of psychotherapy with the elderly, barriers to treatment continue to exist. These include therapeutic pessimism on the part of some mental health professionals, lack of available psychiatric services, hesitancy of primary care physicians to refer elderly patients for psychotherapy, insufficient third-party coverage, and the elderly's own reluctanace to seek psychotherapeutic help.

There continues to be a need for more empirical research that will help answer the perennial question: What type of patient benefits most from what type of treatment in which particular treatment setting?

References

Aldrich CK, Mendkoff E: Relocation of the aged and disabled: a mortality study. J Am Geriatr Soc 1963; 11:185–194

American Medical Associaton: Model Elderly Abuse Reporting Act. Chicago, American Medical Association, 1985

Arnhoff F, Kumbar A: The Nation's Psychiatrists—1970 Survey. Washington, DC, American Psychiatric Association, 1970

Atchley RC: The aging self. Psychotherapy: Theory, Research and Practice 1982; 9:388–396

Beck A, Ruch J, et al: Cognitive Therapy of Depression. New York, Guilford Press, 1979

Benedek T: Parenthood during the life cycle, in Parenthood. Boston, Little, Brown, 1970

Blenkner M: Social work and family relationships in later life with some thought on filial maturity, in Social Structure and the Family: Generational Relations. Edited by Shanas E, Streib GF. Englewood Cliffs, NJ, Prentice-Hall, 1965

Bowlby J: Making and breaking of affectional bonds. Br J Psychiatry 1977; 130:201–210

Butler RN: The life review: an interpretation of reminiscence in the aged. Psychiatry 1963; 26:65–76

Butler RN, Lewis MI: Aging and Mental Health, Positive Psychosocial Approaches. St. Louis, C.V. Mosby, 1973

Cath SH: Functional disorders. An organismic view and attempt at reclassification, in Geriatric Psychiatry. Edited by Bellak L, Karasu TB. New York, Grune & Stratton, 1976

Clark CB: Geriatric abuse—out of the closet. J Tenn Med Assoc 1984; 77:470–471

Council Report—elder abuse and neglect. JAMA 1987; 257:966–971

Davis JM, Fann WE, El-Yousef MK, et al: Clinical problems in treating the aged with psychotropic drugs, in Psychopharmacology and Aging, Advances in Behavioral Biology. London, Plenum Press, 1973

Eisdorfer C, Stotsky BA: Intervention, treatment, and rehabilitation of psychiatric disorders, in The Handbook of the Psychology of Aging. Edited by Birren JE, Schaie KW. New York, Van Nostrand Reinhold, 1977

Erickson EH: The human life cycle, in International Encyclopedia of the Social Sciences. New York, Macmillian, 1968

Fann FE, Lake CR: Drug-induced movement disorders in the elderly: an appraisal of treatment, in Drug Issues in Geropsychiatry. Edited by Fann WE, Maddox GL. Baltimore, Williams & Wilkins, 1974

Feigenbaum E: Ambulatory treatment of the elderly, in Mental Illness in Later Life. Edited by Busse EW, Pfeiffer E. Washington, DC, American Psychiatric Association, 1973

Finkel S: Geriatric psychiatry training for the general psychiatric resident. Am J Psychiatry 1978; 135:101–103

Gallagher D, Thompson LW: Cognitive therapy for depression in the elderly: a promising model for treatment and research, in Depression in the Elderly. Edited by Breslau L, Hang M. New York, Springer, 1982a

Gallagher D, Thompson LW: Differential effectiveness of psychotherapies for the treatment of major depression disorder in older adult patients. Psychotherapy: Theory, Research and Practice 1982b; 19:482–490

Gibson RW: Insurance coverage for treatment of mental illness in later life, in Mental Illness in Later Life. Edited by Busse EW, Pfeiffer E. Washington, DC, American Psychiatric Association, 1973

Goldfarb Al, Turner H: Psychotherapy of aged persons. Utilization and effectiveness of brief therapy. Am J Psychiatry 1953; 19:916–921

Gurel L: A Survey of Academic Resources in Psychiatric Residency Training. Washington, DC, American Psychiatric Association, 1973

Kahana RJ: Geriatric psychotherapy: beyond crisis management, in Treating the Elderly with Psychotherapy: The Scope for Change in Later Life. Edited by Sadavoy J, Leszcz M. New York, International Universities Press, 1987

Kaplitz SE: Withdrawn, apathetic geriatric patients responsive to methylphenidate. J Am Geriatr Soc 1975; 13:6, 271–276

Karusu TB: The specificity versus nonspecificity dilemma: toward identifying therapeutic change agents. Am J Psychiatry 1986; 143:6, 687–695

Kohut H: Forms and transformation of narcissism. J Am Psychoanal Assoc 1966; 14:243–272

Kohut H: The Analysis of the Self. New York, International Universities Press, 1971

Kohut H: Thoughts on narcissism and narcissistic rage. The Psychoanalytic Study of the Child 1972; 27:360–400

Kohut H: The Restoration of the Self. New York, International Universities Press, 1977

Kohut H, Wolf E: The disorders of the self and their treatment: an outline. Int J Psychoanal 1978; 59:413–425

Lawton MP: Geropsychological knowledge as a background for psychotherapy with older people. J Geriatr Psychiatry 1976; 9:221–233

Lazarus LW, Groves L, et al: Brief psychotherapy with the elderly: a study of process and outcome, in Treating the Elderly in Psychotherapy: The Scope for Change in Later Life. Edited by Sadavoy J, Leszcz M. New York, International Universities Press, 1987

Lazarus LW, Newton N: Treatment of the elderly neuropsychiatric patient: psychodynamic psychotherapies, in Advances in Neurogerontology (Volume 5). Edited by Maletta G. 1986

Learoyd BM: Psychotropic drugs in the aging patient. Med J Aust 1972; 1:1131–1133

Lewis MI, Butler RN: Life-review therapy: putting memories to work in individual and group psychotherapy. Geriatrics 1974; 29:11

Lieberman MA: Relationship of mortality rates to entrance to a home for the aged. Geriatrics 1961; 16:575–579

Linden M: Group psychotherapy with institutionalized senile women: studies in gerontologic human relationships. Int J Group Psychother 1953; 3:150–170

Linden M: The significance of dual leadership in gerontological group psychotherapy. Studies in gerontological human relations. Int J Group Psychother 1954; 4:262–273

Meerloo JAM: Psychotherapy with elderly people. Geriatrics 1955; 10:583–587

Meerloo JAM: Modes of psychotherapy in the aged. J Am Geriatr Soc 1961; 9:225–234

Meissner WW: Normal psychology of the aging process revisited: I. Discussion. Presented at the 15th Anniversary Annual Scientific Meeting of the Boston Society of Gerontologic Psychiatry, Boston, 1975

Meyers WA: Dynamic therapy for the older patient. New York, Jason Aronson, 1984

O'Malley TA, Everitt DE, O'Malley HC, et al: Identifying and preventing family-mediated abuse and neglect of elderly persons. Ann Intern Med 1983; 98:998–1005

Pfeiffer E: Psychotherapy with elderly patients. Postgrad Med 1971; 50:254–258

Pfeiffer E: Psychotherapy of the elderly. NAPPHJ 1978; 10:41–46

Rechtschaffen A: Intensive treatment program for state hospital geriatric patients. Geriatrics 1954; 9:28–34

Ripeckyj A, Lazarus LW: Management of old age—psychotherapy: individual, group and family, in Handbook of Studies on Psychiatry and Old Age. Edited by Kay DWK, Burrows GD. Amsterdam, Elsevier, 1984

Schwartz E, Goodman J: Group therapy of obesity in eldely diabetics. Geriatrics 1952; 7:280–283

Shanas E: The unmarried old person in the United States: living arrangements and care in illness, myth and fact. Presented at the International Social Sciences Research Seminar in Gerontology, Markaryd, Sweden, 1963

Silver A: Group psychotherapy with senile psychotic patients. Geriatrics 1950; 5:147–150

Simon A, Lowenthal MF: Crisis and Intervention: The Fate of the Elderly Mental Patient. San Francisco, Jossey-Bass, 1970

Steuer J, Mintz J, et al: Cognitive–behavioral and psychodynamic group psychotherapy in the treatment of geriatric depression. J Consult Clin Psychol 1984; 52:180–189

Sussman MB: Relationships of adult children with their parents in the United States, in Social Structure and the Family: Generational Relationships. Edited by Shanas E, Streib GF. Englewood Cliffs, NJ, Prentice-Hall, 1965

Sussman MB: The family life of old people, in Handbook of Aging and the Social Sciences. Edited by Binstock RH. New York, Van Nostrand Reinhold, 1976

Thompson LW, Gallagher D, Steinmetz-Breckenridge J: Comparative effectiveness of psychotherapies for depressed elders. J Consult Clin Psychol 1987; 55:3, 385–390

U.S. Congress: Elder Abuse: A National Disgrace: Report by the Subcommittee on Health and Long-Term Care of the Select Committee on Aging (Committee Publicaton No. 99-502). U.S. House of Representatives, 1985

Yesavage JA, Karasu TB: Psychotherapy with elderly patients. Am J Psychother 1982; 36:1, 41–55

Wolff K: Group psychotherapy with geriatric patients in a mental hospital. J Am Geriatr Soc 1957; 5:13–19

Chapter 23

Inpatient Treatment of the Older Psychiatric Patient

Alan D. Whanger, M.D.

Introduction

The Role of the Institution in the Treatment of the Older Psychiatric Patient

The part that institutions play and will play in the care of the elderly mentally impaired patient is variable and uncertain, mostly because of funding policies and problems over the years. It was observed years ago by Blenkner that the care of the elderly tends to follow the public dollar (Blenkner 1968). The problems of care frequently are on the front pages of newspapers, where it is pointed out, for instance, that Medicare rules are producing "costogenic morbidity," forcing many of the aged sick to leave the hospital too early and while still too ill, and that others who are "desperately ill never even make it into a hospital bed because Medicare rules say that they are not sick enough." Newspapers report that about two-thirds of elderly Americans living in a nursing home are impoverished in 13 weeks (Fraser and Flaherty 1987; Haglund 1987). The special problems of the aged mentally ill include the discriminatory present Medicare limits of 190 days lifetime allowance for inpatient care in psychiatric hospitals and the $250 per year for outpatient visits for mental illness (Hausman 1987). One of the obvious responses has been a reduction in facilities and programs serving elderly and poor patients (Einzberg 1984).

Presuming that institutional care will remain generally available, this chapter reviews and describes therapeutic situations and interventions that will be or should be reasonably available in such facilities if they are to service adequately those elderly who suffer from various mental disorders. This is approached from the standpoint of a spectrum of health professionals who will be involved in dealing with these problems in a variety of institutional settings.

For many years, virtually the only alternative in the United States for the older individual with a mental disorder who could not be cared for at home was the state mental hospital. The mere fact of being in an institution does not guarantee that any effective treatment is taking place, however, and too often this situation led to custodial warehousing. Both economic and therapeutic considerations eventually led to a greater emphasis on community services. The subsequent discharge and transfer of the patients to other facilities such as nursing homes resulted in a 40 percent decline in the population of the elderly in state mental hospitals between 1969 and 1973 (Butler 1975). Older individuals with psychiatric problems are commonly put into a particular type of institution more as a matter of convenience than because of therapeutic considerations (Eisdorfer and Stotsky 1977). Unfortunately, it is often true that those who once would not have had an alternative to the state mental hospital now have few viable alternatives to the nursing home (Glasscote et al. 1977). There are increasing numbers of psychiatrists who are willing and able to care for older patients, and more are being admitted to recognized psychiatric facilities, but these facilities are still relatively few.

A substantial reservoir of mental illness in the elderly is unrecognized; Stotsky found diagnosable psychoses in over half of nursing home patients without previous psychiatric history (Stotsky 1967). Studies conducted on samples of all the care-giving institutions in a mixed community showed that more than 80 percent of the elderly in nursing care facilities had diagnosable psychiatric problems, indicating a need for increased mental health services (Whanger and Lewis 1975). This is in line with a study in a community nursing home by Rovner et al. (1986) that showed that 94 percent of the residents had mental disorders by criteria from the *Diagnostic and Statistical Manual of Mental Disorders (Third Edition) (DSM-III)* (American Psychiatric Association 1980). While the treatment of mental illness is not a generally recognized function of the nursing home as an institution, it has been found that therapeutic and preventive psychiatric care within nursing care facilities can be an effective and economical approach for both the home and the patients (Sherr and Goffi 1977).

Improvement in the quantity and quality of community services and facilities for the aged is desirable, but institutions will continue to provide important services even with ideal community programs.

Institutional Care in a Historical Perspective

Families or religious institutions generally took care of the mentally or physically impaired older person prior to the 17th century. King Henry VIII in

England began the governmental and secular role in caring for the aged by destroying monasteries and the systems of care in the churches. In 1601, a tax was imposed to set up almshouses and workhouses for custodial care of the poor and elderly in England (Gold 1970; Whanger 1977). By 1790, Pinel was admitting increasing numbers of elderly psychiatric patients to the Salpetriere hospital in France, which provided exercise, nursing care, and environmental manipulation (Hader and Seltzer 1967). In the early 19th century, a number of small and effective psychiatric hospitals were established in the United States and Britain. By the middle of that century, however, large numbers of immigrants swelled the populations of the mentally ill beyond the capacity of the small hospitals, and therefore large state-supported hospitals proliferated. The fact that these understaffed and overcrowded hospitals were used often for the permanent and terminal care of the elderly led many to view them with some justification as warehouses of the dying (Markson 1971). These conditions tended to prevail also in Britain until 1948 when the National Health Service was developed, and the medical specialty of geriatrics was begun (Arie and Isaacs 1978). In the United States, the state mental hospital population peaked at 558,922 in 1955, and has been declining since, although the nursing home population has grown rapidly since that time (Stotsky 1970).

Varieties of Inpatient Facilities

The elderly with psychiatric problems may be institutionalized in a variety of settings. The obvious are private and public psychiatric hospitals and general hospitals with psychiatric wards or units. As mentioned, nursing homes are a huge repository for the mentally impaired elderly. There are several levels of nursing care facilities, namely, continuing care communities that include social activities and room and board in addition to health and personal care; intermediate care facilities, which provide rehabilitative, social, and personal care services in addition to regular nursing care; and skilled nursing facilities providing 24-hour medical care and supervision (National Institute on Aging 1986). Traditionally, long-term care for the aged has been largely synonymous with institutional care, but now a number of the services can be provided in the community. Hopefully, the continuum of need and care of the impaired person can be recognized and matched with the facilities. Goffman long ago recognized the "total institution" as a place where a number of like-situated individuals are cut off from the wider society for an appreciable period of time and lead an enclosed, formally administered round of life (Goffman 1961). There are other varieties of congregate living arrangements for the elderly that are not total institutions or are not considered as health services, and yet still house many psychiatrically impaired elderly. These include foster placements, rest homes, boarding houses, retirement homes, group apartments, and senior citizen hotels and residences (Burack-Weiss 1985).

Criteria for Admission

In order to regulate the numbers of admissions to institutions and to control the costs, various criteria have been established. In 1983, a prospective payment system was established to pay for hospital stays of Medicare beneficiaries, with the level of payment being largely determined by the diagnosis-related group (DRG) into which the patient is classified. Nine of these DRGs are for psychiatric disorders and five are for substance abuse. Actually, psychiatric hospitals as such have been exempt, and certain discrete psychiatric units in general hospitals that met a number of criteria were also exempted (Freiman et al. 1987). Prospective payments, or lack thereof, have had an impact on alcohol, drug abuse, and mental health admissions, but this issue is in such a present state of flux that it is difficult to predict what its outcome will be (McGuire et al. 1987; Mitchell et al. 1987).

With little hope of being able to resolve this difficult issue here, some criteria and factors are presented that I believe are relevant to the admission of elderly psychiatric patients to various institutions.

Severity of illness. In general, those with the following characteristics might appropriately receive care in an institution of some type providing psychiatric care (Whanger 1973; Butler 1977):

1. Those with relatively acute functional psychoses with bizarre or delusional behavior or hallucinations for whom outpatient care is not feasible;
2. Those who are dangerous to themselves or others, with suicidal, assaultive, destructive, self-mutilative, or self-negligent behavior;
3. Those with chronic organic mental disorder or dementia whose behavior, such as escaping, fire setting, or attacking others, is unresponsive to medications and is too disruptive to manage at home or in a less restrictive environment;
4. Those with acute organic mental disorder or delirium, with agitative or potentially destructive behavior;
5. Those with alcoholism or other drug use with such problems as impending delirium tremens, confusion, or other state needing detoxification and rehabilitation;
6. Those unable to perform major activities of daily living because of severe psychiatric symptoms such as panic attacks, psychomotor retardation, agitation, or social isolation;
7. Those with significant toxic effects from therapeutic psychotropic drugs.

Intensity of service. Elderly patients could very appropriately be admitted to psychiatric inpatient facilities when a high level of care is needed that is impractical or impossible on an outpatient basis. Such indications might be as follows:

1. Those needing intravenous or frequent intramuscular psychotropic medications;
2. Those needing close regulation of oral medications, such as individuals with marked drug sensitivities or those requiring titration of medications such as during drug addiction withdrawal or detoxification;
3. Those needing electric convulsive therapy (ECT), at least during the initial series, or frequent treatment;
4. Those needing several intense daily or frequent therapies such as individual and group psychotherapy, drug therapy, occupational therapy, and physical therapy;
5. Those requiring seclusion, restraint, or isolation because of agitated or destructive states.

Criteria for excluding admission. There are a number of situations in which elderly have been admitted to psychiatric facilities in the past, but admission was relatively contraindicated. Some of them are as follows:

1. Those who are acutely physically ill, comatose, or moribund;
2. Those with minor mental symptoms that may be related to medical problems;
3. Those who need mostly adequate living arrangements and support services.

Factors that predispose to and precipitate admissions. Community studies show that about 13 percent of the community-living elderly (over age 65) are suffering from moderately symptomatic to severely impairing mental illness (Blazer and Maddox 1984). This agrees with other studies, such as those by Kay et al. (1964), that indicate that only a minority of elderly persons with functional or organic psychiatric disorders are receiving institutional care. There are several factors, however, that make it more likely that the individuals may wind up in an institution. These include lacking access to personal or community supportive services, having combined mental and physical disabilities, living alone, having no living children, and being white and in a higher economic group (Grauer and Birnbom 1975; Palmore 1976).

Frequently, identifiable events precede and precipitate admissions. These were studied and categorized by Lowenthal and her group (Lowenthal 1964; Lowenthal et al. 1967). In their series, about one-third of the elderly were admitted to psychiatric facilities because of potentially harmful behavior such as wandering or self-neglect; about one-fifth were admitted for actual harmful behavior such as violence, heavy drinking, or fire setting; about one-fourth came in because of environmental factors, such as loss of a caretaker or friends, or at a physician's recommendation; about one-eighth were admitted because of disturbances of thought or feeling such as delirium, incoherence, or depression; and about one-tenth were admitted for physical factors such as feebleness, malnutrition, or strokes. It is recognized that there are substantial variations in reasons for admission and the rate of institutionalization, as illustrated by the study by Preston (1986) in New Zealand, in which it was estimated that approximately 50 percent of the moderately to severely demented individuals are institutionalized.

Coordinating patient and facility. Problems of matching elderly patients with the most appropriate facilities have been aggravated by inaccurate diagnoses, lack of clear admitting criteria, or limited availability of beds. Particular difficulties are often encountered in deciding between a medical or a psychiatric ward, since various studies have shown mixed illnesses to be quite common in elderly patients. Investigations by Langley and Simpson (1970) showed misplacement of older patients to be common, with about 65 percent of the psychiatric patients having physical illness and 63 percent of their physically ill patients having psychiatric disorders. In a study in England, Kidd (1962a) found that 24 percent of older patients in a psychiatric setting had predominantly medical problems, while about 34 percent of those in a medical service had principally psychiatric problems. Those most likely to be misplaced were over age 75, single or widowed, and of low socioeconomic status. Kidd found that the consequences of misplacement included restlessness, disorientation, immobility, reduced staff efficiency, increased incontinence, prolonged hospitalization, and a higher mortality rate (Kidd 1962b).

Screening and preadmission evaluation. A major way of preventing unnecessary admissions or inappropriate placements is for preinstitutionalization screening teams to evaluate the older individuals, preferably in their own home environments. This provides a valuable opportunity to assess realistically the physical and social conditions and the family interaction patterns (Kobrynski and Miller 1970). The team would best consist of a psychiatric or geriatric nurse specialist and a social worker, with back-up availability of a psychiatrist and a geriatrician. This type of team can assess the need for psychiatric institutional care and also help the patient and the family and find alternate arrangements when this would seem more suitable. A study by Wolff (1970) of older people proposed for state mental hospital admission revealed that after screening, only 47 percent required such hospitalization, while 23 percent were sent to nursing care facilities, and 30 percent were returned to their homes and families. Such a preadmission screening visit may ease the transition by informing the patient of what to expect on being institutionalized, thus reducing the shock of the transition as well as enhancing the effectiveness of the treatment program (Whanger 1973).

Therapeutic Modalities in an Inpatient Setting

An effective approach to treating elderly patients with a variety of disorders relies on a useful conceptual approach. Treatment of a single problem in a multiply impaired person will often fail to accomplish much and may often lead to discouragement on the part of both the patient and the therapist. Proper treatment is based on assessment. Especially in institutionalized elderly patients with psychiatric disorders in whom multiple problems are likely present, a biopsychosocial model is essential (Becker and Cohen 1984). A means of assessing the functional status of the individual as well as detecting those diseases and problems that impair the person's ability to perform those activities necessary to an individual's well-being is essential. A systematic multidimensional assessment helps in planning therapeutic and compensatory responses in order to restore and maintain functional status and health as well as possible. Systems of assessment have been developed such as the Older American Resources and Services (OARS) instrument at Duke University (Duke Older Americans Resources and Services 1978; Whanger and Myers 1984; Rubenstein et al. 1983). Neither the assessment techniques nor the therapeutic modalities are limited to inpatient settings, obviously, but they both are important in caring for the more impaired individuals who are likely to be institutionalized.

Milieu Therapy

The concept that the environment and the community in which a psychiatrically impaired person is placed could and should be therapeutic rather than custodial has developed since World War II, first in England and Europe, and later in the United States (Gutheil 1985). Traditional custodial care is seen as detrimental since the patient is expected to play a sick and passive role. The lack of demands on the patient leads to regression, dependency, and deterioration of ego skills (Gottesman 1967). Milieu therapy is based on the principle that all of the elements of the environment (the patients, the staff, the physical setting, and the various treatment programs) should be used as therapeutic agents. The therapeutic community typically has meant the following: a multidisciplinary staff that relates to the patients in several ways, patient participation in decision making, and collective responsibilities for ward events. Some modifications have been necessary to adapt milieu therapy to the elderly, and Coons and her group have been in the forefront of these developments in the United States (Coons 1983). Three major hypotheses underlie their practice. First, patients make the greatest gains when they have opportunity to assume as much as possible the social roles normally available in the community, such as those of citizen, friend, consumer, worker, or user of leisure time. Second, patients do best when the treatment program provides a structured series of meaningful expectations and activities. Third, patients do best when there is a reasonable degree of homogeneity among the individuals regarding their needs and abilities to function independently. Obviously, the application of these principles presents problems and challenges.

In a therapeutic milieu, the specifics of the programs should vary to meet the needs of the older patients and also take into account the resources of the particular institution and the potential of the staff. Thus, the programs should include as much as possible the activities, such as self-care, that make up the patients' everyday life. They should have choices in activities that help them to get pleasure and satisfaction from life and maintain contact with friends, family, and community.

Therapeutic activities help to develop competence, meaning, and responsibility, and provide a realistic appraisal of capabilities (Szekais 1985). These may involve unscheduled self-innovated activities such as clothes washing or bathing, small group activities, discussion and planning groups, craft projects, and even sheltered workshop activities in which tasks are broken down into a structured series of steps allowing the patients to progress to more complex tasks as they succeed at the earlier or simpler ones.

Staff members in a therapeutic milieu are to act as friends, teachers, and therapists rather than just as caretakers. Thus the staff has the primary responsibilities of enhancing the self-actualization and independence of the patients. This requires close communication both with the patients and other staff members and necessitates a team approach to treatment which may break down some of the rigid role boundaries. The patients, on the other hand, are expected to become effective agents in their own treatment and that of other patients. In their multiple social roles, the patients can tie their past life patterns and values with those of the present. Frail patients obviously will be more restricted, but the main objectives for them too are to provide opportunities to get some pleasure out of each day and to continue involvement and relationships as fully as possible.

Various problems have arisen in the application of milieu therapy to elderly psychiatric inpatients. Some have been external, such as cuts in hospital funding that have caused overcrowding and understaffing. Economic pressures have made the rapid turnover and discharge of patients necessary, and the increasing mass of paper work ties up staff time. The characteristics of inpatients often have changed so that there are more seriously ill or demented patients in institutions, or more with severe character disorders who may be disruptive to a therapeutic community (Kleespies 1986). Problems with milieu therapy in aged psychiatric patients were studied by Bok, who found the major sources of difficulties to be lack of patient potential for change, shortage of funds and personnel, rigid attributes of staff members, and a lack of appropriate community alternatives to institutional care (Bok 1971).

Behavioral Therapy Techniques

The various behavioral theories and therapies have several core principles that bind them together. The main concern is problematic behavior, and the premise is that problematic behaviors are learned responses. These are maintained like other behavioral patterns, and more adaptive patterns of behavior can be learned to supplant them (MacDonald and Kerr 1982). In this process, a functional assessment is made, so that there is a clear definition of the problematic behavior as well as the environmental events that surround it. By thus seeing the current role that the dysfunctional behavior serves, a plan of change or modification can be formulated. Some system of continuing assessment is established so that the levels of the problematic behavior can be monitored and alterations or reinforcements made in therapy. A variety of techniques have been used to modify behavior; these include desensitization, extinction procedures, counterconditioning, negative reinforcement, and cognitive mediation.

Although many of the treatment modalities for the older patients involve behavioral modification principles, there are still very few studies of their use specifically among the elderly or of how the results in the elderly might be similar to or different from those in younger people. Appropriate reinforcements, such as money, can modify behavior even in patients with severe organic mental disorder (Ankus and Quarrington 1972). The development of behavioral "prosthetic environments" for geriatric patients was outlined by Lindsley (1964), who used operant conditioning techniques to give maximum support to the patients for behavior and to compensate for behavior deficits in a way analogous to the use of physical prostheses. The use of positive reinforcement techniques in small groups of elderly patients is described by Birjandi and Sclafani (1973). Some particular advantages of behavior therapy in the geropsychiatric inpatient group are its flexible approach, its cost effectiveness in that it can often be used by supervised paraprofessionals, and the fact that the elderly themselves can incorporate the behavioral strategies into their own ongoing treatment programs (MacDonald and Kerr 1982).

Attitude therapy. A systematic approach on the part of the caregivers was developed by Folsom (1966) in order to develop consistency in approach and involvement of all the staff in treatment. Depending on the patient's problem, one of five basic attitudes is prescribed for the patient, although this could be modified as the patient changes. The attitudes are called "kind firmness," for depressed patients; "active friendliness," for apathetic and withdrawn patients; "passive friendliness," for paranoid and suspicious patients; "matter of fact," for alcoholic and sociopathic patients; and "no demand," for destructive patients. A high level of team functioning is critical to the success of this type of therapy.

Habit retraining. Deterioration in personal habits is very frequent among the elderly, especially those in institutions. These changes may be related to the basic physical or mental disorder that the individual has or may be produced by the regression caused by the institutionalization itself. Lack of care and stimulation may lead to immobility, neglect of bathing and personal hygiene, fecal and urinary incontinence, sleep disturbances, or poor eating habits. Problems with incontinence are probably the major ones, since they cause shame, isolation, and dependency, and lead to other problems such as falls or skin problems. It has been estimated that about 50 percent of the elderly in institutions have urinary incontinence to some degree, while about 30 percent have fecal incontinence, as compared with 1 percent of the older people living in the community (Milne 1976).

Urinary incontinence may have multiple physiologic causes, including urinary tract infections, prostatic disease, uterine prolapse, neurologic diseases, or confusion from severe organic impairment. There may also be functional causes of incontinence, such as its being an active expression of rejection and hostility resulting from feelings of neglect and insufficient attention (MacMillan and Shaw 1966).

The management of urinary or fecal incontinence may be undertaken by an alteration in ward or institutional procedure or by biofeedback techniques. A common problem among the elderly is urinary urgency. Incontinence from this can often be helped by having toilets near patient areas with the doors clearly marked with bright colors, and by silhouettes and names so that they can be rapidly identified and located. The problem can be significantly reduced in some patients by taking them to the toilet after meals, every 2 hours during the day, and every 3 hours at night. Bowel regularity and predictability can often be improved by adequate fluid intake, reasonable exercise, and such foods as fruits, bran cereal, and prune juice.

Biofeedback. The systematic use and evaluation of biofeedback have not been done in the elderly. However, the group of Whitehead, Burgio, and Engle reported two well-documented uses of these techniques in the elderly with fairly good results.

First was a series of fecally incontinent patients between ages 65 and 92. After initial evaluation they were put in a habit-training regimen of regular defecation and use of bulk agents or enemas (Whitehead et al. 1985). Since it had been argued that sphincter tone exercises in themselves would help, a program of systematic contraction of the perineal muscles 50 times a day for a month was instituted, prior to the beginning of the actual biofeedback training. A three-balloon rectal probe was used to measure both the contracting of the anal sphincter muscles and the intraabdominal pressure that would indicate inappropriate contractions of the abdominal muscles that would make the incontinence worse. The training was done by having patients view the responses of their anorectal activity on the polygraphs and being instructed in what to strive for. One of the balloons was repeatedly distended to simulate rectal urgency, but the patients were guided in contractions of the appropriate sphincters. They were instructed to do 50 external anal sphincter contraction exercises daily, and a log was kept. The results showed that of those receiving habit training only, 11 percent became continent; of those with sphincter exercises without biofeedback there was no significant improvement either in reduction of incontinence or improvement in sphincter tone. In contrast, the biofeedback program was of significant vaue in 77 percent of the patients, resulting in either continence (or less than one episode of incontinence per month) or a greater than 75 percent reduction in episodes. It was felt that the biofeedback was cost-effective in that the improvements were achieved in an average of 4.1 clinical visits of about 45 minutes each. The gains were generally sustained unless there was intervening major illness.

A similar program was set up to evaluate and treat urinary incontinence in the elderly (over age 60) (Burgio et al. 1985). It was recognized that there were three main types of urinary incontinence, namely, stress incontinence, detrusor muscle instability, and urge incontinence. The study consisted of evaluation, a 1-month habit-training period to gradually increase the voiding interval, and relaxation techniques to cope with the urge to void. Those not benefiting from these procedures were taught continence control exercise with a catheter in the bladder to measure bladder pressure, and a three-balloon rectal probe to measure intraabdominal pressure, as well as external anal sphincter activity, which is a reflection of the external urethral sphincter activity. The patients were able simultaneously to see the polygraph tracings and receive verbal instructions and reinforcements appropriate to the problem. The patients were given instructions in suitable procedures and muscle exercises to use daily between biofeedback sessions. On the average, the patients had 3.5 training sessions, and overall reduced the incontinence frequency by about 85 percent.

There were several limitations in that biofeedback and a behavioral approach to incontinence require active participation by a motivated patient. Thus it is most appropriate for patients with minimal or no cognitive impairment. As far as other psychiatric impairments were concerned, the results of the treatment were better with the less impaired. Those with various organic impairments are much less likely to be suitable candidates.

On the positive side, the behavioral treatments and biofeedback have almost no side effects, making them much more appropriate for the elderly who are at higher risk with either surgical or pharmacologic interventions. Since much of the treatment is self-administered, few training sessions are required, and this is a relatively inexpensive and efficient use of professional time. Considering its rather effective role, it should certainly be used more frequently to help reduce the excessive disability that incontinence inflicts on the institutionalized older person as well as to reduce nursing procedures by those who care for them.

Individual psychotherapy. Traditionally it has been felt that individual psychotherapy was beneficial primarily to the rather young individual, owing, in good part, to Freud's pessimistic belief that psychotherapy with the elderly would be pointless (Freud 1959). However, a number of therapists have found individual psychotherapeutic techniques helpful with their older patients. Some modifications with the elderly are necessary, as summarized by Rechtschaffen (1959). For instance, environmental manipulations may be used, transference and resistance are handled gently, the therapist must be more active, educational techniques may be employed, and therapy is tapered but often not terminated. Many of the psychoanalytically derived techniques are more applicable to the sort of patient who would be more likely to be living in the community than in an institution. Of more value among the latter would be the more supportive and goal-oriented types of therapy. Brief psychotherapy and crisis intervention have been used especially in dealing with major losses like bereavement and physical illness (Kovacs 1977).

Cognitive therapy with a problem-solving orientation dealing with current problems and coping skills has been used with the elderly (Steuer 1982). Those institutionalized with organic mental disorder can often be helped by a technique developed by Goldfarb and Turner (1953). The more severely impaired have a lowered self-esteem because of mental deterioration and tend to look for a strong parent figure, which role the therapist fills. Two short sessions are held the first week to establish a relationship and to allow the expression of hostile and dependent feelings. After that, the patient is seen briefly at intervals for an indefinite period to maintain the patient's sense of having and controlling the therapist but without taxing the patient's cognitive functioning. Thus the patient's dependency needs are gratified and the feelings of security, mastery, and self-esteem are enhanced.

A number of common themes in the psychotherapy of the older individual have been presented by Butler and Lewis (1977). These include awareness and concern with time; desires for new starts and second chances; issues of autonomy and identity; disguised fears of death, grief, and restitution; and guilt and atonement.

Group Therapies in the Inpatient Setting

Characteristics and goals of groups. Since much of a person's life takes place in formal and informal groups, it is appropriate that increasingly groups have been used deliberately as therapeutic tools. Linden has observed that it is unusual in medicine to find a single therapeutic agent that fulfills as many needs, is as appropriate, and manages the total person as well as group psychotherapy does (Linden 1956).

A therapy group differs from other human aggregations in that it is planned; there is at least one leader or therapist; the members of the group share some identifiable concern, disease, or problem; and the group has some formal or informal understanding or contract. The specific goals of any group are dependent on the composition of that particular group and its leaders. Some general goals for geropsychiatric groups might be as follows: alleviation of psychiatric symptoms, improved self-esteem, ability to adjust successfully to a group or institutional setting, and improvement in capacity to make decisions and judgments (Whanger 1980). Groups can assist patients in achieving these goals through alleviation of isolation and loneliness, through role models that they provide, through contact and opportunities for reality testing with peers in a structured situation, and through social contacts and opportunities to help one another (Linden 1953). There are needs and opportunities for a wide variety of therapeutic groups in an institutional setting, and these will be looked at in more detail.

Dynamically oriented psychotherapy groups. A common concept of group therapy is the long-term psychodynamically oriented group to achieve maturity and personality alteration and adjustment. Such groups will be feasible in some institutional settings, but some modifications are usually necessary. Desirable characteristics of such groups would include relative homogeneity of needs, problems, and mental states; regular times and places for meetings; and sexual integration. The size of the group may be variable, depending on the nature of the group and the characteristics and needs of its members. The group should be large enough to provide protection and variation, yet small enough to facilitate interaction and personal involvement by all members. Although 6 to 12 members is often a good size, Horton and Linden (1982) see circumstances that would dictate that a geriatric psychotherapy group be of 3 to 5 members, since the smaller the group, the more control the therapists have over it. This might especially be the case where some of the group members have mild degrees of dementia and hence have more difficulty concentrating on the group discussion unless the therapist could ensure that each member is fully involved. Usually it is desirable to have at least two therapists, a male and a female, who should generally be warm, positive, and fairly active (Verwoerdt 1981).

In institutional settings, groups are usually open ended because of the practical difficulties in maintaining a closed, stable membership group. Although this decreases the group cohesiveness and intensity of interaction, the changes in membership can be used to help the patients learn to deal with change and loss. Inclusion in a psychotherapy group would usually follow the guidelines suggested by Linden (1956): an expressed desire to join the group, relative alertness, fairly good personal hygiene, ability to hear and understand English, some range of affect and empathy, and some degree of previous successful adult adjustment. Criteria for excluding patients from this type of group would include severe dementia, unwillingness to participate, chronic symptoms of paranoid or manic disorders, deafness or inability to understand common language, inability to sit still, and assaultiveness. A number of techniques and goals helpful in establishing and running psychotherapy groups in the institutionalized elderly are given by Horton and Linden (1982) and Klein et al. (1965). Generally it is well to "stack the deck" somewhat in the direction one wishes to go, such as having about two-thirds of the group relatively active and social, if there are several apathetic and withdrawn members.

Outcome studies of geriatric psychotherapy groups are very sparse, and this problem is compounded by the lack of respectable outcome measures as well as the complexity of the patients and phenomena under study. After 3 months of group therapy, Wolff reported better verbalization and controlled feelings, increased activity and communication, better ward adjustment, better grooming, better orientation, decreased anxiety and feelings of isolation, favorable group identification, more appropriate sex role adjustment, and sustained improvement, all of which facilitate adjustment after discharge from the hospital (Wolff 1970). Improvement in disorders of affect and in regressive hostile behavior was noted by Lazarus, who felt that both patients with organic mental disorders and those with functional impairments could benefit from group therapy (Lazarus 1976). Busse and Pfeiffer found that vigorous therapeutic efforts have resulted in improved ward behavior, but that there may be a relapse into the preintervention states when these efforts are stopped. Thus while the group therapies are obviously worthwhile, they may need to be continued in order to sustain the improvements (Busse and Pfeiffer 1969).

Coping groups. Various types of supportive therapy may effectively take place in groups. The goal is not insight, but rather the support of existing or the reacquisition of lost coping mechanisms in the face of current hardships. This method is to help restore the person to a satisfactory and adaptive condition by dealing with resolving external problems, strengthening ego functioning, and enhancing the self-image (Verwoerdt 1981). Such groups may be formed in institutions to help the patients cope with shared problems such as widowhood and the subsequent alterations in life-style. They may also provide opportunities to regain important skills such as cooking or grooming that may have been neglected and thus deteriorated.

Socialization groups. The opportunity to regain social comfort and skills that may have been lost because of illness and isolation may be found in groups that provide chances to discuss with reasonably alert peers such issues as relationships with children, health and financial problems, or more abstract matters such as happiness or politics. These groups may provide an opportunity for older persons to do a certain amount of reminiscence or life review, as described by Lewis and Butler (1974) and by Ebersol (1976), in which the individuals reflect on and share aspects of their past lives and hopes in order to come to better terms with them.

Remotivation. A structured group program was developed to help reawaken and remotivate the interest of very regressed psychotic and apathetic patients in institutions through efforts to reach the healthy and normal aspects of their personalities. The groups consist of 10 to 15 patients, usually led by a nursing assistant, and meet once or twice weekly. There are five steps involved in the meeting: creating a climate of acceptance; building a bridge to reality, such as by reading and discussing poetry or newspaper items; sharing the experiences of the world through discussion of objective topics picked to be of interest to the patients; developing an appreciation of the work of the world, in order to help the patient think about work and activity in relation to himself; and sharing a climate of appreciation (American Psychiatric Association 1965). Through this structured group process, focusing on familiar but not threatening topics in a warm, accepting climate, it is felt that the patients can be drawn out and their interest in the world rekindled in a healthy way (Weiner et al. 1978).

Reality orientation. While evidence would indicate that less than 10 percent of the aged in the community are disoriented or demented, those suffering these problems make up a high percentage of those in many institutions. The studies of Blazer indicated that from 15 to 60 percent of the elderly in mental hospitals and from 35 to 70 percent of these in long-term institutions have signs of organic mental disorders (Blazer 1980). Too often even health care workers tend to view these frequent problems from a very pessimistic standpoint, with little hope for improvement. Of course there are a wide variety of causes for organic mental disorders, but there are also a variety of factors that either mimic or exacerbate organic mental disorders. Among these are withdrawal, apathy and depression, bewilderment and anxiety secondary to events overwhelming the security and self-esteem, identity crisis arising from loss of autonomy and social role, learned helplessness from overprotectiveness, and sensory deprivation, especially if there is recent memory impairment (Lewis 1982).

Programs have been developed to help work with these impaired individuals, and those that seem to be effective have several common features according to Woods and Britton (1977). The effective treatments showed the following characteristics: They were intensive in order to maximize opportunities for learning to occur, they had active patient participation since behavior had to be changed or reinforced, there were rewards and consequences that acknowledged accomplishments in order to develop motivation, and staff were educated and involved in the treatment and in promoting constructive attitudes toward geriatric care.

The best known of these treatment programs is reality orientation (RO) as developed by Folsom (1968). There are two major thrusts of the program, the first being continuous reality orientation, which is a style of verbal interaction. The entire staff is part of the treatment team that addresses confused patients by their names and reminds them of their location, current or upcoming events, time of day, and so forth. Conversations that are rambling or unrealistic are directed back to reality. Sign boards displaying information about the date, the location, the weather, and upcoming activities are placed prominently on the wards so that the patients learn where they can always find this material. Clocks and calendars are available.

The other major aspect of the RO treatment program is reality orientation classes, which are carried out almost daily, usually by nursing or attendant staff, with small groups of patients. The instructor goes over basic information with each patient, dealing with the patient's name, the date, the location, the menu, the weather, and upcoming events, all in a calm, friendly, patient manner. Immediate positive verbal feedback, such as "that's fine," or "good," is given for correct responses. When incorrect responses are given, the instructor provides the correct information in an encouraging, noncritical manner. As the patient progresses, more complex information is added, and more advanced classes may be held for those who are less severely confused (Drummond et al. 1978).

Since few institutions will have all the staff and funds to carry out programs optimally, a reality approach to the establishment and use of a RO program is necessary, such as that worked out by Lewis and her group (Lewis 1982). They set up criteria to identify patients more likely to benefit from RO techniques so that staff could be trained and motivated and procedures could be developed before taking on more difficult patients. Their criteria were as follows: those who were not at a late stage of chronic organic deterioration; those whose problem was not entirely psychiatric, such as catatonics; those who were medically stable; those who did not have severe sensory impairments, such as blindness or deafness; those whose speech was reasonably intelligible; and those whose interpersonal behavior was appropriate enough to function in a small group, without violent or bizarre behavior.

The results of RO are measured in terms of outcomes for both the patients and the staff. In a study of elderly patients in a state hospital, Harris and Ivory (1976) found that patients who had received RO therapy displayed significantly more verbal orientation than a control group. In a controlled study, Woods (1977) showed that those taking part in RO programs of 30 minutes a day for 5 days a week were significantly superior to the control groups as early as 3 weeks into therapy, and this improvement was maintained through the 12 weeks of the study.

The points to be learned by the staff, and that usually could be conveyed to family members and others working with confused people, are as follows:

1. The environment is calm, familiar, predictable, and minimally distracting;
2. Verbal communication is distinct, straightforward, and helpful to the patient;
3. Basic information is repeated frequently during the day to compensate for the patient's faulty memory and attention span;
4. Confused or distorted speech and behavior are immediately interrupted and corrected so as to disrupt spirals of inappropriate behavior and provide realistic guidelines;
5. Staff members learn restraint in not hurrying patients excessively and not doing things for the patient who actually has the capacity to carry out those activities if given time and encouragement;
6. An attitude is developed toward the patient that is sincere, respectful, firm, polite, and adult, and helps maintain the patient's self-esteem; and
7. The techniques and approaches are applied constantly and by all who have contact with the patient (Lewis 1982).

Inspirational groups. Various groups such as Alcoholics Anonymous, religious groups, or Bible study groups may be of considerable benefit to a number of elderly psychiatric patients by providing support, inspiration, hope, and enhancement of values.

Predischarge groups. Especially for those patients who have been institutionalized for a long period of time but who have improved to the point at which discharge or transfer to a less restrictive institution is imminent, groups designed to facilitate this transition can be very helpful. There are many anxieties and problems associated with reentering a community that can be alleviated by group discussions as well as by very practical experiences such as visiting the boarding home, going on shopping trips, or visiting facilities such as the mental health clinic or the department of social services.

Family and marital therapy. While a number of the elderly in institutions may not have viable family relationships because they may have outlived them or because of isolation from them, still about 80 percent of all older people have living children, and of those elderly with children but without a spouse, most live within 30 minutes of at least one child. Thus the extended family of the institutionalized older person is likely to be important both in evaluation and assessment of the patient and in ongoing therapy and placement (Ripeckyj and Lazarus 1984).

In some cases, the family or the spouse may have contributed to the psychiatric problems of the institutionalized older person, but in most cases the illness of the individual will have had a significant deleterious effect on the spouse and the family. For these reasons, family therapy and/or marital therapy is frequently necessary to deal with such issues as accepting the illness of an aged parent, caring for the patient after discharge, repairing a damaged marriage, or helping in successful rehabilitation. There are no strict guidelines in family therapy, but some directions are given by Spark and Brody (1970) and by Grauer et al. (1973). While family therapy groups usually are made of only the immediate family, at times unrelated families with similar problems may meet together.

Rehabilitation Therapies with Inpatients

For the aged ill, good health care should allow enough time for recovery or restoration of functional ability (Kennie 1983), especially since deterioration of mental and physical capabilities and incontinence are principal causes of nursing home placements in elderly patients. Persistent physical disabilities as a result of acute illness are common in hospitalized older adults, as illustrated by Warshaw et al. (1982), who found in a survey of patients over age 70 in a community hospital that 65 percent had problems with mobility, 21 percent were incontinent, and 53 percent had difficulties in self-care. These problems were often not addressed by the primary physician even though they may well have been ameliorated by focused rehabilitation.

An important concept in working with older patients is that many cannot be really rehabilitated, which is, according to Rudd and Margolin (Rudd and Margolin 1968) primarily directed to restoring the patients to physical, mental, social, and economic usefulness commensurate with their abilities or disabilities. They point out that maintenance therapy is also valid, since the point is to encourage the patients within their limitations to enjoy to the fullest extent whatever life has to offer at their current physical or mental levels. Maintenance therapy involves therapeutic measures that will retard deterioration in patients who are chronically ill by either slowing or arresting the processes, even if temporarily. Since many of the therapies are the same regardless of the goal, they will be considered together here. Discrete rehabilitation centers have been shown to have a clearly demonstrated improved outcome of care, as reported by Liem et al. (1986), but there are comparatively few specialized rehabilitation centers available. I shall look at what might be usefully done in other institutions to improve the levels of mental and physical functioning, recognizing that there are a wide variety of rehabilitative therapies, some of which have a more psychosocial approach. It is often helpful to take what Weiner et al. (1978) have called a step-ladder approach to rehabilitation, in which the prescribed programs are used sequentially so that as each one is successfully completed, it leads on to the next.

Physical therapies. Among institutionalized elderly psychiatric patients, physical therapy can have at least three important roles. First, since medical illnesses and physical disabilities are common among psychiatric patients, physical therapy is simply part of the total care of the patient. Both strokes and fractures may cause or compound emotional disorders, and physical therapy is important in both as early as possible to help the victim get mobilized and recover as fully and rapidly as possible. Prolonged immobility of bedridden patients without physical therapy rapidly leads to atrophy and weakness and complicating illness. Even small gains in physical function are important to the psychiatric patient, since these may make the difference as to whether the person will be able to go home after the emotional problems are better or will require continuing care in a long-term institution (Williams 1984).

Second, physical activity and therapy have a direct effect on mental state. Mild daily exercise increases the cognitive abilities and orientation of elderly mental patients, according to Rodstein (1975). Massage and hydrotherapy may be of help in weakness, malaise, or withdrawal. The agitated or restless patient may be calmed by warm baths.

Third, physical therapy provides an opportunity for human physical contact. In contrast to therapy with younger patients, generally physical touch plays an important role in the therapeutic communication with older adults, for as Verwoerdt (1981) points out, physical touch provides a basic, natural way of getting in touch with the patient emotionally as well.

In addition to physical therapy for particular disordered states in the elderly, a regular physical activity program for conditioning older institutionalized patients who are generally able bodied otherwise can be very helpful. The physical therapist is in a good position to translate the results of the patient's initial medical examination into an individualized exercise program to enhance health and help avoid injuries. As Simpson (1986) describes, elderly patients who exercise regularly report more energy, better sleep, less stress, fewer aches and pains, and less craving for stimulants and tranquilizers. In general, exercise for the older patient should have a medical plan for goals with limitations, a very gradual approach to allow for conditioning, warm-up and cool-down times, a warning to stop if pain or faintness occurs, and avoidance of jolting sorts of activities. For instance, jogging is often contraindicated in elderly patients but swimming, walking, or "jarming" (arm exercises) may provide toning without trauma. Motivation for exercise can often be enhanced in a group or institutional setting. Daily morning exercises to music may be a regular part of the institution's activities. As Simpson says, "Those who cannot find time for exercise will very likely find time for illness."

Occupational therapy. For the older institutional patient, occupational therapy is loosely defined, but has the general goals of increased self-confidence and self-esteem and acceptable expression of aggressive feelings through constructive activity suitable to the individual's interests and capacities, often by maintaining or restoring specific skills (Wolff 1970). It may include such varied activities as gardening, cooking, arts and crafts, and taking part in sheltered workshops or other industrial-type activities. Disabilities such as arthritis, impaired vision, or a short attention span may significantly limit the geriatric patients. It was noted by Pincus (1968) that supposed learning deficits in older patients often stem from performance factors such as sensory or psychomotor difficulties, increased response time, or lack of motivation. The motivation to participate can be improved by encouraging the older patients to take part in the selection of the activities that will become a part of their own rehabilitation program (Lewis 1975). Even those elderly who may not be physically or emotionally able to come to an activity area may benefit by an occupational therapy program that goes to the bedside (Wolk et al. 1965).

In some institutions, opportunities for rehabilitation and meaningful activity may be provided by sheltered workshops where contract work is performed by compensation. It has been found that even patients with moderate chronic organic mental disorder could participate successfully in a sheltered workshop (Nathanson and Reingold 1969).

Recreational therapy. Pleasure and relaxation remain as important for physical and mental health in the aged as in the young. For the institutionalized older person, the recreational activities should be more than diversion or merely entertainment, but rather should help to stimulate, revive, or maintain various creative and expressive functions. Card games, ceramics, sewing, reading, painting or drawing, picnics, and parties may be both entertaining and therapeutic (Fish 1971). Music and singing can provide pleasure, help socialization and revive happy memories. Even quite demented patients often remember verses of old songs and hymns. Music has been used as an aid to speech therapy and physical therapy as well as in psychologic rehabilitation (Bright 1972). According to Boxberger and Cotter (1968), music therapy leads to more appropriate behavior; reduction in aggressiveness, incontinence, and undesirable patient noise; less physical and verbal reaction to hallucinations; and improvement in personal appearance in elderly patients.

Less sedentary activities such as walking, gardening, or dancing are beneficial psychologically and physically if undertaken within the patient's physical limitations. Rhythmic movements are a natural accompaniment to music and may facilitate exercise. Dance, both social and creative, can provide a means of increasing expression of feelings and thoughts, of developing more healthy self-awareness, of enhancing socialization, of improving physical endurance, and of promoting communication (Maney 1975).

The line of demarcation among physical, occupational, and recreational therapies is often not sharp when dealing with elderly patients, and this would suggest the value of broadly and specially trained rehabilitation therapists to work with the aged in institutions.

Physical aids and sensory stimulation. The loss of sensory input may contribute to psychopathology as well as restrict participation in rehabilitation programs by the elderly. Virtually all older patients will need glasses in order to participate in many activities or crafts or read printed materials or the lips of people speaking to them. Large-print books, magnifying lenses, and bright lights make reading possible for many elderly with declining vision. Many older patients lose part of their vision by having dirty glasses, so they should be regularly reminded to wash them or have it done for them by the staff or other patients if they are unable.

Hearing problems are very frequent, with Warshaw et al. (1982) finding that 34 percent of those over age 70 in a general hospital had impaired hearing, while 4 percent were almost totally deaf. Many hearing-impaired elderly become withdrawn, suspicious, or hostile when they are unable to perceive clearly what is going on around them. A number may have impacted ear wax blocking their hearing or may be able to benefit by a hearing aid. Speaking slowly and clearly where the patient can see the speaker's face often facilitates communication. An informal hearing aid can be quickly devised by putting the ear pieces of a stethoscope into the patient's ears and then talking into the mouthpiece of the stethoscope. It is well to remember that many older people can hear in a one-to-one situation fairly well but become quite impaired when there are other conversations going on simultaneously.

There is a formal therapy program called sensory stimulation or sensory training which is used for the extremely regressed or organically impaired patient who often is unable to take part in many other rehabilitation programs. The theory behind this program is that part of the confusion and regression seen in such patients is due to sensory deprivation and cerebral disuse atrophy (Bower 1967).

Sensory training has as its goal increasing sensitivity and discrimination of sensation and feelings. It is carried out in a small group, with a series of simple body awareness exercises and with sensory stimuli presented, experienced, reacted to, and understood by the patients (Weiner et al. 1978). Thus the environment becomes more predictable and less confusing, and the interactions with the leader and other patients provide recognition and feedback on behavior that may then be more open to change.

Environmental Considerations in Inpatient Therapy

Age Distribution

The issue of the desirability of age segregation in institutions caring for elderly psychiatric patients is still a debatable topic. Those favoring age segregation feel that the older patients on an age-mixed ward get disproportionately less staff attention and are more at risk from violent younger patients. In addition, it is thought that age segregation provides more appropriate role models and expectations (Kahana 1970). Research has shown, however, that age-homogenous custodial wards are significantly less helpful than age-integrated custodial wards and may even be detrimental to the functional status and behavior of their occupants. Wards that have an active therapeutic program are effective whether age segregated or not (Kahana and Kahana 1970).

Ward Characteristics and Placement

Several types of wards should be available for the most effective treatment of older psychiatric patients, but they would not necessarily all be at the same location and there may be various combinations of these types. Each ward type needs a planned program. In addition, the patient's status and needs must be reassessed periodically so that changes in therapy and location can be carried out to provide adequate care (World Health Organization 1972).

Admission and diagnostic wards. Since comprehensive evaluation of a patient before admission is often impractical or impossible, an admission and diagnostic ward allows for a thorough psychiatric, medical, and social assessment (Kay et al. 1966; Exton-Smith and Robinson 1970; Burrows 1970). Following the assessment, intensive treatment of disorders amenable to correction within 2 or 3 months may be carried out on these wards. It is the policy on some of these units to have a time limit on how long the patient can remain in that ward (Morton et al. 1968). Factors that hinder the effective functioning of such units include inadequate staffing and funding, lack of resources for patients needing long-term care, and problems in transferring patients to appropriate services (Andrews 1970).

Rehabilitation wards. For those patients needing institutional treatment of an intermediate duration as well as for some chronically psychotic patients, rehabilitation wards are the most suitable.

Minimal or self-care wards. Minimal or self-care wards function like a half-way house, providing for patients who are awaiting community placement, and for those patients who are capable of working outside the hospital during the day.

Chronic care wards. Chronic care wards should provide a humane, supportive and protective environment for those with progressive mental deterioration.

Ambulatory senile wards. Since severe degrees of dementing illnesses can occur without psychotic disturbance or marked physical impairment, wards that allow such patients to be active without getting lost or harming themselves are necessary. They generally require a fenced-in area, as well as the ability to lock their doors.

Nursing care facilities. In order to provide care for those elderly who have significant physical deterioration, but who cannot be placed in ordinary nursing homes because of behavioral or other special management problems, nursing care facilities are often needed in larger mental hospitals or other institutions caring for these patients.

Medical wards. Special medical wards are similarly needed in larger institutions for older psychiatric patients who develop medical illnesses requiring intensive treatment or isolation. When major medical illnesses are treated on the psychiatric wards, the result is often less than optimal care for the patient, and is a heavy drain on the nursing staff as well.

Sex Distribution

Although it is common for the wards of many state mental hospitals and other institutions to segregate their older patients on the basis of sex, this is generally not necessary. In fact, sexually integrated wards generally motivate and facilitate the practice of a realistic and appropriate sex role. Grooming, socialization, and manners generally tend to improve on mixed wards, and problems of improper behavior toward members of the opposite sex are rare (Ciarlo and Gottesman 1966).

Structural, Architectural, and Physical Factors

The environment plays a significant role in the behavior of the elderly, perhaps almost equaling the role of the patient's own personal characteristics (Kiernat 1985). The importance of the environment in the treatment process was clearly recognized as early as 1860 when Florence Nightingale observed that the surroundings had a major impact on both the mental and physical functioning of the patient, stating that we know little about the way in which we are affected by form, by color and light, we do know this, that they have an actual physical effect (Nightingale 1969). More recently, some have felt that environmental factors might also be even more critical than personal factors in those with chronic problems or disabilities in determining the outcome of rehabilitation efforts (DeLong 1979). The decreased capacities that come with old age, and especially illnesses that decrease the person's competence further, make the person increasingly dependent on the environmental factors, which Lawton and Simon (1968) have called "environmental docility."

Maladaptive behavior and negative affect is likely to occur either when the environmental demands significantly exceed the patient's mental or physical capacities, or, on the contrary, when the environmental demands are so low that the patient suffers sensory deprivation, dependency, or lethargy.

It is to be hoped that increasing numbers of the institutions caring for older mental patients will incorporate features designed for the convenience, pleasure, and maximal independence of their residents. Wide corridors, handrails, nonslip flooring, doors that open automatically, short corridors, pedestal-type tables, windows that open outward rather than inward, and the absence of thresholds or doorsteps are among features that can reduce the activity restrictions and hazards that result from physical disabilities or limitations. Toilets should be available and clearly marked near dining and activity areas. There should be space provided for rehabilitative therapies, for lounging, for a library, for hair-dressing facilities, for examination and treatment rooms, for laundry machines, and for other needed services. Furniture needs to be arranged to provide adequate room for patients with walkers and wheelchairs, as well as to promote socialization. Carpeting reduces noise, but is often impractical around incontinent patients. Flowers, lamps, tablecloths, upholstered furniture, magazines, books, and a television set help to produce a more home-like atmosphere (McClannahan 1973; American Association of Homes for the Aging 1985).

There is a deleterious effect of varying degree of declining vision on mental functioning and behavior (Snyder et al. 1976). In addition to correcting the patient's vision as much as possible by glasses, the appropriate use of lighting and color is useful for limiting the disability. While glare is a great problem for many older people, the lighting must be bright enough to allow discrimination of color and detail and to facilitate lip reading. Experience would support the recent observations of the importance of high levels of illumination in reducing depression in some people (Rosenthal et al. 1985). Night lights help prevent falls and nocturnal confusion.

Color coding of wards and doors with contrasting wall paints and bright floor tiles is stimulating, contributes to a more cheerful atmosphere, and helps orient confused and visually impaired patients (Agate 1970).

The air temperature and humidity should be controlled, since the ability to adjust to temperature extremes is much reduced in the elderly (Butler and Lewis 1977). Generally the air temperature should be held fairly consistent between 68° and 83° F. The elderly patients on phenothiazines or anticholinergic drugs are especially at risk from excessive heat, since dehydration or hyperpyrexia may develop very rapidly.

People have a sense of both personal space and territorial space that contributes to their sense of personal integrity. Individuals in institutions generally need help in maintaining this sense, or else their energy may be tied up in attempting to preserve their ego integrity rather than in social interaction. Familiar furnishings, pictures, and personal items help many patients with this sense of personal integrity and should be encouraged (Senn and Steiner 1978–1979).

Particular Problems of the Older Psychiatric Inpatient

Institutionalization

Much has been written about the very realistic risks and dangers of the process of institutionalization itself. Institutional care can cause regression and social breakdown, lack of privacy, loss of responsibility for personal decisions, rigid routines, unavailability of supportive and affectionate relationships, lack of intellectual stimulation, and spiritual deprivation. All of this can lead to loss of self-respect, diminished interests and emotional responses, and behavior like that seen in organic mental disorders (Stotsky and Dominick 1969). A syndrome of "institutional neurosis," exhibiting erosion of the personality, overdependence, automatic behavior, expressionless faces, and loss of interest in the outside world was described by Butler and Lewis (1977). Attitudes of the staff may contribute to infantilization and desexualization. Since it is often quicker and easier to do things for patients than to encourage or assist them in taking care of themselves, understaffing problems and misconceptions among the staff regarding appropriate nursing care can foster unnecessary dependency (Leiberman 1973).

Some studies have suggested that the effects of institutional life may be less deleterious than is commonly supposed. The preadmission characteristics or problems that are frequently related to the reasons for the institutionalization, as well as the impact of the changes caused by the entry into the institution, seem to be at least partially responsible for the observed physical and emotional problems of the institutionalized older person (Lieberman 1969). The impact institutionalization has on the amount of social interaction appears to be a more important influence on self-esteem than is the institutionalization itself; thus the institutionalization could actually be helpful to the self-esteem by increasing opportunities for interaction and age-appropriate social roles (Anderson 1967). It has been noted that personality characteristics associated with successful adaptation to institutional life are high activity, high aggression, and a narcissistic body image (Turner et al. 1972).

Of course, many of the therapeutic methods already discussed are applicable to the prevention or improvement of the possible deleterious effects of the institutionalization itself.

Constipation

Problems with constipation and fecal impactions are frequent among elderly psychiatric inpatients and are related to relative inactivity, variable food and fluid intake, alteration of usual bowel habits, modesty in public settings, depression, and the anticholinergic effects of many of the drugs that they may be taking. Agitation, fever, diarrhea, vomiting, walking or sitting bent to one side, lethargy, and increased confusion are among the possible manifestations of an impaction; a rectal examination should be part of the investigation of any of these symptoms. Prevention is done through a judicious combination of bulk in the diet, good fluid intake, adequate activity, stool softeners, and laxatives.

Sleep Problems

Disorders of sleep are discussed elsewhere, but they are frequent among the elderly in institutions. The disorders that brought the patient to the institution may likely cause either physical or emotional pain, or frequent depressions of course often disrupt the sleep cycles. Several factors in the institution itself may contribute to the disturbances of sleep as well, for instance, the strangeness of the place, a hard or saggy mattress or pillow, noises from other patients and the nursing staff, inadequate physical activity during the day, coffee (caffeine) served at supper, too early a bedtime, and an excessive use of hypnotic drugs. A sleep problem in an elderly inpatient should warrant an evaluation of these factors and an appropriate response other than just increasing the sleep medication.

Adverse Drug Reactions

Problems with drug reactions and interactions are certainly not unique to the institutionalized, but various factors lead to a high incidence in this group. They tend to be older, physically sicker, weaker, previously medicated, and in need of something being done about their presenting psychiatric problems, all of which increase the probability of some type of untoward reaction. The side effects and manifestations of adverse drug reactions may be mistaken for worsening psychiatric or physical conditions and therefore may be erroneously treated by adding further medications rather than by reducing or withdrawing the responsible agent (Whanger 1974). The sick elderly are especially vulnerable to hypotensive side effects of psychotropic medications and should have their blood pressure checked in a sitting and standing position for this potentially serious side effect. Drugs given to many chronically institutionalized older patients tend to be perpetuated long after the initial problem has improved, and so a periodic drug review is essential.

Agitated Behavior

Agitation is a major problem of the elderly, for their families, and for their caretakers. It often leads to institutionalization and is a very frequent problem among those who are residents in institutions. The diffuse literature on this subject is well reviewed by Cohen-Mansfield and Billig (1986; also Cohen-Mansfield 1986). They attempt to systematize agitated behavior in order to clarify the problem as well as to better evaluate various proposed methods of management. Agitation is inappropriate verbal, vocal, or motor activity that is not explained by needs or confusion per se. The inappropriateness may be being abusive or aggressive to oneself or others, it may be appropriate behavior done with inappropriate frequency, or it may be inappropriate according to social standards for a particular situation. The incidence and severity will vary since some types of institutions or certain wards within large institutions are more likely to receive the elderly patients with the more severe management problems. A survey by Zimmer et al. (1984) in skilled nursing facilities in New York showed that 64 percent of the residents were identified as having significant behavioral problems, and of these 23 percent were defined as serious problems. The most frequent agitated behaviors (meaning they occurred usually several times a day) were restlessness, constant unwarranted requests for attention, complaining, and wandering. Agitation was often correlated with cognitive decline, and often more than one manifestation of agitation was found in the same individual. The nursing staff felt that agitated behavior would more likely manifest itself under certain circumstances: for instance, when the patient was frustrated at loss of control, especially when some forced activity like bathing or feeding was being done; when the patient's personal space was being invaded; when other patients were agitated; when there was a lack of structure; and when the patient was lonely or depressed. Of course, those who are physically aggressive are most disruptive to ward functionings.

A variety of approaches have been taken to try to control various agitated behaviors. A token economy program was reported to be effective in reducing self-injurious behaviors in elderly long-term mental hospital patients by Mishara and Kastenbaum (1973). Behavioral interventions led to a reduction of agitated utterances in elderly patients, as reported by Davis (1983). More severe agitated behavior usually requires the use of major tranquilizers such as haloperidol, thioridazine, or thiothixene (Risse and Barnes 1986). Even more severe or hazardous agitation may require restraints or seclusion.

Suicidal Behavior

Suicide and suicidal behavior are a major problem with the elderly—it is currently the 10th leading cause of death in the over 65 age group (Blazer et al. 1986). The rate is highest in the 80 to 84 age group, although there is a marked sex and race differential, with the rate of white males in the older age group being about 16 times as great as that for nonwhite females in the same age range. It is expected that suicide in the over-65 age group will probably double over the next 40 years.

Among the young there is a high ratio of suicide attempts (sometimes called parasuicide) to completed suicide, but this ratio is much lower in the elderly. Thus, as Busse and Pfeiffer indicated, when an older person attempts suicide, he almost always fully intends to die. Rescue in the elderly is usually accidental, or a result of bungling the attempt (Busse and Pfeiffer 1969).

This leads to the relevance of inpatient services, since persons in old age attempting suicide should be hospitalized. It is recognized that there are clear-cut risk factors in elderly suicide including unemployment, isolation, poor health, pain, depression, alcoholism, low self-esteem, feeling rejected, and a history of mental illness and previous suicide attempts (Osgood 1985). This group obviously includes those elderly already in institutions, meaning those admitted after suicide attempts or who have major depression or suicidal ideation as well as those more chronic residents who may develop suicidal intents while a patient. In most cases, the patients are mentally ill with a depression, but other problems such as drug dependency, a terminal illness, or dementia may be a major factor (Holding 1984). While elderly people who commit suicide often use a highly lethal method such as a firearm, the already institutionalized older person may attempt indirect suicide by such means as stopping eating or drinking, refusing medications, or refusing various tests and examinations. These actions, especially when combined with an attitude of giving up, may produce a grave situation within a few days.

The prevention of suicide involves the detection and assessment of suicidal ideation. Patients may give direct verbal clues such as the intent to kill themselves (Osgood 1985). These should always be taken seriously in an elderly person, and hospitalization undertaken quickly. More often the elderly give indirect verbal clues such as stating that their family would be better off without them. Behavioral clues are important, such as purchasing a gun, changing a will, showing sudden uncharacteristic actions or agitation, or presenting peculiar somatic complaints to the doctor. The patient should be asked directly about suicidal intent and method. If there is both ideation and significant lethality of intent, measures should be taken immediately to protect the person. The person should not be left alone, and hospitalization should be arranged, by legal commitment if necessary.

The depression should be treated, since in most cases the suicide risk diminishes with the clearing of the depression. Drugs may be satisfactory, but ECT is often indicated in the the elderly person at high risk. Until the depression is definitely improved, the patient must be protected, generally by being on a locked unit with restricted privileges. The patient's belongings should be searched for drugs, razor blades, or other weapons. Frequent checks or a one-to-one nursing situation should be set up. Potential hazards and situations should be avoided, for example, by locking up belts and shoe laces, not having strong hooks on bathroom doors that could be used for a hanging suicide, and having detention screens on the windows.

Of course attempts should be made to improve the home situation as much as possible and to deal with other possible precipitants such as loneliness, ill health, and loss of a spouse or financial security. Arrangements need to be clear for long-term follow-up and care as well. Still, as Holding (1984) indicated, there will remain a proportion of patients under medical and psychiatric care, both as outpatients and inpatients, who will commit suicide.

Psychiatrically Impaired Elderly on Medical and Surgical Inpatient Services

We have already commented on the extremely high incidence of diagnosable psychiatric disorders found in older nursing home patients, which ranges from 80 to 94 percent (Whanger and Lewis 1975; Rovner et al. 1986). Another major issue is the recognition and appropriate treatment of psychiatric impairment among the elderly who are patients on the medical or surgical services of hospitals. The branch of psychiatry that deals with these biopsychosocial issues with medical and surgical patients in a general hospital is known as liaison psychiatry.

The objects of a liaison program have been described by Kaufman and Margolin (1948) as the direct provision of psychiatric services to the hospital population, the teaching and training of both the psychiatric staff and ideally every other member of the hospital staff, and research. Since the majority of those with mental health problems are treated by primary care practitioners rather than by mental health personnel, Brodie has pointed out that these practitioners need adequate training in the psychiatric aspects of patients care (Brodie 1979). There has been no standard method of achieving these goals with adult patients, much less the geriatric group, but Greenhill (1981) points out six models of consultation/liaison programs. These are as follows: the consultation model of patient referral to the psychiatrist for evaluation and care; the liaison model of mental health workers being assigned to selected hospital units to consult, care for, and teach; the milieu model, in which the group processes, the group aspects of patient care, and staff interactions and reactions are focused on; the critical care model, in which the mental health personnel are assigned to critical care units rather than clinical departments; the biologic model, in which the psychiatrist places emphasis on neurosciences and psychopharmacology; and the integral model, which incorporates the whole staff, including psychologic care, as part of all patient care (Greenhill 1981).

Incidence of Illness

There is comparatively little documentation of the extent of psychiatric illness among the elderly inpatients in hospitals. The surveys of Warshaw and Moore and their group of all the patients over age 70 in a general hospital measured functional disability rather than diagnosing specific psychiatric conditions (Warshaw et al. 1982). They found that this group, excluding obstetric and pediatric patients, makes up about one-third of the entire hospital census. They found that 19 percent of the older patients were mildly confused and 31 percent were moderately or severely confused at the time of the survey, and this problem increased with increasing age. Restraints were being used on 19 percent of the patients, and 43 percent were on psychotropic drugs.

A somewhat different approach has been to evaluate those inpatients who are referred for geriatric consultation in a large general hospital, such as those reported by Lichtenstein and Winograd (1984). These geriatricians found that 79 percent of their referrals came from the medical service, 14 percent from surgery, and 7 percent from psychiatry. The most common reason for referral was to evaluate rather nonspecific functional complaints such as anorexia, falls, confusion, gait disorders, incontinence, immobility, or nonspecific deterioration, problems which occur in 55 percent of the patients. Many different diagnoses were reached, since these symptoms reflected a broad range of illnesses, but it was found that 79 percent of all of their referrals had a psychiatric disturbance. These included a delirium in 40 percent, dementia in 38 percent, and depression in 37 percent. They felt that one-third of their referrals had two or more simultaneous psychiatric diagnoses. Complications of hospitalization occurred in 62 percent of the patients, with the problem of medication toxicity being most common.

Another way of getting an idea of the frequency of mental disorders among a general older patient population is to evaluate those who are at the gateway of the institution, namely, the emergency rooms of large general hospitals. One of the earliest of these studies, by Bassuk et al. (1983), showed that those over age 65 made up only 3.9 percent of all those being seen in a psychiatric emergency service. This figure is almost identical with the percentage of older people seen in community mental health clinics in spite of their making up about 11 percent of the total population. They found that the older patients usually described their problems in medical or somatic terms, and they seldom viewed their problems psychologically, interpersonally, or even situationally. Of those seen for psychiatric evaluation and treatment, 64 percent did have documented physical illness in addition to the mental problem. The diagnoses assigned were affective disorder, 22 percent; organic mental syndrome, 18 percent; and situational crises, 16 percent—all markedly higher than in younger psychiatric patients. Among the elderly, problems with drug abuse, assaultive behavior, or suicide were only rare. A number of the older patients came to the emergency room several times during a year, seemingly using the emergency room almost as if it were a primary physician. The investigators noted a persistent lack of teamwork between the medical and psychiatric services, so that the patient was frequently shunted back and forth between the two services until the emotional disorder became unequivocally apparent, and the patient required definitive treatment such as hospitalization or nursing home placement. A major problem was further highlighted by Waxman and his group who found that in their emergency room, the older patients who had complaints that sounded psychiatric were generally quickly referred to psychiatry before a full medical workup was done. Thus, major or even life-threatening illness can be easily misdiagnosed or untreated when the presenting symptoms are predominantly psychiatric and premature transfer is made (Waxman et al. 1984). In another study of emergency psychiatric consultation in a general hospital, Perez and Blouin (1986) noted that most of those over 70 years of age had had their illness longer than 30 days and had been seeing their family physician for the problem, rather than a psychiatrist or a mental health clinic. About 50 percent of these patients were admitted; the three most common reasons for admission were depression, side effects of psychotropic medications, and hallucinations and delusions.

Consultation/Liaison Services

The management of psychiatrically impaired elderly on medical and surgical inpatient services can be carried out in several ways. First, the problem may be largely unrecognized or ignored, running the risk of prolonged morbidity, increased mortality, and unnecessary use of nursing care facilities. Second, consultation may be with an individual psychiatrist who is especially trained in geriatric psychiatry, and who will make recommendations for psychotherapy, drugs, or discharge planning to the primary physician, and then carry out the appropriate parts of it. Third may be the use of an interdisciplinary geriatric consultation service. Fourth may be the development of geriatric assessment units such as those reviewed by Rubenstein et al. (1982) or psychogeriatric assessment units such as have been recommended and developed in Britain (Whanger and Busse 1975).

I shall examine in more detail the interdisciplinary geriatric consultation services that are most likely the ones that could and should respond to patients already in the general hospital on medical and surgical services. One such program, mentioned previously, was developed by Lichtenstein and Winograd (1984). They had the initial physical and mental examination interviews done by a geriatric fellow. An Activities of Daily Living scale was administered, and a nursing assessment was obtained. Social and family data were secured, and all of this was presented to the team. As a consequence, they made a number of new medical and psychiatric diagnoses. Among their recommendations were adjustments (mostly downward) in medications in 62 percent, diagnostic and treatment procedures for psychiatric illness in 59 percent, rehabilitation recommendations in 38 percent, treatment of malnutrition in 30 percent, and coordination of medical and psychitric therapy. They felt that the high incidence of psychiatric disorders in elderly medical patients (79 percent) showed that the medical care of geriatric patients in the hospital is often complicated by the need to treat mental disorders simultaneously.

Frequently, behavioral problems were the major reason for the psychiatric consultation and involvement since the behavior often interfered with the proper diagnosis and treatment of the medical problems. Because most of the patients had multiple problems, they gave priority to treating those conditions whose improvement would improve the patients' ability to care for themselves. In addition, they frequently recommended the aggressive use of rehabilitation services for debilitated elderly patients. They felt they were able to improve the functional capacity of a significant number of their patients so that they were able to return to their own homes rather than go to nursing homes.

Somewhat in contrast were the interdisciplinary geriatric consultation services as a medical unit with a controlled trial, as reported by Campion et al. (1983). They found in consecutive evaluations of all patients over age 75 that 68 percent had moderate to severe cognitive impairment while 15 percent had major depression. In spite of a rather high level of input, they did not find that the intensive additional therapy and intervention helped at all to reduce the high readmission rate that their group as a whole had during the next year. In spite of these results, the consultation team felt that their type of work is useful in that it promotes geriatrics, teaches interdisciplinary teamwork, increases the use of rehabilitative services, and improves the awareness of functional problems of elderly patients (Campion et al. 1983).

Goals and Outcomes of Inpatient Care

Expectations of Inpatient Care

The goals and expectations of inpatient care will vary both with the type of institution or facilities and with the particular patient. The functions of the various institutions such as mental hospitals, nursing homes, boarding homes, or others that provide care to aged patients may overlap, but they are not identical. There have been many cases of patients being mismatched to various institutions, with reports, for example, of 20 to 40 percent of patients in intermediate care facilities receiving unnecessarily high levels of care (Rubenstein et al. 1982). In situations in which a mismatch has occurred, whether because of inadequate assessment and planning or because the most appropriate facility is not available in the region, the goals of the institutionalization may be unclear or difficult to fulfill. In general, the basic goals of the psychiatric hospital are to provide the most effective treatment available for the patients' disorders and to rehabilitate them to their best potential. A mismatch or the inappropriate use of institutional facilities is undesirable for several reasons since it may create further disability by leading to premature labeling of a patient as irremediably sick. It is also wasteful of resources, and incorrect or premature dispositions from hospitals may result in relapses or unnecessary use of nursing homes or other institutions (Rubenstein et al. 1982). It was also noted by Butler (1975) that in inappropriate facilities, the ailing older person may receive incomplete diagnostic evaluations, excessive numbers of prescribed medications, and inadequate rehabilitative services. While many elderly patients may obtain a cure or good remission of their psychiatric disorders, for others the slowing of the rate of their disability or providing humane comfort and support may be valid goals. For some patients, dying with comfort and dignity may be the best achievement possible for them.

Issues Influencing Outcome

In addition to the illness that the older person has, and the structure of the institution in which the individual resides, other factors also affect the outcome. It is difficult to document and quantify outcomes in many ways, although such things as expected discharge rates, the functional status, increased number of diagnoses, use of other facilities, and decrease in amounts of medications are valid and observable. Also of importance, even if they are subjective, are the patient's sense of well-being and improved quality of life (Rubenstein et al. 1982).

Planned and intensive therapy on admission is desirable, since generally those who improve enough to be discharged within 3 months have a much better likelihood of successful return to the community than those who are institutionalized longer (Whanger 1980). A previous good adjustment and an interested family increase the probability of the patient's progress and discharge from the institution. A positive attitude toward the rehabilitation potential of the older individual on the part of the professional and administrative staff and the relatives has an important function, albeit one that is hard to define, in the quality and outcome of care (Kosberg and Gorman 1975).

The Processes of Deinstitutionalization

Leaving an institution, especially after a long stay, may be a very stressful event. Until 1955 when the strong drive to get the chronic patients out of the state mental hospitals began, service planning was rather simple, since most elderly stayed until they died. Now the processes are much more complex, even if more clinically and humanistically focused. Unfortunately, as Bachrach (1986) indicates, the policies, practices, and priorities associated with deinstitutionalization have often resulted in fragmented, decentralized, and complicated programs in which there are large numbers of elderly mentally ill individuals who are virtually estranged from the psychiatric service system.

In terms of programs that will positively facilitate deinstitutionalization, predischarge groups can ease their transition, as might half-way houses for the elderly people. By increasing the sharing of tasks and responsibilities by the patient and lessening the structure of the institutional life so as to decrease dependence, the patients can better prepare for the realities of life in the community. The community itself should have a wide spectrum of services and programs available to assist in the continuing care of the older person, as is discussed in detail in Chapter 24.

At times there may be interinstitutional relocations and transfers that if handled well may decrease depression, alienation, and distress, and improve self-esteem. Recommendations by Mirotznik and Ruskin (1985) have been found to minimize negative psychosocial outcomes. These include maintaining as much integrity in environment and staff as possible; realistically discussing the ways in which the quality of life may be enhanced by the relocation; addressing fears and unrealistic expectations; immediately after the relocation, encouraging the patients to talk about the move and its problems; and resolving actual problems quickly. Useful manuals for deinstitutionalization have been prepared by Grant (1976) and Folsom (1975).

Issues of Placement and Community Care

The effects of placement and moving the elderly in different circumstances are variable, as summarized by Lieberman, who noted that radical environmental changes may cause destructive physical and psychologic effects in some, whereas in others relocation may increase satisfaction and adjustment (Lieberman 1969). In a move from a psychiatric hospital to a nursing home, the early stages of adjustment are the most critical, since crises or mental symptoms that develop during this interval tend to lead to rehospitalization or physical illness unless treated (Stotsky 1970). While the successful adjustment to a nursing home placement depends significantly on psychiatric symptoms and behavioral disturbances, these facilities often seem to be able to handle those patients fairly well (Stotsky 1967). Many schizophrenic patients adjust as well in nursing homes as they do in hospitals. Those with organic mental syndrome tend to show a greater decrease in physical and self-care activities in nursing homes than in the hospitals (Dobson and Patterson 1961). Motivation, determination, and the ability to manipulate a familiar environment help in the successful adjustment to noninstitutional placement (MacLeod 1970).

There are major methodologic problems in comparing patients still in state mental hospitals with those in nursing homes or other facilities, largely because the patients' living circumstances are determined by their clinical conditions. Still, some useful observations were made by Lehman et al. (1986) studying chronically ill, long- or short-term patients in different settings. They found that in general, patients in community nursing homes were better satisfied with their living conditions and were less likely to have been assaulted in them than those still in state hospitals. In addition, those institutionalized for a long period (more than 6 months) tended to be better satisfied than those who had arrived recently. The adequacy of the patient's living situation explained many differences in their sense of well-being, however.

It is important for an older patient being discharged from a psychiatric institution into the community to have access to needed services there. Gaitz analyzed common obstacles interfering with the effective delivery of follow-up service and found them to include poverty, rigidity among the agencies, suspiciousness in the patient, overburdening with red tape and forms, reluctance by physicians to treat older patients, impairment of mobility, resistance from families, tendency to discontinue medications prematurely, problems staying on diets, difficulties in getting to more than one clinic in a day's time, a tendency of some nursing homes to unnecessarily sedate or immobilize their residents, and the simple lack of facilities. A coordinator to facilitate getting to these community resources is often helpful for the patient (Gaitz and Hacker 1970; Gaitz 1970).

In conclusion, we can have mixed feelings about the state of things regarding institutional care of the older patient with mental disorders. Both knowledge of mental disorders and the numbers of trained therapists have increased, but the state of the institutions and programs in which to implement this knowledge is still uncertain. Whatever the politicians and policy-makers decide, there will be older people beleaguered by mental and physical disorders who need good institutional facilities both for acute treatment and for treatment of the chronically ill who lack the capacity to function well outside a highly structured institution. May we continue to remain sensitive to those elderly.

References

Agate JN: The Practice of Geriatrics (Second Edition). Springfield, IL, Charles C. Thomas, 1970

American Association of Homes for the Aging: Guide to Caring for the Mentally Impaired Elderly. Washington, DC, American Association of Homes for the Aging, 1985

American Psychiatric Association: Diagnostic and Statistical Manual of Mental Disorders (Third Edition). Washington, DC, American Psychiatric Association, 1980

American Psychiatric Association: Remotivation Kit. Washington, DC, American Psychiatric Association, 1965

Anderson NN: Effects of institutionalization on self-esteem. J Gerontol 1967; 22:313–317

Andrews J: Psychogeriatric assessment units. Lancet 1970; 1:1004

Ankus M, Quarrington B: Operant behavior in the memory-disordered. J Gerontol 1972; 27:500–510

Arie T, Isaacs AD: The development of psychiatric services for the elderly in Britain, in Studies in Geriatric Psychiatry. Edited by Isaacs AD, Post F. New York, Wiley, 1978

Bachrach LL: Deinstitutionalization: what do the numbers mean? Hosp Community Psychiatry 1986; 37:118–121

Bassuk EL, Minden S, Apsler RE: Geriatric emergencies: psychiatric or medical? Am J Psychiatry 1983; 140:539–542

Becker PM, Cohen HJ: The functional approach to the care of the elderly: a conceptual framework. J Am Geriatr Soc 1984; 32:923–929

Birjandi PF, Sclafani MJ: An interdisciplinary team approach to geriatric patient care. Hosp Community Psychiatry 1973; 24:777–778

Blazer DG: The epidemiology of mental illness in late life, in Handbook of Geriatric Psychiatry. Edited by Busse EW, Blazer DG. New York, Van Nostrand Reinhold, 1980

Blazer DG, Maddox GL: The use of epidemiologic survey data in planning for geriatric mental health services, in Mental Health and Therapeutic Intervention with Older Adults. Edited by Whanger A, Meyers A. Rockville, MD, Aspen, 1984

Blazer DG, Bachar JR, Manton KG: Suicide in late life: review and commentary. J Am Geriatr Soc 1986; 34:519–525

Blenkner M: The place of the nursing home among community services. J Geriatr Psychiatry 1968; 1:135–144

Bok M: Some problems in milieu treatment of the chronic older mental patient. Gerontologist 1971; 11:141–147

Bower HM: Sensory stimulation and the treatment of senile dementia. Med J Aust 1967; 1:1113–1119

Boxberger R, Cotter VW: Music therapy for geriatric patients, in Music in Therapy. Edited by Gaston ET. New York, Macmillan, 1968

Bright R: Music in Geriatric Care. Sidney, Australia, Halstead Press, 1972

Brodie HKH: Mental health and primary care. Psychosomatics 1979; 20:658–659

Burack-Weiss A: Long-term-care institutions, in Handbook of Gerontological Services. Edited by Monk A. New York, Van Nostrand Reinhold, 1985

Burgio K, Whitehead WE, Engel BT: Urinary incontinence in the elderly. Ann Intern Med 1985; 104:507–515

Burrows HP: Psychogeriatric assessment units. Lancet 1970; 1:1004

Busse EW, Pfeiffer E: Functional psychiatric disorder in old age, in Behavior and Adaptation in Late Life. Edited by Busse EW, Pfeiffer E. Boston, Little, Brown, 1969

Butler RN: Why survive? Being old in America. New York, Harper & Row, 1975

Butler RN, Lewis MI: Aging and Mental Health (second edition). St. Louis, C.V. Mosby, 1976

Campion EW, Jette A, Berkman B: The interdisciplinary geriatric consultation service: a controlled trial. J Am Geriatr Soc 1983; 3:792–796

Ciarlo JA, Gottesman LE: The effects of differing treatment milieus upon the ward behavior of geriatric mental patients. Paper presented at the annual meeting of the American Psychological Association, New York, 1966

Cohen-Mansfield J: Agitated behaviors in the elderly: II. Preliminary results in the cognitively deteriorated. J Am Geriatr Soc 1986; 34:722–727

Cohen-Mansfield J, Billig N: Agitated behaviors in the elderly: I. A conceptual review. J Am Geriatr Soc 1986; 34:711–721

Coons DH: The therapeutic milieu: social-psychological aspects of treatment, in Clinical Aspects of Aging. Edited by Reichel W. Baltimore, MD, Williams & Wilkins, 1983

Davis A: Back on their feet: behavioral techniques for elderly patients. Nurs Times 1983; 43:26

DeLong G: Independent living: from social movement to analytic paradigm. Arch Phys Med Rehab 1979; 60:435

Dobson WR, Patterson TW: A behavioral evaluation of geriatric patients living in nursing homes as compared to a hospitalized group. Gerontologist 1961; 1:135–139

Drummond L, Kirchhoff L, Scarbrough DR: A practical guide to reality orientation: a treatment approach for confusion and disorientation. Gerontologist 1978; 18:568–573

Duke Older Americans Resources and Services: Multidimensional Function Assessment: The OARS Methodology—A Manual (Second Edition). Durham, NC, Duke University, Center for the Study of Aging and Human Development, 1978

Ebersole PP: Reminiscing and group psychotherapy with the aging, in Nursing and the Aged. Edited by Burnside IM. New York, McGraw-Hill, 1976

Eisdorfer C, Stotsky BA: Intervention, treatment, and rehabilitation of psychiatric disorders, in Handbook of the Psychology of Aging. Edited by Birren JE, Schaie KW. New York, Van Nostrand Reinhold, 1977

Exton-Smith AN, Robinson KV: Psychogeriatric assessment units. Lancet 1970; 1:1292

Fish HU: Activities Program for Senior Citizens. West Nyack, NY, Parker, 1971

Folsom GS: Life Skills for the Developmentally Disabled: An Approach to Accountability in Deinstitutionalization (Volumes 1, 2, and 3). Washington, DC, George Washington University, 1975

Folsom JC: Attitude Therapy and the Team Approach. Tuscaloosa, AL, Veterans Administration Hospital, 1966

Folsom JC: Reality orientation for the elderly mental patient. J Geriatr Psychiatry 1968; 1:291–307

Fraser J, Flaherty M: Succor for the ailing elderly becomes a promise broken. Scripps Howard News Service release, April 15, 1987

Freiman MP, Mitchell JB, Rosenbach ML: An analysis of DRG-based reimbursements for psychiatric admissions to general hospitals. Am J Psychiatry 1987; 144:603–609

Freud S: On psychotherapy, in Collected Papers, Vol 1; The International Psycho-Analytical Library, No. 7. Edited by Jones E. New York, Basic Books, 1959

Gaitz CM: The coordinator: an essential member of a multidisciplinary team delivering health services to aged persons. Gerontologist 1970; 10:217–220

Gaitz CM, Hacker S: Obstacles in coordinating services for the care of the psychiatrically ill aged. J Am Geriatr Soc 1970; 18:172–182

Ginzberg E: The financial support of health care for the elderly and the indigent: economic perspectives, in Health Care for the Poor and Elderly: Meeting the Challenge. Edited by Yaggy D. Durham, NC, Duke University Press, 1984

Glasscote R, Gudeman JE, Miles D: Creative Mental Health Services for the Elderly. Washington DC, American Psychiatric Association and the Mental Health Association, 1977

Goffman E: ASYLUMS: Essays on the Social Situation of Mental Patients and Other Inmates. Garden City, Anchor Books, 1961

Gold JG: Development of care of the elderly: tracing the history of institutional facilities. Gerontologist 1970; 10:262–274

Goldfarb AI, Turner H: Psychotherapy of aged persons: II. Utilization and effectiveness of "brief" therapy. Am J Psychiatry 1953; 109:916–921

Gottesman LE: The response of long-hospitalized aged psychiatric patients to milieu treatment. Gerontologist 1967; 7:47–48

Grant FE: Rehabilitation and placement programs for psychogeriatric treatment, in Catawba Hospital Handbook for Facilitators. Ann Arbor, MI, Institute of Gerontology, 1976

Grauer H, Birnbom F: A geriatric functional rating scale to determine the need for institutional care. J Am Geriatr Soc 1975; 23:472–476

Grauer H, Betts D, Birnbom F. Welfare emotions and family therapy in geriatrics, J Am Geriatr Soc 1973; 21:21–24

Greenhill MH: Liaison psychiatry, in American Handbook of Psychiatry (Volume 7). Edited by Arieti S, Brodie HKH. New York, Basic Books, 1981

Hader M, Seltzer HA: La Salpetriere: an early home for elderly psychiatric patients. Gerontologist 1967; 7:133–135

Haglund K: MDs bare "costogenic" morbidity. Med Tribune 1987; 28:1,10

Harris SC, Ivory PBCB: An outcome evaluation of reality orientation therapy with geriatric patients in a state mental hospital. Gerontologist 1976; 16:496–503

Hausman K: New Medicare cap proposed for psychiatric hospitalization. Psychiatric News 1987; 22:1,11

Holding TA: Suicidal behavior in the elderly, in Handbook of Studies on Psychiatry and Old Age. Edited by Kay DWK, Burrows GD. New York, Elsevier, 1984

Horton AM Jr, Linden ME: Geriatric group psychotherapy, in Mental Health Interventions for the Aging. Edited by Horton A Jr. New York, Praeger, 1982

Kahana B: Changes in mental status of elderly patients in age-integrated and age-segregated hospital milieus. J Abnorm Psychol 1970; 75:177–181

Kahana E, Kahana B: Therapeutic potential of age integration. Effects of age-integrated hospital environment on elderly psychiatric patients. Arch Gen Psychiatry 1970; 23:20–29

Kaufman MR, Margolin SG: Theory and practice of psychosomatic medicine in a general hospital. Med Clin North Am 1948; 611–616

Kay DWK, Beamish P, Roth M: Old age mental disorders in Newcastle upon Tyne. Br J Psychiatry 1964; 110:146–158

Kay DWK, Roth M, Hall MRP: Special problems of the aged and the organization of hospital services. Br Med J 1966; 2:967–972

Kennie DC: Good health care for the aged. JAMA 1983; 249:770–773

Kidd CB: Criteria for admission of the elderly to geriatric and psychiatric units. J Ment Sci 1962a; 108:68–74

Kidd CB: Misplacement of the eldery in hospital. Br Med J 1962b; 2:1491–1495

Kiernat JM: Environmental aspects affecting health, in Care of the Elderly: A Health Team Approach. Edited by Maguire G. Boston, Little, Brown, 1985

Kleespies PM: Hospital milieu treatment and optimal length of stay. Hosp Community Psychiatry 1986; 37:509–512

Klein WH, Leshan EJ, Furman SS (eds): Promoting Mental Health of Older People Through Group Methods. New York, Manhattan Society for Mental Health, 1965

Kobrynski B, Miller AD: The role of the state hospital in the care of the elderly. J Am Geriatr Soc 1970; 18:210–219

Kosberg JI, Gorman JF: Perceptions toward the rehabilitation potential of institutionalized aged. Gerontologist 1975; 15:398–403

Kovacs AL: Rapid intervention strategies in work with the aged. Psychotherapy: Theory, Research and Practice 1977; 14:368–380

Langley GE, Simpson JH: Misplacement of the elderly in geriatric and psychiatric hospitals. Gerontologia Clinica 1970; 12:149–163

Lawton MP, Simon B: The ecology and social relationships in housing for the elderly. Gerontologist 1968; 8:108

Lazarus LW: A program for the elderly at a private psychiatric hospital. Gerontologist 1976; 16:125–131

Lehman AF, Possidente S, Hawker F: The quality of life of chronic patients in a state hospital and in community residences. Hosp Community Psychiatry 1986; 37:901–907

Lewis CA: Facilitating a better reality: a treatment approach for the confused and disoriented, in Mental Health Interventions for the Aging. Edited by Horton A Jr. New York, Praeger, 1982

Lewis MI, Butler RN: Life review therapy: putting memories to work in individual and group psychotherapy. Geriatrics 1974; 29:165–169, 172–173

Lewis S: A patient-determined approach to geriatric activity programming within a state hospital. Gerontologist 1975; 15:146–149

Lichtenstein H, Winograd CH: Geriatric consultation: a functional approach. J Am Geriatr Soc 1984; 32:356–361

Lieberman MA: Institutionalization of the aged: effects on behavior. J Gerontol 1969; 24:330–340

Lieberman MA: Crises of the last decade of life: reactions and adaptations, in Community Mental Health and Aging: An Overview. Edited by Feldman AG. Los Angeles, University of Southern California, 1973

Liem PH, Chernoff R, Carter WJ: Geriatric rehabilitation unit: a 3-year outcome evaluation. J Gerontol 1986; 41:44–50

Linden ME: Group psychotherapy with institutionalized senile women: II: Study in gerontologic human relations. Int J Group Psychother 1953; 3:150–170

Linden ME: Geriatrics, in The Fields of Group Psychotherapy. Edited by Slavson SR. New York, International Universities Press, 1956

Lindsley OR: Geriatric behavioral prosthetics, in New Thoughts on Old Age. Edited by Kastenbaum R. New York, Springer, 1964

Lowenthal MF: Lives in Distress. New York, Basic Books, 1964

Lowenthal MF, Berkman PL, Brissett GG, et al: Aging and Mental Disorder in San Francisco. San Francisco, Jossey-Bass, 1967

MacDonald ML, Kerr BB: Behavior therapy with the aging, in Mental Health Interventions for the Aging. Edited by Horton A Jr. New York, Praeger, 1982

MacLeod RD: Unrealistic discharges. Gerontologia Clinica 1970; 12:31–39

Macmillan D, Shaw P: Senile breakdown in standards of personal and environmental cleanliness. Br Med J 1966; 2:1032–1037

Maney J: A class in creative movement for residents of an in-hospital halfway house within a geriatric therapeutic community. Ann Arbor, MI, Institute of Gerontology, 1975

Markson E: A hiding place to die. Transactions, December, 1971; 48–54

McClannahan LE: Therapeutic and prosthetic living environments for nursing home residents. Gerontologist 1973; 13:424–429

McGuire TG, Dickey B, Shively GE, et al: Differences in resource use and cost among facilities treating alcohol, drug abuse, and mental disorders: implications for design of a prospective payment system. Am J Psychiatry 1987; 144:616–620

Milne JS: Prevalence of incontinence in the elderly age groups, in Incontinence in the Elderly. Edited by Willington EL. London, Academic Press, 1976

Mirotznik J, Ruskin AP: Inter-institutional relocation and its effects on psychosocial status. Gerontologist 1985; 25:265–270

Mishara BL, Kastenbaum R: Self-injurious behavior and environmental change in the institutionalized elderly. Int J Aging Hum Dev 1973; 4:133

Mitchell JB, Dickey B, Liptzin B, et al: Bringing psychiatric patients into the Medicare prospective payment system: alternatives to DRGs. Am J Psychiatry 1987; 144:610–615

Morton EVB: Barker ME, MacMillan D: The joint assessment and early treatment unit in psychogeriatric care. Gerontologia Clinica 1968; 10:65–73

Nathanson BF, Reingold J: A workshop for mentally impaired aged. Gerontologist 1969; 9:293–295

National Institute on Aging: When you need a nursing home. Age Page, November 1986. (U.S. Government Printing Office Publication No. 491–280/40003)

Nightingale F: Notes on Nursing: What It Is and What It Is Not. New York, Dover Publications, 1969 (Originally published 1860)

Osgood NJ (ed): Suicide in the Elderly. Rockville, MD, Aspen, 1985

Palmore E: Total chance of institutionalization among the aged. Gerontologist 1976; 16:504–507

Perez EL, Blouin J: Psychiatric emergency consultations to elderly patients in a Canadian general hospital. J Am Geriatr Soc 1986; 34:91–94

Pincus A: New findings on learning in old age: implications for occupational therapy. Am J Occup Ther 1968; 22:300–303

Preston GAN: Dementia in elderly adults: prevalence and institutionalization. J Gerontol 1986; 41:261–267

Rechtschaffen A: Psychotherapy with geriatric patients: a review of the literature. Gerontology 1959; 14:73–84

Ripeckyj AJ, Lazarus LW: Management of old age—psychotherapy: individual, group, and family, in Handbook of Studies on Psychiatry and Old Age. Edited by Kay DWK, Burrows GD. New York, Elsevier 1984

Risse SC, Barnes R: Pharmacologic treatment of agitation associated with dementia. J Am Geriatric Assoc 1986; 34:368–376

Rodstein M: Challenging residents to assume maximal responsibilities in homes for the aged. J Am Geriatr Soc 1975; 23:317–321

Rosenthal NE, Sack DA, Carpenter CJ, et al: Antidepressant effects of light in seasonal affective disorders. Am J Psychiatry 1985; 142:163–170

Rovner BW, Kafonek S, Filipp L, et al: Prevalence of mental illness in a community nursing home. Am J Psychiatry 1986; 143:1446–1449

Rubenstein LZ, Rhee L, Kane RL: The role of geriatric assessment units in caring for the elderly: an analytic review. J Gerontol 1982; 37:513

Rudd JL, Margolin RJ: Maintenance Therapy for the Geriatric Patient. Springfield, IL, Charles C. Thomas, 1968

Senn BJ, Steiner JR: Don't tread on me: ethological perspectives on institutionalization. Int J Aging Hum Dev 1978–1979; 9:177

Sherr VT, Goffi MT Sr: On-site geropsychiatric services to guests of residential homes. J Am Geriatr Soc 1977; 25:269–272

Simpson WM Jr: Exercise: prescriptions for the elderly. Geriatrics 1986; 41:95–100

Snyder LH, Pyrek J, Smith KC: Vision and mental function of the elderly. Gerontologist 1976; 16:491–495

Spark GM, Brody EM: The aged are family members. Fam Proc 1970; 9:195–210

Steuer J: Psychotherapy with the elderly, in Psychiatr Clin North Am 1982; 5:199–213

Stotsky BA: Psychiatric disorders common to psychiatric and nonpsychiatric patients in nursing homes. J Am Geriatr Soc 1967; 15:664–673

Stotsky BA (ed): The Nursing Home and the Aged Psychiatric Patient. New York, Meredith Corporation, 1970

Stotsky BA, Dominick JR: Mental patients in nursing homes: I. Social deprivation and regression. J Am Geriatr Soc 1969; 17:33–44

Stotsky BA, Frye S: Comparison of psychiatric and nonpsychiatric patients in nursing homes. J Am Geriatr Soc 1967; 15:355–363

Szekais B: Using the milieu: treatment-environment consistency. Gerontologist 1985; 25:15–18

Turner BF, Tobin SS, Lieberman MA: Personality traits as predictors of institutional adaptation among the aged. J Gerontol 1972; 27:61–68

Verwoerdt A (ed): Clinical Geropsychiatry (second edition). Baltimore, MD, Williams & Wilkins, 1981

Warshaw GA, Moore JT, Friedman SW, et al: Functional disability in the hospitalized elderly. JAMA 1982; 248:847–850

Waxman HM, Dubin W, Klein M, et al: Geriatric psychiatry in the emergency department: II. Evaluation and treatment of geriatric and nongeriatric admissions. J Am Geriatr Soc 1984; 32:343–349

Weiner MB, Brok AJ, Snadowsky AM: Working with the Aged: Practical Approaches in the Institution and Community. Englewood Cliffs, NJ, Prentice-Hall, 1978

Whanger AD: When should a mentally ill older person be sent to the hospital?, in Mental Illness in Later Life. Edited by Busse EW, Pfeiffer E. Washington, DC, American Psychiatric Association, 1973

Whanger AD: Drug management of the elderly in state hospitals, in Drug Issues in Geropsychiatry. Edited by Fann WE, Maddox GL. Baltimore, MD, Williams & Wilkins, 1974

Whanger AD: The history and development of geriatric psychiatry. Career Directions 1977; 5:2–11

Whanger AD: Treatment within the institutions, in Handbook of Geriatric Psychiatry. Edited by Busse EW, Blazer DG. New York, Van Nostrand Reinhold, 1980

Whanger AD, Busse EW: Care in hospitals, in Modern Perspectives in the Psychiatry of Old Age. Edited by Howells JG. New York, Brunner/Mazel, 1975

Whanger AD, Lewis P: Survey of institutionalized elderly, in Multidimensional Functional Assessment: The OARS Methodology. Edited by Pfeiffer E. Durham, NC, Duke University, 1975

Whanger AD, Myers AC (eds): Mental Health Assessment and Therapeutic Intervention with Older Adults. Rockville, MD, Aspen, 1984

Whitehead WE, Burgio KL, Engel BT: Biofeedback treatment of fecal incontinence in geriatric patients. J Am Geriatr Soc 1985; 33:320–324

Williams TF: Rehabilitation in the aging: philosophy and approaches, in Rehabilitation and the Aging. Edited by Williams TF. New York, Raven Press, 1984

Wolff K: The Emotional Rehabilitation of the Geriatric Patient. Springfield, IL, Charles C Thomas, 1970

Wolk RL, Seiden RB, Wolverton B: Unique influences and goals of an occupational therapy program in a home for the aged. J Am Geriatr Soc 1965; 13:989–997

Woods RT, Britton PG: Psychological approaches to the treatment of the elderly. Age Aging 1977; 6:104–112

World Health Organization: Psychogeriatrics (World Health Organization Technical Representatives Series No. 507). Geneva, World Health Organization, 1972

Zimmer JG, Watson N, Treat A: Behavioral problems among patients in skilled nursing facilities. Am J Pub Health 1984; 74:1118–1121

Chapter 24

The Continuum of Care: Movement Toward the Community

George L. Maddox, Ph.D.
Thomas A. Glass, M.A.

In recent decades public discussion of care for older persons has continually concentrated on what has come to be called "the alternatives issue." The attention of congressional committees initially focused on alternatives to institutionalization, particularly nursing home care, because older persons consume public health and related welfare resources at a higher rate than adults generally and nursing home care is an expensive component of total cost. Older persons therefore provide a very visible illustration of a general problem of securing quality care at bearable cost. What have clearly concerned the U.S. Congress about care of older people are the very high cost of services that appear to be poorly distributed and inappropriate care of debatable quality (U.S. Senate, Special Committee on Aging, 1977). However, public discussion of efficient and effective alternative forms of care for older people, while generating a great deal of rhetoric, has produced little definitive evidence that would inform choices among a bewildering array of competing options.

At the beginning of 1970s discussion focused on alternatives to institutionalization. A consensus among both professionals and laity emerged that too many older people were inappropriately and unnecessarily institutionalized in mental hospitals and nursing homes. This consensus unquestionably had some basis in fact; however, since no definitive consensual procedures existed for determining appropriate levels and locales for care, estimates of the number of older people inappropriately institutionalized or receiving too much care varied from as little as 6 percent to as much as 40 percent or more. The confidence that too many people were receiving care, and perhaps too much care, in the wrong care settings, was matched by confident assertions that care in the community and, if possible, at home, provided obviously preferable alternatives at obviously lower cost. The obviousness of these conclusions has repeatedly been confronted by a troublesome fact: The efficiency and effectiveness of alternatives to the current organization of services continue to be asserted rather than systematically demonstrated. Some relevant evidence has accumulated, however; options have been more clearly defined, and systematic evaluation is increasingly possible. Yet in the 1980s some of the current issues have the familiar look of old questions that have not been definitively resolved. The search for the optimal solution in organizing and financing long-term care has not been rewarded. An important observation about the organization and financing of health care in democratic, market-oriented societies is suggested by this outcome. The dominant values in the civic culture of a society—or at least those who are empowered to make decisions for the society—determine the political feasibility of arrangements proposed by the planners of health and welfare services. The technical feasibility of a plan to organize health and welfare services for older adults is not the only or even the prime consideration. Assessment of political feasibility is a major consideration. In our view, the relevant dimensions of the civic culture include strong preferences for individual responsibility for personal welfare, for decentralization in decision making, for location of care services in the private sector, and for the provision of health care services primarily by physicians. In such a political environment, comprehensive planning for care services and consensus about who needs what services at whose expense are unlikely (Maddox 1971; Rodwin 1984).

Structuring the Issues

The development of scientific knowledge, the transfer of that knowledge to professionals through training, and the translation of knowledge into professional practice take place in the context of organizations. An understanding of the delivery of care to a population therefore benefits from a sociologic understanding of how organizations define the roles and rules that structure the interactions of the professional helpers and those they help, and how societies and communities allocate resources among organizations.

More than two decades ago Charles Perrow (1965) wrote a very insightful sociologic analysis of key factors that influence the behavior of organizations whose product is personal care. His analysis provides a conceptual structure for thinking about some basic issues in the organization of helping resources. Perrow concentrated on three interactive societal factors: (1) the *cultural system* of a society embodying values and beliefs that influence the setting of legitimate organization goals, (2) the available *technology* that determines the means for goal attainment, and (3) the *social structure* of organizations in which specific techniques are embedded in ways that facilitate or inhibit goal attainment. Perrow's illustration of these three factors focused on care in mental hospitals. His basic argument, however, is broadly applicable to an understanding of how care is organized in response to impairment generally.

Culture is a shared, socially transmitted construction of reality. The concept refers broadly to the goals members of a society value and pursue; to the rules and roles that structure social life; and to the technologies and the material and symbolic products of group life. Through processes of socialization and social control, most individuals' cultural expectations are transmitted from generation to generation. Consequently, conformity to social expectations is the common experience of everyday life. Most members of most social groups want to become and be what they are expected to become and be. Dissents, conflict, and nonconformity do occur and are considered normal in democratically organized societies. When they do occur, cultural belief systems provide plausible explanations and suggest corrective measures to ensure an acceptable level of social integration and cohesion. Illness is a case in point. Illness has social as well as personal significance in all societies. This is so because illness typically impairs the performance of social roles. There are, therefore, social as well as personal reasons for limiting the impact of illness. Illness typically evokes temporary exemption from usual role obligations and helpful social response, but usually with the expectation that the sick individual wants to limit the debilitating effects of illness as much as possible. Modern societies attach considerable importance to controlling the effects of illness. In American society, for example, one of our largest industries, to which we devoted in the 1980s more than 10 percent of our annual Gross National Product (GNP), is health care. Scientific medicine and its related technologies, manpower, and organization are integral parts of our culture. This is so much the case that some observers refer to belief in the "Great Equation," that is, medical care equals health (Wildavsky 1977). Others refer to the dominance of physicians in the provision and control of health care as "medicalization of care" (Fox 1977).

There is no question that in the last half-century advances in medical technology have raised public expectations regarding the conquest of disease. Average life expectancy has increased dramatically (Maddox 1977). Sick people, for the most part, expect to receive care and be cured. Unfortunately, very high expectations encounter substantial obstacles. Health resources, particularly primary health care, are not equally distributed geographically and hence are not equally accessible. Moreover, as Wildavsky contends, the Great Equation is probably wrong; medical care does not equal health (Ingelfinger 1978; Saward and Sorensen 1978). The medical system—doctors, other health professionals, hospitals, and drugs—may account for and deal with only a small proportion of the factors affecting health. A much larger proportion appears to be determined by factors over which the medical system has little or no control—factors such as life-style (smoking, eating, drinking, worrying, inactivity); social conditions (income, inheritance); and social environment (air, water, noise, safety). This is why Wildavsky and others (Maddox 1971; Ingelfinger 1978; Saward and Sorensen 1978; Enthoven 1980; Rodwin 1984) feel that a medical system cannot ensure health at any cost, much less at a bearable cost. Even in a society becoming accustomed to high inflation generally, the total cost of health care is escalating more rapidly than other services (Culliton 1978; Walsh 1978). The result is a widespread sense of concern that reflects, according to public opinion polls, less a crisis in confidence in the value of medical care than in the belief that appropriate care will not be received at a bearable cost (Lewis et al. 1976). Or, in terms of the three interacting factors stressed by Perrow, cultural beliefs and expectations about health care are mismatched with both the available technology and the organization of care for achieving shared goals for ensuring health care. Medical technology available for diagnosis and treatment is impressive, although it is directed primarily toward acute illness. The organization for health care delivery concentrates on medical care dependent on high technology controlled by highly specialized personnel centralized in or near hospitals. Financing of health care is directed primarily to medical care and to care that must be certified by medical practitioners. There is a growing body of opinion that Wildavsky's extreme conclusion regarding the important but modest contribution that medicine can make in ensuring health is more right than wrong (Ingelfinger 1978; Saward and Sorensen 1978). Hence, increasing amounts of resources poured into health services as they are currently organized are likely to produce a decreasing marginal return on investment and less satisfaction with the outcome. In regard to health services, doing better in many ways but feeling worse (Knowles 1977) has been the outcome. Problems related to the health care of older persons are specific and instructive illustrations of why there is a sense of crisis regarding our capacity to achieve adequate health care at a bearable cost and a continuing interest in "alternatives to institutionalization" (Kane and Kane 1978; Maddox 1977; Meltzer et al. 1981; Vogel and Palmer 1983; Harrington et al. 1985).

Health Care for Older Persons

The cultural beliefs and values regarding the care of older persons in the United States are most accurately described as complex, ambiguous, and contradictory. All citizens, including older ones, have a right to the best available care. What is *best* tends to be associated with high technology, that is, sophisticated equipment operated by specialized personnel, centralized in hospitals and medical centers. In recent decades the short-stay hospital has come to be associated with curative therapies, which tends to evoke a positive image. This positive image has been tempered somewhat by concerns about the high cost of care. Long-stay institutions, on the other hand, evoke a very negative image, as indicated by public attitudes toward mental hospitals and nursing homes. Such institutions have been the focus of social concern and have provided the illustrations of unnecessary and inappropriate custodial, as distinct from curative, service. Nursing homes as they have developed extensively in this country since the advent of Medicare and Medicaid programs are clearly extensions of a medical model of care. Access to and continuation in nursing homes is contingent on both medical certification and, for many older adults, eligibility for Medicaid. In addition, critics of the very extensive development of nursing homes (more than 26,000 homes, 1.5 million beds, and a $30 billion annual cost in 1982) usually comment that the care provided does not emphasize the social components of care enough. Nursing homes suffer from the perception of being second rate, understaffed, and underfunded hospitals (Kane and Kane 1978).

Deinstitutionalization of the mentally ill, including many older persons, has been the intention of public policy as well as cultural preference in this country for more than two decades (Maddox 1972, 1975). Both public policy and cultural preference regarding deinstitutionalization reflect evidence as well as emotion. Media coverage of dramatic events involving older persons in long-term care institutions—events such as deaths resulting from fires, incidents involving abuse and inadequate care, and evidence of fiscal mismanagement—provide fuel for strong emotional response. But there is also evidence of what appears to be unnecessary institutionalization, dependency-producing overcare, and questionable effectiveness of high-cost services (Kane and Kane 1978; Maddox 1972). A large number of persons, including many older persons, have been removed from mental institutions. Hospital censuses and length of stay have been reduced. Between 1955 and 1980, for example, the censuses of state hospitals declined nearly 75 percent (Goldman et al. 1983). There is little definitive evidence, however, with regard to the selection procedure used to determine who will be placed in the community, the fate of older individuals who have been so placed, or the impact of this placement on neighborhoods and communities. The best evidence indicates that many of the "deinstitutionalized" are reinstitutionalized in less publicly visible long-term care facilities in the community (Kane and Kane 1978). Some observers suggest that the reimbursement structure of Medicaid is an important factor in a process that is better described as a transfer between institutions than as deinstitutionalization (Gronfein 1985). Occasionally those who rally behind the philosophy of deinstitutionalization make extravagant claims about the proportion of older individuals who are inappropriately institutionalized, with estimates running as high as 40 percent. In fact, we do not have definitive evidence on this point. There is some evidence indicating that the great majority of individuals in, for example, nursing homes are significantly impaired, that 13 to 14 percent might be cared for appropriately in a situation providing less intensive care, and that perhaps another 10 percent who probably benefit from institutionalization overall receive more care than their functional impairments require (Maddox 1977; Laurie 1978).

In the absence of a definitive technology in long-stay institutions that gives reasonable assurance of achieving the restoration of functioning, the inference is invited not only that such institutions are primarily custodial, focusing on maintenance rather than rehabilitation, but also that the organization of life within them unnecessarily increases the dependence of residents. Unlike hospitals and medical centers, where high cost at least is associated with the hope for restoration of function, high cost in long-stay institutions has come to be associated with the expectation of increased dependence in a custodial environment. The organization of long-term care in the United States continues to be dominated by and to suffer from comparison with what has been called "a medical model" of care, a model symbolized by a specialized physician in a hospital supported by technicians and technology. While the continuing dominance of a medical model of long-term care might be interpreted as additional evidence of medicine's control of health care, this dominance does reflect continuing hope that current medical technology and organizaton of care can effect cures for the chronically ill in the face of discouraging evidence to the contrary. The continuing search for alternatives to institutionalization and a preference for deinstitutionalization of health care for older persons are therefore hampered by the lack of demonstrably effective, efficient, and adequately distributed organizations for care in communities whose performance is superior to the overall performance of medical institutions (see, e.g., Lamb 1981).

Nevertheless, both professional and public opinion increasingly reflect a belief in the desirability as well as the feasibility of more long-term care in the community rather than institutional settings. This opinion is buttressed with increasing experience of satisfactory care outside institutions that is, at least, no more expensive than institutional care and possibly less expensive (Maddox 1977; Hurtado et al. 1971; U.S. Department of Health and Human Services 1986). The United States has consequently entered an era in which experimenting with alternative organization and financing of care will continue to increase. The actual transformation of the care system to emphasize community-based rather than hospital-based care has moved slowly and will probably move slowly, at least in the foreseeable future (Leader 1986; Kavesh 1986; Koren 1986). This is the case, in part, because reliable and valid procedures for determining the proper level and locale for care and for measuring outcome are inadequately developed and neither routinely available nor consistently applied even when available (Maddox 1972; Maddox and Karasik 1975; Maddox and Dellinger 1978; Meltzer et al. 1981). The implications of a substantial reorientation of care to emphasize community-based services for professional training and manpower development are also not yet well understood. It is not at all clear that public preference for high-technology medicine will be significantly reduced by the addition of opportunities for care in the community or that the total cost of care will be reduced by additional forms of care unless the alternative forms are a substitute for existing forms. Some evidence indicates that an increasing number of highly technical medical procedures are being introduced into community care (Koren 1986) and hospice care, which in its initial stages of development was strongly antitechnology, is under pressure to become more like mainstream institutional care (Paradis and Cummings 1986). And, finally, although we have learned that more and better formal care does not diminish the commitment of kin and friends to care for older adults for whom they are responsible, we understand too little about the impact on kin and friendship networks of placing more responsibility for care in the community (Maddox 1975; Laurie 1978; George and Gwyther 1986). But these constraints notwithstanding, extensive development of community-based care for older persons will continue to be an issue in health care policy in the foreseeable future. Some observers believe that alternative forms of long-term care will be *the* dominant issue in the organization and financing of health care (e.g., Vogel and Palmer 1983).

The Case for Community-Based Care

The case for increasing the probability that the locale for care will be outside institutions and that the care offered will stress social and psychologic as well as medical components is outlined briefly here and developed in the sections that follow. In brief, it is argued first that community and home care for impaired older persons are commonsense responses to common problems of dependency in late life. Historically, these forms of care preceded institutionalization and continue today to provide most of the services required. Community and home care are old ideas that are currently being rediscovered (Maddox 1975, 1977). Public attitudes and public policy regarding appropriate sources and location of care have typically reflected high regard for professional expertise and limited confidence in the competence and responsibilities of families to deal with impaired members. The transfer of presumed responsibility for impaired members of families from families to professional family surrogates has been pronounced (Fox 1977). Nevertheless, a substantial majority of the care provided to impaired older persons is provided not by public agencies, but by a network of kin and friends (Maddox 1975; Laurie 1978; Health Policy Analysis Program 1978). Community and home care are hardly novel ideas or unusual experiences.

Second, a wide array of community and home services (e.g., home health and home help in the public and private sector) already exist (Health Policy Analysis Program 1978; Comptroller General of the United States 1977a, 1977b; Medicus Systems Corporation 1977; Weiler and Rathbone-McCuan 1978; Vogel and Palmer 1983). The feasibility of establishing a wide variety of community-based services is not at issue. However, services for community and home care, like health and social services, generally are fragmented, uncoordinated, and not routinely accessible to or used by a majority of impaired adults (National Center for Health Statistics 1986).

Third, discussions of the economics of community and home services continue to be inconclusive. Intuitively, offering services outside institutions where high technology is concentrated ought to achieve economies. This has not been demonstrated to be the case, particularly when the quality and quantity of professionally prescribed services are also considered (Mor and Kidder 1985; U.S. Department of Health and Human Services 1986). In any case, the crucial economic issue in assessing alternative types of care services is the total cost of all services to the care system of acceptable levels and quality of care, not the cost of a discrete subset of services. The reduction of total service system cost attributable to community and home services has not been demonstrated (Maddox 1977; Hurtado et al. 1971; Sager 1977; U.S. Department of Health and Human Services 1986).

Fourth, concentration of public discussion on the cost-effectiveness of community and home services probably is an interesting diversion from a more basic issue. The basic issue is the fragmented, unsystematic organization of care and of the public financing of care. Only comprehensive, integrated care delivery systems at local levels offer any prospect for achieving cost-effectiveness for community and home care. And the most significant contribution of community and home care to the achievement of economy, according to some analysts, may be the removal of patients from exposure to high-technology, high-cost health care centers (Enthoven 1978; Ball 1978) and the requirement that care organizations deliver specified services for fees set prospectively (Enthoven 1980; Harrington et al. 1985).

Fifth, achieving an appropriately comprehensive, integrated system of care delivery at the local level will probably take the form of current proposals for a type of care system illustrated by health maintenance organizations (HMOs) (Garfield 1970; Lewis et al. 1976). This type of care system may continue to emphasize the medical as distinct from social and psychologic aspects of care for older persons. Yet the emerging tradition of the HMO may offer a significant opportunity for melding the strengths of medical and social–psychologic components of care in a manner that is publicly and politically appealing and viable. Current evaluations of social health maintenance organizations are expected to provide useful information about the cost-effectiveness of melding social and medical models of prepaid care for older adults. The HMO offers an opportunity for local variations in the specific organization of a care system while providing for both prepayment and a relatively comprehensive, integrated, and controllable system of care. Manpower development and training, financing, and procedures for assignment to alternative types of care within any care system are critical problems whose solutions will determine how adequate, effective, and efficient that system of care will be. Recent evidence has suggested that the use of HMOs for geriatric care is not, however, risk free or automatically effective (Iglehart 1987).

Rediscovering Community and Home Care

Scientific medicine in the United States and optimism about the beneficial effects of exposure to physicians and hospitals date only from the second decade of this century (Ingelfinger 1978). Care of impaired individuals in general and of elderly individuals in particular tended to be a family, a neighborhood, or a community responsibility. Until World War II, federal spending for health care was largely confined to investment in traditional public health activities such as immunization. In the postwar era, a change in public attitudes and policy occurred, resulting in federal programs of increasing variety and scale. Prior to 1965, the federal investment in health care for the aged and poor was $4.4 billion. By 1977 that investment was $49.6 billion, of which Medicare and Medicaid accounted for $35.7 billion and the Department of Defense and the Veterans Administration for another $6 billion (Walsh 1978). The financing of long-term care by Medicare and Medicaid was a prime factor in promoting the development of a nursing home industry, which, by the mid-1980s, included some 26,000 nursing homes with 1.5 million beds at a cost of more than $30 billion annually (Rabin and Stockton 1987). Long-term care beds are occupied by very elderly impaired persons— 75 percent of them are over the age of 75, most having multiple impairments and more than half having significant mental impairment. In the 1970s persons age 65 and older accounted for an average of 64 million hospital days annually, and on average, each visited a physician almost seven times annually, and the total health cost to older persons was about three times higher than that of adults generally (U.S. Department of Health, Education and Welfare 1977a; Shanas and Maddox 1977). In the 1980s older adults continue to use various health services at a rate higher than that of other adults. Personal annual per capita dollar expenditures for hospital care, physicians' visits, and drugs tend to average about three times higher for adults over age 65 compared with younger adults (U.S. Senate, Special Committee on Aging, 1985). About 5 percent of persons age 65 and older tend to be institutionalized at any point in time in the United States in recent decades, and the estimated probability of a period of long-term institutionalization in late life is about 25 percent (Palmore 1976).

These widely quoted statistics are impressive and invite the incorrect inference that medical and institutional care have supplanted traditional community and home care. This is far from the case. Epidemiologic surveys provide evidence that while an estimated 80 percent of older adults have at least one chronic condition, about 60 percent of older persons are not significantly impaired in five important dimensions of functioning—social support networks, economic security, physical health, mental health, and the capacity for performing basic physical and management activities of daily living (Comptroller General of the United States 1977a; Maddox and Dellinger 1978; National Center for Health Statistics 1983). More than 9 out of 10 older adults will live most of their later years in the community. And for the approximately 12 to 15 percent of older persons in the community who are seriously impaired, approximately 80 percent of the services they receive are provided by kin and friends, not a public agency (Comptroller General of the United States 1977b; Health Policy Analysis Program 1978).

The fact that currently an estimated 20 percent of health and social services provided to seriously impaired older persons have a public source of financing surely constitutes a change and a historical trend worth noting. Federal funding of total national health expenditures increased from 13 percent in 1965 (the year Medicare was enacted) to 23 percent 2 years later and to 29 percent of total expenditures by 1983 (Rabin and Stockton 1987). This change challenges both a cultural and a political preference for asserting the primacy of familial responsibility for older persons and activates anxieties about the weakening of family ties and related social obligations. Social theorists have accentuated this concern with discussions of what may be called the "consequences of modernization" thesis, which contends that the inevitable price of industrialization, urbanization, and rapid social change is the weakening of familial and community ties. The dependent old, in turn, would obviously be vulnerable to isolation, social irrelevance, and neglect. There is evidence that family structure and function have changed in recent decades. The divorce rate is high, single parent families are now common; alternative family life-styles are more visible; and families have access to and use an increasing array of experts to help in solving personal and familial problems. Yet the fact remains that most older people are not isolated from kin and friends; impressive majorities of adult children indicate a continuing willingness to care for an older adult family member (Maddox and Wiley 1977; Maddox 1972; Kane and Kane 1978; U.S. Department of Health and Human Services 1986). In sum, community and home care of dependent, impaired older persons have been and continue to be the rule, not the exception. Therefore, current discussions of community and home care most appropriately stress a long-established pattern that may be in need of redis- covery and revitalization but which is certainly not a daring new adventure.

Proliferation of Community Services

Community and home services, both public and voluntary, have been widely available and widely used in Western European countries for many years. In European settings, particularly those with comprehensive care systems, pub- lic debate focuses not on whether community and home services are feasible and desirable, but on how to increase their availability to underserved and unserved populations. On the basis of such experience, a considerable body of documentation and expertise exists regarding the organization, training, staffing, and performance of noninstitutional services for older persons. In general such services have high social visibility, are integrated into comprehensive care systems, and are reasonably well financed. Experience in Europe suggests that one community or home care worker to help with household maintenance and personal care is required for every 100 older persons, a rate that is currently approximated in the Nordic countries. The United Kingdom has achieved a rate of one worker per 750 older persons. In the United States the current rate is about one worker per 5,000 older persons (Maddox 1977).

Contemporary health care in the United States is characterized by a high degree of specialization of information, personnel, therapeutic procedures, and locales for delivering services (Vogel and Palmer 1983). This specialization includes community and home care (Leader 1986; Kavesh 1986; Koren 1986). The permutations and combinations of specialized people, activities, and locales have no known limits and therefore generate acute problems of fragmentation, require organizational coordination, and tend to have gaps in coverage (Harrington et al. 1985). The proliferation of specialized components in health care illustrates one logical outcome of disaggregating health care into its specialized components. Early in this century health care was considerably less specialized in terms of knowledge, personnel, techniques, and locale of service. Hence, one encountered general practitioners and general nurses offering services primarily in homes and incidentally in hospitals. If one disaggregates the process of general medical care into specialized components, the logical possibilities are numerous—medical specialists, physician extenders, hospital nurses, public health nurses, practical nurses, home health aides, home helpers, and so on. Similarly, if one observes a family caring for an impaired older member, this holistic process can be disaggregated into a large number of basic components, each of which can be the basis for a specialized activity for one or another category of professional or quasi-professional persons.

Let us assume that a society concludes (1) that a number of impaired older persons need supportive health and welfare services, (2) that these services can be and should be offered outside institutions (i.e., in the community or at home), and (3) that there should be some public support for these services when individuals do not have the informal social support ordinarily provided by kin and friends. What one would expect to develop is what one currently observes—a specialized service system that reflects the disaggregation of the holistic process into components and the development of specialized programs to deal with these components. Specialized systems of public community and home care are emerging for each element of service ordinarily provided by kin and friend networks, for example, adult family homes, day care, day health, personal care, continuing supervision, congregate care, meals/nutrition, household maintenance, home health, social interaction/recreation, physical therapy, education, housing, transportation, information and referral, special income maintenance, and protective services (Health Policy Analysis Program 1978; Weiler and Rathbone-McCuan 1978). The process of disaggregation could logically go on and on. The availability and use of such services is relatively limited currently: Less than 1 percent of Medicare expenditures in the 1970s and less than 3 percent currently have been, for example, directed to community and home care (U.S. Department of Health, Education and Welfare 1977b; Leader 1986). Nevertheless, many components of a noninstitutional care system are already present.

One or more of these types of specialized noninstitutional services currently exists in most communities in the United States, complex combinations of services exist in many communities, and, in a few communities, a comprehensive range of services is found. There is no question that a case can be made for the feasibility and desirability of each type of service, although how much and for whom are very much in doubt. In the typical instance, each discrete service has developed its own justification, manpower estimates, training procedures, and clienteles. Certification and state surveillance of community-based services are minimal. In the typical community, moreover, adequate provision is made neither for coordinating the discrete programs administratively and financially nor for articulating them with the dominant health care delivery system. The principal issues regarding community and home services is, therefore, not their feasibility and desirability, but rather their efficiency, effectiveness, financing, and coordination with other elements of the care system.

The Cost-Effectiveness and Efficiency of Alternatives

Public discussions of alternative care programs have concentrated increasingly on the key issues of cost-effectiveness and the effective integration of noninstitutional services into the existing care system. Conclusions regarding costs have continued to be inconclusive not only because the definitive evidence is lacking but also because the questions being asked are typically the wrong questions. The question typically asked is, "Are community and home alternatives cheaper than institutionalization?" The intuitive answer would certainly be in the affirmative. This answer is misleading, however, because it avoids the issue of the cost implications of particular services for the total system of care and ignores issues of access and of quality of care. It is intuitively obvious, for example, that individuals with moderate functional impairments requiring limited support services could be maintained in a community or home setting more cheaply than in an institutional setting. This is true, to a considerable degree, because noninstitutional care costs are shifted from the public sector to the private sector, specifically to family and friends (Comptroller General of the United States 1977b; Sager 1977). It is also intuitively obvious that a minimally impaired person who is for some reason in an institution that provides more than the required care could be managed more economically as well as more appropriately elsewhere. Enthoven (1978), Luft (1978), and Ingelfinger (1978) all note the operation of "the technologic imperative" in health care institutions; the specialized health care professionals in high-technology settings have professional, ethical, and legal reasons for trying one or more tests or procedures. These observers are convinced that, in high-technology settings, the marginal utility of medical treatment, in both a medical and an economic sense of benefits in relation to investment, is frequently reached and often exceeded. Insofar as community and home care removes an individual from the technology typically found in institutional settings, reduction in the cost of care should follow. Health maintenance organizations apparently reduce the total cost of care through rationing access to hospitals (Luft 1978), and proponents of the hospice movement are explicit in emphasizing care of dying patients that minimizes use of costly medical technology and maximizes use of relatively more economical psychosocial supportive therapy (Berdes 1978). The appropriateness and defensibility of such a removal, however, is clearly a debatable quality-of-care issue that would require far more evidence than is currently available (Donabedian 1978; Frazier and Hiat 1978; Tancredi and Barondess 1978; Breslow 1978). Recent evidence from a review of the cost-effectiveness of hospice care after such care became covered under Medicare has not been reassuring (Mor and Kidder 1985; Paradis and Cummings 1986).

The more severe the functional impairment of the individual, the less intuitively obvious the cost-effectiveness of community and home care becomes. A critical issue in assessing the cost effectiveness of alternative forms of health and social services is, therefore, a determination of degree of functional impairment and the minimal number and quality of services that would meet acceptable standards of care for persons with a known degree and kind of impairment in ability to perform normal social roles. In exploring such an issue, one can imagine an experimental or quasi-experimental design in which at least four categories of older persons emerge: (1) those whose impairments are so severe that, by professional and public consensus, they would need to be in an institutional setting; (2) those whose impairments are moderate and for whom the consensus of professionals is that they might be appropriately managed in either institutional or noninstitutional settings; (3) those whose impairments require supportive services, but clearly in noninstitutional settings; and (4) those whose degree of well-being requires no special services. The second category is the critical one for testing hypotheses about comparative costs of alternative types of care (Smyer 1977). The first and third categories raise different questions. For example, if a person in the first category were found in the community or a person in the third category were found in a long-stay institution, we would be interested primarily in explaining an inappropriate placement. The issue of the difference in cost of maintaining third-category persons in the community or in an institution is uninteresting because it has a predetermined answer; such persons are almost certainly misplaced in institutions. A person in the first category living in the community or a person in the fourth category residing in an institution is certainly misplaced. With degree of functional impairment specified and reasonable consensus achieved regarding the type and amount of required services specified, one can imagine relatively definitive comparative research that might address the issue of cost-effectiveness of alternative care programs for impaired older persons. A few research studies reflect an understanding of and a response to these necessary conditions for drawing conclusions regarding the relative cost of alternative systems of care. These are discussed below.

The General Accounting Office in Cleveland, Ohio, designed a study to assess the impact of defined services on the well-being of a random sample of persons age 65 and older in that city (Comptroller General of the United States 1977a, 1977b). The design incorporated a methodology developed at the Duke University Center for the Study of Aging and Human Development (Maddox 1972, 1985; Maddox and Dellinger 1978). The Duke methodology has three elements: (1) a reliable, valid multidimensional assessment of functional status; (2) a procedure for identifying the number, quantity, and cost of basic components of commonly used services; and (3) a matrix that relates the services actually received by persons of known functional status initially to their functional status at some subsequent time.

The Cleveland study found that 60 percent of the older individuals surveyed had minimal impairments that required no special intervention or required, at most, services like transportation, help with housing, social and recreational opportunities, and occasionally home help. At the other extreme, 10 percent of the sample were severely impaired and required and were receiving an extensive range of supportive services. Of the 60 percent relatively unimpaired, the average individual received the equivalent of $349 in services each month, with 60 percent of this amount being provided by family and friends. Of the 10 percent who were extremely impaired, the average cost per month for services received was estimated to be $845, of which 80 percent was provided by family and friends. This $845 is considerably above the $597 that was the average monthly cost of nursing home care in Ohio at that time. These data suggest several conclusions:

1. A large number of extremely impaired older persons are maintained in the community;
2. The extremely impaired are maintained in the community at a cost well above the cost of nursing home care;
3. The high cost of noninstitutional care is borne primarily by kin and friends rather than public agencies.

For the extremely impaired older persons in the Cleveland study living in the community, total cost of care in a noninstitutional setting was not less than institutional care, but it was less costly to the public treasury, which was responsible for only 20 percent of the bill. What about the estimated cost of care for the 30 percent of older persons lying between the classifications "unimpaired" and "extremely impaired"? Such persons in Cleveland were receiving services valued at an average of $323 per month, 70 percent of which was provided by kin and friends. The total cost of services for this category was about half the cost of nursing home care, even if it had been paid entirely from public resources. Since some persons living in nursing homes —possibly 12 to 14 percent (Laurie 1978; Health Policy Analysis Program 1978)—have an intermediate degree of functional impairment, this category is clearly critical in assessing the potential cost savings that would come from ensuring that needed care is provided outside institutions.

The estimate of 12 to 14 percent of older persons in nursing homes whose functional impairments might be managed in noninstitutional settings is a plausible and conservative estimate based on admittedly limited data. Estimation of persons inappropriately institutionalized or receiving more than required care in institutions has varied considerably from study to study, depending on the procedures used to assess impairment and to determine appropriateness of care in relation to the degree of impairment assessed. Some estimates of inappropriate care in institutions have ranged as high as 40 percent (Health Policy Analysis Program 1978). Current evidence does not permit a resolution of the reported variance in estimates. The consensus is only that the rate of unnecessary institutionalization and the inappropriately high levels of care are significant. Further research is clearly needed. Several existing studies do, however, provide relevant illustrations of the problems of producing definitive information and present some suggestive findings.

Hurtado et al. (1971) at the Kaiser facility in Portland, Oregon, have reported the economic effects of introducing an extended-care facility and a home care service into a comprehensive prepayment health plan with a history of low hospitalization use among subscribers. The effect on Medicare subscribers was of particular interest. The authors demonstrated that with these new services administratively and spatially an integral part of the comprehensive care organization, hospital use by Medicare patients was reduced by 27 percent. Most of the observed reduction was attributable to the use of the extended care facility rather than the home care service. Moreover, the total cost of the services to Medicare patients outside the hospital service was greater than the savings from the reduced hospitalization; that is, while hospital days were reduced, less expensive extended care and home services were used for longer periods of time, thus tending to equalize the cost of illness episodes managed primarily inside or outside the hospital service.

Similarly, Weiler and Rathbone-McCuan (1978), who are advocates of community-based care for older persons, summarize research on the cost of 10 day care facilities that variously emphasized rehabilitation or social support services. The observed range of average daily cost was from $11 to $61, and an average for the 10 facilities was about $25. This average cost for adult day care was above the national average cost of about $10 per day for nursing home care at the time of the comparison. It is important to note that the day care program reported by those authors did not include an estimate of the out-of-pocket cost-of-living expenses of program participants.

Alan Sager (1977) has provided an imaginative pilot study of the cost of alternative forms of care for impaired older persons that illustrates the problems of cost estimation. Working with a sample of individuals at the point of discharge from a hospital, he had nine professionals experienced in discharge planning estimate whether home or nursing care would be the more appropriate assignment. Home care was estimated to be more appropriate for 12 percent. The assessors then proposed detailed care plans. Reasonable consensus was achieved among planners for each individual and the estimated cost of implementing the recommended care plans was determined. The average daily cost of the estimated home care plans, with maintenance cost of board and lodging factored in, was about $52. Assessors were also asked to prescribe an alternative care plan for each individual if the person were institutionalized. The estimated cost of the services proposed for delivery in a nursing home proved to be almost exactly the same as for home care. By happenstance, nine subjects for whom home care and nursing home care plans had been developed were in fact institutionalized; the actual average cost per day was about $60.

The conceptualization of Sager's study warrants special comment. First, careful attention was given to establishing professional consensus on appropriate service requirements regardless of the service site chosen. Second, total cost of services, whether public or private, was estimated. Third, experienced professional service planners proposed alternative care plans in both nursing home and home settings that proved to have the same total cost, although the actual cost of nursing home care proved to be above the estimated cost. And, fourth, at the point of discharge from the hospital, a large majority (almost 90 percent) of older patients considered for inclusion in the study were judged to be inappropriate for home care.

Medicus Systems Corporation (1977), under a federal contract, attempted to implement an ambitious controlled trial of the outcome of assigning appropriately selected individuals being discharged from hospitals to day care or home care programs, to a combination of both, or to a "no special care" control condition. The cost of additional services for the experimental subjects assigned to day care or home service was provided by special federal financial arrangements. For various reasons the research study did not meet the stringent conditions of a controlled clinical trial because true random alternative assignment of subjects proved to be difficult, services received by controls could not be monitored carefully, and cost determination was inadequate. However, within these constraints, considerable variation in cost of services between presumably similar programs was observed. The general conclusion was that extended benefits available to participants in noninstitutional programs did appear to lower the use of traditional health services appreciably. There was some indication that total cost of care increased on the average. These conclusions are similar to those reached by

Hurtado et al. (1971) in their Portland, Oregon, study.

The most recent evidence on the cost-effectiveness of community-based care comes from the National Long-Term Care Demonstration (known informally as the Channeling Project) which was initiated in September, 1980, by three divisions of the U.S. Department of Health and Human Services. Its objective was to assess the effects of compehensive case management of community care on cost containment in long-term care without sacrificing quality of care for needy, impaired elderly (U.S. department of Health and Human Services 1986). The demonstration was designed to finance some direct services and to arrange for waiver of some financial restrictions on some types of community care; but the demonstration did not include direct control over medical and nursing home care. Case management in the basic demonstration of how an existing service system might be effectively coordinated consisted in the Channeling Project of seven features: (1) outreach, (2) standard eligibility screening, (3) comprehensive assessment, (4) initial care planning, (5) service arrangement, (6) monitoring, and (7) periodic assessment. An alternative financial control model made it possible for health care managers in some demonstration sites to expand the range of services offered, to offer services on the basis of need rather than eligibility, to pool resources for strategic allocation to particular services, and to require partial copayment by recipients in some cases. The five sites selected to test each model were operational in 1982 and continued fully operational through June 1984.

Over the life of the demonstration, 11,769 applicants were screened and 9,890 were identified as eligible. Of these, 6,341 were randomly assigned to demonstration or control categories. Several data sources were used in the evaluation of the program's effects. In addition to telephone screening interviews, an extensive in-person survey was administered to both treatment and control groups at baseline and then at 6, 12, and (for half the sample) 18 months. Contact was subsequently made by telephone with a subset of informal caregivers at 6 and 12 months. Service use and cost data were collected from Medicare, Medicaid, and channeling records, and from providers directly.

Principal findings from the Channeling Project demonstration include the following:

1. Channeling's selection criteria did identify an extremely vulnerable group of older adults. Twenty-two percent were unable to perform any of five activities of daily living; more than 90 percent were IADL (Instrumental Activities of Daily Living)-impaired; 53 percent were incontinent; there was evidence of cognitive impairment; one-third lived alone; and more than half reported incomes of below $500 a month.
2. The demonstration, whose design was implemented essentially as planned, provided an evaluation of the effects of coordination of basic and

slightly enriched services for older adults; these effects included the following:

a) Channeling increased formal community service use;
b) Neither type of demonstration (basic or financial model) reduced or had any major effects on the informal care being provided to participants;
c) In spite of identifying a group of elderly persons living in the community who were at high risk for institutionalization, the demonstration did not identify the subpopulation at highest risk or reduce nursing home use;
d) The channeling interventions did not reduce the relatively heavy use of physicians and medical services among these high-risk older adults;
e) The costs of expanded case management and community services were not offset by reductions in nursing home and other costs;
f) In general, the demonstration increased client and informal caregiver confidence and satisfaction with life; and
g) The demonstration did not significantly affect client functioning or risk of mortality.

The Channeling Project was an expensive demonstration and reconfirmation of several general observations repeatedly made about the organization of health care in the United States over many years. Manipulations of the system of formal care services do not appear ordinarily to reduce the availability of informal support. In the case of the Channeling Project, both the persons receiving care and their caregivers responded positively to efforts to improve care for the elderly persons for whom they were responsible. The presumption that a large number of persons in nursing homes do not need to be there has persisted for a long time without the benefit of definitive evidence. The estimates based on data generated by the Duke Older Americans Resources and Services Program and the U.S. General Accounting Office (Maddox 1985) are worth noting again because they suggest that the number of nursing home residents who might, on medical grounds, be treated more appropriately elsewhere may be 10 percent. On the other hand, in our estimation, possibly an equal percent of community-dwelling elderly may be so disabled as to benefit from nursing home placement. In demonstrations like the Channeling Project, which emphasized comprehensive screening, it would be reasonable to assume, therefore, that some screening of community residents would lead to a recommendation *for* rather than *against* institutionalization. In any case, the demonstrated failure of the well-conceived Channeling Project to reduce institutionalization and medical care usage illustrates how such projects may add to rather than reduce or moderate total system cost for the care of older populations. Research suggests that the most likely way in which total system cost can be reduced is through a capped organizational budget that covers inpatient, outpatient, and community care services

(Enthoven 1980; Harrington et al. 1985; Maddox 1977; Evans 1985). In such cases the issue becomes one of suballocation of a specified total budget to these various services and the decentralization of health planning and delivery. Budget capping has technical merit as a cost control strategy but is politically quite controversial as illustrated by recent assessment of the merits of using HMOs to provide medicare-financed care for older adults (Iglehart 1987).

The most adequate information on the cost of community and home programs designed as alternatives to institutionalization, while clearly not definitive, does not confirm the hopes of the advocates of alternative forms of care. The assertion that community and home care lowers average daily cost or total system cost is not confirmed when there is some control for the level of functional impairment of the older individual involved and for the cost accounting procedures used. It is also evident that community and home care appears most favorable in comparison with institutional care only when public cost is considered and basic maintenance cost and other nonpublic contributions are not factored in. Further, and this is a critical issue, such evidence as there is does not indicate that total system cost is reduced by community-based care programs. On the contrary, total cost appears to be the same or perhaps slightly higher (e.g., Hurtado et al. 1971; U.S. Department of Health and Human Services 1986).

The current evidence on cost-effectiveness of community care does not provide a decisive argument against such care. Economic cost is not necessarily the only or the most important consideration. It is quite possible, for instance, that cost being equal, community and home care provide good value for money invested because the care provided is more appropriate than institutional care, is of better quality, or is more effective in the long run. Or the long-run implications may be more favorable for noninstitutional care than short-term studies have indicated. Or public policy might favor noninstitutional care, not because its total cost is less than institutional care, but because noninstitutional care transfers a significant part of the cost to the private sector. Or, by removing impaired individuals from high-technology environments, public policy that emphasizes noninstitutional care may reduce long-run system cost through reducing the use of high-cost interventions of questionable value. Each and all these explanations are plausible and future research must sort out the facts. Concentration on cost may, however, divert attention from what many observers believe to be the more salient problem—the organization of care.

The Organizational Context of Health Care

We have argued above that community and home care for impaired older persons is needed and feasible and that such care is not demonstrably more economical than institutional forms of care when degree of functional impairment is controlled and total cost is determined. However, the cost-effectiveness of noninstitutional care is probable, we have argued, for perhaps 30 percent of older persons who are moderately but not severely impaired. Essential evidence does not exist that cost-effective noninstitutional care of appropriate quality can be provided for this significant category of impaired elderly within the care system as presently organized. This is so primarily for two reasons. First, currently the care system and its financing have a decidedly medical and institutional emphasis. That is, the care system is most easily accessed by individuals with a medically certifiable impairment and access to some community services has often been contingent on the individual's having been institutionalized. Community and home services, while recognized in Medicare legislation, continue to be a small (about 3 percent) fraction of the services financed. The concepts of preventive care and social support services are essentially foreign to Medicare and mental health services and payment for these services is limited (Blazer and Maddox 1977; Glasscote 1976; Glasscote et al. 1977; Berger 1978).

Contemporary discussions of health usually stress the desirability of taking a broad view of health in terms of functional capacity and the total well-being of individuals. That is, a philosophic interest in the social components of health and well-being is frequently expressed, and strong cases have been made for preferring social models of care to medical models (Breslow 1978; Kane and Kane 1978; Saward and Sorensen 1978). Philosophic preferences aside, the dominant care system available to older persons has a decidedly medical focus. Second, the dominant care system is highly specialized, fragmented, uncoordinated, and without a single point of entry to provide systematic, comprehensive assessment of impairment and assignment to appropriate services. One result is that each segment of the care system competes for public resources that are known to be limited. Hence, each additional service program tends to add to total system cost rather than to substitute for the cost of some other service. A striking characteristic of the care system of the United States is that its implied total annual budget is in essence unlimited and is determined retrospectively by the cumulative cost of all care programs, and total cost is known only after the costs have been incurred. This is in contrast to nationalized systems and, in fact, the prepaid comprehensive programs in this country, which assume a fixed annual budget that must be allocated among the alternative components of the system.

In 1971 the U.S. Department of Health, Education and Welfare (now Department of Health and Human Services) distributed an analysis of what was described as "the crisis of health care." This document asked whether the perceived crisis was produced by (1) inferior health care as reflected in the assessed well-being of citizens; (2) the absence of essential resources; or (3) both of these. The answer in each case was negative. While indications of health like mortality and morbidity statistics and life expectancy rates in this country are not the best in the world, they are tolerable by most standards and are most distinctively different from other countries in regard to variations in health indicators by race, socioeconomic status, and locale of residence. Health indicators of white, middle-class, urban populations in this country generally compare quite favorably with European populations; nor does this country lack resources. Our health personnel/population ratios are favorable, our hospital bed/population ratios are favorable, and our committed percentage of GNP to health (more than 10 percent) is among the highest in the world. Again the most evident problem is maldistribution of resources, particularly primary care resources, rather than absence of resources. For example, 82 active physicians per 100,000 population might be found in Mississippi, whereas 228 active physicians per 100,000 population might be found in New York. Large metropolitan areas average 2½ times more physicians per unit population than rural areas. In recent decades the proportion of primary care physicians has declined to the point that, at the beginning of this decade, more than 6 in 10 active physicians were in specialty practice. The report concluded that the crisis is best described as organizational. The nation suffers, according to this analysis, from excessive fragmentation and poor coordination of existing resources. Significantly, the report did not comment directly on what Wildavsky calls the Great Equation (medical care equals health), although this idea is implicit. For instance, the report does stress the importance of environmental factors that affect health, preventive care, and health education. The central illustration of a possible solution to the organizational problem identified was HMOs. This preference was justified in the report by evidence then available that HMOs are cost effective, a conclusion supported also by current evidence (U.S. Department of Health, Education and Welfare 1977b).

Following the report by the U.S. Department of Health, Education and Welfare, legislation intended to foster HMOs emerged. The concept has been politically controversial, has had limited public acceptance, and has generated a considerable amount of rhetoric for and against (Lewis et al. 1976). Articles by Enthoven (1978) and Luft (1978) that summarized the issues and the evidence a decade ago remain surprisingly current. Enthoven correctly noted the absence of controlled trials in comparing alternative care systems and the consequent inability to draw definitive conclusions regarding the cost-effectiveness and quality of care provided by competing alternatives. He reviewed the incentive structures of alternative care systems and concluded that fragmented, uncoordinated systems lack any obvious incentive for control of cost. Further, if a fragmented, uncoordinated collection of health care programs is dominated by high-technology institutions, the probability is high that a "technological imperative" will operate. That is, the availability of technology encourages high rates of use even in the face of evidence that its use has low marginal utility. This conclusion led Enthoven to argue that within a total system of care, there should be alternative care sites, some of which remove individuals from the high-technology care centers. Such removal reduces the opportunity, and the inclination, to introduce types of care whose return in terms of increased functioning is demonstrably low. By implication, then, Enthoven argued that community and home care might achieve economies precisely because individuals in such settings are not, and presumably are appropriately not, at risk for high-technology therapeutic intervention. Enthoven did, however, introduce the caution that his general argument for alternative forms of care is not an endorsement of any specific form of care in the absence of controlled trials that take into consideration quality as well as cost.

It is worth noting in this context that some proponents of the hospice movement appear to have reached a similar conclusion (Berdes 1978). In high technology settings, there are a variety of incentives—professional, ethical, and legal—to make extraordinary efforts to extend life by any available means and at any cost. Proponents of hospices commonly argue that such efforts are not only patently artificial but also, in the final analysis, inhumane. This conclusion leads to the deliberate exclusion of advanced technology from the hospice to a specific emphasis on the social and behavioral rather than medical components of care. Medical technology is emphasized in the hospice movement, if at all, in connection with the reduction of pain rather than with the extension of life. The promises of hospice have not been fulfilled automatically, as recent evidence indicates (Mor and Kidder 1985; Paradis and Cummings 1986). The cost of hospice as an alternative to hospitalization for terminal care is not automatically cheaper. Over time, hospice care has tended to become more like the institutional care it was designed to replace.

An article by Luft (1978) reviewed the rhetoric and the evidence regarding the reputed savings attributed to HMOs and concludes that the claimed economies are probably real and substantial. These reported savings in the total cost of care apparently were then and are now attributable primarily to the lower rates of hospitalization in HMOs and not to differences in the use of ambulatory care services or length of stay in hospitals. The studies Luft reviewed are relatively compelling because they are methodologically adequate, taking into consideration standardized age and sex rates and case mixes. Luft was not altogether certain why the apparent cost-effectiveness is consistently observed. Possibly, he argued, the HMO client is less sick or differently disposed to use available care, although most evidence suggests that this is not the case; on the contrary, some evidence suggests that prepaid plans tend to attract a disproportionate number of chronically ill persons. Or perhaps HMOs undertreat their patients, although evidence that this is so is lacking. It should be recalled here that the research of Hurtado et al. (1971) did not find cost savings in an experiment with alternative forms of service within a particular comprehensive prepaid medical plan. One recent experience in the prepayment of HMOs for care of older adults under Medicare suggests that the established organizational strengths of HMOs in the cost-effective delivery of health care cannot compensate for poor fiscal management of a particular HMO (Iglehart 1987).

Constructing the Future

As noted earlier in the discussion of Perrow's analysis of the three factors that affect service delivery organizations, cultural and ideologic factors dominate when the technology for achieving preferred social goals is unavailable and when existing organizational structure adversely affects the application of such technology. Many people, including many expert observers, believe that community and home care are forms of noninstitutional service delivery that are both desirable and feasible. This belief is bolstered by a number of factors, including evidence from this country and abroad that (1) programs of care for older persons outside institutional settings can be efficient and effective; (2) care in institutional settings not only is very expensive but also provides too much service for some older people and not enough for others who could benefit from minimal supportive care; and (3) appropriate technology and model organizational forms of community-based care exist that provide the basis for future development of an adequate comprehensive care system.

Beliefs, Technology, and Organization

In spite of the attractiveness of these beliefs, community and home care services have been developed slowly and with considerable cautiousness in the United States. The explanation of this apparently contradictory trend is suggested by Perrow's analysis. At the cultural level, the attractiveness of low-technology community and home care is matched by the appeal of high-technology medical care. In the abstract, both health care providers and consumers would surely respond favorably to the prospect of more noninstitutional forms of care of high quality and at low cost. In the concrete, it is not at all clear that either would respond affirmatively to more noninstitutional care if this meant fewer hospital beds, rationed access to hospitals and physicians, or reduction in the specialized tests and therapeutic procedures that are at the heart of contemporary diagnosis (Fox 1977). That is, if given the choice of a fixed amount of money to be allocated to health and welfare with more community care resulting in less institutional care, it remains to be seen where public beliefs lie.

The critical question is not whether reallocation of resources to alternative forms of care is possible. Most countries in Western Europe provide illustration of successful community care programs as integral components of their systems of care. The question is also not whether the health of populations suffers intolerably from extensive use of noninstitutional services. It does not. Every country in Western Europe has gross indicators of mortality and morbidity that compare favorably with our own (U.S. Department of Health, Education and Welfare 1971; Rabin and Stockton 1987; Raffel 1985).

The question is whether health care personnel and the people of the United States they serve can live with the implications of a changed health care system in which access to medical and hospital care would be rationed and the autonomy, perceived or real, of both professionals and their patients/clients would be reduced (Chapman 1978; Enthoven 1980). The evidence and the speculation are variable and suggest that American values and attitudes regarding health care are essentially contradictory. Some social survey evidence suggests that a majority of adult Americans perceive a crisis in health care delivery and identify the inaccessibility of primary care and the cost of health care as their primary concerns (Lewis et al. 1976). Fox (1977) argues that while Ivan Illich's radical critique of "medicalization" of society and his plea for "demedicalization" have some merit, health remains a central preoccupation of this society. Saward and Sorensen (1978) document the continuing societal preoccupation with curative rather than preventive medicine.

Individuals continue to resist modifying behavior and life-styles that increase the risk of morbidity and mortality—cigarette smoking, overeating, physical inactivity, and nonuse of auto seat belts, for example. Of special interest are indications that social controls intended to modify risky behavior or noxious environmental factors are widely interpreted as infringements on personal freedom. It is as though, these authors conclude, freedom from regulations is more dear than life itself. Wildavsky's caustic, pessimistic essay "Doing Better, Feeling Worse" (Knowles 1977) is preoccupied with the contradictory, the ironic, indeed what he believes to be the pathologic aspects of health care in this country. In addition to persistent belief in the wrongheaded Great Equation, he notes the "paradox of time: past success leads to future failure" (p. 106). For example, increased longevity is a human triumph that precipitates the crisis of an aging society. To save our shaky belief that investment in medicine ensures health, we displace our goals; interest in curing is displaced by interest in caring, and caring becomes equated with demonstrating we have access to ineffective services. Every move to increase equality in one dimension of health care increases inequality in another dimension. No society is willing and no care system is able, Wildavsky argues, to provide as much care as a population is willing to consume. We are driven by a technologic imperative; there is always one more procedure to try. Cost of health care inevitably rises to a total that is provided by private insurance and federal subsidy. One is hardly surprised by the bottom line of Wildavsky's diagnosis: The politics of health care in the United States can only be described as conflicted, ambivalent, pathologic. The prognosis is not encouraging. No definitive treatment is available for our ambivalent feelings and contradictory preferences.

Perrow's analysis suggests that the persistent ideologic quality of contemporary discussion about health care constitutes evidence of the inadequacy of available technology and organizational arrangements for ensuring either curing or caring at a tolerable social cost. Our love affair with medical technology apparently is not over, but it is pursued with less enthusiasm than before. The evidence of decreasing marginal utility of costly applications of medical technology is simply too great to be ignored (Ingelfinger 1978; Saward and Sorensen 1978; Frazier and Hiat 1978; Tancredi and Barondess 1978; Enthoven 1980). Yet there are few signs that continued discussion of "the crisis of health care" portends a radical reorganization and reallocation of health resources. After all, there is not yet even consensus about legislation on one or another form of national health insurance (Hurtado et al. 1971) or the objectives to be pursued in a national policy for long-term care of older adults (Meltzer et al. 1981).

Perrow's analysis is also helpful in sensitizing the observer to an additional consequence of a plurality of ideologic views about the organization and financing of health care. The policy-making arena clearly contains multiple key players, and some of the players hold a disproportionate share of the kind of organizational power to affect the direction of policy flow. So while consumers of health care services may hold a clear preference for noninstitutional forms of care, their interests may compete with the interests of health planners, politicians, health care administrators, and physicians. The analysis of Robert Alford documents how health care resources may be underallocated to groups whose interests are subordinate to those of dominant groups (Alford 1975). His analysis of the relative underdevelopment of occupational health demonstrates that the preferences and needs of workers may be eclipsed by a dominant medical model that determined the kinds of health care provided during most of this century. What is of particular interest here, however, is that the balance of power is clearly changing in the health policy arena today. A new actor, the health administrator, has entered the field and has claimed an unprecedented share of the decision-making power. The health care administrator, whose language is that of economics and not of medical science, has altered the rules and format of the game. Stated more formally, the predominant shift in health policy in the last decade has been a move from professional control to the predominance of administrative control. Partly the result of key legislation, and partly the result of naturally occurring economic forces that have produced an unacceptable level of inflation of health care costs, it is clear that the bottom line in health planning in the 1990s will continue to focus on cost. The implications of this modulation or transfer of organizational power for the future of community-based care is, as we have argued, not entirely clear. What is clear is that decision-making processes and the decision makers are changing.

For the foreseeable future, for better or worse, the United States seems destined to tinker incrementally with its fragmented, uncoordinated nonsystem of care. Incrementalism—a euphemism for only minor modifications of existing programs that the British call "muddling through"—has some merit in stable, democratically controlled societies (Maddox 1971). Several incremental changes at selected points in the current system of care affecting older persons do warrant at least some basis for guarded optimism about the future.

Adaptive Responses

Policy-making is not the only sphere in which the control of health care by physicians has been challenged. Public acceptance of unconditional professional autonomy and a medical monopoly of health care resources has been increasingly challenged. The origins of this challenge lie in the distant past as Chapman (1978) has documented. The legal basis of laws regarding professional malpractice can be traced to the 14th century. In the intervening centuries public challenge of uncontrolled professional autonomy and monopoly has been expressed through laws dealing with due process, licensure, restraint of trade, and quality control. Willingness of legislatures to limit the autonomy of medical professionals has been clearly demonstrated. Physicians, hospitals, and long-term care institutions will continue to play a vital role in the continuum of care that older persons require and in decisions about the allocation of resources to various components of the care system. The issue therefore is not the involvement of physicians and medical institutions in designing health care for the future, but the increasing involvement of nonmedical professions and nonmedical, community-based facilities in designing that future. Legislators have been reluctant to control access to high-technology medicine and to limit the proliferation and geographic concentration of highly specialized health personnel. They have also been slow to develop a plan for national health insurance and to involve government as a prudent buyer and not just an insurer of desired health and social services with emphasis on preventive and primary care. Research and demonstrations assessing alternative compehensive, prepayment care systems integrating health and social services have not produced definitive conclusions. Orientation of consumers to realistic assessment of the relative merits of hospital and community-based health care has been minimal. Although belief in the desirability and feasibility of more community-based services is increasing, nothing approximating a national consensus regarding the reorganization and financing of a comprehensive health care system designed to serve older persons is evident.

Organizational Development

Pragmatic, incremental experience with the organization of care in the United States has produced an outcome that, while not altogether satisfactory, is satisfactory enough to mitigate any inclination toward radical reorganization of care delivery in the immediate future. This same pragmatic, incremental orientation does, however, permit experimentation and model building that can provide public standards for assessing effectiveness and efficiency. In this country elaboration of the HMO concept appears to have particular merit for responding to needs of older persons for comprehensive care.

The cost-effectiveness of HMOs has been reasonably established, and this effectiveness is usually attributed not to restriction of access to care generally but to reduction of institutionalization (Luft 1978). The HMO concept also emphasizes comprehensiveness of care within a fixed budget. Consider, for example, Figure 1 (Garfield 1970). In this figure health is defined broadly as well-being, and attention is given to social as well as medical aspects of care and to preventive maintenance as well as sick care. An integral and important aspect of this care system is the availability of initial screening for purposes of triage, although there is provision for bypass of screening when alternative assignment to health care, preventive maintenance, or sick care is clearly indicated. Another striking feature of this conceptualization of a care system is that while traditional medical services are considered basic, social and psychologic dimensions of care are equally basic and integral to the system. Given the origins of HMOs within the dominant medical model of care, one is hardly surprised that reference is made to *paramedical* staff and services with *medical* supervision. No violence is done to the concept by the substitution of such concepts as *paraprofessional* staff with *professional* supervision in order to transform this conventional medical model into a professional model that can include experts in social and psychologic dimensions of care. Special attention is called in Figure 1 to programs of health education, exercise, and psychologic counseling in the health care center component of the model; to provision of extended care, which could include community and home care for the impaired elderly, in the sick care component; and to geriatric clinics in the preventive maintenance component.

The HMO model of a comprehensive health mainenance organization is similar to the system of geriatric care that has operated in Glasgow, Scotland, for several decades (McLachlan 1971; Kane and Kane 1978). The Scottish model has as its focal point a primary care health center staffed by general practitioners, visiting nurses, and social workers who have been trained to work as a team. The health center personnel in this setting have access to an impressive continuum of alternative care settings, including in-home services, day care, day hospitals, sheltered housing, and in-patient hospital services with both general and specialized hospital wards, including geriatric psychiatry. Moreover, in Glasgow, community programs supplement the health services by providing special health education and a health examination coincident with retirement and a variety of community support programs. The Scottish Home and Health Service, as a part of the British National Health Service, has a long tradition of integrating medical and social services and is, by definition, a comprehensive, prepaid care system. In Glasgow, professionals appear to use alternative placement of older persons judiciously and to place the impaired elderly at sites where the most appropriate care is

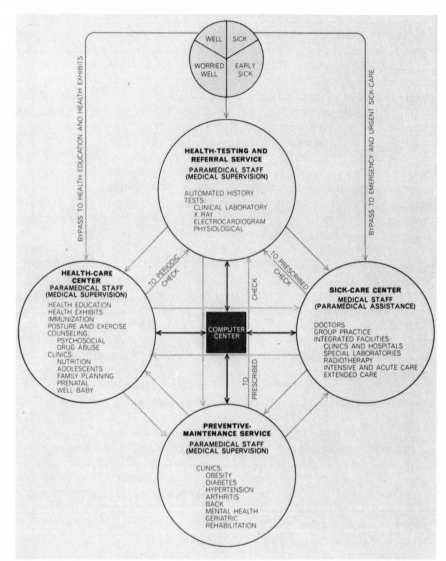

Figure 1. Initial concept of integrated care in a health maintenance organization. (Reprinted with permission from Garfield SR: The delivery of medical care. Sci Am 1970; 222:15–23.)

available. Although detailed information about the cost of a comprehensive service such as that in Glasgow is not available, in general the British investment in the delivery of care runs about 2 percent of GNP less than in the United States.

A systematic investment of governmental resources in the development of model HMOs to include assessment, health care, sick care, and preventive maintenance care for older persons appears to be indicated and is to be recommended. Such a decision would not preclude alternative investments in other forms of care. Yet the existence of a comprehensive system of care could provide a specific context for comparing the efficiency and effectiveness of alternative programs. In fact, the Health Care Financing Administration funded in the early 1980s a comparative study of the cost-effectiveness of social health maintenance organizations in six sites in the United States. The final report of findings has not been released. However, the apparent applicability and desirability of such a plan, as Perrow suggests, may or may not be sufficient to overcome existing organizational commitments and ideologic preferences. In health planning, the best idea often turns out to be the politically feasible idea and the one that pleases those who have the authority to decide and to allocate resources.

Technologic Development

Our national fascination with technology and its implementation could appropriately be directed increasingly to problems of special relevance to caring for older persons. In the interest of serving older persons more effectively, primary attention might be given to the implementation and specific applications of two existing types of technology. Badly needed are (1) a reliable, valid, economical procedure for identifying the existence and pattern of functional impairment among older persons (Institute of Medicine 1977); and (2) the development of information systems that will facilitate the monitoring and evaluation of the efficiency and effectiveness of alternative systems of care (Donabedian 1978; Frazier and Hiat 1978; Breslow 1978; Maddox and Dellinger 1978; Maddox 1978, 1985). Assessment of the effectiveness and efficiency of care in alternative settings is contingent on the appropriateness of matching level and type of functional impairment with resources intended to maintain or restore function. Adequate procedures for systematic, comprehensive assessment of functioning exist, but the available procedures are not widely available or consistently applied. As one might expect in the fragmented, uncoordinated array of services that characterizes the situation in the United States, there is no tradition of single points of entry into the care system that could provide assessment, triage, and monitoring of the outcomes of services. Experiments that provide assessment of alternative systematic assessment, triage, and monitoring of older adult populations are clearly feasible and warranted in spite of the discouraging findings of the Channeling Project described earlier. Case coordination is not the sole strategy for producing cost-effective geriatric care.

While explicit experiments in new forms of comprehensive care delivery for older persons are feasible and warranted, the opportunity to benefit from existing care programs should not be underestimated. Legislated governmental programs of care constitute social experiments from which important information can be derived (Maddox and Dellinger 1978; Tancredi and Barondess 1978; Schoolman and Bernstein 1978; Maddox 1985) if several conditions can be met. The efficiency and effectiveness of any service program can be assessed if (1) the functional status of participants can be measured at several points in time, and (2) the components of service to which participants are exposed can be specified. There is no longer any question that these conditions can be met in reasonably economic ways and in ways that are based on the types of information care programs routinely gather or could gather.

The implications of legislation in 1983 which instituted a diagnosis-related group (DRG) strategy for estimating prospectively the cost of hospitalization for Medicare recipients will be followed with interest. Consciously designed as a cost containment measure, the DRG strategy has in fact since 1983 helped reduce the average stay in hospitals for older patients by almost one day. Shortened hospital stays should increase interest in the increased need for and use of community-based care and in whether total Medicare costs are reduced. The evidence to date is not definitive, but in 1987 use of nonhospital services increased slightly but without evidence that this increase reduced the total Medicare bill.

As a sense of crisis about the cost and effectiveness of care for older persons escalates in the years ahead, experimentation with alternative systems of care will increase. The nation has the resources and the technology to develop an effective and efficient system of care for older persons at a bearable cost. Our capacity to develop an adequate system will hinge on our ability to reorganize the resources already at our disposal.

References

Alford R: Health Care Politics: Ideological and Interest Group Barriers to Reform. Chicago, University of Chicago Press, 1975

Ball RM: National health insurance: comments on selected issues. Science 1978; 200:864–870

Berdes C: Social Services for the Aged Dying and Bereaved in International Perspective. Washington. International Federation on Aging, 1978

Berger PA: Medical treatment of mental illness. Science 1978; 200:974–981

Blazer D, Maddox G: Developing Geriatric Services in a Community Mental Health Center: A Case History of a University-Based Affiliate Clinic. Durham, NC, Duke University Center for the Study of Aging and Human Development, 1977

Breslow L: Risk factor intervention for health maintenance. Science 1978; 200:908–912

Chapman CB: Doctors and their autonomy. Science 1978; 200:851–855

Comptroller General of the United States: The Well-being of Older People in Cleveland, Ohio. A Report to the Congress, April 19, 1977. Washington, DC, U.S. General Accounting Office, 1977a

Comptroller General of the United States: Home Health—The Need for a National Policy to Better Provide for the Elderly. A Report to the Congress, December 30, 1977. Washington, DC, U.S. General Accounting Office, 1977b

Culliton BJ: Health care economics: the high cost of getting well. Science 1978; 200:883–885

Donabedian A: The quality of medical care. Science 1978; 200:856–863

Enthoven AC: Cutting cost without cutting the quality of care. N Engl J Med 1978; 298:1229–1238

Enthoven AC: Health Plan. Reading, MA, Addison-Wesley, 1980

Evans R: Strained Mercy: The Economics of Canadian Health Care. Toronto, Butterworths, 1985

Fox C: The medicalization and demedicalization of American society, in Doing Better and Feeling Worse: Health in the United States. Edited by Knowles JH. New York, W.W. Norton, 1977

Frazier HS, Hiat HH: Evaluation of medical practices. Science 1978; 200:875–879

Garfield SR: The delivery of medical care. Sci Am 1970; 222:15–23

George L, Gwyther L: Caregiver well-being: a multidimensional examination of family caregivers of demented adults. Gerontologist 1986; 26:253–259

Glasscote R: Old Folks at Home: A Field Study of Nursing and Board and Care Homes. Washington, DC, Joint Information Service of the American Psychiatric Association and the National Association of Mental Health, 1976

Glasscote R, Gudeman JE, Miles D: Creative Mental Health Services for the Elderly. Washington, DC, Joint Information Service of the American Psychiatric Association and the Mental Health Association, 1977

Goldman H, Adams N, Taube C: Deinstitutionalization: the data demythologized. Hosp Community Psychiatry 1983; 34:129–134

Gronfein W: Incentives and intentions in mental health policy: a comparison of Medicaid and community mental health programs. J Health Soc Behav 1985; 26:126–206

Harrington C, Newcomer R, Estes C, et al: Long-Term Care of the Elderly: Policy Issues. Beverly Hills, Sage Publications, 1985

Health Policy Analysis Program: Long Term Care for the Elderly in Washington. Seattle, WA, University of Washington, Department of Health Services, 1978

Hurtado A, Greenlick A, Saward E: Home and Extended Care in a Comprehensive Prepayment Plan. Chicago, Hospital and Research Educational Trust, 1971

Iglehart JK: Second thoughts about HMOs for Medicare patients. N Engl J Med 1987; 316:1487–1492

Ingelfinger FJ: Medicine: meritorious or meritricious? Science, 1978; 200:942–945

Institute of Medicine: The Elderly and Functional Dependency. Washington, DC, National Academy of Science, 1977

Kane RL, Kane RA: Care of the aged: old problems in need of new solutions. Science 1978; 200:913–918

Kavesh W: Home care, in Annual Review of Gerontology and Geriatrics (Volume 6). Edited by Eisdorfer C. New York, Springer, 1986

Knowles JH (ed): Doing Better and Feeling Worse. New York, W.W. Norton, 1977

Koren MJ: Home care—who cares? N Engl J Med 1986; 314:917–920

Lamb R: What did we really expect from deinstitutionalization? Hosp Community Psychiatry 1981; 32:105–109

Laurie WF: Employing the Duke OARS methodology in cost comparisons: home services and institutionalization. Duke University Center Reports in Advances in Research 1978; 2:2

Leader S: Home Care Benefits Under Medicare. Washington, DC, Public Policy Institute, American Association of Retired Persons, 1986

Lewis CE, Fein R, Mechanic D: A Right to Health: The Problem of Access to Primary Medical Care. New York, Wiley, 1976

Luft HS: How do health maintenance organizations achieve their "savings"? N Engl J Med 1978; 298:1336–1343

Maddox GL: Muddling through: planning for health care in England. Medical Care 1971; 9:439–448

Maddox GL: Interventions and outcomes: notes on designing and implementing an experiment in health care. Int J Epidemiol 1972; 1:339–345

Maddox GL: Families as context and resource in chronic illness, in Long-Term Care: A Handbook for Researchers, Planners, and Providers. Edited by Sherwood S. New York, Spectrum, 1975

Maddox GL, Karasik R: Planning Services for Older People. Durham, NC, Duke University Center for the Study of Aging and Human Development, 1975

Maddox GL: Community and home care: the unrealized potential of an old idea, Care of the Elderly: Meeting the Challenge of Dependency. Edited by Exton-Smith AN, Evans JG. New York, Grune & Stratton, 1977

Maddox GL, Wiley J: The scope, concepts, and methods in the study of aging, in Handbook of Aging and the Social Sciences. Edited by Binstock R, Shanas E. New York, Van Nostrand Reinhold, 1977

Maddox GL: Aging, social change and social policy, in Major Social Issues: A Multidisciplinary View. Edited by Yinger M, Mausch H, Cutler S. New York, Free Press, 1978

Maddox GL: An information system for planning and evaluating geriatric care: the Duke Older Amerians Resources and Services Program, in Collecting Evaluation Data: Problems and Solutions. Edited by Bernstein L, Freeman H, Rossi P. Beverly Hills, Sage, 1985

Maddox GL, Dellinger DC: Assessment of functional status in a program evaluation and resources allocation model. Annals of the American Academy of Political and Social Sciences 1978; 438:59–70

McLachlan G: Problems and Progress in Medical Care. Oxford, Oxford University Press, 1971

Medicus Systems Corporation: Evaluation of Day Care and Homemaker Demonstrations: Executive Summary: Report No. 36. Chicago, Medicus Systems Corporation, 1977

Meltzer J, Farrow F, Richman H: Policy Options in Long-Term Care. Chicago, University of Chicago Press, 1981

Mor V, Kidder D: Cost savings in hospice: final results of the national hospice study. Health Services Research 1985; 20:407–422

National Center for Health Statistics: Physical and home management activities. Advancedata 1983; 93

National Center for Health Statistics: Aging in the 1980s: use of community services. Advancedata 1986; 124

Palmore E: Total chance of institutionalization. The Gerontologist 1976; 16:504–507

Paradis L, Cummings S: The evaluation of hospice in America toward homogeneity. J Health Soc Behav 1986; 27:370–386

Perrow C: Hospitals: technology, structure, goals, in Handbook of Organizations. Edited by March JG. Chicago, Rand McNally, 1965

Rabin D, Stockton P: Long-Term Care for the Elderly: A Factbook. New York, Oxford University Press, 1987

Raffel M: Comparative Health Systems. University Park, PA, Pennsylvania State University Press, 1985

Rodwin V: The Health Care Planning Predicament. Berkeley, University of California Press, 1984

Sager A: Estimating the Cost of Diverting Patients from Nursing Homes to Home Care. Waltham, MA, Levinson Policy Institute, Brandeis University, 1977

Saward E, Sorensen A: The current emphasis on preventive care. Science 1978; 200:889–894

Schoolman HM, Bernstein LM: Computer use in diagnosis, prognosis, and therapy. Science 1978; 200:926–930

Shanas E, Maddox GL: Aging, health and the organization of health resources, in Handbook of Aging and the Social Sciences. Edited by Binstock R, Shanas E. New York, Van Nostrand Reinhold, 1977

Smyer MA: Differential usage and differential effects of services for impaired elderly. Duke University Center Reports on Advances in Research 1977; 1:4

Tancredi LR, Barondess JA: The problem of defensive medicine. Science 1978; 200:879–883

U.S. Department of Health and Human Services: The Evaluation of the National Long-Term Care Demonstration: Final Report. Washington, DC, U.S. Department of Health and Human Services, 1986

U.S. Department of Health, Education and Welfare: Towards a Comprehensive Health Policy for the 1970s. Washington, DC, U.S. Department of Health, Education and Welfare, 1971

U.S. Department of Health, Education and Welfare: Current estimates from the health information survey, United States, 1975. Vital and Health Statistics. 1977a; 10:115

U.S. Department of Health, Education and Welfare: Medicare: utilization of home services, 1974. Health Insurance Statistics, November 2, 1977b

U.S. Senate Special Committee on Aging. Older Americans: The Alternatives Issue, I and II. Washington, DC, U.S. Government Printing Office, 1977

U.S. Senate Special Committee on Aging: Aging America: Trends and Projections, 1985–86 Edition. Washington, DC, U.S. Department of Health and Human Services, 1985

Vogel RJ, Palmer HC (eds): Long-Term Care: Perspectives from Research and Demonstrations. Washington, DC, Health Care Financing Administration, U.S. Department of Health and Human Services, 1983

Walsh J: Federal health care spending passes the $50-billion mark. Science 1978; 200:886–888

Weiler PG, Rathbone-McCuan E: Adult Day Care: Community Work with the Elderly. New York, Springer, 1978

Wildavsky A: Doing better and feeling worse: the political pathology of health policy, in Doing Better and Feeling Worse: Health in the United States. Edited by Knowles JH. New York, W.W. Norton, 1977

Looking to the Future

Chapter 25

The Future of Geriatric Psychiatry

Ewald W. Busse, M.D.
Dan G. Blazer, M.D., Ph.D.

The Path to Geriatric Psychiatry in the United States

The relatively recent emergence of geriatric psychiatry in the United States is based on two centuries of interest and work by both Americans and non-Americans. Europeans, during the 18th and 19th centuries, greatly influenced American medical and lay leaders. This review will touch on the identification and contribution of a few such public leaders as well as behavioral scientists and physicians whose contributions have been basic to the development of geriatric psychiatry. Some of these individuals have escaped the notice of modern geriatric psychiatrists whose attention is understandably focused on the rapidly expanding science and practice related to aging and the care of the elderly.

Among his many interests and talents, Benjamin Franklin (1706–1790) maintained a strong belief that science would eventually discover the aging processes and be able to control them and rejuvenate people. He apparently was convinced that if the patriarchs of the antediluvian era could achieve extended life spans, so could the human of the future. Franklin had considerable interest in thunder and lightning, and this interest led to his invention of the lightning rod. Franklin also explored the possibility that lightning might influence the resurrection of deceased animals and people. Another of his inventions may actually contribute to the well-being of the elderly, and that is the Franklin stove (Gruman 1966).

Franklin was convinced that science would eventually extend life and improve health. Such thoughts prompted him to say that it "occasions my regretting sometimes that I was born too soon." In referring to restoration of life, he stated, "We live in an age too early and too near the infancy of science to hope to see an art brought, in our time, to its perfection" (Gruman 1966, p. 84).

Benjamin Rush (1745–1830), a famous American physician, patron of the American Psychiatric Association (APA), and signer of the Declaration of Independence, wrote extensively and lucidly on a variety of subjects. In 1805 he published "An Account of the State of the Body and Mind in Old Age; With Observations on Its Diseases and Remedies" (Butterfield 1976).

G. Stanley Hall (1846–1924) was a psychologist who founded one of the first psychology departments in a university in this country at Johns Hopkins University. He was president of Clark University and was responsible for organizing a conference inviting Sigmund Freud to the United States. Hall is also credited for coining the word *adolescence*. In 1922 he published a book entitled *Senescence: The Last Half of Life*. Hall organized the scattered studies and theoretical speculations concerned with the aging adult and problems of the aged. One of Hall's innovations was the study of old people's religious beliefs and fears of death by means of a questionnaire. Hall found that people did not necessarily show an increase in religious interest as they grew older. He also discovered that the old in his sample had not become more fearful of death.

The invention of the telephone by Alexander Graham Bell (1847–1922) is linked to his efforts to teach the deaf to speak. Among his many interests were the subjects of heredity and longevity.

Sir William Osler (1849–1919), the distinguished physician of McGill University, the University of Pennsylvania, Johns Hopkins University, and the University of Oxford, was a contemporary of G. Stanley Hall. Osler believed that aging was closely related to the state of blood vessels in the body and maintained that if the brain did change with aging, it was the result of hardening of the arteries.

In the 1930s increased interest focused on aging research. Walter R. Miles and his associates developed a project known as the Stanford Greater Maturity Project with the object of investigating systematically the psychologic aspects of aging. Medical research was enhanced by the publication of Edmond B. Cowdry, who brought together physical and health-related problems in a volume entitled *Problems in Aging* (1938). Cowdry played a major role in organizing the American Geriatrics Society, the Gerontological Society of America, and the International Association of Gerontology. Also in the late 1930s two important sociologists, Leo Simmons and Ernest W. Burgess, independently developed considerable activity and interest in the social aspects of the aging adult. In 1945 Simmons published a pioneer study of aging concerned with 70 preliterate societies (Simmons 1945). In 1948 Otto

Pollak reviewed the activities of the Social Science Research Council and released a publication, "Social Adjustment in Old Age." Ernest Burgess and his associates at the University of Chicago developed a number of instruments to measure personality adjustment in old age. In 1946, the American Psychological Association created the division of later maturity and old age. In the same year the first issue of *The Journal of Gerontology* was published by the Gerontological Society of America. The first national conference held in 1950 was followed by several White House Conferences. The first occurred in 1956, the second in 1971, and the third in 1981. Also in 1950 the International Association of Gerontology was formally organized in Liege, Belgium. International conferences have been held in St. Louis (1951), London (1954), Merano and Venice (1957), San Francisco (1960), Copenhagen (1963), Vienna (1966), Washington, DC (1969), Kiev (1972), Jerusalem (1975), Tokyo (1978), Hamburg (1981), and New York (1985).

The 1917 issue of the *Medical Review of Reviews* was dedicated to I.L. Nascher, "The father of geriatrics in America." Dr. Nascher inaugurated a department devoted to the diseases of the aged. According to Freeman (1961), Nascher not only was the father of American geriatrics, but coined the word *geriatric* and published a text under the title. This text, *Geriatrics: The Diseases of Old Age and Their Treatment,* was published in 1914 (second edition in 1916). Nascher was born in Vienna in 1863 and was brought to the United States as an infant. He graduated in pharmacy from Columbia University in 1882 and in 1885 received his medical degree from New York University. At the age of 24 Nascher entered medical practice. He published many known works of concern for the field of aging including an article, "Longevity and Rejuvenescence," in 1909 when he was 49 years of age. He lived until December 25, 1944. "The Aging Mind" was published a month before his death. In this paper, Nascher tabulated the characteristics of chronic brain syndrome and suggested that it was a primary change of senescence and that it must have a familial determinant since he had observed the disease occurring in a mother and a daughter at approximately the same age. He believed that accelerated primary aging was a feature of heredity.

Edward J. Stieglitz (1943) edited a publication entitled *Geriatric Medicine: Diagnosis and Management of Disease in the Aging and in the Aged.* A psychiatrist and President of the APA, Winfred Overholser was a professor of psychiatry at George Washington University School of Medicine, Superintendent of Saint Elizabeth's Hospital, and a member of the National Advisory Committee on Gerontology of the National Institutes of Health. Overholser contributed a section on the disorders of the mind and nervous system. Carl D. Camp, professor of neurology at the University of Michigan, contributed a chapter on the organic diseases of the brain, spinal cord, and peripheral nerves.

One of the first American books on aging and psychiatry appeared in 1969. This book, *Behavior and Adaptation in Late Life,* was edited by Ewald

W. Busse and Eric Pfeiffer. Busse in 1971 became President of the APA. He was Vice President of the APA from 1966 to 1967. Busse and Pfeiffer edited a second book in 1973. Prior to the appearance of these two books, among the best known of those in the English language was Felix Post's *The Clinical Psychiatry of Late Life* (1965). Another early publication was *Aging and the Brain* edited by Charles M. Gaitz (1972). Gaitz's publication was the proceedings of the Fifth Annual Symposium held at the Texas Research Institute of Mental Sciences. Similarly, Zinberg and Kaufman (1963) edited *Normal Psychology of the Aging Process*. This volume was the first annual scientific meeting of the Boston Society for Gerontological Studies, Inc. It appears that the Boston Society was probably the first psychiatric group interested in aging that was organized and productive.

American Psychiatric Association Council on Aging

Authorized by the constitution of the APA, the APA Council on Aging was established in 1979 with the following rationale:

> The APA represents a body of knowledge, experience, and skills indispensable to the identification, treatment, relief, and prevention of mental disorders in the aging population. The APA identified six specific areas of activity including evaluation and diagnosis, training, interface problems between psychiatry and other disciplines in geriatric care, design of services and third-party payment for psychiatric treatment of the elderly, decisions made by government that influence the mental health of the aged, and lastly identifying and implementing research into the problems of geriatric psychiatry. (APA 1981, pp. 71–72)

The Council on Aging is composed of nine psychiatrists and is responsible for developing and maintaining liaison with the appropriate non-APA organizations involved in the mental health care of aging Americans, with federal agencies similarly involved, and with other APA components so involved. Between May 1981 and May 1982, three Council task forces were operating. These included a Task Force on Fellowships and Career Development in Geriatric Psychiatry, a Task Force on the White House Conference on Aging, and a Task Force on Psychiatric Services for the Elderly. In addition, the APA Council on Research in 1979 established the Task Force on the Treatment of the Dying Patient and Family. The Council on Research of the APA also has had a Task Force on Research on Aging since 1974. The APA can take pride in the roles its members have played in the development of geriatrics.

The Group for the Advancement of Psychiatry (GAP) was organized in 1946. By 1950 its membership was composed of approximately 150 psychiatrists divided into 17 working groups. In 1950 the Committee on Hospitals published *The Problem of the Aged Patient in the Public Psychiatric Hospital,* GAP's Report No. 14. In 1966 GAP established the Committee on Aging, and this committee has been active ever since, publishing a number of reports.

Psychiatrists have played leadership roles in the activities of two major United States societies concerned with aging—the Gerontological Society of American (GSA) and the American Geriatrics Society (AGS). The GSA, founded in 1945, is a multidisciplinary organization with four distinct sections. In recent years, three psychiatrists have served as president of this important organization. The AGS, established in 1942, is composed largely of physicians and members of the health care professions. Psychiatrists have also led this medical society, which for over the last 20 years has given the Edward B. Allen Award for contributions to geriatric psychiatry. The American Association for Geriatric Psychiatry (AAGP) was founded in 1978. Its membership now exceeds seven hundred. This association has taken a significant role in the effort to obtain the recognition of geriatric psychiatry as a subspecialty.

The impacts of the National Institute on Aging (NIA) and the Administration on Aging (AoA) on gerontology in the United States cannot be overestimated. The AoA was created in 1965 to develop and coordinate research and service programs for the elderly. The AoA was originally a component of the U.S. Department of Health, Education and Welfare. Its mission was and is in many respects quite different from those of the NIA and the National Institute of Mental Health (NIMH).

The Center for Studies of the Mental Health of the Aging was established at NIMH in 1975. In 1977 it received funds to support and coordinate research, research training, and clinical training projects. Its efforts in the area of geriatric psychiatry have been focused on two general areas. Clinical training has focused on developing specialty-training fellowship programs; on establishing a faculty development program, as yet unfunded; and on continuing education, in-service training, and demonstration training and curriculum projects. The second area of focus is research training. A new research career program (Geriatric Mental Health Academic Award) has just been announced in this area. While the future of training projects supported by clinical training funds is highly uncertain, training initiatives from research and research training funds are likely to increase (Cohen 1987).

The NIA was established in May 1974 as part of the NIMH. The first director of the NIA was a psychiatrist, Robert N. Butler. The establishment of NIA represented the culmination of 20 years of effort to gain government recognition and support for research on aging. Enabling legislation designated NIA as the chief federal agency responsible for promoting, coordinating, and supporting basic research and training relevant to the aging process and to the diseases and problems of the elderly. A unique aspect of NIA's mandate was that it was the first component of the National Institutes of Health to be formally charged by Congress with conducting research in the biologic, biomedical, behavioral, and social sciences. This broad research mandate has resulted in activities that are different from those of the other national health research institutes. Since 1974 NIA basic research funding has tripled, grant applications have more than doubled, and more than 100 new researchers have been in training (Kawecky CA: Legislative and Administrative History. National Institute on Aging, draft document not for circulation).

For many years, medical and health care education related to geriatrics received little attention. The first training program in geriatric psychiatry supported by NIMH was established at Duke University Medical Center in 1965 and was the only such program for almost a decade. There is now a rapidly increasing number of geriatric psychiatry fellowship programs. In the last few years, federal and state agencies have provided financial support for training in geriatrics in the medical fields of internal medicine, family practice, psychiatry, and neurology. While the American Board of Medical Specialties has discouraged the formation of separate subspecialty boards such as geriatric psychiatry, it does favor certification in subspecialties by primary specialty boards. The American Board of Psychiatry and Neurology, for instance, certifies diplomates who obtain and can demonstrate special competence or special qualifications in a subspecialty, for example, child psychiatry and child neurology.

For several years the American Board of Psychiatry and Neurology has been demonstrating increasing interest in geriatric psychiatry. At the July 1987 meeting of the Board, unanimous approval was given to the concept of training and acknowledgment of added qualifications in geriatric psychiatry.

The training required would be an additional year after the basic 4 years of psychiatric training. Many of the existing programs utilize fourth and fifth years for geriatric psychiatry. This is similar to the pattern in child psychiatry. At the present time the NIMH is funding 17 geriatric training programs. The fellows usually are trained for 2 years—the fourth and fifth years. There are actually 30 geriatric psychiatry training programs existing in the United States. Obviously, a number of them are funded by sources other than the NIMH. As to the curriculum guidelines in such programs, the GAP Report of 1983 is the one usually employed. However, the 17 programs funded by the NIMH recently had a planning committee for the purpose of developing a core curriculum.

Funding for Training

Cohen (1987) believes that the "clinical training support at the NIMH is at a critical juncture" (p. 3). In recent years support for clinical training in medicine and the related health professions in general, has been losing financial support from the U.S. Congress. This is in direct contrast to funding for research in aging, which continues to receive favorable support from the U.S. Congress.

Public Law 99-660 was passed by Congress in November 1986. This law authorized major services research programs in the area of Alzheimer's disease and related dementias. In order to ensure communication and cooperation between various funding agencies within the government, this legislation mandated a Council on Alzheimer's Disease as well as a Panel on Alzheimer's Disease. The Council consists entirely of federal members, while the Panel is composed of 15 members representing at least five categories. The Panel was appointed by the Office of Technology Assessment, an arm of Congress. The Council began its work early in 1987 while the Panel was scheduled to begin activity in the fall of 1987.

The need for geriatric psychiatry training and qualification is emphasized by a number of studies.

Supply, Demand, and Training

A recent report was issued by a committee of the Institute of Medicine of the National Academy of Sciences. One of the important recommendations made by this committee is that by the year 2000, medical schools in the United States will require 2,100 faculty members training in geriatrics. As of 1987 there were only about 100 physicians a year who completed fellowships in geriatric medicine or geriatric psychiatry. If the objective of expanding faculty ranks is to be attained, it will be necessary to at least double the number of geriatric trainees. Obviously there will be a need for the well-trained geriatrician. In the foreseeable future, the professional demands will be intense and the major emphasis will be on the training of academicians.

Some professional and lay persons advocate developing a specialty in geriatrics, pointing to Great Britain where a more or less distinct hospital-based specialty of geriatrics has emerged. Although there have admittedly been some gains in Britain, there have also been some losses, particularly because the specialty is hospital based. Moreover, the emergence of the geriatrics specialty in the United Kingdom has spanned a period of 25 years and is tied to a system of health insurance and social assistance that has not been acceptable in the United States. The following summarizes the current status of geriatric training and official recognition in the United States and Canada.

Added Qualifications in Geriatrics in the United States

The recent announcement (Scherr 1987) of a mutual effort by the American Board of Internal Medicine and the American Board of Family Practice to implement joint standards for recognition of achievement in geriatrics and to insist on similar standards for training is a remarkable and sensible advancement. As of 1988, the Amerian Board of Internal Medicine and the American Board of Family Practice will each offer certificates of added qualifications in geriatrics. This will be accomplished by a one-day, multiple-choice examination which will include a jointly prepared written examination for all candidates and all candidates will adhere to the same passing score. For the next 5 years internists and family practitioners who are certified will be able to take this examination. Thereafter, it will be available to those who have completed training in an accredited and standard program.

According to Lawrence Scherr of the American College of Physicians, impressive plans have been developed for these training programs. Both disciplines must have completed their respective accredited residencies. Emphasis will be placed on the physiology of aging, the pathophysiology of related disease, the functional assessment of the elderly, and overall treatment and management. Furthermore, these training programs will give special attention to the behavioral aspects of illness, socioeconomic factors, and ethical and legal considerations of medical management. In order to accomplish this training mission, there will be multiple sites for training including acute hospitals, long-term care institutions, home care, day care, and ambulatory settings. This enormous step forward pioneered by internal medicine and family practice should be emulated by neurology and psychiatry. In any training program devised for a geriatric psychiatrist, he or she must be moving toward becoming a neuropsychiatrist.

Geriatric Psychiatry in Canada

The Royal College of Physicians and Surgeons of Canada carries the major responsibility for setting and enforcing standards for training programs of all medical and surgical specialties. Training in geriatric medicine in Canada emerged between 1973 and 1977 when the clinical medicine section of the Canadian Association on Gerontology, under the supervision of Jack Mac-Donell, prepared a statement seeking recognition of geriatric medicine as a subspecialty of internal medicine. This was submitted to the Royal College of Physicians and Surgeons. In 1981, the first examination for certification of special competence in geriatric medicine was held in Canada. Prior to this time, the College had developed criteria for training programs. Candidates for the certificate of special competence in geriatric medicine must have completed training in internal medicine and must have passed examinations in both clinical medicine and geriatric medicine. Between 1981 and 1986, 39 individuals sat for the examination in geriatric medicine; 23 of the candidates were successful. These now form a nucleus of well-qualified internists/geriatricians who are developing academic medicine programs in geriatric medicine in Canadian medical schools.

The College also recognized in 1981 that it was necessary to develop programs in geriatric psychiatry (Reichenfeld 1987). Since 1983, the College has mandated that all psychiatric programs include a psychogeriatric experience. The oldest division of geriatric psychiatry was established prior to the action of the college. In 1978 a division of geriatric psychiatry was established at the University of Toronto and used a variety of clinical settings for their training activity (Cape and MacDonell 1986).

Geriatric Medicine in the United Kingdom

Geriatric consultants have served in the British health service for many years. A geriatric consultant is not a primary care physician and sees patients by referral usually from general practitioners (Brocklehurst 1978). The geriatric consultant is likely to be hospital based. The objectives of the geriatric physician are twofold. The first is to maintain old people living independently in the community by early treatment, rehabilitation, and day care hospitals and services. The second objective is the management of patients requiring long-term care. All geriatric long-term care beds are under the charge of geriatricians; however, psychogeriatric long-term beds are increasing in number. Usually a consultant psychiatrist specializing in the psychiatry of old age is responsible for the psychogeriatric long-term beds.

Diploma in Geriatric Medicine in the United Kingdom

In 1985 the Royal College of Physicians of London conducted their first examination of candidates for a diploma in geriatric medicine. The examination was declared not to be intended for those aiming to be consultants in geriatric medicine. Rather, the examination is intended for doctors wishing to contribute to the geriatric services of their districts in a nonconsultant capacity, in particular, general practitioners wishing to do sessions as clinical assistants or hospital practitioners in geriatric medicine.

The Board of Examiners of the College includes representatives from general practice and from psychogeriatrics. The examination is held twice a year and includes both written and clinical sections. The emphasis in both sections of the examination is on the practicalities of patient management, particularly in the community and primary care settings.

The move toward a diploma in geriatric medicine was influenced in part by the fact that consultants in geriatric medicine are primarily hospital based, which often limits the scope of their medical practice.

Geriatric psychiatry is thus a relatively new area of concentration. Its clinical and scientific development has not been clearly traced or documented, and its future as an area of specialization is not yet entirely certain. Personality and development theories of aging are complicated by the fact that as human beings pass through life experiences, they become increasingly different rather than increasingly similar. This life span divergence is largely related to the wide array of possible learning and life experiences and, to an unknown degree, to late-onset genetic influences (Busse 1981). Psychiatrists with a strong commitment to geriatrics and gerontology have been in the forefront of those whose efforts are directed toward improving the health and care of the elderly and toward maintaining and increasing their life satisfaction.

Geriatric Medicine and Geriatric Psychiatry as Specialties

For the past several decades, psychiatry has been experiencing what is called by many an identity crisis. This crisis in identity centers on the sphere of professional activity that is the proper task of psychiatrists and whether their activity provides a source of self-esteem to the psychiatrists (Busse 1972; Detre 1987). The geriatric psychiatrist in relationship both to the general psychiatrist and the geriatrician is making a significant contribution to resolving this so-called identity crisis.

The geriatric psychiatrist assumes in many ways the role of primary care. He must not only maintain a proficiency in general medicine, but must apply the special knowledge of epidemiology, and behavioral and social aspects of patient care. For example, geriatric psychiatrists have no alternative but to recognize that many of the disorders that they treat cannot be cured or prevented, but the resulting suffering can be relieved and the disability reduced. Recognizing this fact alone may not be inherently rewarding; however, it does encourage the clinician to make observations that contribute to a better understanding of the course of chronic illness and to look for more hidden clues that can lead to investigations which may in the future bring improved convalescence or even erradication of such disorders if recognized earlier in their course.

To achieve the goal of effective care of the chronically ill older adult with psychiatric problems, geriatric psychiatrists must broaden their skills to include proficiency in geriatric medicine, neurology, and the neurosciences as well as focus their skills on advances in geriatric psychiatry. The proficient geriatrician and geriatric psychiatrist must be aware of aging changes that affect the human organism's capacity to respond to stress, disease, and trauma and eventually may result in death (Busse and Blazer 1980). Specific procedures of therapy, such as the treatment of a urinary tract infection, moderate hypertension, and peripheral edema, should not require the geriatric psychiatrist to consult an internist or geriatrician for appropriate management. Though the role of the geriatric psychiatrist may be such that specialty consultation is frequent and combined management of the patient is effected by a geriatrician and geriatric psychiatrist (such as in a tertiary care center), the skill of the geriatric psychiatrist should be proficient so that, in the absence of the geriatrician, adequate medical care can be administered.

At the same time, significant advances in the epidemiology, pathophysiology, diagnosis, and treatment of the most frequently encountered psychiatric disorders in late life have emerged. These disorders span at least the range described in this volume, though even a "short list" must include the dementias, the affective disorders, the anxiety disorders, the schizophrenic-like disorders, and psychologic and social factors affecting physical conditions. Advances in the neuroscience and clinical management of primary degenerative dementia alone illustrate the substantial knowledge base on which geriatric psychiatry is practiced. Previous trends have been such that when a biologic etiology has been identified for a behavioral disorder, that disorder is passed from psychiatry to another specialty, usually neurology. Surely this cannot be tolerated in the future by geriatric psychiatrists. For example, geriatric psychiatrists must maintain a central role in the clinical management of the dementia patient. To do so, however, the skills of the psychiatrist must be such that they are not overshadowed by other geriatric physicians.

The identity crisis faced by geriatric psychiatry emerges in another arena—patient referrals. Though geriatric psychiatry in theory is a broad-based specialty, in practice it is rarely the recipient of primary referrals. Patients do not usually consider the psychiatrist the coordinator or the provider of general medical care. For the most part, geriatric psychiatry depends for patient flow on referrals. These referrals may come from family physicians, internists, and geriatricians or specialty providers (neurology as well as the other medical specialties). A major concern regards the point at which a primary care physician refers a patient to the geriatric psychiatrist. For example, if a patient with major depression is treated with an antidepressant medication, and the results are unsuccessful, should that patient then be referred or should a second medication be tried?

Another common problem facing the geriatrician is a problem of psychosis in dementia. These psychoses are undoubtedly poorly treated at present. They are seen most frequently in nursing home settings. Should geriatric psychiatrists be regular consultants to long-term care facilities treating dementia patients? A third, quite common (5 percent of the population) disorder for which geriatric psychiatrists can contribute uniquely to patient care is moderate to severe generalized anxiety. Many older adults are prescribed benzodiazepines and sedative–hypnotic agents inappropriately for anxiety symptoms. The geriatric psychiatrist also would appear to have a role in the treatment of hypochondriacal older adults.

Involved discussion regarding "a proper time for referral" will not establish the geriatric psychiatrist firmly within the medical community nearly as effectively as quality provision of the psychiatric care. Psychiatry in general, and geriatric psychiatry in particular, have advanced to the point that no apology is necessary for the effectiveness of diagnostic and treatment methods. At the same time, these advances are often sophisticated enough to warrant the existence of a specialty; that is, the complexity of treatment extends beyond the usual competence of a primary care physician. Unfortunately, the very terminology used in psychiatry, such as "depression," can seduce other physicians and nonphysicians into believing they intuitively possess skills to treat the impaired elder. Geriatric psychiatrists can enhance their status in the medical community by producing methodologically sound, data-based, clinical research at scientific meetings that demonstrates the scientific sophistication of the specialty as well as the expanding knowledge base from which it is practiced.

Given the expanded knowledge base of geriatric psychiatry, there is an ever increasing need to coordinate the delivery of psychiatric care within the context of interdisciplinary care. At a time when psychiatrists possessed fewer therapeutic tools, they were more likely to develop their skills as a team leader and treatment coordinator. The team concept of health care delivery is no less essential today for health care delivery than it was 10 years ago, though there are many competing priorities.

The Geriatric Psychiatrist and Public Health

There is an ever increasing number of older persons in North America, and resources are limited for the psychiatric care of these elders. Therefore, the geriatric psychiatrist in the future must have an interest in and understanding of the prevalence and distribution of psychiatric disorders in the population and the delivery of psychiatric services to these older adults. Most older adults suffering from a psychiatric disorder do not receive any care for the disorder. The majority of those who do receive the care from a primary care physician (German 1985).

In planning for a more effective and efficient delivery of psychiatric services to older adults, the geriatric psychiatrist must consider intervention at one of three points in the natural course of a disorder. These points correspond to the three classic types of prevention described by public health specialists, that is, primary, secondary, and tertiary prevention (Last 1980). Primary prevention means preventing the occurrence of disease or injury. Secondary prevention means early detection and intervention. Tertiary prevention means minimizing the effects of disease and disability.

The geriatric psychiatrist can affect primary prevention by identifying potential events and elements in the environment of the older adult, both social and physical, that contribute to the onset of a psychiatric disorder. For example, forced isolation and the absence of effective communication with the older adult contribute to the onset of major depression and paranoid psychoses. The education of physicians in the appropriate use of psychotropic medications may prevent the occurrence of acute organic brain syndromes in an older adult who is bereaved. Early supportive intervention has been demonstrated to prevent the onset of major depression.

Secondary prevention requires the geriatric psychiatrist to intervene early enough in the course of an illness to facilitate the prescription of effective treatment to prevent a complicated convalescence. It is at this level that the geriatric psychiatrist may achieve the greatest success, given limited resources available. For example, early diagnosis of major depression permits the psychiatrist to attempt a rational course of antidepressant therapy as an outpatient, prior to the complication of excess medication or neglect of physical health that may ensue during the course of a depressive illness.

Tertiary prevention is directed toward preventing the disability that may result from mental illness. Rehabilitation techniques are well known and important in long-term care facilities, especially in the management of the dementia patient (e.g., reality orientation, adequate hygiene). Though the activities themselves may not be the direct responsibility of the geriatric psychiatrist, the development of a comprehensive treatment and rehabilitation plan must involve the geriatric psychiatrist.

Funding for the geriatric psychiatrist to engage in these preventive health activities is inadequate at present. Unfortunately, there is great pressure at present on the federal government to provide many services that it cannot afford. A simple complaint that "more money is needed for psychiatric care" will undoubtedly fall on deaf ears. Rather, specific recommendations are needed by the geriatric psychiatrist to help mold the health care policy for older adults in the future.

For example, recent statements by the APA and the AGS are related to funding of psychiatric services for the elderly. The first of these is catastrophic health insurance. The catastrophic health insurance bill, before Congress at this writing, includes an expanded outpatient psychiatric benefit. The $2,000 benefit per year with a 50 percent copayment (instead of a $500 benefit) means the amount Medicare will pay increases after 20 years from $250 to $1,000 (APA 1987). The implementation of this increased outpatient coverage would be a significant step toward remedying the most blatant gap in the psychiatric care of older adults, and in turn may alleviate unnecessary hospitalization.

Medicare coverage of mental illness, in general, has not changed since the beginning of the program in the 1960s. At present, there is a $250 limit (as noted above) for outpatient treatments per year. According to the APA, this benefit is worth about $57 in constant dollars (compared with its value at inception) and would need to be established near $2,200 to provide the beneficiary the purchasing power equal to what was available in the 1960s. Only one change has occurred in Medicare reimbursement for psychiatric disorders in recent years, and that is the realignment of Alzheimer's disease as a medical illness worthy of rehabilitative and treatment reimbursement in long-term care facilities.

In addition, there is a 190-day lifetime limit on psychiatric inpatient care. For conditions such as Alzheimer's disease for which psychiatric care may be needed for periods of time throughout the illness—an illness that can last 10 to 15 years and that is manifested primarily by behavioral problems through most of its course—the 190-day limit precludes reasonable clinical care. This shortcoming is magnified with the recognition that the life expectancy of older adults in general has increased for the 65 + age group (see Chapter 9) and especially for the 85 + age group. If Medicare continues to provide the core medical care reimbursement for all persons age 65 and older (a policy that may require change), this 190-day limit for Alzheimer's disease is unreasonable.

Another disorder that may lead to extended hospitalizations is a rapid-cycling affective disorder. Though not the usual case, there is a significant minority of older adults suffering from major depression who require recurrent hospitalizations (sometimes two or three times per year for 2 or 3 weeks at each admission) and some of these individuals must be treated with electroconvulsive therapy. The 190-day limit precludes reimbursement for the "catastrophe" of recurrent and treatment-resistant affective illness. Hospital care is essential to the humane management of these difficult treatment cases.

The geriatric psychiatrist also must be concerned with the relative benefits of home care versus institutional care. Though the issue is of less relevance to the delivery of psychiatric care, if and when home care becomes more accessible, approaches to the management of psychotic behavior in home settings will be necessary. At present, Medicare pays for only 100 days of skilled nursing care and there have been repeated programs to attempt to develop incentives for maintaining frail and impaired older adults in the community. Medicaid generally will undertake the reimbursement for routine nursing home care in most states when Medicare benefits have expired and when the financial status of the older adult meets appropriate requirements for Medicaid.

Ginzberg (1987) recently stated, "It is highly unlikely that the prevailing discrimination against psychiatric patients by Medicare and commercial insurance will be reduced or removed" (p. 725). Ginzberg observes that the two principal payers for health care, government and corporations, are looking, largely unsuccessfully, to contain the expenditures for health care costs. Though there is some minor encouragement in the changing reimbursement pattern for Alzheimer's disease, pressures on the government to contain costs bode poorly for improved reimbursement for the psychiatrically impaired elder. Geriatric psychiatrists in conjunction with corporations and third-party providers must explore alternative means of financial support for appropriate health care. Unfortunately, older adults frequently are no longer contributors to the economic growth of society, live on fixed incomes, and therefore are at greatest risk for neglect in a "pay as you go" society. The development of private insurance to cover long-term care, for example, has proved particularly anemic despite the increasing demands for such care and the recognition by a significant portion of older adults of the need of such insurance. Actuarial tables that would provide guidelines to third-party carriers in developing such programs are surprisingly limited in their scope.

Yet the psychiatrist who cares for the older adult must not despair regarding the economic disincentives for entering such a practice. Problems faced in reimbursement for appropriate care of the psychiatrically impaired elder are part of the central problem in providing humane medical care to our society overall. For example, the balance between high-technology diagnostic procedures and low technology but intense personal services in the management of the patient with Alzheimer's disease illustrates a generic problem in medicine, especially within the United States. A recent decision by Medicare not to reimburse for cardiac transplantation is a first attempt to make those decisions that high technology and limited resources require.

In addition, much of the suffering experienced by older adults derives from disorders for which there is no quick and easy solution. Though diagnostic-related groups were developed to encourage efficient medical care, the variance around the mean number of days required for a psychiatric hospitalization in late life is dramatic, and the individual who exceeds the mean may be the very person who can benefit most from a hospitalization. For example, an older person with multiple medical problems admitted for the treatment of a depressive disorder may require a week to 10 days for a thorough diagnostic workup and assessment of physical functioning before treatment of the depressive disorder can be implemented. These persons cannot be admitted to a medical service (in that no problem is severe enough to warrant admission under Medicare), yet they cannot be treated immediately on a psychiatric ward because of the medical complications. One potential solution is a step down and step up in levels of care within the hospital setting to accommodate different requirements for intensity of service through the course of an extended hospitalization.

There has been much talk but little adequate demonstration of lower "levels" of care for the psychiatrically impaired older adult. A major breakthrough would be the development of a cost-efficient yet effective long-term treatment program for the dementia patient. Such dementia units would undoubtedly be nursing units and might require minimal, if appropriate, medical intervention. Once again, as private entrepreneurs become more involved in the delivery of comprehensive care, geriatric psychiatrists should work with these individuals in the development of appropriate treatment facilities.

Legal and Ethical Issues

In recent years medical ethics and legal issues associated with medical science and practice have been receiving increased attention by the news media, by religious and human rights organizations, by the legal profession, and by governments. The medical profession has not only responded to such pressure, but also has been attempting to foresee the emergence of new ethical problems and develop applicable guidelines.

The reasons for this increased activity cannot be attributed to the existence of major defects within the generally accepted code of medical ethics, but rather results from rapid changes in social values and major advances in science and technology including the extension of the length of life. History clearly demonstrates that professional ethics are constantly evolving. How and why such changes or shifts occur should be understood by physicians, patients, and the public (King 1982; Konold 1977).

Accepted principles of ethical conduct or good behavior are not homogenous throughout the world. There are a limited number of universal norms, such as the incest taboo, but heterogeneity of ethical principles is the rule. There are groups of people who promote and attempt to explain standards of behavior.

Ethical issues that commonly occur in the practice of geriatric psychiatry are not necessarily confined to this age group. However, elderly mentally ill patients are likely to be different from younger adult patients. A 65-year-old or older person is likely to have three to six chronic diseases and physical disabilities that impair, to varying degrees, work and other activities. In addition, the social and economic situation for the elderly may not be as favorable as that of younger persons. The adverse circumstances of late life make more complex certain ethical issues.

Some ethical issues of geriatric psychiatry and child psychiatry are similar but reversed—a mirror image. Dependency on another person for protection, support, and survival is a shared condition of children and frail elderly. But there is a substantial difference. The child is moving to greater independence while the frail elderly person will become increasingly dependent on others. Decisions regarding long-term care are influenced by this difference.

The geriatric psychiatrist can look forward to many years of exciting advances in scientific knowledge and improvement of the health and well-being of the elderly. All advances are complicated by the need to evolve new and modified ethical and legal issues. For the geriatric psychiatrist, progressive and irreversible mental decline, varying from mild to severe, is not only a serious clinical problem, but a very complex ethical matter. Ethical and legal issues that are particularly relevant to dementia are (1) informed consent, (2) the concept of the patient's "right to know," (3) competency and the appointment of a guardian or some alternative, (4) the withdrawal of life-support systems, (5) a living will, and (6) testamentary capacity. These and other legal and ethical issues are often intertwined, for example, the legal status of mental competence is a required condition for informed consent.

The concept of informed consent implies a highly rational process (Busse 1985). It requires that the source and the content of the communication be clear and complete and that the patient be an intelligent, rather stable individual capable of questioning any point requiring clarification. Unfortunately, the geriatric psychiatrist often recognizes that an elderly individual is beginning to show signs of brain deterioration or may actually fluctuate in his or her ability to understand and communicate. Consequently, the geropsychiatrist will want to double-check questionable patients. Another alternative is to have present an advocate for the patient.

Informed Consent and the Right to Know

Informed consent and the concept of the patient's "right to know" are almost synonymous. The right to know is inherent in consent. Furthermore, mental competence is a required condition for informed consent. Decisions that are made by a so-called normal person as well as decisions made by a "sick" person are influenced by a number of interacting determinants. These include intelligence, inherent and acquired (education); response to situation stress; biologic defects, particularly of the central nervous system, or perhaps perceptual changes; current emotional status; personal and social values; loyalties and religious convictions; legal constraints and consequences; and socioeconomic factors and environmental factors (Busse 1985).

There are many intelligent elderly patients with impaired perception who may make faulty interpretations because of their failure to hear or see properly. Some elderly do not admit to defects; consequently, such patients should have provided to them not only verbal information, but also written statements and illustrated material. When perceptual difficulties are evident, a valuable person is a family member who, through experience, knows when to assist the patient.

There are individuals who are limited in capacity to deal with informed consent but are legally competent. The autonomy of the individual, which is central to informed consent, is a status that is not always welcomed by the patient. There are patients who prefer the physician maintain a paternalistic attitude. Their approach is "father knows best," and they believe the physician will make a correct decision. Similarly, there are professionals and lay persons who believe that a patient who has detailed, accurate knowledge of his or her disease may experience considerable stress and suffering because of this knowledge. Therefore, they believe that such extensive, accurate knowledge is not actually in the best interest of the patient.

There are times when a patient is not able to fully participate in the process of informed consent, since he or she lacks the ability necessary to understand complex medical problems. The question then arises as to the obligation of the physician to either (1) take the time to educate the person to a level of complete understanding or (2) present the complex situation in a simplified manner that expedites the patient's decision. The first approach can be time consuming, while the second contains a strong element of paternalism.

The term *fiduciary* describes an important relationship between the patient and the physician, the lawyer and the client, or the clergyman and the parishioner. A fiduciary relationship is based on confidences and trust. A fiduciary is a person who stands in a special relationship of trust, confidence, or responsibility in his or her obligation to another person or persons. A fiduciary relationship is the essence of informed consent (Dyer 1982).

It is becoming increasingly apparent that informed consent, which was originally an ethical concept, is becoming an important and changing legal issue (Gutheil 1987). Gutheil reports that in a 10-year study performed at the Risk Management Foundation, out of 1,200 cases only 159 had an informed consent component. However, he feels that this component will become an increasingly important forensic problem. Gutheil believes that this hindsight allegation results from the patient's actually experiencing the harm and bad outcome and then claiming in retrospect that he or she was not adequately informed.

The failure to provide informed consent has been recognized by the courts as a complex information process focusing on the medical matters under question. The courts have recognized that there are difficulties in communication of scientific information by the trained physician to the untrained patient and almost limitless risks in any proposed treatment. Consequently, the legal position has been that what the patient has a right to know must be harmonized with patient recognition that an undue burden should not be placed on the physician. However, the physician owes to the patient the duty to disclose any reasonable matter or significant medical information that the physician possesses or reasonably should possess that is material to an intelligent decision by the patient whether to undergo a proposed procedure. Furthermore, the legal stance has been that an informed physician should possess that knowledge which is held by the average qualified physician or, in the case of a specialty, by the average qualified physician specialist. The court standard, therefore, has been a peer group comparison and not a patient-centered standard.

It appears that the court now has decided that the physician must provide medical information that is "material to the intelligent decision by the patient" (Gutheil 1987, p. 5). The physician is expected to know or "should know" of the patient's position in regard to the disclosed risk or risks that are associated with the decision to submit or not submit to surgery or treatment. This new court interpretation emphasizes the importance of a physician's empathetic judgment.

Although it is not yet explicitly recognized by the court, it is evident that the ability of a "reasonable person" to make a complicated decision is influenced by numerous personal attitudes, values, and experiences. Many such influences may be essentially unknown (i.e., may reside in the unconscious of the patient) and may not be apparent to the physician. These new legal developments emphasize the importance for the geriatric psychiatrist to include in his or her clinical records an adequate summary of the process of informed consent reviewing the medical information that has been given to the patient and the patient's reaction to this information, particularly pertinent questions and responses.

Competence and Incompetence

The terms "incompetent" and "competent," as legally used in the United States, do not necessarily designate extreme or opposing points along a continuum. A competent individual has the quality or condition that makes him or her capable of participating in certain legally recognized activities. In addition, a competent person is responsible for his or her acts. A person is considered competent until declared incompetent. Incompetence is a generally used term to denote the lack of capacity to legally consent or make a contract.

In addition, there are specific areas in which a person can be declared incompetent. A person may be unable to give informed consent; to have testamentary capacity, that is, to execute a last will and testament; or to be held responsible for certain illegal acts. If an individual is incompetent in one area, it does not necessarily make that person incompetent in other areas.

Competence is not an all-or-nothing mental condition and may be limited and/or intermittent. Competence is usually an accepted condition in which it appears that an individual has the capacity to cope with common events of everyday life. Unfortunately, the degree of competence is subject to greater variation when the individual is faced with a new, acute situation that requires a solution.

Alzheimer's disease and related progressive dementias are held to be a steady deterioration devoid of periods of plateau or actual periods of restoration. Longitudinal studies suggest that in many individuals there are episodes of organic mental impairment, that is, exacerbation and remission. Consequently, there are fluctuations in the mental competence of such patients. Observers at different times may justifiably reach opposing conclusions.

Geriatric psychiatrists are advised to be thoroughly acquainted with the laws of the state in which they reside or practice. In many states an incompetent adult or child is one who lacks a mental capacity to manage him- or herself and his or her affairs or who lacks sufficient capacity to make or communicate important decisions concerning person, family, or property. An overview (APA 1986) of legal issues in geriatric psychiatry notes that there are two types of competence. *De facto competence* is based on a person's understanding of what is being proposed—medical treatment, hospitalization, and so on. Psychiatrists are asked to give their opinions about patients' de facto competence as a prelude to formal legal review. De facto competence differs distinctly from *de jure competence*, which is competence due to a status under the law; that is, the person has not been declared legally incompetent and therefore is presumed to be competent for a variety of purposes, unless the person has legally been found to be incompetent for a specific purpose. By definition of the law, de jure competence is not given to children or adolescents since they are incompetent up to specified ages.

Consequently, because of age alone, under certain circumstances, they are unable to make contracts, marry, purchase alcoholic beverages, or decide various aspects of their medical care. In an adult, de jure *in*competence is established after a legal hearing designed to decide that specific issue.

Unfortunately, many state laws are complex and confusing. It is possible for an individual to be incompetent in one area, but competent in another. A person may be unable to give informed consent, but may be able to execute a last will and testimony. Again, the geriatric psychiatrist must be alert to the fact that a person at one time may seem to be alert and understanding and other times may be confused and unable to pay attention. Observers should make certain that they see the patient several times and at different times of the day and week. All of this should be duly noted in a permanent record by the geriatric psychiatrist.

It is sometimes necessary for the geriatric psychiatrist to become involved in legal procedure to determine the status of competency and, if the person is declared incompetent, for the court to appoint a guardian. Guardians may be divided into several classes: a guardian of the estate, a guardian of the person, or a general guardian of both the estate and person. Guardianship ad litem permits a person appointed by the court to represent the interests of a person lacking in capacity in a particular procedure or for a particular purpose. All states have laws that allow a guardian to be appointed if a person is no longer able to manage his or her affairs. This usually becomes obvious when he or she is unable to handle property or financial affairs. The laws in most states require that a concerned individual file for a procedure to be carried out that establishes a guardianship. This usually involves a hearing of some sort. Some states require that the patient be examined by professionals prior to the court hearing. These are often designated by the court. Unfortunately, hearings can be very embarrassing, particularly if the mentally impaired individual does not want to have a guardian. Although the procedure varies from state to state, often the judge or presiding legal authority will recognize that the hearing can be a very traumatic procedure and will structure the hearing to reduce the trauma to the individual and to the family or interested parties.

A further complication is that family members themselves may disagree that a guardian is necessary, and this results in a very unfortunate situation. It is strongly recommended that the geriatric psychiatrist be aware of the various views held by a family. The recommendation of a guardian should be a unanimous family decision.

Most geriatric psychiatrists are quite familiar with a commitment procedure to an institution. Most state laws require that a person who is committed to an institution have a mental illness that causes the individual (1) to be an immediate danger either to him- or herself or to others, or (2) to be unable to care for him- or herself. Again, hearings are often held within the facility where the person is being cared for. Most states provide a temporary commitment followed by reviews at regular intervals to prevent any misuse of the commitment procedure.

A person who has been declared incompetent can be assigned into a hospital or a facility as a voluntary patient with the written approval of the person's guardian. This can be done whether or not the patient is willing. In many states, getting a person declared incompetent and having a guardian appointed is a complicated and traumatic procedure. Consequently, alternative procedures that are less traumatic are certainly desirable. The preferred solution is that of power of attorney. The power of attorney must be given freely, and when given, the person must be competent. The power of attorney limits the authority that is set forth in the document. In most states, a power of attorney given by a competent person immediately becomes nonfunctional when the person becomes incompetent. All of these types of power of attorney are revocable. If an older person is at risk for becoming mentally incapacitated in the future, it is desirable to set up what is referred to as a durable power of attorney.

In many states, protective services for the elderly are in place. Again the geriatric psychiatrist is advised to be fully informed about the existence of protective services. Although they are designed to protect the older person and avoid the traumatic experience of declaring the person incompetent, there do exist instances when the procedure has been questioned since a fiduciary relationship did not exist. Protective services may not include a requirement for notice to the client for the filing of the petition nor does the client have to be present at the hearing.

It should also be noted that the term conservatorship denotes a condition in which the court provides control over a person's property or person. Consequently this term is confused with that of a guardianship.

Testamentary capacity (not testimonial capacity) is the capacity to make a will. This requires that the individual understand the approximate monetary value and nature of his or her estate. The person should know the natural heirs to his or her bounty, that is, spouse or blood-related persons to whom the estate should ordinarily be expected to go; the person should know what kind of an instrument he or she is signing (that it is, in fact, his or her will); and the person should know the beneficiaries of the will.

A penultimate or "living" will has been declared a legal instrument and procedure in many states. A living will is a written document prepared and signed by a person while mentally competent. A living will specifies the circumstances under which a person will permit the cessation of extraordinary treatment to prolong life and allow death to occur in accordance with the natural progression of the person's disease. A penultimate will can include instructions that in the event that the individual becomes mentally incompetent, he or she is willing to participate in research activity that has little or no likelihood of therapeutic benefit to him- or herself but would add to the understanding of the disease process and may benefit the lives of others. A written living will is an important component of a medical record, particularly for those who are terminally ill. Obviously, it must be properly signed and in conformity with state laws. The existence of such a document not only is of great comfort to the patient, but permits the physician to behave in accord with the desires of the patient and considerably reduces the burden and emotional conflict for the nursing and supporting staff of a facility and for the patient's loved ones.

Acquisition of Moral and Ethical Values:
Can Ethics Be Taught?

When attempting to teach ethics it is necessary to start with a definition. Ethics is concerned with personal and social values that result in behavior that is acceptable to oneself and to others. Consequently, ethics includes a consideration of one's personal well being and the needs and rights of others as individuals and as a society (Ethics Resource Center 1980). Further, behavior becomes unethical when it favors a special-interest group or a special person out of proportion to and without consideration for the interests of society as a whole or for another individual. It is held that altruism and reciprocal altruism are essential. Gray areas do exist, since it is almost impossible to find an example of altruistic behavior that, under certain peculiar circumstances, can't inadvertantly hurt another individual or group.

Religion, undoubtedly, includes moral values and ethics, while science per se is nonmoral. The application of scientific knowledge does include the concepts of moral values and ethics.

Relevant to the teaching of ethical values to psychiatrists and to geriatric psychiatrists is an understanding of how the individual develops moral values and how such values can be altered. This is very understandable when one realizes that one cannot teach higher mathematics unless the individual understands basic mathematics. Similarly, it is highly unlikely that geriatric psychiatrists can fully appreciate complex ethical issues unless they have an understanding and adherence to an appropriate value system. Although no definite answers exist requiring the teaching of professional ethics, attention must be given to this critical matter. Socrates recognized this lack of definite answers when he admitted to Meno that he did not know how virtue is acquired—whether it can be taught or even what it really is (National Institute of Child Health and Human Development [NICHHD] 1968). The studies that have been attempted suffer from a consistent lack of a definition of "moral values."

A further complication occurs during periods of rapid social change. Individuals must go through endless processes of psychologic experimentation and altering patterns of behavior in a search for inner stability and consistent moral values.

Lawrence Kohlberg (NICHHD 1968), the developmental psychologist, believes that the acquisition of moral values passes through six stages that follow each other in the same order in all cultures. As in psychoanalytic theory, Kohlberg believes that each stage is more differentiated and at the same time integrated than the preceding ones. The final stage is considered maturity, although individuals can be arrested at any of these stages and may never attain maturity.

Social scientists believe that societies go through developmental stages similar to those of individuals. When an individual moves more rapidly than the society of which he or she is a part, the individual may be rejected or punished by society. Certainly in a rapidly changing society there are not only individuals but significant groups of people who do not have the capacity to move ahead.

References

American Board of Internal Medicine: Report to Subspecialty Board Members. ABIM Newsletter, March 1986; 2

American Psychiatric Association: A Psychiatric Glossary, fifth edition. Washington, DC, American Psychiatric Press, 1980

American Psychiatric Association: Operations Manual of the APA. Washington, DC, American Psychiatric Association, 1981

American Psychiatric Association: An Overview of Legal Issues in Geriatric Psychiatry, Task Force Report 23. Washington, DC, American Psychiatric Press, 1986

American Psychiatric Association: Legislative Newsletter. APA, Division of Government Relations. August 20, 1987, p. 1

Brocklehurst JC: The evolution of geriatric medicine. J Am Geriatr Soc 1978; 26:433–439

Busse EW: The future of psychiatry—a Hobson's choice? Psychiatr Q 1971; 46:329–342

Busse EW: The presidential address: there are decisions to be made. Am J Psychiatry 1972; 129:33–41

Busse EW: Old age, in The Course of Life, Vol III. Edited by Greenspan SI, Pollock GH. Washington, DC, Department of Health and Human Services, 1981

Busse EW: Ethical issues in geriatric psychiatry, in Psychiatry, Vol 8. Edited by Pichot P, Berner P, Wolf R, et al. New York, Plenum, 1985

Busse EW, Blazer DG: The theories and processes of aging, in Handbook of Geriatric Psychiatry. Edited by Busse EW, Blazer DG. New York, Van Nostrand Reinhold, 1980

Busse EW, Pfeiffer E (eds): Behavior and Adaptation in Late Life. Boston, Little, Brown, 1969; second edition 1977

Busse EW, Pfeiffer E (eds): Mental Illness in Later Life. Washington, DC, American Psychiatric Association, 1973

Butterfield LH: Harvard Medical Alumni Bulletin 1976; 50(4):16–22

Cape RDT, MacDonell JA: Integrated university training program in geriatric medicine accredited and evaluated by the Royal College of Physicians and Surgeons of Canada. J Am Geriatr Soc 1986; 34:787–789

Cohen GD: Update. American Association of Geriatric Psychiatry Newsletter 1987; 9(3):3

Committee on Aging, Group for the Advancement of Psychiatry: Mental Health and Aging: Approaches to Curriculum Development, publication number 114. New York, Mental Health Materials Center, 1983

Committee on Hospitals, Group for the Advancement of Psychiatry: The Problem of the Aged Patient in the Public Psychiatric Hospital, Report No. 14. Topeka, Kansas, 1950

The Commonwealth Fund: Problems facing elderly Americans living alone. January 1987

Cowdry EV: Problems of Aging: Biological and Medical Aspects. Baltimore, Williams & Wilkins, 1938

Detre T: The future of psychiatry. Am J Psychiatry 1987; 144:621–625

Dyer AR: Assessment of competence to give informed consent, in Proceedings: Conference on Senile Dementia and Related Diseases—Ethical and Legal Issues. Washington, DC, National Institute on Aging, 1982

Ethics Resource Center: Common Sense and Everyday Ethics. Washington, DC, American Viewpoint, 1980

Freeman JT: Nascher: excerpts from his life, letters and works. Gerontologist 1961; 1(1): 17–26

Gaitz CM (ed): Aging and the Brain. Proceedings of the Annual Symposium of Texas Research Institute of Mental Sciences, Houston, October 1971. New York, Plenum, 1972

German PS, Shapiro S, Skinner EA: Mental health of the elderly: use of health and mental health services. J Am Geriatr Soc 1985; 33:246–252

Ginzberg E: Psychiatry before the year 2000: a long view. Hosp Community Psychiatry 1987; 38:725–728

Gruman GJ: A History of Ideas About the Prologation of Life: The Evolution of Prolongevity Hypotheses to 1800. Transactions series, Vol 56, Part 9. Philadelphia, The American Philosophical Society, 1966

Gutheil TG: Forensic psychiatry. American Association of Geriatric Psychiatry Newsletter 1987; 9(3):4–5

Hall GS: Senescence: The Last Half of Life. New York, Appleton, 1922

King LW: The old code of medical ethics and some problems it had to face. JAMA 1982; 248:2329–2333

Konold DE: The history of the codes of medical ethics, in Encyclopedia of Bioethics. Edited by Reich WT. New York, Free Press, 1977

Last JM (ed): Public Health and Preventive Medicine (11th edition). New York, Appleton-Century-Crofts, 1980

Nascher IL: Geriatrics: The Diseases of Old Age and Their Treatment. Philadelphia, P Blokiston's Son, 1914

Nascher IL: Longevity and rejuvenescence. New York Medical Journal 1909; 89: 795

Nascher IL: The aging mind. Medical Record #157 1944; p. 669

National Institute of Child Health and Human Development: The Acquisition and Development of Values: Perspectives on Research. Bethesda, MD, National Institute of Child Health and Human Development, 1968

Pollak O: Social Adjustment in Old Age. New York, Social Science Research Council, 1948

Post F: The Clinical Psychiatry of Late Life. Oxford, Pergamon Press, 1965

Reichenfeld HF: Geriatric psychiatry north of the border. American Association of Geriatric Psychiatry Newsletter 1987; 9(3):11–12

Rowe JW, Grossman E, Bond E, et al: Academic geriatrics for the year 2000. N Engl J Med 1987; 316(22):1425–1428

Scherr L: Advances in geriatrics: common ground for cooperation. The ACP Observer, June 1987; 2

Simmons LW: The Role of the Aged in Primitive Societies. New Haven, Yale University Press, 1945

Stieglitz EJ: Geriatric Medicine: Diagnosis and Management of Disease in the Aging and in the Aged. Philadelphia, WB Saunders, 1943

Zinberg NE, Kaufman I: Normal Psychology of the Aging Process. New York, International Universities Press, 1963

INDEX

697